Fluid and Electrolyte Balance

Nursing Considerations

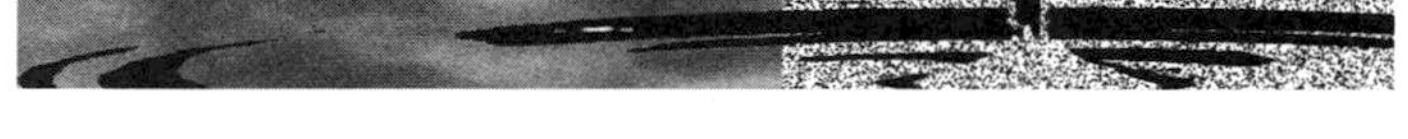

Fluid and Electrolyte Balance

Nursing Considerations

Third Edition

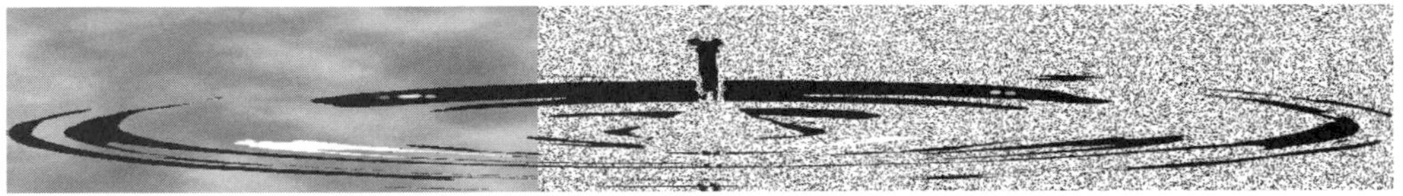

NORMA M. METHENY, PHD, RN, FAAN
Professor of Nursing
Saint Louis University School of Nursing
St. Louis, Missouri

WITH 14 CONTRIBUTORS

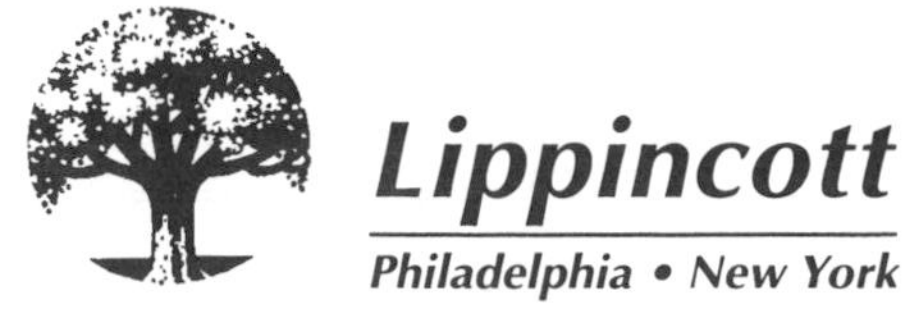

Lippincott
Philadelphia • New York

Acquisitions Editor: Lisa Stead
Editoral Assistant: Brian MacDonald
Production Editor: Molly E. Dickmeyer
Production Service: Berliner, Inc.
Cover Designer: Lou Fuiano
Printer/Binder: Courier/Kendalville
Cover Printer: Lehigh Press

Third Edition

Library of Congress Cataloging-in-Publication Data

Fluid and electrolyte balance: nursing considerations / [edited by]
Norma M. Methany ; with 14 contributors.—3rd ed.
p. cm.
Includes bibliographical references and index.
ISBN 0-397-55191-6
1. Body fluid disorders. 2. Body fluid disorders—Nursing.
I. Methany, Norma Milligan.
[DNLM: 1. Water-Electrolyte Imbalance—nurses' instruction.
2. Water-Electrolyte Balance—nurses' instruction. WD 220 F646
1996]
RC630.F556 1996
616.3'9—dc20
DNLM/DLC
for Library of Congress 95-49883
CIP

The material contained in this volume was submitted as previously unpublished material, except in the instances in which credit has been given to the source from which some of the illustrative material was derived.

Any procedure or practice described in this book should be applied by the health-care practitioner under appropriate supervision in accordance with professional standards of care used with regard to the unique circumstances that apply in each practice situation. Care has been taken to confirm the accuracy of information presented and to describe generally accepted practices. However, the authors, editors, and publisher cannot accept any responsibility for errors or omissions or for any consequences from application of the information in this book and make no warranty, express or implied, with respect to the contents of the book.

The authors and publisher have exerted every effort to ensure that drug selection and dosage set forth in this text are in accordance with current recommendations and practice at the time of publication. However, in view of ongoing research, changes in government regulations, and the constant flow of information relating to drug therapy and drug reactions, the reader is urged to check the package insert for each drug for any change in indications and dosage and for added warnings and precautions. This is particularly important when the recommended agent is a new or infrequently employed drug.

Materials appearing in this book prepared by individuals as part of their official duties as U.S. Government employees are not covered by the above-mentioned copyright.

9 8 7 6 5 4 3 2 1

This book is dedicated to Virginia Henderson
for her great and sustained contributions to nursing practice

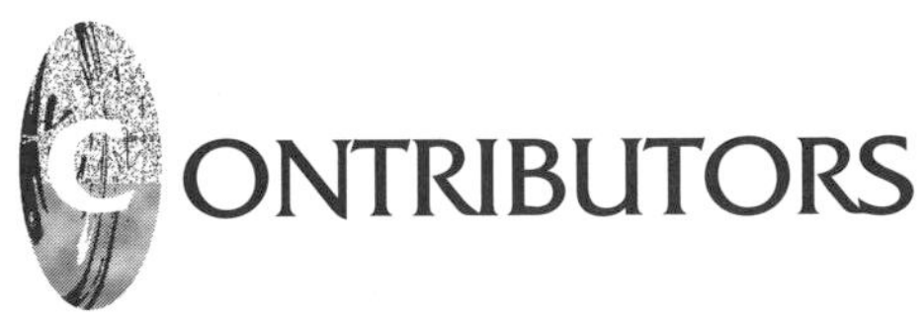

CONTRIBUTORS

Charold L. Baer, PhD, RN, FCCM, CCRN
Professor
Oregon Health Sciences University
School of Nursing
Portland, Oregon
CHAPTER 17: Renal Failure

Linda K. Book, RN, BSN
Burn Nurse Clinician
St. John's Mercy Burn Center
St. Louis, Missouri

Donna C. Casperson, RN, MSN, OCN
Oncology Clinical Nurse Specialist
Deaconess Health System
St. Louis, Missouri
CHAPTER 22: Oncologic Conditions

Susan Cole, RN, MSN, CCRN
Clinical Nurse Specialist
St. Francis Hospital
Cape Girardeau, Missouri
CHAPTER 21: Cirrhosis with Ascites

Mary Ellen Grohar-Murray, PhD, RN
Associate Professor
Saint Louis University School of Nursing
St. Louis, Misouri
CHAPTER 19: Fluid Balance in the Brain-Injured Patient

Marilyn Hackenthal, RN, MSN
Professor of Nursing
Lewis and Clark Community College
Alton, Illinois
CHAPTER 20: Acute Pancreatitis

Mary Kay Macheca, RN, MSN(R), CDE
Diabetes Clinical Nurse Specialist
Barnes Hospital at Washington University
St. Louis, Missouri
CHAPTER 18: Diabetic Ketoacidosis and Hyperosmolar Syndrome

Kathryn Neunaber, RN, BSN, CCRN, CEN
Surgical/Trauma Intensive Care Unit
Saint Louis University Health Sciences Center
St. Louis, Missouri
CHAPTER 15: Hypovolemic Shock in Trauma and Postoperative Patients

Catherine C. Powers, MSN(R), RN, CCRN
Cardiovascular Clinical Nurse Specialist
Barnes Hospital at Washington University
St. Louis, Missouri
CHAPTER 16: Heart Failure

Lisa Reed, RN, MSN(R)
Research Associate
Saint Louis University Health Sciences Center
St. Louis, Missouri
CHAPTER 15: Hypovolemic Shock in Trauma and Postoperative Patients

Irene I. Riddle, PhD, RN
Professor and Director of Doctoral Program in Nursing
Saint Louis University School of Nursing
St. Louis, Missouri
CHAPTER 24: Fluid Balance in Infants and Children

Sherry Robinson, MSN, RNCS
Gerontological Clinical Nurse Specialist
Decatur Memorial Hospital
Decatur, Illinois

CHAPTER 25: Fluid Balance in the Elderly Patient

Patsy L. Ruchala, RN, DNSc
Assistant Professor
Coordinator, Perinatal Nursing Master's Specialty
Saint Louis University School of Nursing
St. Louis, Missouri

CHAPTER 23: Pregnancy

Marilyn Schallom, RN, MSN, CCRN
Critical Care Clinical Nurse Specialist
Deaconess Health System
St. Louis, Missouri

CHAPTER 14: Fluid Balance in the Surgical Patient

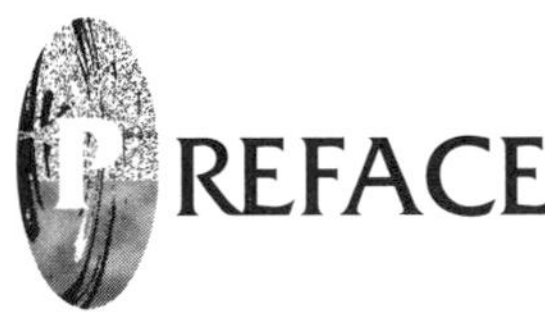

PREFACE

The third edition of *Fluid and Electrolyte Balance: Nursing Considerations* carries on in the tradition established by the prior editions of this textbook. It provides current and comprehensive information related to the nursing care of patients with fluid, electrolyte, and acid–base imbalances in a readable and user-friendly manner. Because concepts of fluid and electrolyte balance apply to a broad spectrum of patient problems, the book's scope is wide. While written simply, to promote ease of understanding for students, it contains enough information to stimulate the interests of advanced practitioners. The most current research findings related to conditions affecting fluid and electrolyte balance are integrated throughout the text. All chapters have been completely revised and updated with an increased emphasis on providing care to patients in long-term and ambulatory care settings.

ORGANIZATION

The basic organization remains unchanged. As in prior editions, the first three units present concepts fundamental to understanding the clinical chapters that follow. Unit I—Basic Concepts—includes a chapter on fundamental concepts and definitions, and a completely revised nursing assessment chapter. Unit II—An Overview of Fluid and Electrolyte Problems—provides chapters on fluid volume imbalances, sodium imbalances, potassium imbalances, calcium imbalances, magnesium imbalances, phosphorus imbalances, and acid–base disturbances. Case studies are included to enhance understanding of specific imbalances. Unit III—Parenteral and Enteral Nutrition—has been completely revised and updated to reflect the latest developments in parenteral fluid administration as well as in parenteral and enteral nutrition. Unit IV—Clinical Situations Associated with Fluid and Electrolyte Problems—contains the bulk of the clinical chapters. Included are chapters on gastrointestinal problems, fluid balance in surgical patients, hypovolemic shock in trauma and postoperative patients, heart failure, renal failure, diabetic ketoacidosis and hyperosmolar syndrome, fluid balance in the brain-injured patient, acute pancreatitis, cirrhosis with ascites, oncologic conditions, and pregnancy. The final unit (Unit V)—Special Considerations in Children and the Elderly—offers a concise explanation of special fluid and electrolyte problems in the very young and the very old.

The book retains its strong nursing focus to help facilitate integration of the information into nursing practice. In all chapters, pathophysiology is discussed to promote an understanding of rationales for nursing interventions. Assessment of fluid and electrolyte balance, based on an understanding of pathophysiology, is integrated throughout the textbook. Because monitoring for the occurrence or worsening of imbalances is an integral part of the nurse's role, patients at risk for specific imbalances are identified throughout the text, as are the common indicators of these problems. Examples of nursing diagnoses related to fluid and electrolyte problems are presented when appropriate, followed by a description of nursing interventions. By their nature, these interventions often involve manipulation of fluid and nutrient intake; therefore, the electrolyte content of common beverages and foods is included as appropriate.

NEW TO THIS EDITION

Each chapter has been completely reviewed, revised, and updated to reflect the latest developments in the study of fluid and electrolyte balance. Extensive reference lists are provided to allow the reader to pursue particular areas of interest. These references include the most recent nursing and medical research related to fluid and electrolyte balance, as well as classic work that provides the foundation for current practice. For example, the most current research findings regarding the management of sodium imbalances in postoperative and neurological patients is included.

The book's layout and design have been updated to promote easy access to material. Information on providing care in the home and community has been integrated throughout the book. Clinical tips are highlighted for easy identification when information is needed in a hurry.

Additional case studies in a variety of areas have been added with an eye toward supporting critical concepts with immediate clinical relevance. Examples of new material are case studies on postoperative shock due to hemorrhage and trauma, sodium imbalances in premenopausal women, safe intravenous sodium administration, hyperphosphatemia from hypertonic sodium phosphate enemas in an elderly patient, multiple electrolyte imbalances in an adolescent with anorexia nervosa, pH disturbances associated with vomiting and diarrhea, postoperative hyponatremia, postoperative hypocalcemia following neck surgery, and imbalances associated with congestive heart failure, renal failure, uncontrolled diabetes mellitus, head injuries, pancreatitis, cirrhosis of the liver, pregnancy, and oncologic conditions. Other case studies include diarrhea in an infant and hypernatremia in an elderly patient with Alzheimer's disease.

A new chapter, "Hypovolemic Shock in Trauma and Postoperative Patients," is included in this edition, reflecting the complex nature of this topic. In addition, the nursing assessment chapter (Chapter 2) has been extensively revised to include information on sophisticated monitoring of physiological changes with pulmonary artery catheters. More information on the care of geriatric patients has been integrated throughout the text, as well as in the geriatric chapter, to help the reader deal with the growing elderly population. Information pertaining to patients receiving parenteral and enteral nutrition has been increased, with the addition of extra tables to help the reader locate important information quickly. Also, information to help nurses provide care for home patients with fluid and electrolyte problems has been integrated throughout the text. For example, sick day rules for diabetic patients have been updated, and information related to the safe use of laxatives and enemas has been included to allow nurses to prevent fluid and electrolyte imbalances through education of home patients and their families.

I wish to acknowledge the skilled master clinicians who have thoroughly revised their chapters to reflect current practice, and also the contributors to prior editions. Because of these individuals' high level of expertise, the information presented in their clinical chapters is pragmatic and ready for application to practice.

Fluid and Electrolyte Balance: Nursing Considerations, third edition, was written with the intent of fostering critical thinking in those providing care to patients with potential or actual fluid and electrolyte disturbances. Designed for students and practicing nurses, it provides the necessary information to deliver safe, effective, scientifically based nursing care.

Norma M. Metheny

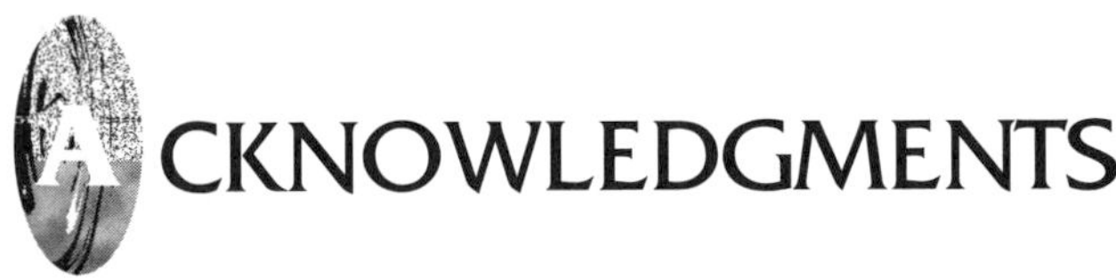

ACKNOWLEDGMENTS

The author wishes to thank the following individuals who helped to make the third edition of *Fluid and Electrolyte Balance: Nursing Considerations* possible:

Lisa Stead, *Associate Editor*
Brian MacDonald, *Nursing Editorial Assistant*
Nancy Berliner, *Project Coordinator*

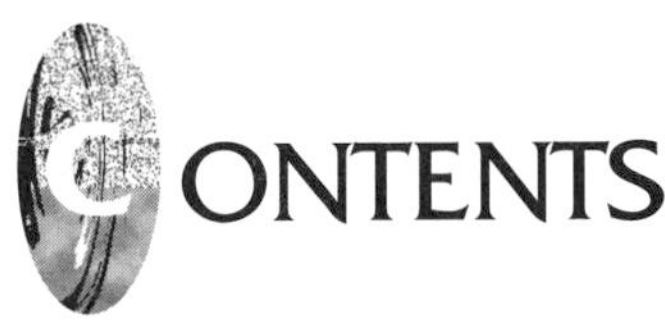

CONTENTS

UNIT FIVE
Special Considerations in Children and the Elderly

Fluid and Electrolyte Balance

Nursing Considerations

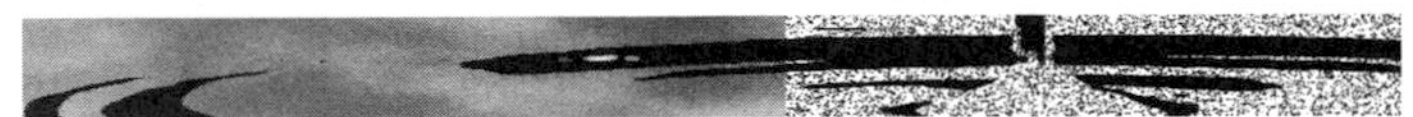

I

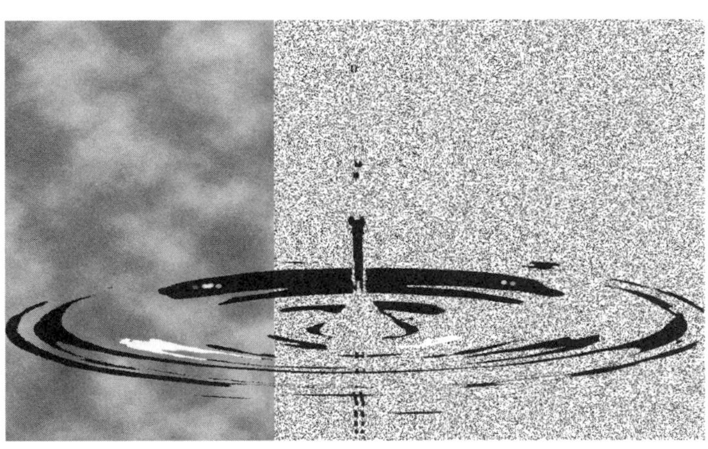

Basic Concepts

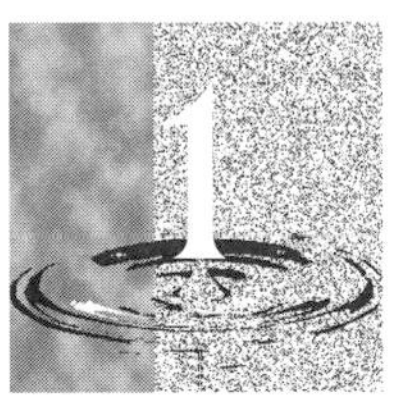

Fundamental Concepts and Definitions

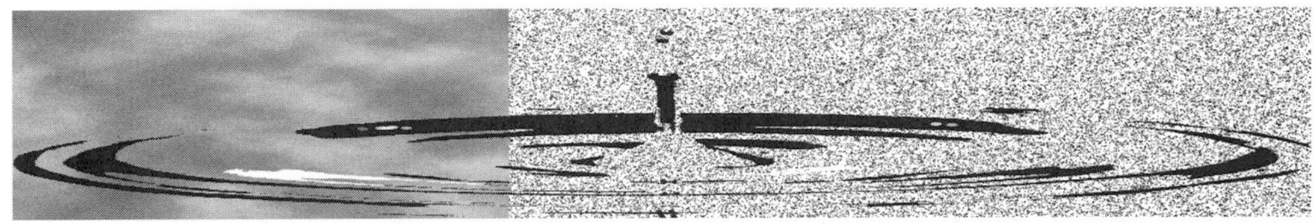

- **DISTRIBUTION OF BODY FLUIDS AND ELECTROLYTES**
- **UNITS OF MEASURE FOR ELECTROLYTES**
- **FUNCTIONS OF BODY FLUIDS**
- **REGULATION OF BODY FLUID COMPARTMENTS**
  - OSMOSIS
  - DIFFUSION
  - FILTRATION
  - SODIUM–POTASSIUM PUMP
- **ROUTES OF GAINS AND LOSSES**
  - LUNGS
  - SKIN
  - GASTROINTESTINAL TRACT
  - KIDNEYS
- **HOMEOSTATIC MECHANISMS**
  - KIDNEYS
  - HEART AND ATRIAL NATRIURETIC FACTOR
  - LUNGS
  - PITUITARY GLAND
  - ADRENAL GLANDS
  - PARATHYROID GLANDS

DISTRIBUTION OF BODY FLUIDS AND ELECTROLYTES

In the typical adult, approximately 60% of weight consists of *fluid* (water and electrolytes). This fluid is either *intracellular* (within the cells) or *extracellular* (outside the cells). Extracellular fluid (ECF) is further subdivided into *intravascular fluid* (plasma) and *interstitial fluid* (fluid lying between the cells, or tissue fluid) (see Fig. 1-1). Also part of the ECF are transcellular fluids, primarily representing secretions from epithelial cells and having ionic compositions different from the plasma and interstitial fluids. Examples of transcellular fluid include secretions in the salivary glands, pancreas, liver, and biliary tract, as well as fluid in the gastrointestinal and respiratory tracts, sweat gland ducts, cavities of the eyes, cerebrospinal fluid, and kidneys.[1] In adults, two-thirds of the body fluid exists in the intracellular space (primarily in the skeletal muscle mass). The remaining one-third is primarily found between the cells and in the plasma space. Microscopically, one might visualize the body fluids as in Figure 1-2.

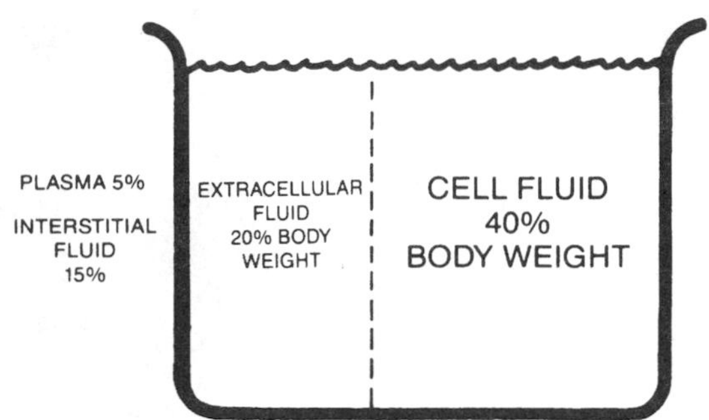

Figure 1–1. Total body fluid, 60% body weight.

Total body water content varies with body fat content, sex, and age. Fat cells contain little water, whereas lean tissue is rich in water. Thus, women have less body fluid than men because they have proportionately more body fat. The elderly have less body fluid than their younger counterparts for the same reason. Obese individuals, in general, have considerably less fluid than those of lean build (see Fig. 1-3).

Infants have a high body fluid content (approximately 70% to 80% of their body weight). In addition to having proportionately more body fluid than adults, infants have relatively more ECF. Indeed, more than half of the newborn's body fluid is extracellular, whereas in the adult only a third or less is extracellular. Because ECF is more readily lost from the body than is cellular fluid, infants are more vulnerable to fluid volume deficit. As infants become older, their total body fluid percentage decreases; the change is most rapid during the first 6 months of life. By the end of the second year, the total body fluid approaches the adult percentage of approximately 60% (36% cellular and 24% extracellular). At puberty, the adult body composition is attained (40% cellular and 20% extracellular). For the first time there is a sex differentiation in fluid content. (See Table 1-1.)

After 40 years of age, mean values for total body fluid in percentage of body weight decrease for both men and women; however, the sex differentiation remains. After 60 years of age the percentage may decrease to approximately 52% in men and 46% in women (even less in obese persons). Again, the reduction in body fluid is explained by the fact that with aging there is a decrease in lean body mass in favor of fat. Variations in total body fluid with age are listed in Table 1-1.

Body fluid is composed primarily of water and electrolytes. An *electrolyte* is defined as a substance

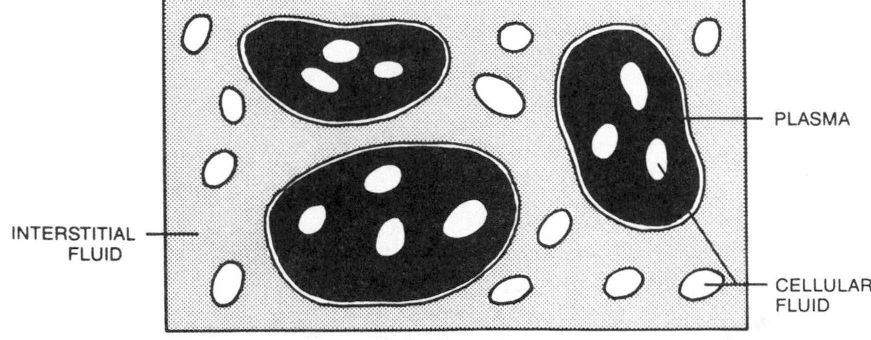

Figure 1–2. Microscopic visualization of body fluid distribution.

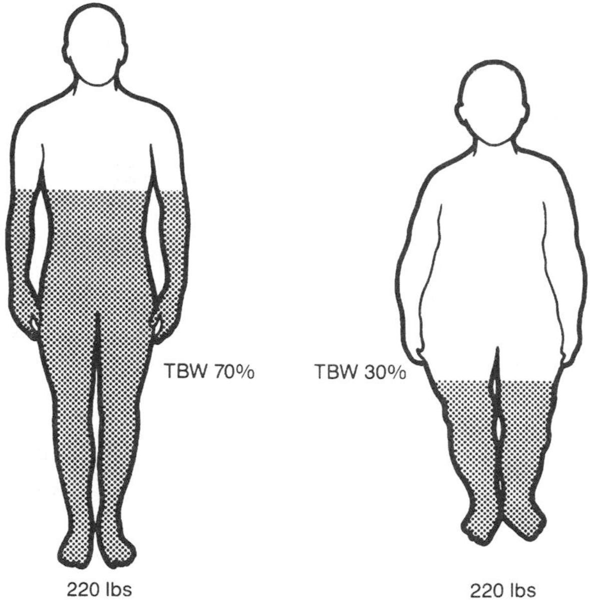

Figure 1–3. Body composition of a lean and an obese individual. Adapted from Statland H: Fluid & Electrolytes in Practice, 3rd ed. Philadelphia, JB Lippincott, 1963; with permission.

TABLE 1–2

Plasma Electrolytes

ELECTROLYTES	mEq/L
Cations	
Sodium (Na^+)	142
Potassium (K^+)	5
Calcium (Ca^{2+})	5
Magnesium (Mg^{2+})	2
Total cations	154
Anions	
Chloride (Cl^-)	103
Bicarbonate (HCO_3^-)	26
Phosphate (HPO_4^{2-})	2
Sulfate (SO_4^{2-})	1
Organic acids	5
Proteinate	17
Total anions	154

that develops an electrical charge when dissolved in water. Examples of electrolytes are sodium, potassium, calcium, chloride, and bicarbonate. Those that develop a positive charge in water are called *cations*; for example, sodium (Na^+), potassium (K^+), calcium (Ca^{2+}), and magnesium (Mg^{2+}). Electrolytes that develop negative charges when dissolved in water are called *anions*; for example, chloride (Cl^-) and bicarbonate (HCO_3^-). In all body fluids, anions and cations are always present in equal amounts, as positive and negative charges must be equal (an electrochemical fact).

The electrolyte content of intracellular fluid (ICF) differs significantly from that of ECF. Table 1-2 lists the electrolytes in plasma (ECF) and Table 1-3 lists

TABLE 1–1

Approximate Values of Total Body Fluid as a Percentage of Body Weight in Relation to Age and Sex

AGE	TOTAL BODY FLUID (% BODY WEIGHT)
Full-term newborn	70%–80%
1 year	64%
Puberty to 39 years	Men: 60% Women: 52%
40 to 60 years	Men: 55% Women: 47%
More than 60 years	Men: 52% Women: 46%

TABLE 1–3

Approximation of Major Electrolyte Content in Intracellular Fluid

ELECTROLYTES	MEq/L
Cations	
Potassium (K^+)	150
Magnesium (Mg^{2+})	40
Sodium (Na^+)	10
Total cations	200
Anions	
Phosphates Sulfates	150
Bicarbonate (HCO_3^-)	10
Proteinate	40
Total anions	200

those in ICF. Because special techniques are required to measure the concentration of electrolytes in the ICF, it is customary to measure the electrolytes in the ECF, namely plasma. Plasma electrolyte concentrations are used in assessing and managing patients with electrolyte imbalances. Some tests are performed on *serum* (the portion of plasma left after clotting); for practical purposes, the terms *serum electrolytes* and *plasma electrolytes* are used interchangeably.

The major electrolytes in the ECF are sodium (Na^+) and chloride (Cl^-), with a great preponderance of sodium ions (142 mEq/L) compared with other cations. About 90% of the ECF osmolality (concentration) is determined by the sodium concentration. Sodium is of primary importance in regulating body fluid volume; it is recognized that retention of sodium is associated with fluid retention. Whenever excessive quantities of sodium are lost, body fluid volume tends to decrease.

The electrolyte content of interstitial fluid is not measured in clinical situations; however, it is essentially the same as that of plasma, except that it contains less proteinate. (Recall that plasma protein is necessary to maintain oncotic pressure and keep the intravascular fluid inside the blood vessels.)

The major electrolytes in the ICF are potassium and phosphate. Because the ECF can tolerate only small potassium concentrations (approximately 5 mEq/L), release of large stores of intracellular potassium through cellular trauma can be extremely dangerous.

The body expends a great deal of energy maintaining the extracellular preponderance of sodium and the intracellular preponderance of potassium. It does so by means of cell membrane pumps, which exchange sodium and potassium ions.

UNITS OF MEASURE FOR ELECTROLYTES

Concentrations of solutes can be expressed in several ways, for example, milligrams per deciliter (mg/dL), milliequivalents per liter (mEq/L), or millimoles per liter (mmol/L). Because all of these units may be used in clinical settings, a brief review of their meanings is appropriate. *Milligrams per 100 mL (deciliter)* expresses the weight of the solute per unit volume. In contrast, a milliequivalent is a measure of chemical activity. The milliequivalent related to combining power with H^+.[2] By definition, a *milliequivalent of an ion* is its atomic weight expressed in milligrams divided by the valence. This measure is most favored in the United States for expressing the small concentrations of electrolytes in body fluids because it emphasizes the principle that ions combine milliequivalent for milliequivalent, not millimole for millimole or milligram for milligram. Also, the important concept of *electroneutrality* is clarified when using milliequivalents, because milliequivalents of cations and anions exist in equal numbers in the body fluids (see Fig. 1-4). This obligatory relationship is not evident if the ionic concentrations are measured in millimoles per liter or in milligrams per deciliter. Because electrolytes in body fluids are active chemicals (anions and cations) that unite in varying combinations, it is considered more logical to express their concentration as a measure of chemical activity rather than as a measure of weight. Consider this analogy: when a hostess creates a guest list for a dance, she does not invite 1000 pounds of boys per 1000 pounds of girls, she invites the same number of boys and girls.

Countries using the Système Internationale (S.I.) units express electrolyte content in body fluids in millimoles. To understand millimoles, it is necessary to review the definition of a mole. One *mole* (mol) of a substance is defined as the molecular (or atomic) weight of that substance in grams. For example, a mole of sodium is equivalent to 23 g (the atomic weight of sodium is 23). A *millimole* is one thousandth of a mole, or the molecular or atomic weight expressed in milligrams. Thus, a millimole of sodium is equivalent to 23 mg. Univalent elements, such as sodium (Na^+), chloride (Cl^-), and potassium (K^+), have identical numbers for milliequivalents and millimoles; that is, 140 mEq of Na^+ = 140 mmol of Na^+ and 5 mEq of K^+ = 5 mmol of K^+. However,

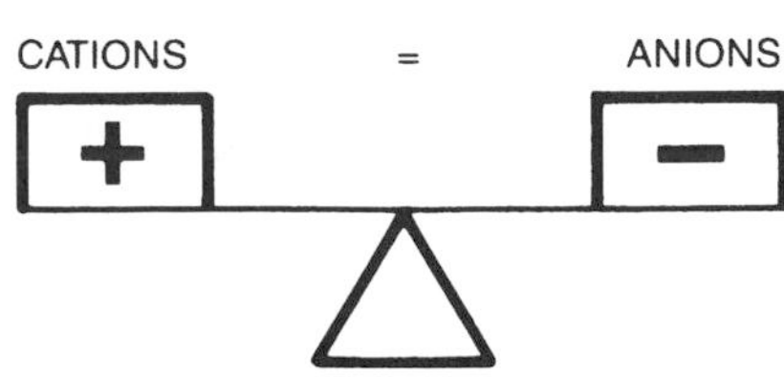

Figure 1–4. Number of cations equals number of anions.

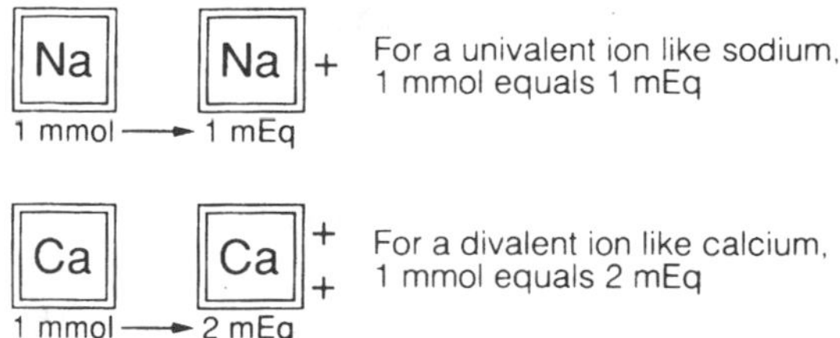

Figure 1–5. Millimoles versus milliequivalents for univalent and divalent ions.

different numbers are required for electrolytes that are not univalent. To convert from units of millimoles per liter to milliequivalents per liter, use the following formula: mEq/L = mmol/L × valence. For example, because the valence of calcium is 2, 1 mmol of calcium = 2 mEq of calcium[3] (see Fig. 1-5). Although the milliequivalent is not an S.I. unit, it is so widely used and conceptually useful that it is likely to be used for some time.

FUNCTIONS OF BODY FLUIDS

Body fluids are in constant motion, maintaining healthy living conditions for body cells. The ECF interfaces with the outside world and is modified by it, but the ICF remains stable. Nutrients are transported by the ECF to the cells, and wastes are carried away from the cells by means of the capillary bed. Approximately 10 billion capillaries with a total surface area close to the size of a football field provide this function for the entire body.[4]

Normal movement of fluids through the capillary wall into the tissues depends on two forces: hydrostatic pressure (exerted by pumping of the heart) and oncotic pressure (exerted by nondiffusible plasma proteins, primarily albumin). At the arterial end of the capillary, fluids are filtered through its wall by a hydrostatic pressure that exceeds the oncotic pressure exerted by plasma proteins. In contrast, because oncotic pressure is greater than hydrostatic pressure in the venous end of the capillary, fluids re-enter the capillary here (see Fig. 1-6).

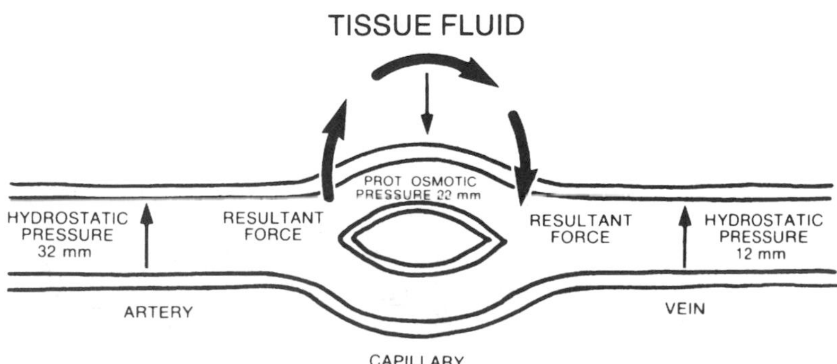

Figure 1–6. Fluid movement at capillary bed.

REGULATION OF BODY FLUID COMPARTMENTS

OSMOSIS

When two different solutions are separated by a membrane impermeable to the dissolved substances, a shift of water occurs through the membrane from the region of low solute concentration to the region of high solute concentration until the solutions are of equal concentration (see Fig. 1-7). The magnitude

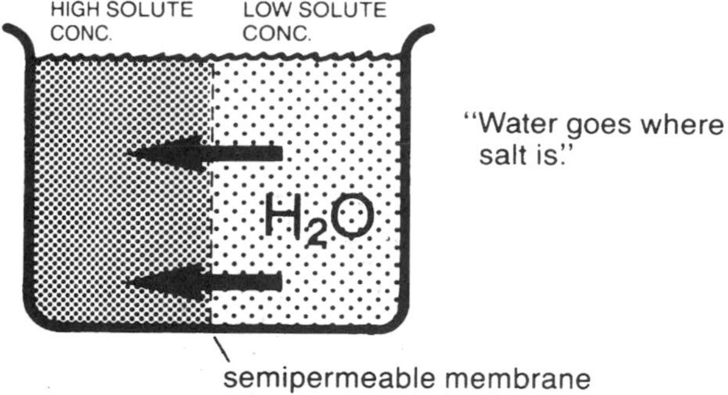

Figure 1–7. Osmosis.

of this force depends on the number of particles dissolved in the solutions and not on their weights.

The number of dissolved particles in a unit of water determines the solution's concentration, and can be expressed as either osmolality or osmolarity. *Osmolality* refers to the number of osmoles per kilogram of water; thus, the total volume will be 1 L of water plus the relatively small volume occupied by the solute.[5] On the other hand, *osmolarity* refers to the number of osmoles per liter of solution. In this instance, the volume of water is less than 1 L by an amount equal to the solute volume. Because of the very low solute concentration in body fluids, the difference between osmolality and osmolarity is negligible. Nonetheless, osmolality is the correct term to use when referring to body fluids because osmotic activity in the body depends on the concentration of active particles per kilogram of water.[6] The term *tonicity* is sometimes used instead of osmolality. Solutions may be termed isotonic, hypotonic, or hypertonic. Isotonic solutions have the same effective osmolality as body fluids (close to 285 milliosmolal [mOsm]). An example of an isotonic fluid is 0.9% sodium chloride. In contrast, a hypotonic solutions has a lower osmolality than body fluids; an example of a hypotonic fluid is 0.45% sodium chloride. Finally, a hypertonic solution has an effective osmolality greater than that of body fluids; an example of a hypertonic fluid is 3% sodium chloride.

DIFFUSION

The continual movement of molecules among each other in liquids, or in gases, is called *diffusion*.[7] An example of diffusion is the exchange of oxygen and carbon dioxide (CO_2) between the alveoli and capillaries.

FILTRATION

Filtration is the transfer of water and dissolved substances from a region of high pressure to a region of low pressure; the force behind it is hydrostatic pressure. An example of filtration is the passage of water and electrolytes from the arterial capillary bed to the interstitial fluid; in this instance, the hydrostatic pressure is furnished by the pumping action of the heart.

SODIUM–POTASSIUM PUMP

The sodium concentration is greater in the ECF than in the ICF, therefore, there is a tendency for sodium to enter by diffusion. This tendency is offset by the *sodium–potassium pump*, which is located in the cell membrane and, in the presence of adenosine triphosphate (ATP), actively moves sodium from the cell into the ECF. Conversely, potassium is the predominant cation in the ICF, therefore, the high intracellular potassium concentration is maintained by pumping potassium into the cell. Active transport occurs to move other ions (such as calcium and hydrogen) from areas of lesser concentration to areas of greater concentration. By definition, active transport implies that energy expenditure must take place for the movement to occur against a concentration gradient.

ROUTES OF GAINS AND LOSSES

Water and electrolytes are gained in various ways. In healthy humans, fluids are gained by drinking and eating (much of solid food is actually fluid). In illness, fluids may be gained by the parenteral route (intravenously or subcutaneously) or by means of an enteral feeding tube in the stomach or intestine. Organs of fluid loss include the lungs, skin, gastrointestinal tract, and kidneys. When fluid balance is critical, *all routes of gain* and *all routes of loss* must be recorded and the volumes compared. For critically ill patients, even small gains of fluid (such as that provided by humidifiers) must be considered.

LUNGS

The lungs normally eliminate water vapor (*insensible loss*) at a rate of approximately 300 to 400 mL/day. The loss is much greater with increased respiratory rate, depth, or both. Losses from the lungs are dependent on external factors, such as humidity and oxygen concentration.

SKIN

Visible water and electrolyte loss through the skin occurs by sweating (*sensible perspiration*). Sweat is a hypotonic fluid containing several solutes; the chief ones are sodium, chloride, and potassium. Actual sweat losses vary according to environmental temperature (from 0–1000 mL or more an hour). Significant sweat losses occur if the patient's body temperature exceeds 38.3 °C (101 °F) or if room temperature exceeds 32.2 °C (90 °F).

Continuous water loss by evaporation (approximately 600 mL/day) occurs through the skin as *insensible perspiration*, a nonvisible form of water loss. The presence of fever greatly increases insensible water loss through the lungs and the skin. Loss of the natural skin barrier in major burns also increases water loss by this route.

GASTROINTESTINAL TRACT

Each day, the healthy small intestine absorbs fluids that are ingested as well as those that are secreted into the gastrointestinal tract. Thus, although in adults approximately 8 L of fluid circulate through the gastrointestinal tract (GI) system every 24 hrs (the "GI circulation"), only about 100 to 200 mL are lost through the GI tract each day. Obviously, very large losses can be incurred from the GI tract if abnormal conditions occur such as diarrhea, fistulas, or vomiting. Diarrheal fluid losses tend to be isotonic with the extracellular fluid; however, diarrheal losses from the terminal part of the large intestine are hypotonic and reflect losses of free water.[8] Not only does vomiting cause fluid loss by the ejection of ingested and secreted fluids in the stomach and upper small intestine, it is usually associated with nausea that further limits oral intake of fluid.

KIDNEYS

While losses from the lungs, skin, and GI tract are determined by changing environmental events, losses from the kidney can be regulated by homeostatic organs. As such, the kidneys play a crucial role in the regulation of ECF volume in healthy and disease states.

The usual urine volume in the adult is between 1 and 2 L/day. A general rule of thumb is approximately 1 mL of urine per kilogram of body weight per hour (1 mL/kg/hr), with boundaries of 0.5 to 2 mL/kg of body weight per hour.[9]

Of note, Table 2-1 shows that in a healthy adult the average 24-hr intake and output of water is approximately equal.

HOMEOSTATIC MECHANISMS

The body is equipped with homeostatic mechanisms to keep the composition and volume of body fluid within narrow limits of normal. Organs involved in this mechanism include the kidneys, lungs, heart, blood vessels, adrenal glands, parathyroid glands, and pituitary gland.

KIDNEYS

The kidneys are vital to the regulation of fluid and electrolyte balance. They normally filter 135 to 180 L of plasma a day in a normal adult, while excreting only 1.5 L of urine.[10] They act both autonomously and in response to blood-borne messengers, such as aldosterone and antidiuretic hormone (ADH).

Major functions of the kidneys in fluid balance homeostasis include:

- Regulation of ECF volume and osmolality by selective retention and excretion of water and electrolytes. The juxtaglomerular apparatus (JGA) located within the kidney monitors both renal perfusion and solute excretion. The JGA, made up of specialized renin-secreting cells in the afferent glomerular arteriole and highly differentiated cells in the distal tubule (macula densa), is stimulated to release renin when there is a decrease in wall tension in the afferent arteriole or a decrease in salt delivery to the macula densa.[11] Renin converts angiotensinogen to angiotensin I, which is further metabolized to angiotensin II. In addition to being a vasoconstrictor, angiotensin II is a potent antinatriuretic hormone (causing sodium to be retained by the kidney). Also, angiotensin II stimulates aldosterone secretion, which enhances sodium reabsorption in the distal tubule.
- Regulation of electrolyte levels in the ECF by selective retention and excretion. The quantity of solutes and water in urine are highly variable according to the intake of these substances. For example, a person who has ingested a large quantity of sodium will excrete more sodium than will an individual who has been on a low-sodium diet.
- Regulation of acid–base balance. The kidneys must excrete the 50 to 100 mEq of noncarbonic

acid generated each day. In addition, they are responsible for reabsorbing virtually all of the filtered HCO_3^-.[12] (It should be remembered that loss of HCO_3^- in the urine is equivalent to adding hydrogen ions [H^+] ions to the body.)

- Excretion of metabolic wastes (primarily acids) and toxic substances. Urine contains high concentrations of uncharged molecules, particularly urea (allowing metabolic end products to be excreted, rather than accumulating in the body).[13]

Renal failure results in multiple fluid and electrolyte problems (see Chapter 17).

HEART AND ATRIAL NATRIURETIC FACTOR

Plasma must reach the kidneys in sufficient volume to permit regulation of water and electrolytes. The pumping action of the heart provides circulation of blood through the kidneys under sufficient pressure for urine to form; of course, renal perfusion makes renal function possible.

A hormone known as atrial natriuretic factor (ANF) or atrial natriuetic peptide (ANP) is released in the right atrium. The primary stimulus for release of ANF is atrial distention, which is associated with an increased venous return that increases right atrial pressure and stretch. This hormone acts on the kidney to cause a diuresis of sodium and water, thereby decreasing the intravascular volume. In addition, ANF is a direct vasodilator, which lowers the systemic blood pressure.[14]

The clinical significance and pharmacologic use of ANF is as yet unclear. For congestive heart failure patients, the diuretic effect of ANF appears to be most beneficial in acute heart failure; however, there appears to be a blunted renal response to ANF in chronic congestive heart failure patients.[15]

LUNGS

The lungs are also vital in maintaining homeostasis. Alveolar ventilation is responsible for the daily elimination of approximately 13,000 mEq of H^+, as opposed to only 40 to 80 mEq excreted daily by the kidneys.

Under control of the medulla, the lungs act promptly to correct metabolic acid–base disturbances by regulating the level of CO_2 (a potential acid) in the ECF. For example, to compensate for metabolic alkalosis, the lungs hypoventilate to retain CO_2; the increased acidity helps correct excess alkalinity of the body fluids. Just the opposite occurs with metabolic acidosis; the lungs hyperventilate to remove CO_2, which helps decrease the excess acidity of body fluids.

Pulmonary dysfunction can produce a rapid change (matter of seconds) in the plasma H^+ concentration (acid–base balance). Hypoventilation causes respiratory acidosis; hyperventilation causes respiratory alkalosis. When the lungs are at fault, the kidneys must compensate for the pH disturbances. Acid–base regulation is discussed in depth in Chapter 9.

The lungs also remove approximately 300 mL of water daily through exhalation (insensible water loss) in the healthy adult. Abnormal conditions, such as hyperpnea or continuous coughing, increase this loss; mechanical ventilation with excessive moisture decreases the loss.

PITUITARY GLAND

Specialized cells located in the hypothalamus manufacture a substance known as *antidiuretic hormone* (ADH), which is stored in the posterior lobe of the pituitary gland and released as needed. ADH is also known as arginine vasopressin. Because ADH makes the body retain water, it is sometimes referred to as the "water-conserving" hormone. Without the water-conserving effects produced by ADH, body water losses would be lethal.

The amount of water retained or excreted by the kidneys is partially regulated by ADH. ADH attaches to specialized receptor sites in the collecting and distal renal tubes, causing decreased urine output and increased urine osmolality.[16] Thus, as ADH secretion increases, renal water retention increases. The opposite occurs when there is decreased ADH production; that is, there is increased urinary output of dilute urine. Minor changes in body fluid osmolality constantly occur during normal living and lead to minor physiological changes in ADH production. A rising plasma osmolality, such as occurs with salt intake, increases ADH production and therefore, water retention; a falling plasma osmolality, such as occurs with water intake,

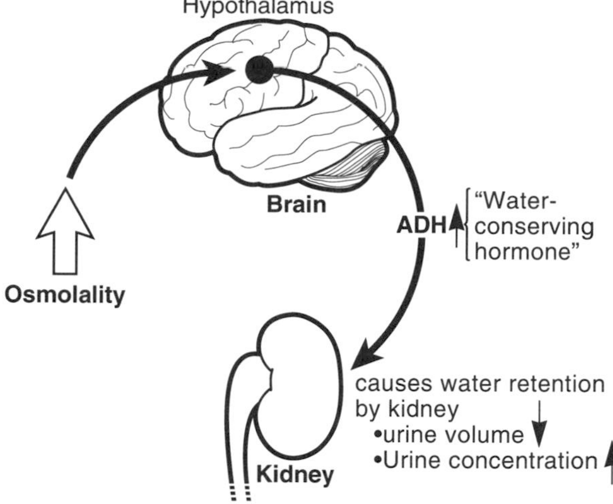

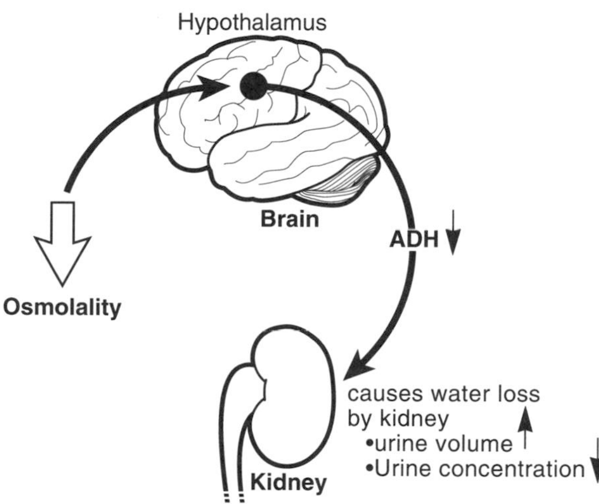

Figure 1–8. Effect of serum osmolality on ADH release and urine output.

decreases ADH production and enhances water excretion (see Fig. 1-8). Therefore, plasma osmolality and ADH are in constant interaction. In the presence of a falling blood volume, ADH secretion and subsequent water retention are stimulated by volume stimuli (probably arising from sensors in the heart and great vessels).

Syndrome of inappropriate antidiuretic hormone (SIADH) and *diabetes insipidus* (DI) are disorders of water balance due to ADH disturbances at opposite ends of a continuum. In SIADH, excessive ADH secretion causes water retention. The opposite happens in DI, which is characterized by large urine volumes due to inadequate amounts of ADH. These pathological states are discussed further in Chapters 4 and 19.

ADRENAL GLANDS

The primary adrenocortical hormone in the influence of fluid balance is *aldosterone*, a mineralocorticoid secreted by the outer zone of the adrenal cortex. This hormone acts chiefly on the distal tubules of the kidney to promote Na^+ reabsorption in exchange for K^+ and H^+ ions (which are excreted). Thus, aldosterone production causes sodium retention and expansion of the ECF, along with renal excretion of potassium. Occurrences that can stimulate aldosterone secretion include a fall in the plasma sodium concentration or an increase in the potassium concentration. However, the primary regulator of aldosterone secretion appears to be angiotensin II, which is produced by the renin-angiotensin system. A decreased blood volume or flow activates this system and increases aldosterone secretion. The aldosterone, in turn, increases renal retention of sodium (along with water) to correct the volume deficit (see Fig. 1-9). The opposite happens when a state of volume overexpansion exists.

Cortisol, another adrenocortical hormone, has only a fraction of the mineralocorticoid potency of aldosterone. However, secretion of cortisol in large quantities can produce sodium and fluid retention, and potassium deficit.

PARATHYROID GLANDS

Most persons have four parathyroid glands (see Fig. 1-10). These pea-sized glands, embedded in the corners of the thyroid gland, regulate calcium and phosphate balance by means of parathyroid hormone (PTH). Control of calcium ion concentration by PTH is largely due to this hormone's effect on bone reabsorption. Fall in calcium ion concentration stimulates PTH secretion. This, in turn, acts directly on the bones to increase reabsorption of bone salts, releasing large amounts of calcium into the ECF. Conversely, when the extracellular calcium level is too high, PTH secretion is depressed so that almost no bone reabsorption occurs. Long-term control of calcium ion concentration results from the effect of PTH on calcium reabsorption from the

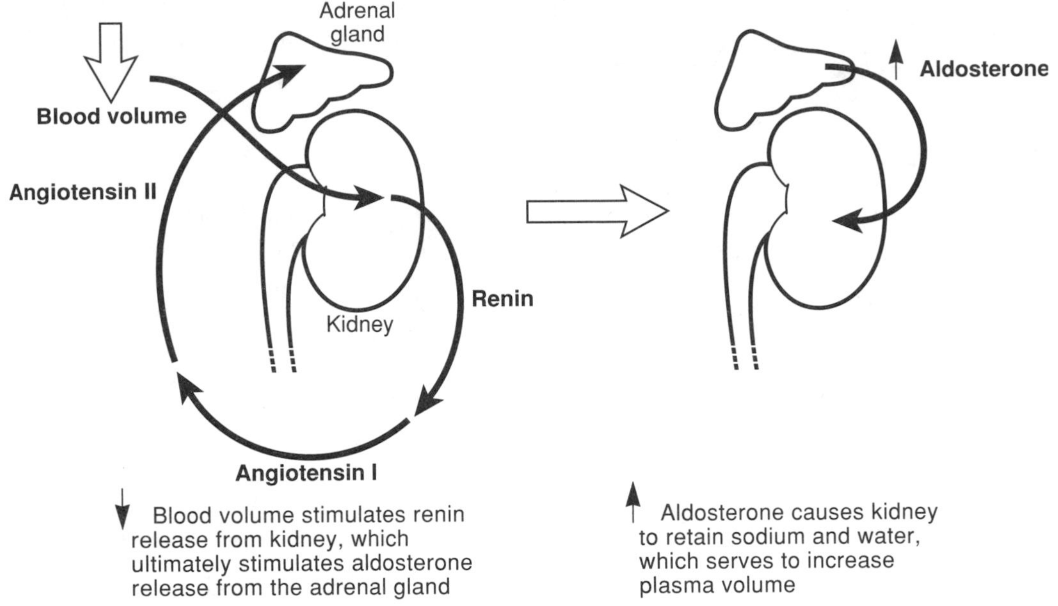

Figure 1–9. Effect of hypovolemia on the renin-angiotensin-aldosterone system.

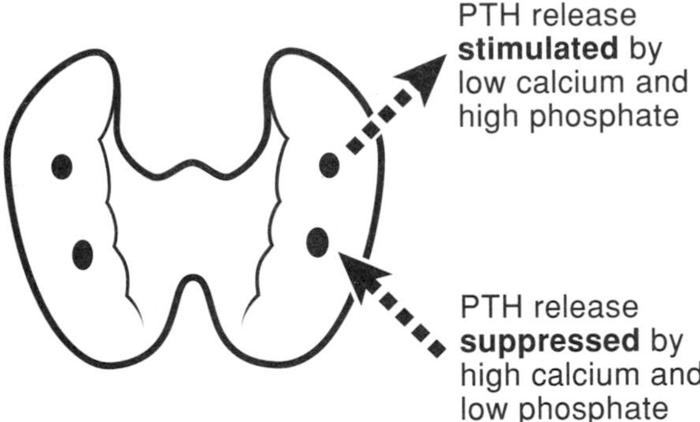

Figure 1–10 Effect of serum calcium and phosphorus on PTH release.

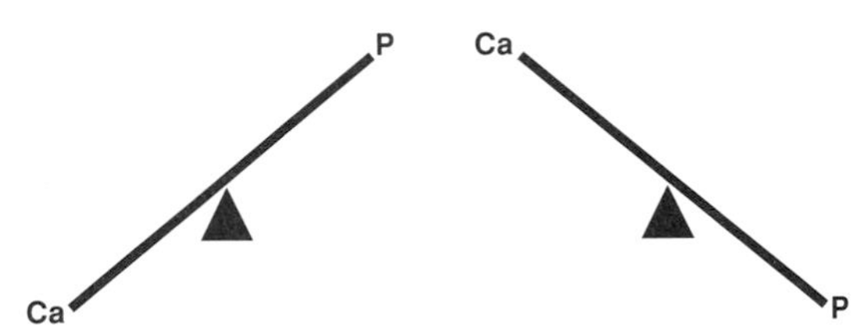

Figure 1–11. Reciprocal relationship between calcium and phosphorus.

kidney tubules and calcium absorption from the gut through the GI mucosa. Both of these effects are significantly increased by PTH.

A reciprocal relationship exists between extracellular calcium and phosphate levels in that an elevation of one usually causes a depression of the other (see Fig. 1-11). Thus, a high extracellular phosphate concentration causes a secondary depression of extracellular calcium; as a result, PTH release is stimulated (a condition often seen in renal failure).

Another hormone that bears consideration in the regulation of calcium is calcitonin, a substance secreted by the thyroid gland. Calcitonin's action on calcium is opposite to that of PTH; calcitonin reduces plasma calcium concentration. At high concentrations, calcitonin inhibits osteoclastic bone resorption.[17] Its effect on plasma calcium concentration is relatively stronger in children than in adults because the action of calcitonin involves bone remodeling, which is more rapid in children.[18] Pharmacological use of calcitonin in the treatment of hypercalcemia is discussed in Chapters 6 and 22.

REFERENCES

1. Narins R (ed): Maxwell & Kleeman's Clinical Disorders of Fluid and Electrolyte Metabolism, 5th ed, p 11. New York, McGraw-Hill, 1994
2. Ibid, p 1088
3. Smith K, Brain E: Fluids and Electrolytes: A Conceptual Approach, 2nd ed, p 14. New York, Churchill Livingstone, 1991
4. Guyton A: Textbook of Medical Physiology, 8th ed, p 170. Philadelphia, WB Saunders, 1991
5. Smith, p 18
6. Smith, p 19
7. Guyton, p 39
8. Smith, p 4
9. Pestana C: Fluids and Electrolytes in the Surgical Patient, 4th ed, p 223. Baltimore, Williams & Wilkins, 1989
10. Rose B: Clinical Physiology of Acid-Base and Electrolyte Disorders, 4th ed, p 7. New York, McGraw-Hill, 1994
11. Szerlip H, Goldfarb S: Workshops in Fluid and Electrolyte Disorders, p 3. New York, Churchill Livingstone, 1993
12. Rose, p 12
13. Ibid, p 303
14. Ibid, p 12
15. Toto K: Endocrine physiology. In: Endocrine and Metabolic Disturbances in the Critically Ill, p 647. Crit Care Nurs Clin N Am December, 1994
16. Ibid
17. Bell T: Diabetes insipidus. Endocrine and Metabolic Disturbances in the Critically Ill, p 676. Crit Care Nurs Clin N Am December, 1994
18. Narins, p 281

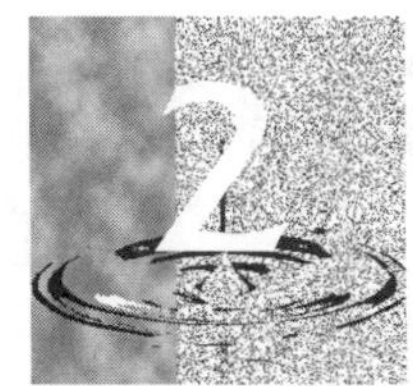

Nursing Assessment

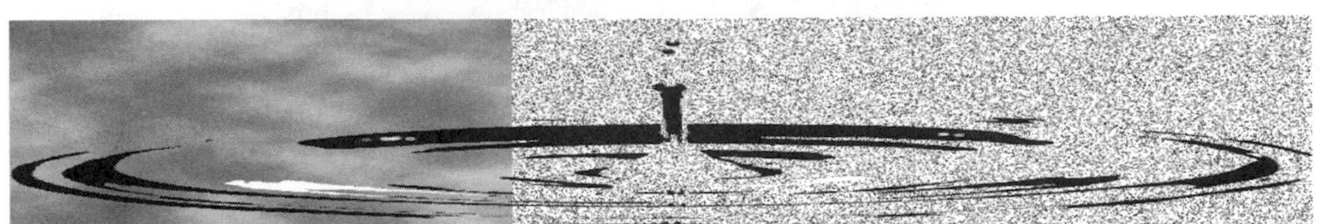

Nurses are responsible for monitoring patients for actual or potential fluid and electrolyte problems. It is logical for nurses to assume this vital role, as nurses are directly responsible for hospitalized patients 24 hrs a day and often they are the primary contact for patients both in extended-care facilities and in the home setting. Monitoring for fluid balance disturbances involves more than simple observations, and is based on an understanding of normal physiological mechanisms as well as of the indicators of disrupted fluid balance. As with many conditions, a high level of suspicion is necessary to detect fluid and electrolyte problems. The suspicion that an electrolyte abnormality exists is strengthened by the presence of clinical features known to occur, and often by the results of laboratory tests and electrocardiographical findings.

Nursing assessment of fluid balance requires a review of the patient's history and laboratory data, as well as careful clinical observation. In summary, one must know "what to look for," "where and how often to look," and "when to expect certain changes as a result of interventions" (outcome criteria).

HISTORY

The following questions should be considered in the nursing history:

1. Is there a disease process or injury state present that can disrupt fluid and electrolyte balance? (Examples might include diabetes mellitus, pancreatitis, and bowel obstruction.) In what type of imbalance(s) does this condition usually result?
2. Is the patient receiving any medication or treatment that can disrupt fluid and electrolyte balance? (Examples include steroids, diuretics, and total parenteral nutrition [TPN].) If so, how might this therapy upset fluid balance?
3. Is there an abnormal loss of body fluids and, if so, from what source? What types of imbalances are usually associated with the loss of these fluids?
4. Have any dietary restrictions (for example, a low-sodium diet) been imposed? If so, how might fluid balance be affected?
5. Has the patient taken adequate amounts of water and other nutrients orally or by some other route? If not, how long has the inadequate intakc bccn present?
6. How does the total intake of fluids compare with the total output of fluid?

CLINICAL ASSESSMENT

After the history described above has been reviewed, one should be able to identify potential problems related to fluid and electrolyte imbalances. At this point, a thorough nursing assessment is indicated. Of course, nursing assessment is not a "one-time" procedure but must be done at regular intervals to detect changes.

INSPECTION/EXAMINATION

Facial Appearance

An individual with a severe fluid volume deficit (FVD) has a pinched facial expression. A significant FVD causes decreased intraocular pressure; thus, the eyes appear sunken and feel soft to the touch.

Moisture in Oral Cavity

A dry mouth may be the result of FVD or of mouth breathing. If it is due to FVD, all of the oral tissues will be dry. In contrast, if the dryness is due to mouth breathing, the areas where the gums and cheek membranes meet will remain moist. Dry, sticky mucous membranes are noted with sodium excess (hypernatremia).

Thirst

Thirst is a subjective sensory symptom that has been defined as an awareness of the desire to drink. It has been reported to occur at a serum osmolality level of 295 mOsm/kg (at the point where antidiuretic hormone [ADH] secretion has been maximally stimulated).[1] An increased concentration of the extracellular fluid will osmotically pull fluid from the cells in the thirst control center and stimulate thirst. In general, any factor that causes intracellular dehydration will cause the sensation of thirst.

It has been shown that drinking and the presence of water in the stomach of a person with thirst usually produces satiety (long before any significant absorption has taken place). Gastric distention is affected by the temperature and osmotic properties of the consumed liquids.[2] For example, cold liquids tend to delay gastric emptying more than warm fluids; therefore, smaller volumes of cold liquids are required to achieve thirst satiation and small drinks of cold liquids are more likely to quench the thirst of patients on restricted fluid intake.[3]

The sense of thirst is so protective of the normal serum sodium level that hypernatremia virtually never occurs unless thirst is impaired or rendered ineffective because of unconsciousness or inaccessibility of water. In adults, hypernatremia is most often seen in persons older than 60 years of age, partially because age is associated with diminished osmotic stimulation of thirst.[4]

Thirst is prominent in patients who have increased water losses (such as occur in hyperglycemia, high fever, or diarrhea). An infant can be tested for thirst by offering water, although the presence of nausea may mask the symptom. Unfortunately, patients with altered states of consciousness do not experience normal thirst. Also, many patients are debilitated and unable to respond to thirst. It is no wonder that hypernatremia is a relatively common imbalance on neurologic units.

In addition to fluid volume changes, thirst can be affected by electrolyte balance. For example, thirst and polyuria are prominent and early signs of hypercalcemia. Also, long-standing hypokalemia can cause a type of diabetes insipidus and result in polyuria and thirst.

Tearing and Salivation

Tearing and salivation are decreased in patients with FVD. These signs are particularly helpful in pediatric patients to detect FVD.

Tongue Turgor

In a healthy person, the tongue has one longitudinal furrow. In the person with FVD, there are additional longitudinal furrows, and the tongue is smaller (due to fluid loss). Unlike skin turgor, tongue turgor is not appreciably affected by age and therefore is a useful assessment for all age groups. Note that sodium excess causes the tongue to appear red and swollen.

Filling of Neck Veins

The jugular veins provide a built-in manometer to follow the changes in central venous pressure (CVP). No invasive maneuvers are required and the procedure can be reliable when done correctly (see Fig. 2-1). The vein on the right side is preferred for assessment because the right internal jugular vein is nearly a direct conduit to the right atrium. The left internal jugular vein is less desirable because the brachycephalic vein may be compressed by the aortic knob, resulting in false elevation of CVP.[5]

Changes in fluid volume are reflected by changes in neck vein filling, provided the patient is not in heart failure. Normally, with the patient supine, the external jugular veins fill to the anterior border of the sternocleidomastoid muscle. Flat neck veins in the supine position indicate a decreased plasma volume. With the patient positioned sitting at a 45-degree angle, the venous distentions normally should not extend higher than 2 cm above the sternal angle. Elevated venous pressure is indicated by neck veins distended from the top portion of the sternum to the angle of the jaw; this is often seen in severe heart failure.

To estimate jugular venous pressure, the nurse should do the following:

1. Position the patient in a semi-Fowler's position (head of bed elevated to a 30- to 60-degree angle), keeping the neck straight.
2. Remove any of the patient's clothing that could constrict the neck or upper chest.

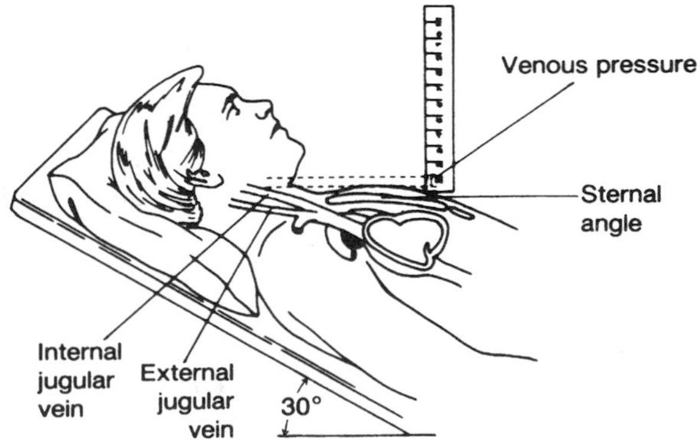

Figure 2–1. Assessment of jugular vein pulsations. Adapted from Smeltzer S, Bare B: Brunner & Suddarth's Textbook of Medical–Surgical Nursing, 7th ed, p 625. Philadelphia, JB Lippincott, 1992.

3. Provide adequate lighting to visualize effectively the external jugular veins on each side of the neck.
4. Measure the level to which the veins are distended on the neck above the sternal angle. The vertical distance between this point and the sternal angle is measured and reported as centimeters above or below the sternal angle.

Appearance and Temperature of Skin

Severe FVD causes the skin to be pale and cool because of peripheral vasoconstriction, which occurs to compensate for hypovolemia. Metabolic acidosis can cause warm, flushed skin due to peripheral vasodilatation.

Skin Turgor

In a healthy person, pinched skin will immediately fall back to its normal position when released. This elastic property, referred to as turgor, partially depends on the interstitial fluid volume. In an individual with a FVD, the skin flattens more slowly after the pinch is released, and may remain elevated for several seconds.

Tissue turgor is best measured by pinching the skin over the sternum, in the inner aspects of the thighs, or on the forehead (see Fig. 2-2), although some nurses prefer to test skin turgor in children over the abdominal area and on the medial aspects of the thighs.

Although the purpose of the skin turgor test is to measure only interstitial fluid volume, it also measures skin elasticity. It is common for persons older than 55 to 60 years of age to have reduced skin turgor because they have less skin elasticity relative to younger persons. Skin turgor may be difficult to assess in elderly patients or in those with recent weight loss and is not diagnostic in the absence of other signs of FVD.

In children, skin turgor begins to diminish after 3% to 5% of the body weight is lost. However, severe malnutrition, particularly in infants, can cause depressed skin turgor even in the absence of fluid depletion. Obese infants with FVD may have skin turgor that is deceptively normal. Infants with hypernatremia may have firm skin that feels thick.

In summary, tissue turgor can vary with age, nutritional state, and even race or complexion. Observations are most meaningful if done sequentially before the development of a fluid balance abnormality.

Edema

Edema is defined as an excessive accumulation of interstitial fluid (the body fluid that bathes the cells). Edema usually does not become clinically apparent

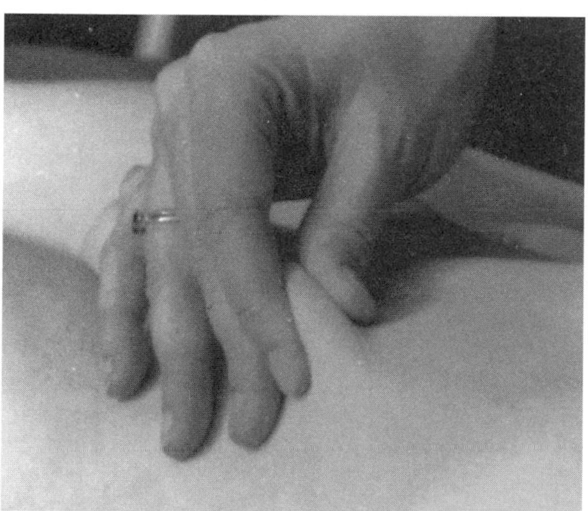

Figure 2–2A. Testing skin turgor on the abdomen of a well-hydrated infant. From Bates B: A Guide to Physical Examination, 6th ed, p 582, 1995.

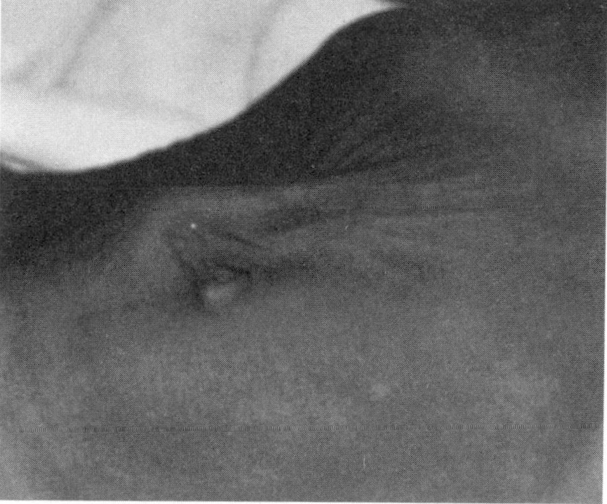

Figure 2–2B. Tenting of skin on abdomen of a dehydrated patient. From Bates B: A Guide to Physical Examination, 6th ed, p 582, 1995.

until the interstitial volume has increased by at least 2.5 to 3 L.[6]

Causes of edema include (1) increased capillary permeability, which allows fluid to leak into the interstitium (as in burns or localized trauma); (2) increased capillary hydraulic pressure, which forces fluid into the interstitium (as in heart failure or venous obstruction); (3) decreased plasma oncotic pressure of hypoalbuminemia, which fosters the transfer of fluid into the interstitium (particularly when the plasma albumin level is less than 2 g/dL); and (4) lymphatic obstruction, which permits local edema (as in node enlargement of malignancy).[7]

Edema formation may be either localized (as in thrombophlebitis) or generalized (as in heart failure and the nephrotic syndrome). An excess of interstitial fluid accumulating predominantly in the lower extremities of ambulatory patients and in the presacral region of bedridden patients is referred to as *dependent edema*. *Generalized edema* is spread throughout the body, and may accumulate in periorbital and scrotal regions because of the relatively lower tissue hydrostatic pressure in these regions. Edema related to salt retention is generally pitting and can be manifested by pressing one's finger into the soft tissues (see Fig. 2-3). After the pressure is removed, the "pit" gradually disappears. Barely perceptible pitting edema indicates that total body sodium content has increased by approximately 400 mEq (2.7 L of saline).[8]

Describing peripheral edema by appearance is somewhat subjective. For example, it is sometimes indicated by using plus signs to represent the amount, ranging from +1 to +4, with +1 indicating barely perceptible, +2 and +3 moderate, and +4 severe edema. Measuring an extremity or body part with a millimeter tape in the same area each day is the most exact method.

There is little or no peripheral edema with only water retention (as occurs in excessive secretion of ADH). Instead, there is cellular swelling that sometimes can be detected by pressing one's finger over the sternum (or other bony prominence) and producing a visible fingerprint.

Pulmonary Edema

Pulmonary edema results from excessive shifting of fluid from the vascular space into the pulmonary interstitium and air spaces. Such accumulation of extravascular water (EVW) affects pulmonary functioning and gas exchange to varying degrees depending both on the site of accumulation (interstitial versus alveolar) and on the quantity of fluid involved. Cardiogenic causes of increased EVW usually result in alveolar fluid, and noncardiogenic causes in interstitial edema.[9]

Clinical symptoms of EVW result primarily from either one or both of two phenomena: (1) fluid entering the air spaces and (2) increased interstitial pressure impinging on bronchioles and blood vessels, which results in increased airway and vascular resistances, leading to abnormal distribution of perfusion and ventilation.[10]

Capillary Refill

Capillary refill can be checked by applying pressure to a fingernail for 5 sec and then releasing the pressure and noting how rapidly the normal color returns.[11] Color will return in less than 1 to 2 sec in a healthy person. A delayed capillary refill could indicate constriction of the peripheral vessels, decreased cardiac output, or anemia. Other factors that reduce capillary refill time include cold temperatures and cigarette smoking.

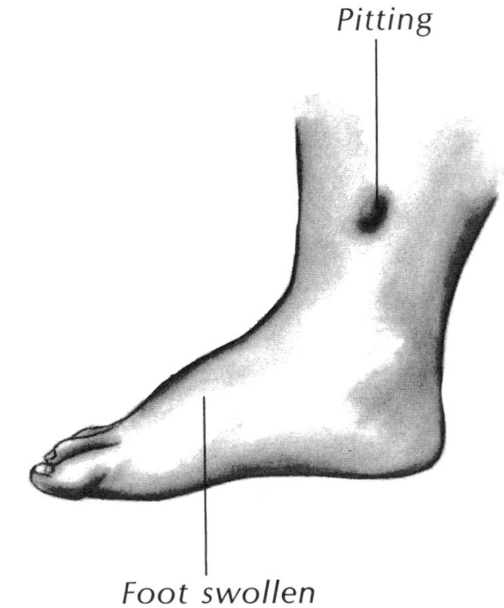

Figure 2–3. Pitting edema of foot. From Bates B: A Guide to Physical Examination, 6th ed, p 447, Table 16-4, 1995.

Neuromuscular Irritability

It is sometimes necessary to assess patients for increased or decreased neuromuscular irritability, particularly when imbalances in calcium, magnesium, and sodium are suspected.

The nurse may, as necessary, check for Chvostek's sign and Trousseau's sign; also, deep tendon reflexes can be tested to monitor neuromuscular irritability.

To test Chvostek's sign, the facial nerve should be percussed about 2 cm anterior to the earlobe. A positive response shows a unilateral twitching of the facial muscles, including the eyelid and lips. Chvostek's sign is indicative of hypocalcemia or hypomagnesemia. However, it is not specific for these conditions as it is present in about 25% of healthy adults.[12]

To test for Trousseau's sign, place a blood pressure cuff on the arm and inflate above systolic pressure for 3 min. A positive reaction is the development of carpal spasm (Fig. 2-4). This sign is also not specific for hypocalcemia as it is present in about 4% of the normal population and may be negative in 30% of patients with latent tetany.[13]

The common deep tendon reflexes include the biceps, triceps, brachioradialis, patellar, and Achilles reflexes. A deep tendon reflex is elicited by briskly tapping a partially stretched tendon with a rubber percussion hammer, preferably over the tendon insertion of the muscle. The broad head of the hammer is used to stroke easily accessible tendons (eg, the Achilles) and the pointed end for less accessible tendons (eg, the biceps). The response in the prospective muscle is a sudden contraction. The muscle being tested should be slightly stretched (by the position of the limb), and the patient should be relaxed. With too little or too much muscle stretch the reflex cannot be elicited.

The reflexes are usually graded on a 0 to 4+ scale

0 = no response
1+ = somewhat diminished, but present
2+ = normal
3+ = brisker than average and possibly but not necessarily indicative of disease
4+ = hyperactive

Deep tendon reflexes may be hyperactive in the presence of hypocalcemia, hypomagnesemia, hypernatremia, and alkalosis. They may be hypoactive in the presence of hypercalcemia, hypermagnesemia, hyponatremia, hypokalemia, and acidosis. Of course, many factors other than electrolyte disturbances can produce abnormalities in deep tendon reflexes. As with most other signs, deep tendon reflexes should be evaluated in light of other clinical signs, patient history, and laboratory data.

Other Signs

Other areas to consider in clinical assessment include changes in

- Behavior
- Sensation
- Fatigue level

Because these changes are often vague, they are best evaluated in context with specific imbalances (see Chapters 3 through 9).

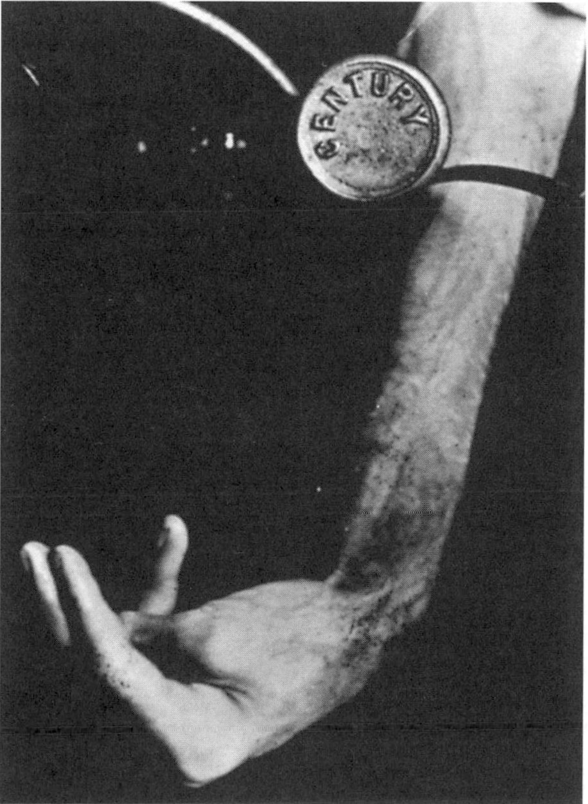

Figure 2–4. Carpopedal attitude of hand. From Ezrin C: Systematic Endocrinology, 2nd ed, p 510. Hagerstown, MD, Harper & Row, 1979.

VITAL SIGNS AND HEMODYNAMICS

Body Temperature

Changes in body temperature as *symptoms* of fluid and electrolyte imbalances may include:

1. Elevation in body temperature in hypernatremia may occur due to excessive water loss.[14] The elevated body temperature is probably related to lack of available fluid for sweating. Also, dehydration probably has a direct effect on the hypothalamus.
2. In a cool room, a patient with an isotonic FVD may be slightly hypothermic (probably related to the decreased basal metabolic rate). After partial correction of the FVD, the temperature generally increases to an appropriate level. With moderate FVD, temperature taken rectally may be 36.1 °C (97 °F) to 37.2 °C (99 °F); with severe FVD, it may be 35 °C (95 °F) to 36.7 °C (98 °F).[15]

Body temperature changes do not reflect only fluid balance problems. Fever can *cause* fluid balance problems if not promptly recognized and treated. Fever causes an increase in metabolism rate and, as a result, in formed metabolic wastes, which require fluid to make a solution for renal excretion; therefore, fluid loss is increased. Fever also causes hyperpnea, an increase in breathing rate resulting in extra water vapor loss through the lungs. Because fever increases loss of body fluids, temperature elevations must be detected early and appropriate interventions taken.

A temperature elevation between 38.3 °C (101 °F) and 39.4 °C (103 °F) increases the 24-hr fluid requirements by at least 500 mL, and a temperature higher than 39.4 °C (103 °F) increases it by at least 1000 mL.[16]

Pulse

Tachycardia is usually the earliest sign of the decreased vascular volume associated with FVD. It may also be associated with deficits of magnesium or potassium. Conversely, excesses of magnesium or potassium can cause decreased pulse rate. Irregular pulse rates also occur with potassium imbalances and magnesium deficit. Pulse volume is decreased in FVD and increased in fluid volume excess (FVE).

Respirations

Deep, rapid respirations may be a compensatory mechanism for metabolic acidosis or a primary disorder causing respiratory alkalosis. Slow, shallow respirations may be a compensatory mechanism for metabolic alkalosis or a primary disorder causing respiratory acidosis.

Weakness or paralysis of respiratory muscles is likely in severe hypokalemia or hyperkalemia and in severe magnesium excess (the respiratory center may be paralyzed at a serum magnesium level of 10–15mEq/L). Moist rales, in the absence of cardiopulmonary disease, indicate FVE.

Blood Pressure

A sensitive method for detecting volume depletion is measurement of the blood pressure and pulse with the patient in a lying and then standing position. Standing from a supine position causes an abrupt drop in venous return, for which sympathetically mediated cardiovascular adjustments normally compensate. In the healthy individual, cardiac return is maintained by increased peripheral resistance and a slight increase in heart rate; systolic pressure falls only slightly and diastolic pressure may actually rise a few millimeters of mercury. In contrast, a fall in systolic pressure greater than 15 mmHg or an increase in the pulse rate greater than 15 beats/min is suggestive of intravascular volume deficit.[17] When hypovolemia is suspected, it is helpful to measure the blood pressure in three positions (supine, sitting, and standing); a repeat reading after 2 to 3 min may identify orthostatic hypotension missed by earlier readings.[18] Of course, conditions associated with autonomic neuropathy (such as diabetes) can also produce these orthostatic blood pressure and pulse changes, as can sympatholytic antihypertensive medications.

Hypotension may occur with magnesium excess, perhaps first occurring at a level of 3 to 5 mEq/L. Hypertension can occur with magnesium deficit and with FVE.

Nursing observations must be *interpreted*, using one's knowledge of the patient's history and pathophysiological condition, to determine whether the information gained from the assessment suggests normal or abnormal signs or measurements, and to what degree. Then, the appropriate nursing action(s) must be determined. One must also know when medical intervention is required.

Central Venous Pressure

Central venous pressure refers to pressure in the right atrium or vena cava and provides information about the following parameters: blood volume, effectiveness of the heart's pumping action, and vascular tone. When CVP is measured with a water manometer, pressure in the right atrium is usually 0 to 4 cm of water and pressure in the vena cava is approximately 4 to 11 cm of water. When CVP is measured with a transducer system, the normal range is approximately 0 to 7 mm Hg. A *low* CVP may indicate:

- Decreased blood volume,
- Drug-induced vasodilation (causing pooling of blood in peripheral veins), or
- Condition that reduces venous return to the heart

In contrast, a *high* CVP may indicate:

- Increased blood volume,
- Heart failure, or
- Vasoconstriction (causing the vascular bed to become smaller)

More important than absolute values are the upward or downward trends; these trends are determined by taking frequent readings (often every 30–60 min). It is always important to evaluate the CVP in reference to other available clinical data such as:

- Blood pressure
- Pulse
- Respirations
- Breath and heart sounds
- Fluid intake
- Urinary output

Example: A rise in CVP paralleling that of systolic blood pressure (BP) in a previously hypotensive patient is an indication of adequate fluid volume replacement. A low CVP persisting after fluid volume replacement may be a sign of continued occult bleeding.

In those patients with normal cardiac function and relatively normal pulmonary function, the CVP remains an acceptable guide to blood volume. Patients with acute cardiopulmonary decompensation require more extensive hemodynamic monitoring with a device that reflects pressures in both sides of the heart.

Rate of Fluid Administration

Sometimes the rate of an infusion is titrated according to the patient's CVP; when this is necessary, the physician should designate the desired limits so that the nurse can adjust the flow rate accordingly. For example, in acute hypercalcemia, the physician may order isotonic saline at a rate of 250 mL/hr, provided that the CVP does not exceed 10 cm of water. As long as urinary output remains adequate and the CVP does not change significantly, it can be assumed that the heart is accommodating the amount of fluid being administered. On the other hand, if the CVP begins to fall despite fluid administration, hypovolemia must be suspected and is an indicator for more rapid fluid administration.

Methods of Measuring CVP

CVP can be measured with a water manometer (Fig. 2-5) or a pressure transducer system (Fig. 2-6). The water manometer is most often used in the nonintensive care settings, whereas the pressure transducer system is usually used for patients in an intensive care unit.

WATER MANOMETER The manometer is a fluid-filled tube that relays the patient's pressure reading without the use of electrical equipment. It is connected to the patient's intravenous infusion system; in turn, this connects to the central venous catheter. Take the following steps to read the CVP:

1. First, turn the stopcock so that the solution will flow from the container to the manometer (see Fig. 2-5, System 2).
2. Second, turn the stopcock to direct manometer flow to the patient (see Fig. 2-5, System 3). The fluid level should drop, reaching a reading level in about 15 sec.
3. Third, record the reading at the upper level of the respiratory fluctuation of fluid in the manometer (fluid falls slightly on inspiration and rises slightly on expiration).

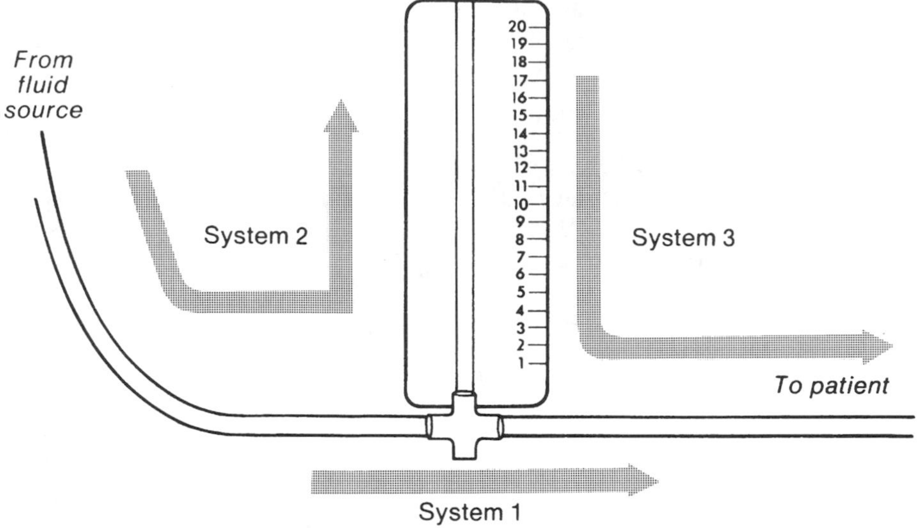

Figure 2–5. Fluid flow systems in central venous pressure measurement. System 1 allows flow from the container to the patient (routine infusion). System 2 allows flow from the container to the manometer (allows manometer to fill). System 3 allows flow from the manometer to the patient (allows reading of CVP). From Hudak et al: Critical Care Nursing, 5th ed, p 122. Philadelphia, JB Lippincott, 1990.

Transducer System A single transducer is connected to the central catheter lumen, which is connected to the monitor. The pressure is measured by the transducer and converted to a numerical value that is continuously displayed on the monitor (see Fig. 2-6). (Halck et al.[19] reported a close linear correlation between CVP measurements performed with water manometrics and electric equipment.)

Nursing Considerations

1. Measure CVP with the patient lying flat in bed if this position can be tolerated. If not, have the patient in the same position each time CVP is measured. Indicate the patient's position on the chart when recording the pressure. Place the zero point of the manometer at the level of the patient's right atrium (see Fig. 2-7). The point

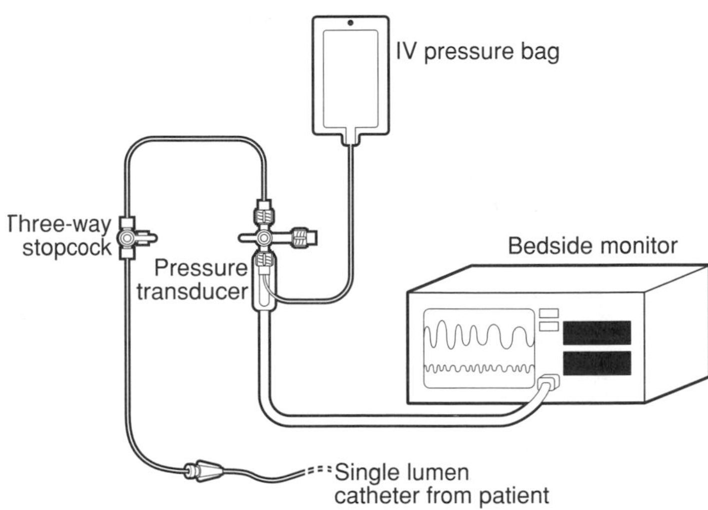

Figure 2–6. Transducer system. The transducer is an instrument that is used to sense physiological events and transform them into electrical signals. If central venous pressure is the only measure needed, a single lumen catheter may be used and connected to a water manometer or a transducer system. The transducer system is also used with pulmonary artery catheters.

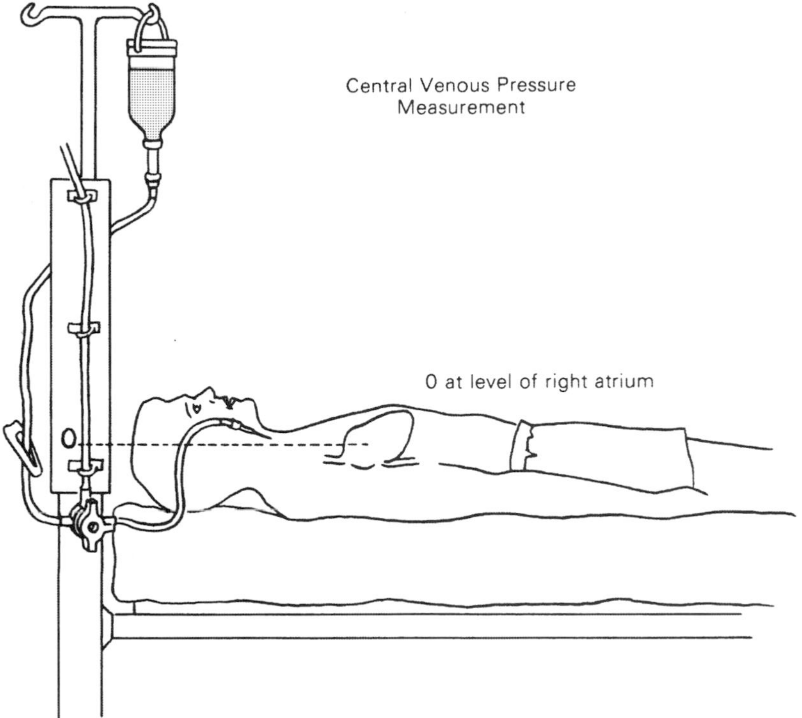

Figure 2–7. Central venous pressure measurement with zero point of manometer at level of right atrium. From Huda, et al: Critical Care Nursing, 5th edit, p 122. Philadelphia, JB Lippincott, 1990.

selected may be marked on the patient's side so that the zero mark may be used consistently.

2. Be aware that a falsely high reading will result if the patient is being ventilated on a respirator.[20] When recording the measurement, be sure to note that it was made during artificial ventilation.
3. Be aware that the fluid should fluctuate 3 to 5 cm in the manometer with respirations when the catheter is patent and properly positioned in the vena cava.

Pulmonary Artery and Pulmonary Artery Wedge Pressures

At times, CVP measurements are not adequate for evaluating the patient's clinical status or for determining proper flow rates. It may be necessary to use more invasive hemodynamic monitoring to adequately assess heart function.

The appropriate indications for pulmonary artery (PA) catheter monitoring have been debated for more than a decade. The potential benefits of using such a device include:

- It allows more accurate determination of the hemodynamic status of critically ill patients than is possible by clinical assessment of CVP alone.
- It can be helpful in assessing fluid status in patients with confusing clinical pictures, especially those for whom errors in fluid management and drug therapy have major consequences.

Proper usage of PA catheters can assist clinicians in achieving better patient outcomes.[21] Unfortunately, there are indications that nurses need more education on using PA catheters and properly interpreting results. For example, a group of nurses attending a recent American Association of Critical Care Nurses' National Teaching Institute conference performed poorly (mean score of 48.5%) on a 37-item test regarding interpretation of PA catheter results.[22] This indicates that current teaching practices regarding the PA catheter may need to be reevaluated and specific credentialing policies need to be considered.

Description of PA Catheter

The PA catheter is used to monitor pressures in the right side of the heart and in the pulmonary vasculature. These catheters have variable numbers of lumens (two to five). A four-lumen catheter is depicted in Figure 2-8. Two of these four lumens are connected to the transducer and yield waveforms.

- The proximal lumen monitors the CVP (or right atrial pressure). It also carries the injectate into the right atrium for cardiac output (CO) measurement. It can be used for blood sampling or for infusions of saline or dextrose solutions between measurements.
- A second lumen is the balloon lumen for inflation and deflation of the balloon to measure pulmonary capillary wedge pressure (PCWP). PCWP is obtained by inflating the catheter balloon. The balloon occludes a branch of the PA and indicates the presence and degree of pulmonary congestion, as well as the performance of the left ventricle.
- A third lumen is for the thermistor, which contains temperature-sensitive thermistor wires to determine CO. Cardiac output is the amount of blood ejected with each heartbeat (measured in liters per minute). Computer programs are now available that measure CO continuously; however, the most commonly used method is the "thermodilution" method in which a known solution (iced or room temperature) is injected in the right atrium port. As venous mixing occurs, the change in temperature of the injectate is measured. Some catheters will automatically calculate the cardiac index (CI), provided the patient's height and weight have been entered into the computer. Cardiac index is

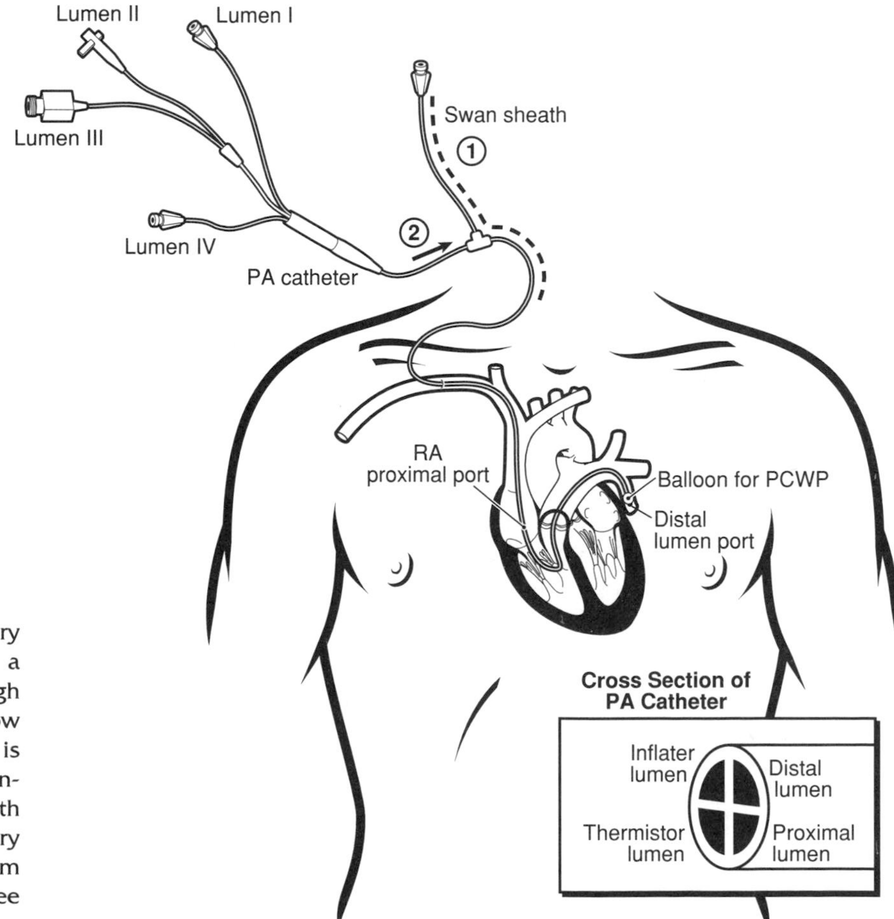

Figure 2–8. Pulmonary artery catheter. (1) Swan sheath is a short 7 or 8.5 Fr device through which the longer, more narrow pulmonary artery catheter is inserted. Fluids may be administered through the sheath catheter. (2) Pulmonary artery catheter (approximately 110 cm in length) has four lumens (see text).

equal to CO per square meter of body surface area. This measure helps individualize treatment; for example, a small person requires less circulating blood and would have a lower CO.

- The PA or distal lumen terminates at the tip of the catheter. When connected to a monitor, the PA pressures give an estimate of the venous pressure within the lungs and the mean filling pressure of the left atrium and ventricle. A normal PA pressure is 25/10 mmHg with a mean of 15 mmHg. Pulmonary artery systolic (PAS) pressure reflects right ventricular contraction and pulmonary artery diastolic (PAD) pressure reflects the resistance to flow by small arterioles and pulmonary capillaries. When there is no pulmonary vascular obstruction, PAD pressure should be approximately the same as the PCWP. The distal lumen also gives mixed venous oxygen saturation (SvO_2)—a measure of the degree to which tissues of the body are using oxygen and the adequacy of oxygen supply.

Insertion of PA Catheter

Before insertion of the PA catheter, the lumens of the catheter are connected to a transducer system (the transducers convert pressures of the heart and PA into electrical energy, which is reflected on the monitor as numbers and waveforms). The catheter may be inserted by a brachial, subclavian, jugular, or femoral vein and is advanced into the right atrium, through the tricuspid valve into the right ventricle, and finally out the pulmonic valve into the pulmonary artery (see Fig. 2-8). During insertion, the PA port is used to check catheter location as the catheter is advanced. The monitor that the catheter is connected to reflects different waveforms according to catheter position in the heart (see Fig. 2-9).

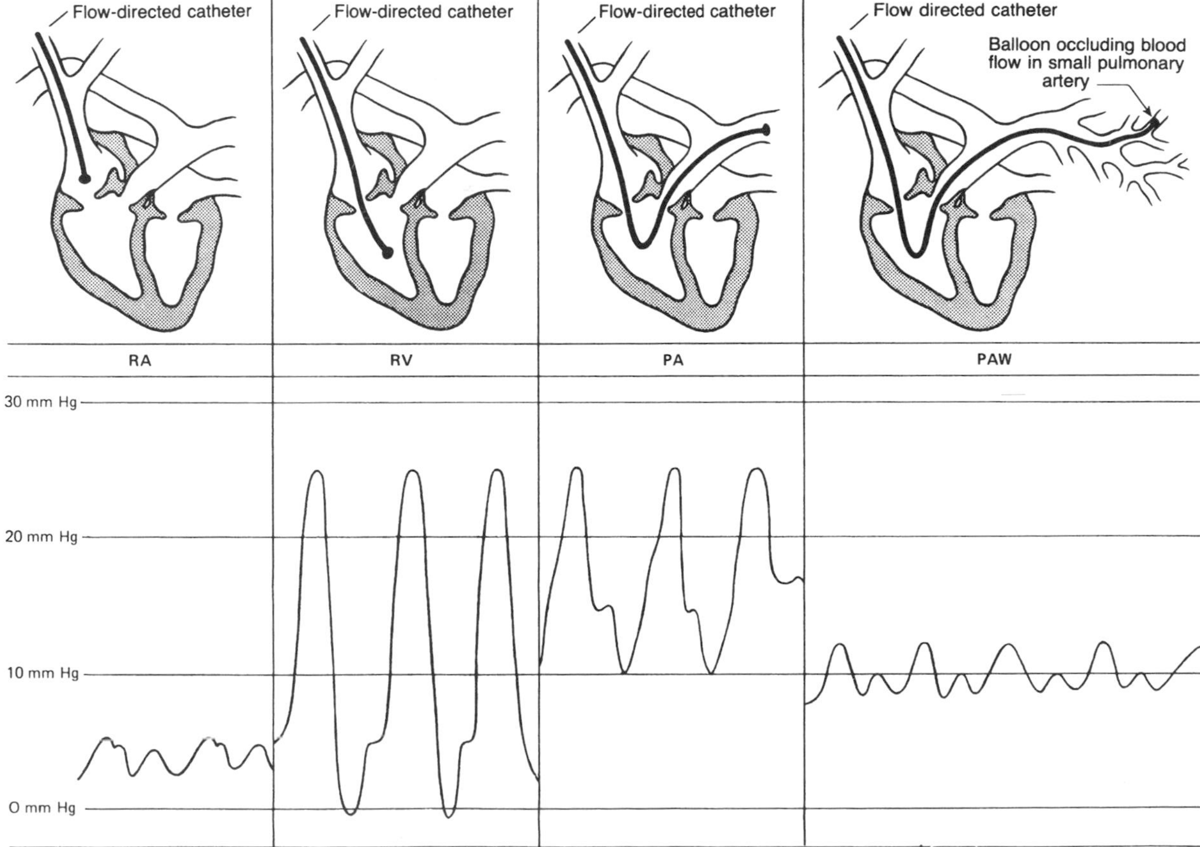

Figure 2–9. Flow-directed catheter positions with corresponding pressure tracings. (RA, right atrium; RV, right ventricle; PA, pulmonary artery; PAW, pulmonary artery wedge). As the catheter is passed through each chamber, the waveform will change.

Reference Level and Hemodynamic Readings

To reference the catheter, the bed is positioned so that the patient is in a zero to 45-degree, supine position.[23] Next, the phlebostatic axis is determined by locating the fourth intercostal space on the edge of the sternum and drawing an imaginary line along the fourth intercostal space laterally, along the chest wall. Then a second line is drawn from the axilla downward, midway between the anterior and posterior chest wall. Where these two lines intersect is the phlebostatic axis (level of the right atrium).

After the catheter has been referenced, it must be zeroed (calibrated). Zeroing is performed by opening the system to air to establish atmospheric pressure as zero. The needed frequency of this procedure is not clearly defined. Some institutions have protocols where this is done every 4 hrs; however, other hospitals require this only after the system has been disconnected from the monitor to change lines or transport the patient off the division. A recently reported study concerning zeroing of 388 disposable transducers suggests that zeroing needs to be performed only once, unless the transducer is disconnected from the monitor; however, this study needs to be replicated.[24]

Hemodynamic readings must be made with the appropriate reference point (see above). A number of research studies have supported taking PA pressures in a supine position, with the head of the bed elevated.[25–27] The taking of readings with the head of the bed at greater than 45 degrees has been studied, but further research is needed. Research on lateral positioning for PA and PCWP readings remains controversial.[28,29] Further research is needed in this area to guide nurses on how and when to take pressure measurements when the patient is in a lateral position.[30] It is difficult to determine the exact position of the phlebostatic axis when the patient is positioned laterally.

Bridges and Woods[31] developed a research-based protocol for PA pressure measurement; they indicate that removal of ventilated patients from the ventilator for PA pressure measurement is generally not warranted.

URINE VOLUME AND CONCENTRATION

Urine Volume

As a general rule of thumb, the normal urinary output is about 1 mL/kg of body weight per hour, with boundaries of 0.5 to 2 mL/kg/hr.[32] Table 2-1 shows that the usual urine volume in adults is approximately 1500 mL/day (range, 1000–2000 mL/day). This is equivalent to approximately 40 to 80 mL/hr in the typical adult. Urine volume in children is less, and is dependent on age and weight.

During periods of stress, the 24-hr urine volume in the adult may diminish to 750 to 1200 mL/day (or 30–50 mL/hr). Urine volume is somewhat less during periods of stress because of increased aldosterone and ADH secretion.

A low urine volume suggests FVD, and a high urine volume suggests FVE. Several factors can alter urinary volume, including:

- Amount of fluid intake
- Losses from skin, lungs, and gastrointestinal tract

TABLE 2–1

Average Intake and Output in an Adult for a 24-hr Period

INTAKE		OUTPUT	
Oral liquids	1300 mL	Urine	1500 mL
Water in food	1000 mL	Stool	200 mL
Water produced by metabolism	300 mL	**Insensible:**	
Total	2600 mL	Lungs	300 mL
		Skin	600 mL
		Total	2600 mL

- Amount of waste products for excretion (Urine volume is increased in conditions with high solute loads, such as diabetes mellitus, high-protein tube feedings, thyrotoxicosis, and fever.)
- Renal concentrating ability (When concentrating ability is diminished, urine volume is increased to allow adequate solute excretion.)
- Blood volume (Hypovolemia causes decreased renal perfusion and thus oliguria; hypervolemia causes increased urinary volume if the kidneys are functioning normally.)
- Hormonal influences (primarily aldosterone and ADH)

Nursing Considerations

1. Maintain input and output (I&O) records on all patients with real or potential fluid balance problems. Measure all fluid gains and losses according to routes.
2. Be alert for fluid intake greatly exceeding fluid output, or fluid output greatly exceeding fluid intake. Totals of I&O records for several consecutive days should be obtained for a clearer understanding of fluid balance status.
3. Be aware that the usual urine output in adults is 1 to 2 L/day (or approximately 750–1200 mL/day during periods of stress).
4. Be aware that the usual urine output in adults is 40 to 80 mL/hr (or 30–50 mL/hr during periods of stress).
5. Use a device calibrated for small volumes of urine when hourly urine volumes must be measured (see Fig. 2-10).
6. Be aware that patients taking in high-solute loads (as in high-protein tube feedings) need extra water to aid in solute elimination.
7. Be aware that individuals with diminished renal concentrating ability (such as the aged) need more fluid to excrete solutes than do those with normal renal function.
8. Be aware that a low urine volume with a high specific gravity (SG) indicates FVD.
9. Be aware that a low urine volume with a low SG is indicative of renal disease.
10. Evaluate I&O levels and urinary SG in relation to other clinical signs.
11. Be aware of common sources of errors in I&O measurements (see Clinical Tip: Overcoming Common Errors in Measuring Intake and Output).

Urine Concentration

Urinary SG measures the kidneys' ability to concentrate urine. In this test, the concentration of urine is compared with the 1.000 SG of distilled water. Because urine contains electrolytes and other substances, its SG is greater than 1.000. The range of SG in urine is from 1.003 to 1.035; most random specimens are between 1.012 and 1.025. Typical urine osmolality (another measure of urine concentration) ranges from 500 to 800 mOsm/kg; extreme ranges are from 50 to 1400 mOsm/kg.

Urinary SG is elevated when there is a FVD, as the healthy kidney seeks to retain needed fluid, thus excreting solutes in a small concentrated urine volume. However, one should be aware that heavy molecules not normally present in large quantities in urine can falsely affect SG readings. For example, glucose, albumin, or radiocontrast dyes will elevate urinary SG out of proportion to the actual concentration. Therefore, it is more accurate to measure urine osmolality in patients with glycosuria, proteinuria, or recent use of radiopaque dyes.

Specific gravity can be measured with a refractometer, a dipstick that has a reagent area for SG, or with a urinometer. Freshly voided urine specimens at room temperature are desirable for testing SG.

(text continues on page 30)

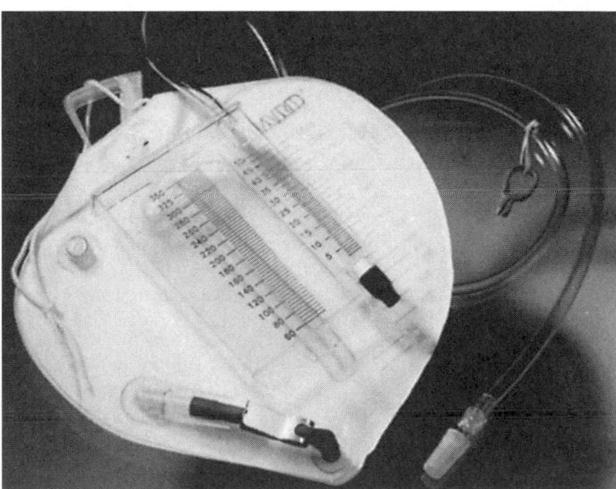

Figure 2–10. Device suitable for measuring small urine volume. (350-mL urine meter bag). Courtesy of Bard Urological Division, Covington, GA.

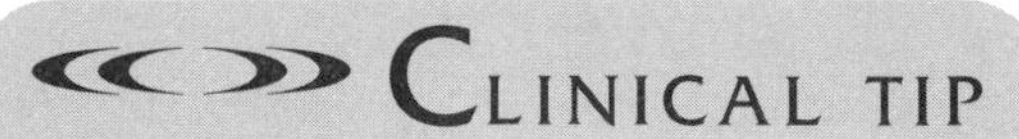

Overcoming Common Errors in Measuring Intake and Output

COMMON ERRORS	SUGGESTIONS
Errors Involving Both Intake and Output:	
Failure to communicate to the entire staff which patients require intake–output measurement (Body fluids are often discarded without being measured, and oral fluids are not recorded, merely because staff members are not aware of the patients on intake–output.)	1. A "measure intake–output" sign should be attached to the patient's bed to serve as a reminder. 2. A list of all patients requiring intake–output measurement should be posted in a convenient work area for quick reference. 3. Also, for quick reference, the card file should contain a list of all patients requiring intake–output measurement. 4. An adequate patient report should be given to all personnel.
Failure to explain intake–output to the patient and family (Most patients will cooperate *if* they know what is expected of them.)	1. Both the patient and the family should receive a simple explanation of why intake–output measurement is necessary. 2. Careful instructions are necessary to acquaint the patient and family with their role in helping to achieve an accurate intake–output record.
Well-meaning intentions to record a drink of water or an emptied urinal at a later, more convenient time are often forgotten.	Measurements should be recorded at the time they are obtained.
Failure to measure fluids that can be directly measured because it takes less time to guess at their amounts	Measure *all* fluids amenable to direct measurement—guesses should be reserved for fluids that cannot be measured directly.
Errors Related to Intake:	
Failure to designate the specific volume of glasses, cups, bowls, and other fluid containers used in the hospital (Each person may ascribe a different volume to the same glass of water.)	The bedside record should list the volumes of glasses, cups, bowls, and other fluid containers used in the hospital.
Failure to obtain an adequate measuring device for small amounts of oral fluids (Patients frequently drink small quantities of fluids; the amounts must be estimated unless a calibrated cup is available—frequent estimates increase the margin of error.)	Small calibrated paper cups should be kept at the bedside for such a purpose.
Failure to consider the volume of fluid displaced by ice in iced drinks frequently causes an overstatement of ingested oral fluids	Only small amounts of ice should be used for iced drinks so that the accurate amount of fluid ingested can be recorded.

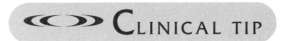

Overcoming Common Errors in Measuring Intake and Output (cont.)

COMMON ERRORS	SUGGESTIONS
Overstatement of fluid volume given as ice chips; note that the liquid volume of a glass of ice chips is only about half a glass	Record fluid intake from ice chips as approximately half of the ice chips volume (for example: an ounce of ice chips is approximately 15 mL of water).
Failure to consider that parenteral fluid bottles are overfilled; a 1000-mL bottle may actually contain 1100 mL; a 500-mL bottle may contain 550 mL	Run excess fluid through tubing during set-up, or record actual volume infused.
Assuming that the contents of empty containers were drunk by the patient	The patient should be asked what fluids were drunk.
(Patients sometimes give their coffee or juice to a visiting relative or other patients in the room; they may forget to tell the person checking the tray.)	
Errors Related to Output:	
Failure to estimate fluid lost as perspiration	1. An attempt should be made to describe the amount of clothing and bed linen saturated with perspiration—it has been estimated that one necessary bed change represents at least 1 L of lost fluid. 2. Some intake–output records require the nurse to estimate perspiration as +, + +, + + +, or + + + + (+ represents sweating that is just visible, and + + + + represents profuse sweating).
Failure to estimate "uncaught" vomitus (Frequently, "uncaught" emesis is recorded merely as a lost specimen.)	The amount of fluid lost as vomitus should be estimated and recorded as an estimate—it is better to guess than to give no indication at all as to the amount.
Failure to estimate the amount of incontinent urine (Intake–output records often indicate the number of incontinent voidings but give no indication of the amounts; obviously, such records are of little value.)	The amount of incontinent urine should be estimated—it is helpful to note the amount of clothing and bed linen saturated with urine.
Failure to estimate fluid lost as liquid feces	1. The patient should be encouraged to use the bedpan or a measuring device over the toilet so that the fluid loss can be directly measured. 2. The amount of fluid lost in incontinent liquid stools should be estimated.
Failure to estimate fluid lost as wound exudate	1. The amount of drainage on a dressing should be measured and charted—this can be done by measuring the width of the stained area and determining the thickness of the dressing. 2. If extreme measures are necessary, the dressing can be weighed before application and again when removed. 3. If a fistula is present, a stoma bag should be applied to catch the drainage.

(continued)

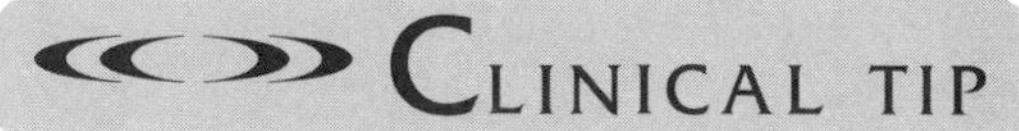

Overcoming Common Errors in Measuring Intake and Output (cont.)

COMMON ERRORS	SUGGESTIONS
Failure to check a urinary catheter for patency when there is decreased drainage of urine (It is sometimes too quickly assumed that decreased drainage from a catheter is due to decreased urine formation.)	Decreased drainage from a urinary catheter is an indication to check for patency before charting the absence of, or decrease in, urinary output.
Failure to obtain an adequate measuring device for hourly or more frequent checks on urinary output (An error of even 10 mL could be significant when dealing with small amounts of urine.)	A collecting device calibrated to measure small amounts of urine should be used (see Fig. 2-10).
Failure to record the amount of solution used to irrigate tubes and the amount of fluid withdrawn during the irrigation	1. One method for dealing with this problem is to add the amount of irrigating solution to the intake column, and the amount of fluid withdrawn to the output column. 2. Another method is to compare the amount of irrigating solution used with the amount of fluid withdrawn during the irrigation—if more fluid was put in than was taken out, the excess is added to the intake column; if more fluid was taken out than was put in, the excess is added to the output column.

Refrigerated samples may have falsely elevated readings, as may specimens exposed to excessive heat and dryness (a result of evaporation). Ideally, urinary SG should be measured immediately after the specimen is collected; however, in some situations this is not possible.

To determine the variability in specimens tested immediately after voiding and at intervals up to 4 hrs after voiding, a study of 20 ill infants with disposable diapers was conducted.[33] Urine was aspirated from each diaper immediately after voiding and tested with a refractometer. Subsequently, the diaper was folded, rolled, and taped so that the urine was not exposed to air, heat, or light. Specific gravity measurements of urine aspirated from each diaper at up to 4-hr intervals after voiding were not significantly different from those obtained at the time of urination.

INTAKE/OUTPUT AND BODY WEIGHT

Comparison of Intake and Output

Many serious fluid balance problems can be averted by maintaining a careful vigil on the patient's I&O and keeping accurate records. (Totals for several consecutive days should be compared.) If the total intake is substantially less than the total output, it is obvious that the patient is in danger of FVD. On the other hand, if the total intake is substantially more than the output, the patient is in danger of FVE (or, in the case of inappropriate secretion of ADH, water excess). To understand abnormal states better, it is helpful to review the 24-hr average I&O in a normal adult (see Table 2-1).

Balance of I&O is desirable only in steady-state conditions. In pathophysiological conditions, therapy is directed at promoting recovery. For example, in hypovolemic shock, as much as three times the volume of blood lost must be infused if the replacement fluids are crystalloids (such as isotonic saline or lactated Ringer's solution) to restore plasma volume to acceptable levels.[34]

It is important to initiate I&O records for any patient with a real or potential water and electrolyte problem: do not wait for an order from the physician.

1. Intake should include all fluids taken into the body (oral fluids, foods that are liquid at room temperature, intravenous fluids, subcutaneous fluids, fluids instilled into drainage tubes as irrigants, tube feeding solutions, water given through feeding tubes, and even enema solutions in patients requiring strict fluid intake recording, such as those in renal failure).
2. Output should include urine, vomitus, diarrhea, drainage from fistulas, and drainage from suction apparatus. Perspiration should be noted and its amount estimated. The presence of prolonged hyperventilation should also be noted as it is an important route of water vapor loss. Drainage from lesions (such as from large decubitus ulcers) should be noted and estimated.
3. The I&O record should include the time of day and the type of fluid gained and lost. This information is necessary in planning therapy.
4. The type of I&O record used often depends on the patient's condition. Patients with a severe fluid balance problem may require an hourly summary of their fluid gains and losses so that the fluctuating needs can be dealt with quickly. Many patients require only 8-hr summaries of their fluid gains and losses. A record suitable for this purpose, listing the volumes of containers used, should be available at the bedside.

Although it is not technically difficult to measure fluid I&O or to record the measurements, persistent effort is required if one is to achieve an accurate account. There are innumerable possibilities for error in the measurement and recording of fluid gains and losses; however, some errors occur much more frequently than others. Common errors and suggestions for overcoming them are shown in the Clinical Tip.

Pflaum[35] examined the accuracy of a routine I&O technique in a general hospital and found it lacking; when compared with measurement of body weight, the mean daily error was 800 mL. From her results Pflaum concluded that measurement of I&O is of little value and that a more accurate indicator, body weight, should be adopted. Although it is generally recognized that I&O records are often sorely lacking, one should use I&O measurements and body weights to best evaluate a patient's fluid balance status. Unfortunately, body weight measurements are also often inaccurate. Kilfoy-Perez[36] reviewed the charts of 100 hospitalized patients on general medical divisions to compare acute fluid gains and losses to body weight changes. Only 52 of the 100 charts contained sufficient data to make these comparisons. Most of the 48 unusable charts were deficient in I&O recordings, but a few also lacked recordings of daily body weight measurements. Of the 52 usable records, a statistically significant, positive correlation was found between net differences in fluid and weight changes over a 48-hr period.

Body Weight Variations

Weighing patients with potential or actual fluid balance problems daily is of great clinical importance for the following reasons: (1) Accurate body weight measurements are usually easier to obtain than accurate fluid I&O measurements; and (2) Rapid variations in weight, when measured correctly, reflect changes in body fluid volume.

When analyzing changes in a patient's weight, it is important to consider factors that may hinder the accuracy of weight measurement. For example, there may be errors in the weighing technique or in the recording of results, or the scales themselves may be faulty. A recent report, by means of a Quality Improvement program in which staff were held accountable for achieving accurate body weight measurements, showed a significant increase in both the number of weights performed as well as their accuracy; the improvements were attributed to use of written standards for the weighing procedure in addition to education programs on the topic.[37] Another recent study indicated that a small but significant percentage of scales in clinical use are inaccurate and imprecise to a clinically important degree.[38] The investigators perceived the problem to be related to breakage and wear rather than manufacturing defects. To minimize inaccuracies in weight measurements, medical institutions should test the accuracy of their clinical scales periodically. Before obtaining the patient's weight, it is helpful to test one's own weight on the scale to note any obvious discrepancy. Indicators of an inaccurate scale may include the following: one's own weight seems to be in error, a change greater than 1 lb occurs when one's weight is shifted on the scale's platform, the platform is wobbly, or other defects in the scale's structure are apparent.

The following practices should be followed in weighing patients:

1. Use the same scale each time, as there may be significant variation among scales. Because this may present a problem when the patient is transferred from unit to unit, the need for accurate scales throughout an institution is obvious. This point emphasizes the need to test the accuracy of clinical scales routinely.
2. Measure weight in the morning before breakfast and after voiding.
3. Be sure the patient is wearing the same or similar clothing each time and that the clothing is dry.
4. If the patient is unable to stand for weighing on a small portable scale or a stand-on scale, use a sling-type scale. Wheelchair and under-bed scales are also commercially available.

Body weight as an index of fluid balance is based on the assumption that the patient's dry weight remains relatively stable. Over a short period (hour-to-hour), this assumption is valid, and changes in body weight reflect changes in body fluid volume rather than tissue mass changes. To assess these small hourly changes, it is necessary to use extremely accurate metabolic scales, which are not available on most patient care units.

Long-term (day-to-day) body weight variations reflect changes in tissue mass as well as body fluid volume. Thus, factors affecting tissue mass (caloric intake and metabolic status) must also be evaluated. Tissue loss occurs in catabolic states (such as severe stress) and tissue mass gain occurs in anabolic states. It is generally assumed that a relative deficit of 3400 calories is needed to lose 1 lb of tissue mass; this deficit can be the result of inadequate caloric intake, increased metabolic rate, or both.

Body weight loss will occur when the total fluid intake is less than the total fluid output. A rapid 2% loss of total body weight indicates mild FVD, whereas a 5% loss represents moderate FVD and a rapid loss of 8% or more represents severe FVD. Conversely, body weight gain will occur when the total fluid intake is greater than the total fluid output. A rapid 2% gain of total body weight indicates mild FVE, whereas a 5% gain represents a moderate FVE and an 8% or greater gain a severe FVE.

A rapid body weight gain or loss of 1 kg (2.2 lb) is approximately equivalent to the gain or loss of 1 L of fluid (or expressed another way, a gain or loss of 500 mL of fluid is equivalent to a gain or loss of 1 lb). A patient may have a severe FVD, although body weight is essentially unchanged or even increased, when there is a "third-space" shift of body fluid (see Chapter 3).

A group of researchers recently reported the use of bioelectrical impendance analysis (BIA) in a group of postoperative cardiac patients as a method to assess fluid balance.[39] The principle of the BIA method is based on passing an imperceptible electrical current through the patient's body fluids (between surface electrodes applied to the patient's hand and foot). Adjacent electrodes measure the voltage drop across the body. Conductivity of the electrical current is far greater through the fat-free mass that contains most of the body's water than it is through fat (which is relatively anhydrous). Because bioelectrical conduction is related to water and its ionic distribution within the body, changes in body water or its electrolyte composition influence total body impedance. The researchers simultaneously measured fluid I&O and body weights. They found that changes in the BIA readings correlated better with fluid I&O findings than did changes in body weight readings. In summary, the researchers report that the speed and simplicity of this noninvasive bedside technique (which does not require active participation by the patient) and the information gained are the greatest assets of BIA.

EVALUATION OF LABORATORY DATA

Data from laboratory tests provide the nurse with valuable information about the patient's fluid and electrolyte status. However, it is important that specimens be collected properly to obtain valid results and that the findings be evaluated in light of the patient's history and clinical status. Treatment for an abnormality reported on an improperly performed laboratory test can be quite serious. For example, assume that the laboratory erroneously reports a serum potassium level of 8.0 mEq/L (due to an accidentally hemolyzed blood sample) in a patient with an actual serum potassium of 4.0 mEq/L. Initiation of aggressive treatment for nonexistent hyperkalemia could reduce the serum level to dangerously low levels. When in doubt, it is wise to confirm a grossly abnormal test result.

OBTAINING SPECIMENS

Venous Blood Samples

Several general principles should be kept in mind when obtaining venous blood samples:

1. *Avoid drawing blood samples from a site above an infusing intravenous (IV) line.* Data indicate that specimens for serum biochemical and hematologic profiles should be drawn from the opposite arm or *below* the IV while it is infusing or out of the IV needle after the IV fluids have been stopped for 2 min.[40]
2. Take measures to prevent hemolysis of sample. This is particularly disruptive when the test is for serum potassium, magnesium, or phosphate levels. (Recall that these electrolytes are primarily found *intra*cellularly; rupture of the blood cells causes a falsely high reading of serum levels.) Measures to avoid hemolysis at the time of blood collection include[41]:
    - Allowing the alcohol applied to the skin to dry before performing the venipuncture
    - Avoiding over-vigorous mixing of the blood in the collection tube
3. Avoid prolonged use of tight tourniquets and opening and closing of the patient's hand when drawing blood for potassium levels. Tight tourniquet application in combination with excessive arm exercise before venipuncture may cause a spurious elevation in potassium concentration.[42]
4. Repeated clenching and unclenching of the fist after the tourniquet has been applied is sometimes done in an attempt to make the veins more apparent; however, it may have a contributory role in artifactually elevating the plasma potassium concentration by as much as 1 to 2 mEq/L because exercise causes potassium to be released from the cells.[43]
5. Be aware that the blood-drawing procedure should be performed as skillfully and as atraumatically as possible. Watson et al. [44] suggest that when there is difficulty with phlebotomy, test results may show great variation and should be reviewed with care. The major cause of pseudohyperkalemia is mechanical trauma during venipuncture, resulting in the release of potassium from red blood cells. (When this occurs, the serum will have a characteristic red tint as hemoglobin is also released.)[45]

Urine Samples

Twenty-Four-Hour Specimens

Because 24-hr urine specimens are often indicated in the measurement of urinary excretion of electrolytes, it is helpful to review the steps in the procedure:

1. Obtain a collection bottle from the laboratory; if a preservative is needed, it should be obtained with the bottle.
2. Follow directions from the laboratory with regard to any special preparation of the patient (for example, some tests may require dietary modifications or the withholding of certain drugs).
3. To begin collection, ask the patient to void and discard the specimen; note the exact time on the lab slip.
4. Save *all* urine for the next 24 hrs and pour it into the collection bottle (omission of even one specimen invalidates the test).
5. Include a final voiding as close as possible to 24 hrs after the initiation of the test (record exact finish time on lab slip).
6. For infants, obtain specimens in pasted-on collection devices.
7. Be sure to explain the test to the patient and gain his or her cooperation. This is imperative for any successful 24-hr test (for example, patients who are using bedpans should be instructed to void before having a bowel movement, and not to place toilet paper in the collection container).
8. Remind the staff and patient (with signs) of the importance of saving all urine.

Single Urine Specimens

For a single urine specimen, the first voided morning specimen is ideal because of its greater concentration. However, a fresh specimen collected at any time is reliable for most purposes. To avoid false readings, the specimen must be collected in a clean container. If a specimen is kept more than 1 hr before analysis, it should be refrigerated to avoid changes in the urine.

INTERPRETING TESTS USED TO MEASURE FLUID BALANCE

Blood and urine tests that can be used to assess fluid and electrolyte status are listed in Tables 2-2 and 2-3. Usual reference ranges for the tests and significance of variations are also included. Commonly used units of measures are reported with Système Internationale (S.I.) units in parentheses.

Laboratory reports in the chart should be reviewed at regular intervals to note the patient's current status and to detect trends in the data. Because normal ranges for laboratory tests vary slightly from institution to institution, it is necessary to evaluate results according to those listed by the laboratory performing the tests. Also, one must consider variables that can affect the results of specific tests.

TABLE 2–2

TEST	USUAL REFERENCE RANGE	COMMENTS
Serum potassium	3.5–5.0 mEq/L (3.5–5.0 mmol/L)	Alterations in acid–base balance significantly affect potassium distribution: • Acidosis results in a shift of potassium out of the cells, causing serum potassium concentration to increase • Alkalosis results in a shift of potassium into the cells, causing a decrease in serum potassium • On the average, every 0.1-unit change in pH causes a reciprocal change of 0.5 mEq/L in plasma concentration.[46] There are a number of causes of factitious hyperkalemia: • Tight tourniquet around an exercising extremity (as in opening and closing the hand) can elevate potassium by shifting potassium from the cells to the serum • Hemolysis of sample (as in traumatic venipuncture) releases potassium from blood cells into the serum, thus elevating the serum potassium level • Leukocytosis in the range of 100,000/mm^3, as in leukemia, or platelet counts greater than 400,000/mm^3, as in thrombocytosis. (Leukocytes and platelets, which are rich in potassium, may release their large intracellular potassium stores during the clotting process.) In these conditions, there may be spurious elevations in the serum potassium concentration to as high as 9 mEq/L.[47]
Serum sodium	135–145 mEq/L (135–145 mmol/L)	Serum sodium level is closely related to body water status: • For the adult, it can be roughly estimated that each 3 to 4 mEq elevation of serum sodium above normal range represents a deficit of approximately 1 L of body water.[48]

TABLE 2–2 (cont.)

TEST	USUAL REFERENCE RANGE	COMMENTS
Serum sodium (cont.)		• An elevated plasma glucose level pulls water out of the cells into the extracellular fluid; by dilution, this lowers the plasma sodium concentration. In theory, every 62 mg/dL increment increase in plasma glucose will draw enough water out of the cells to dilute the plasma sodium concentration 1 mEq/L.[49] • The measured plasma sodium concentration may be artifactually reduced when marked hyperlipidemia is present.
Serum calcium	*Total calcium:* 8.9–10.3 mg/dL (2.23–2.57 mmol/L) Total calcium in serum is the sum of the ionized (47%) and nonionized (53%) calcium components. The nonionized portion consists of calcium bound to albumin (40%) and the portion (13%) chelated to anions (such as citrate and phosphate).	• Total calcium is the test performed in most clinical settings. To evaluate the actual calcium level, the clinician must first know the serum albumin level to apply the following rule: In the noncritically ill, the total serum calcium may be corrected for variations in the serum albumin by estimating that a change in the serum albumin of 1.0 g/dL (10 g/L) will change the total serum calcium by 0.8 mg/dL (0.2 mmol/L).[50] • The above estimation is not valid when situations are present that affect pH (which changes the percentage of ionized calcium) or the quantity of substances available to bind with calcium is altered. Alkalosis increases the binding of calcium to albumin, as does an increased free fatty acid level (common in stressed patients). Other factors that can acutely lower ionized calcium are increased levels of lactate, bicarbonate, citrate, phosphate, and some substances in radiographic contrast media.[51]
Serum	*Total calcium*	Although many attempts have been made to mathematically correct the total serum calcium concentration for alterations in pH and circulating albumin, total serum calcium and calculated ionized calcium levels have been poor predictors of the actual physiologically active ionized calcium.[52]
	Ionized calcium 4.6–5.1 mg/dL (1.15–1.27 mmol/L)	Many laboratories now have the capability to directly measure the ionized calcium level. This is desirable, especially in critically ill patients, as it is the ionized level that is physiologically active and is clinically important. Variations in the sample collection technique can affect the results. For example, variations in the amount of heparin in the collecting device and acid–base changes from prolonged tourniquet application can both artifactually alter the measured Ca^{2+}.
Serum magnesium	1.3–2.1 mEq/L (0.65–1.05 mmol/L)	Hemolysis of the sample will invalidate the results by releasing magnesium from the red blood cells into the serum (recall that magnesium is primarily an intracellular ion).

(continued)

TABLE 2–2 (cont.)

TEST	USUAL REFERENCE RANGE	COMMENTS
Serum chloride	97–110 mEq/L (97–110 mmol/L)	• Less than normal concentration indicates hypochloremia (commonly associated with hypokalemia and metabolic alkalosis). • Greater than normal concentration indicates hyperchloremia, which may be associated with excessive administration of isotonic saline.
Carbon dioxide content	22–31 mEq/L (22–31 mmol/L)	• This test measures total bicarbonate and carbonic acid in venous blood and is a general measure of the degree of alkalinity or acidity. It should not be confused with the partial pressure of carbon dioxide, PCO_2, obtained from arterial blood gas analysis.) • A level below normal indicates metabolic acidosis. • In the absence of chronic obstructive pulmonary disease, an elevated level indicates metabolic alkalosis.
Serum phosphate	2.5–4.5 mg/dL (0.81–1.45 mmol/L)	• Hemolysis of the sample will invalidate the results by releasing phosphate from the red blood cells into the serum (recall that phosphate is primarily an intracellular ion). • Phosphate levels are evaluated in relation to calcium levels since there is an inverse relationship between the two (eg, an increased phosphorus level causes the calcium level to decrease). • Phosphate levels normally higher in children than in adults. • Drugs containing high phosphate levels may temporarily increase the serum phosphate level for several hours after the dose. • Insulin promotes entry of extracellular phosphorus into cells. • Intravenous glucose running before or at the time of the test causes a lowered serum phosphorus level (due to carbohydrate metabolism).
Plasma ammonia	11–35 μmol/L (reported values vary according to laboratory)	• The body is less able to handle high ammonia levels when the serum potassium is low or when alkalosis is present. • Ammonia level varies with protein intake and is affected by some antibiotics.
Serum osmolality	280–295 mOsm/kg Can be measured by lab or can be calculated by the following formula: pOsm = $2(Na) + \frac{G}{18} + \frac{BUN}{2.4}$	• Serum osmolality is determined mainly by serum sodium concentration (recall that serum sodium makes up 90% of the osmotic pressure generated by plasma). • Finding is increased in dehydration (hypernatremia). • Finding is decreased in overhydration (hyponatremia). • Finding is increased in hyperglycemia and in presence of elevated BUN.
Anion gap	12 ± 2 mEq/L $AG = Na - (Cl + HCO_3)$	• Anion gap is useful in ascertaining cause of metabolic acidosis. • A level >14 mEq/L indicates presence of excessive organic acid (as in diabetic ketoacidosis, lactic acidosis, uremic renal failure, and salicylate intoxication). • Normal anion gap acidosis may be due to diarrhea, ureterostomies, excessive chloride administration, and distal tubular acidosis.

TABLE 2–2 (cont.)

TEST	USUAL REFERENCE RANGE	COMMENTS
BUN	8–25 mg/dL (2.9–8.9 mmol/L)	• Elevated BUN can be due to reduced renal blood flow secondary to fluid volume deficit (causing reduced urea clearance). • Excessive protein intake can elevate BUN by increasing urea production. • Increased catabolism due to trauma, starvation, bleeding into the intestines, or catabolic drugs can also increase the BUN by increasing urea production. • A low BUN is often associated with overhydration and may also be associated with low protein intake.
Creatinine	0.6–1.5 mg/dL (53–133 μmol/L)	• As an indicator of renal disease is more specific and sensitive than BUN since nonrenal causes of elevation are few. • In patients with large muscle mass of acromegaly, it may be slightly above normal. • A slightly elevated creatinine level may occur in severe fluid volume depletion, which results in a reduced glomerular filtration rate. • Spurious elevations in serum creatinine may occur with the administration of cefoxitin (which interferes with the Jaffe reaction used in assaying creatinine) and cimetidine (which interferes with tubular secretion of creatinine; exaggerated increases in serum creatinine also occur with rhabdomyolysis (due to sudden release of large quantities of muscle creatine phosphate that is converted to creatinine).[53]
BUN/ creatinine ratio	10:1 (approximate)	This ratio is useful in evaluating hydration status: • When the ratio increases in favor of the BUN (ratio >10:1), conditions such as hypovolemia, low perfusion pressures to the kidney, or increased protein metabolism may be present. • When the ratio is <10:1, conditions such as low protein intake, hepatic insufficiency, or repeated dialysis may be present. • When both the BUN and creatinine level rise, maintaining the 10:1 ratio, the problem is likely intrinsic renal disease (although it may also be seen when fluid volume depletion results in reduction in the glomerular filtration rate).
Hematocrit (%)	Male: 44–52 Female: 39–47	• Hematocrit determines the percentage of red blood cells in plasma. • Changes are interpretable in terms of fluid balance only when no changes in the red blood cell mass (such as bleeding or hemolysis) are occurring. • Hematocrit is elevated in fluid volume deficit (because red blood cells are contained in a relatively smaller plasma fluid volume). • Hematocrit is decreased in fluid volume excess (because the red blood cells are contained in a relatively larger plasma fluid volume).

(continued)

TABLE 2–2 (cont.)

TEST	USUAL REFERENCE RANGE	COMMENTS
Fasting plasma glucose	65–110 mg/dL (3.58–6.05 mmol/L)	A markedly elevated glucose level in bloodstream causes osmotic diuresis and resultant fluid volume deficit. • Results will be elevated above baseline if patient is receiving parenteral glucose (regardless of site from which the specimen is drawn).[54]
Plasma lactate (venous blood)	0.6–1.7 mEq/L (0.6–1.7 mmol/L)	• Lactic acidosis is considered to be present if the plasma lactate level is greater than 4 to 5 mEq/L in an acidemic patient.[55] • Most cases of lactic acidosis are due to marked tissue hypoperfusion. • Venous specimens are usually used for convenience, even though they may yield higher results than arterial specimens. Venous and arterial levels are virtually alike if the patient remains at complete bedrest before sample collection; hand clenching can significantly raise blood lactate levels.[56]
Albumin	3.5–4.8 g/dL (35–48 g/L)	• Decreased serum albumin level causes reduced colloidal osmotic pull in intravascular space, allowing fluid to shift to the interstitial space and produce edema. • It is important to know the albumin level when evaluating total calcium values.

TABLE 2–3

Urine Tests Used to Evaluate Fluid and Electrolyte Status

TEST	USUAL REFERENCE RANGE	COMMENTS
Urinary sodium	No fixed normal values—kidneys vary rate of excretion to match dietary intake Sodium excretion in urine is usually 30–280 mmol/24 hours[57] Random specimen usually contains >40 mEq/L[58]	• Urinary sodium is helpful in assessing volume status, diagnosis of hyponatremia and acute renal failure, and assessing dietary compliance in patients on sodium-restricted diets • Less than 20 mEq/L in hypovolemic states, reflecting renal sodium conservation to maintain blood volume.[59] • Greater than 40 mEq/L in hypovolemic states associated with the following:[60] — Underlying renal disease — Osmotic diuresis — Hypoaldosteronism • Greater than 40 mEq/L in SIADH[61] • Important to record dietary intake during 24-hr period because measurement of urinary sodium without knowledge of dietary intake is of limited value. • Urinary sodium levels must be evaluated in light of total clinical picture.

TABLE 2–3 (cont.)

TEST	USUAL REFERENCE RANGE	COMMENTS
Urinary potassium	No fixed normal values. Kidneys vary rate of excretion to match dietary intake and endogenous production Random specimen usually >40 mEq/L[62] If potassium depletion occurs, urinary potassium excretion can fall to a minimum of 5–25 mEq/24 hours[63]	• Primary use of 24-hr urine measurement of potassium is to assess cause of hypokalemia. • Low value suggests nonrenal potassium loss (usually from the gastrointestinal tract) or diuretic use (if urine collected after diuretic effect has worn off). • In contrast, if more than 25 mEq are excreted in the urine of a hypokalemic patient, there is at least a component of renal potassium wasting.[64]
Urinary chloride	110–250 mEq/24 hr (110–250 mmol/24 hr) Varies with salt intake	• Usually similar to that of sodium in hypovolemic states because sodium and chloride are generally reabsorbed together[65] • Helpful in differentiating between types of metabolic alkalosis[66]: — Less than 25 mEq/L when metabolic alkalosis is due to vomiting, gastric suction, or diuretic use (late). — Usually greater than 40 mEq/L when metabolic alkalosis is due to mineralocorticoid excess, profound (<2.0 mEq/L) hypokalemia, or early diuretic use.
Urinary calcium (quantitative)	100–300 mg/24 hr in adults (depends on dietary intake)[67]	• Increased in hypercalcemia associated with metastatic tumors • May be quite low when hypocalcemia present
Urinary specific gravity (SG)	Varies from 1.003 to 1.035[68] 1.016–1.022 (with normal intake)[69]	• SG depends on the state of hydration and varies with the urine volume and solute load to be excreted. • SG is elevated in fluid volume deficit as the normal kidney seeks to retain needed fluid and thus excreted solutes in a small concentrated urine volume. • Urines <1.007 SG are called hyposthenuria.[70] • SG fixed at 1.010 signals significant renal disease (isothenuria). • Heavy molecules such as glucose, albumin, or radiocontrast dyes will elevate SG out of proportion to the actual concentration. Thus, it is more accurate to measure urine osmolality in patients with glucosuria, proteinuria, or recent use of radiopaque dyes.

(continued)

TABLE 2–3 (cont.)

TEST	USUAL REFERENCE RANGE	COMMENTS
Urine osmolality	Maximally diluted and concentrated urine shows osmolalities between 50–1400 mOsm/L[71] Correlates fairly well with urinary SG unless larger molecules (such as glucose or albumin) are present[72]: SG 1.000 Osmolality 0 mOsm/L SG 1.010 Osmolality 350 mOsm/L SG 1.020 Osmolality 700 mOsm/L SG 1.030 Osmolality 1050 mOsm/L	• Simultaneous measurement of serum and urine osmolality is a more accurate way to measure renal concentrating ability than is urinary SG.
Urinary pH	4.6–8.0[73] (average is 6.0)	• Urine pH reflects serum pH and helps confirm the presence of acidosis or alkalosis (with the exception of paradoxical aciduria in hypokalemic alkalosis, alkaline urine due to urea-splitting infections, and alkaline urine in renal tubular acidosis). • Urine pH is increased with use of alkalinating agents such as sodium bicarbonate and potassium citrate. • Urine pH is decreased with the use of acidifying agents such as ascorbic acid, sodium acid phosphate, and methenamine mandelate. • Urine pH fluctuates throughout the day. • Specimen should be examined soon after collection because urine that is left standing too long becomes alkaline due to bacterial-induced splitting of urea into ammonia.

REFERENCES

1. Baylis P, Thompson C: Osmoregulation of vasopressin secretion and thirst in health and disease. Clin Endocrinol 29:549–576,1988
2. Porth C: Physiology of thirst and drinking: Implications for nursing practice. Heart Lung 21:273–284, 1992
3. Ibid
4. Phillips P, Bretherton M, Johnston C, Gray L: Reduced osmotic thirst in healthy elderly men. Am J Physiol 261:R166,1991
5. Willis P: Inspection of the neck veins. Heart Dis Stroke 3:9–15,1994
6. Rose B: Clinical Physiology of Acid-Base and Electrolyte Disorders, 4th ed. p 447. New York, McGraw-Hill, 1994
7. Ibid, p 450
8. Condon R, Nyhus L: Manual of Surgical Therapeutics, 8th ed, p 177. Boston, Little, Brown, 1993
9. Askanazi J, Starker P, Weissman C: Fluid and Electrolyte Management in Critical Care, p 235. Boston, Butterworths, 1986
10. Ibid
11. Sims L, D'Amico D, Stiesmeyer J, Webster J: Health Assessment in Nursing, p 467. Redwood City, CA, Addison-Wesley, 1995
12. Hoffmann E: The Chvostek's sign: A clinical study. Am J Surg 96:33,1958
13. Martinez-Maldonado M, Garcia A: Hypo- and hypercalcemia, Chapter 3. In Martinez-Maldonado M (ed): Handbook of Renal Therapeutics. New York, Plenum Press, 1983
14. Schwartz S, Shires T, Spencer F: Principles of Surgery, 6th ed, p 66. Baltimore, Williams & Wilkins, 1994
15. Ibid
16. Condon, Nyhus, p 183
17. Kokko J, Tannen R: Fluids and Electrolytes, 2nd ed, p 72. Philadelphia, WB Saunders, 1990
18. Bates B: A Guide to Physical Examination and History Taking, 6th ed, p 279. Philadelphia, JB Lippincott, 1995
19. Halck S, et al: Reliability of central venous pressure measured by water column (Letter). Crit Care Med 18:461–462,1990

20. Hudak C, Gallo B, Benz J: Critical Care Nursing, 5th ed, p 123. Philadelphia, JB Lippincott, 1990
21. Task Force on Guidelines for Pulmonary Artery Catheterization: Guidelines for pulmonary artery catheterization. Anesthesiology, 78:380–384,1993
22. Iberti T, et al: Assessment of critical care nurses' knowledge of the pulmonary artery catheter. Crit Care Med 22:1674–1678,1993
23. Boggs R, Wooldridge-King M: Hemodynamic monitoring, Chapter 10. AACN Procedure Manual for Critical Care, 3rd ed, p 290–291. Philadelphia, WB Saunders, 1993
24. Ahrens T: Ask the experts. Crit Care Nurse 14(6):98, 1994
25. Ahlberg et al: PA pressure measurement in pulmonary hypertension (Abstract). Heart Lung 18(3): 300–301,1989
26. Laulive J: Pulmonary artery pressures and position changes in the critically ill adult. Dimens Crit Care Nurs 1(1):28–34,1982
27. Woods S, et al: Effect of backrest position on pulmonary artery pressure in critically ill patients. J Cardiovasc Nurs 28:19,1982
28. Osika C: Measurement of pulmonary artery pressures: Supine versus side-lying head elevated position (Abstract). Heart Lung 18(3):298–299,1989
29. Keating D, et al: Effect of sidelying positions on pulmonary artery pressures. Heart Lung 15(6):605–610, 1986
30. Boggs, Wooldridge-King, p 290
31. Bridges E, Woods S: Research-based protocol. Pulmonary artery pressure measurement: State of the art. Heart Lung 22:99–111,1993
32. Pestana C: Fluids and Electrolytes in the Surgical Patient, 4th ed, p 223. Baltimore, Williams & Wilkins, 1989
33. Stebor A: Posturination time and specific gravity in infants' diapers. Nurs Res 38(4):244,1989
34. Condon, Nyhus, p 6
35. Pflaum S: Investigation of intake-output as a means of assessing body fluid balance. Heart Lung 8:495,1979
36. Kilfoy-Perez L: Comparison of acute fluid gains and losses to body weight changes. Unpublished master's thesis: Saint Louis University School of Nursing, 1994.
37. Savage S, Wilkinson M: Patient weights: From physician complaints to improved nursing practice through quality improvement. Gastroenterol Nurs 16(6)264–268,1994
38. Schlegal-Pratt K, Heizer W: The accuracy of scales used to weigh patients. Nutr Clin Pract 5(6):254,1990
39. Mequid M, Lukaski H, Tripp M, Rosenburg J, Parker F: Rapid bedside method to assess changes in postoperative fluid status with bioelectrical impendance analysis. Surgery 112:502–508,1992
40. Watson K, O'Kell R, Joyce J: Data regarding blood drawing sites in patients receiving intravenous fluids. Am J Clin Pathol 79:119,1983
41. Henry J: Clinical Diagnosis & Management by Laboratory Methods, 18th ed, p 76. Philadelphia, WB Saunders, 1991
42. Narins, p 707
43. Rose, p 827
44. Watson et al, p 119
45. Rose, p 827
46. Condon, Nyhus, p 165
47. Rose, p 827
48. Condon, Nyhus, p 177
49. Rose, p 668
50. Olinger M: Disorders of calcium and magnesium metabolism. Emerg Med Clin North Am 7(4):798, 1989
51. Ibid
52. Zaloga G, Chernow B: Divalent ions: Calcium, magnesium, and phosphorus, Chapter 46. In Chernow B (ed): The Pharmacologic Approach to the Critically Ill Patient, 3rd ed, p 779. Baltimore, Williams & Wilkins, 1994
53. Henry, p 1181
54. Watson et al, p 119
55. Rose, p 555
56. Henry, p 186
57. Ibid, p 129
58. Condon, Nyhus, p 179
59. Rose, p 398
60. Ibid
61. Ibid, p 674
62. Condon, Nyhus, p 179
63. Rose, p 383
64. Ibid
65. Rose, p 490
66. Ibid
67. Henry, p 1373
68. Henry, p 125
69. Ibid, p 1375
70. Ibid, p 396
71. Ibid, p 125
72. Rose, p 648
73. Henry, p 1373

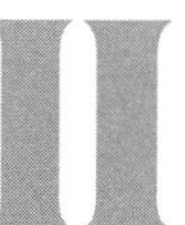

II

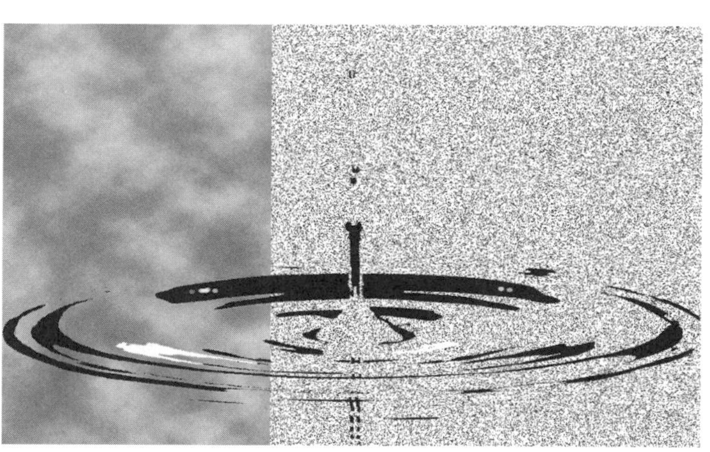

Overview of Fluid and Electrolyte Problems: Nursing Considerations

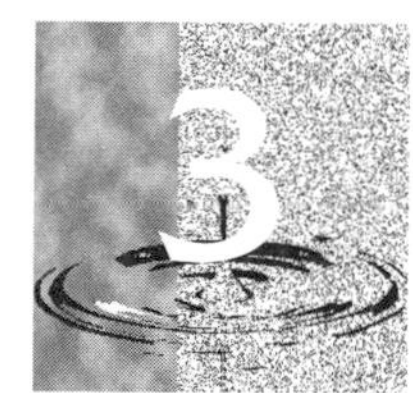

Fluid Volume Imbalances

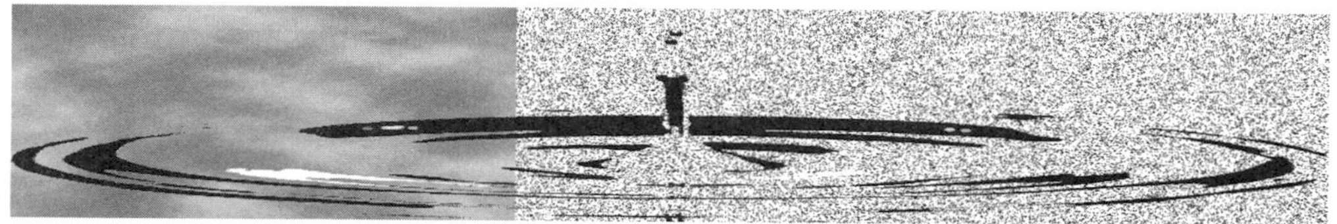

Fluid volume imbalances are commonly seen in nursing practice. Although they may occur alone, they most frequently occur in combination with other imbalances. Thus, events leading to fluid volume disturbances also frequently lead to electrolyte problems. For the purposes of this chapter, however, fluid volume imbalances are discussed in their "pure" form, that is, without the presence of other disturbances. There is much the nurse can do to prevent the occurrence of fluid volume imbalances, or at least decrease their severity. This chapter describes assessment for fluid volume disturbances and explains rationales for nursing interventions.

ISOTONIC FLUID VOLUME DEFICIT

Fluid volume deficit (FVD) results when water and electrolytes are lost in an isotonic fashion (see Fig. 3-1). It should not be confused with the term "dehydration," which refers to a loss of water alone (leaving the patient with sodium excess). FVD may occur alone or in combination with other imbalances. Unless other imbalances are present concurrently, serum electrolyte levels remain essentially unchanged.

ETIOLOGICAL FACTORS

FVD is almost always due to loss of body fluids and occurs more rapidly when coupled with decreased intake for any reason. It *is* possible to develop FVD solely on the basis of inadequate intake, provided the decreased intake is prolonged.

Losses of Gastrointestinal Fluids

In review, many liters of gastrointestinal (GI) secretions are produced each day; most of these secretions are reabsorbed in the ileum and proximal colon, leaving only approximately 150 mL of relatively electrolyte-free fluid to be excreted daily in the feces. When any abnormal route of loss is present, such as vomiting, diarrhea, GI suction, fistulas, or drainage tubes, it becomes evident how large losses can occur (resulting in FVD).

Fluids trapped in the GI tract, as is the case with intestinal obstruction, are physiologically outside the body (third-space effect). Indeed, any condition that interferes with the absorption of fluids from the GI tract can cause serious FVD.

Polyuria

Any condition that causes excessive urine formation can produce FVD. This situation is commonly seen in patients with profound hyperglycemia, as either diabetic ketoacidosis or nonketotic hyperosmolar coma. To excrete a large solute load, the kidneys must also excrete a large urine volume. One also sees polyuria associated with a large solute load in patients receiving hyperosmolar tube feedings. No matter what the cause of the high solute load, absence of sufficient exogenous fluid to allow for excretion of the solute will cause fluid to be "pulled in" from the plasma, tissue space, and even from the cells.

Fever

An elevated body temperature can cause FVD if extra fluids are not supplied as indicated. Fever causes an increase in metabolism and as a result, in formed metabolic wastes, which require fluid to make a solution for renal excretion; in this way, fluid loss is increased. Fever also causes hyperpnea, an increase in breathing resulting in extra water vapor loss through the lungs.

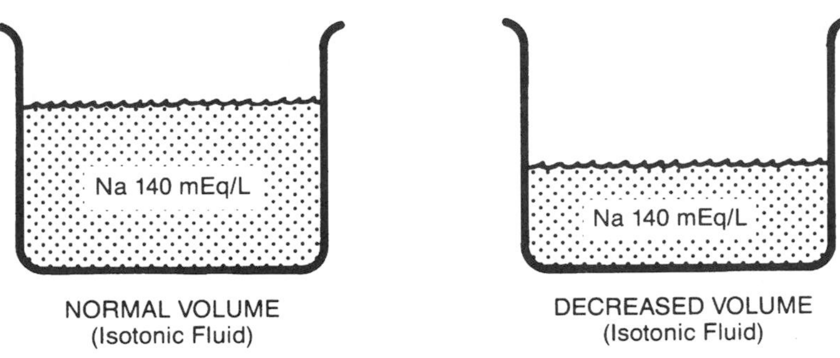

Figure 3–1. Fluid volume deficit.

A temperature elevation between 38.3 °C (101 °F) and 39.4 °C (103 °F) generally increases the 24-hr fluid requirement in adults by at least 500 mL, and a temperature higher than 39.4 °C (103 °F) increases it by at least 1000 mL.[1] A respiratory rate greater than 35 per minute further increases fluid needs.[2] Individual patients must be assessed clinically to determine precise fluid requirements.

Sweating

Recall that sweat is a hypotonic fluid containing primarily water, sodium, chloride, and potassium. Sweat can vary in volume from 0 to 1000 mL/hr, or more. Thus, it is conceivable that a person can become volume-depleted from severe perspiration in the absence of adequate fluid replacement. Frequently, a sodium imbalance is superimposed on the volume depletion (either hyponatremia if excessive water is ingested, or hypernatremia if no liquids are consumed).

Third-Space Fluid Losses

Because third-space fluid losses are unique in character, a separate section has been devoted to this subject immediately after the discussion of FVD.

Decreased Intake

Unfortunately, several circumstances can interfere with normal fluid intake. Among these are anorexia, nausea, and fatigue. Patients unable to swallow because of neurological impairment are frequently noted to have at least some degree of FVD. Others prone to this condition are those patients who are reluctant to swallow because of oral or pharyngeal pain or those individuals unable to gain access to fluids because of decreased mobility. Depression can be so severe as to interfere with normal fluid intake.

DEFINING CHARACTERISTICS

A FVD can develop slowly or with great rapidity, and can be mild, moderate, or severe, depending on the degree of fluid loss. Important characteristics of FVD are discussed below and listed in the Summary of Fluid Volume Deficit.

Weight Loss

Rapid weight loss reflects loss of body fluid because fluctuations in lean body mass do not occur quickly. For example, it has generally been assumed that it takes a caloric deficit of approximately 3400 kcal to lose 1 lb (0.45 kg) of weight.[3] Theoretically, therefore, a typical adult on bedrest with a normal metabolism would have to take in zero calories to achieve a "real" weight loss of 1 lb in 2 days. On the other hand, a 1 L of fluid weighs approximately 2 lbs; this amount of fluid can easily be lost in a short period. Indeed, some patients can quickly lose much more than this.

Decreased Skin and Tongue Turgor

In most healthy persons, pinched skin will immediately fall back to its original position when released. This elastic property, or turgor, is partially dependent on interstitial fluid volume. In a person with FVD, the skin may remain slightly elevated for many seconds after being pinched, indicating a deficit of fluid in the interstitial compartment (one segment of extracellular fluid [ECF]). It is important to remember that, because tissue turgor also reflects the degree of skin elasticity, it is less valid as a sign of FVD in persons older than 55 to 60 years (because skin elasticity decreases with age). Although reduced skin turgor is an important finding, it is possible that turgor will appear normal in some individuals with fluid deficit (for example, this may occur when the deficit is mild or in obese patients with fat stores that interfere with turgor assessment).

In a person with FVD, the tongue is smaller and has additional longitudinal furrows, again reflecting loss of interstitial fluid. Fortunately, tongue turgor is not affected appreciably by age and thus is a useful assessment for all age groups. In a recent study of 55 emergency room patients (ranging in age from 61 to 98 years), tongue dryness and increased longitudinal tongue furrows were found to be good indicators of FVD (as were dry oral mucous membranes, sunkenness of eyes, confusion, speech difficulty, and upper body muscle weakness).[4]

Decreased Moisture in Oral Cavity

A dry mouth may be due to FVD or to mouth breathing. If due to FVD, all of the oral tissues will be dry. In contrast, if the dryness is due to mouth breathing, the areas where the gums and cheek membranes meet will remain moist. If the serum sodium is elevated in conjunction with FVD, the mucous membranes will be dry and sticky.

Decreased Urinary Output

Decreased urinary output reflects inadequate perfusion of the kidney because there is not enough ECF to bring the requisite amount of plasma to the glomeruli. A urine volume less than 30 mL/hr in an adult is cause for concern if it persists. One must be constantly aware that persistent oliguria in the severely volume-depleted patient can result in renal tubular damage (discussed later in this chapter).

Increased Urinary Specific Gravity

Elevation of urinary specific gravity (SG) is a reflection of compensatory fluid conservation by the kidneys. Recall that urinary SG can range from 1.003 to 1.035 in normal situations. Thus, a healthy renal response would be one toward the upper limits of normal.

Disrupted Blood Urea Nitrogen/Creatinine Ratio

The blood urea nitrogen (BUN) level rises slowly out of proportion to the serum creatinine with a long-standing FVD of sufficient magnitude to reduce glomerular filtration rate, thus interfering with clearance of nitrogenous wastes.

Changes in Vital Signs

Body temperature is subnormal (sometimes as low as 35 °C [95 °F]), due to decreased metabolism, unless infection is present. In contrast, note that body temperature is often elevated in patients with water deficit (hypernatremia), also referred to as "dehydration."

Postural hypotension and increased pulse rate are signs of hypovolemia. On changing from a lying to an upright position, a drop in systolic pressure greater than 15 mmHg or an increase in the pulse rate greater than 15 beats/min suggests intravascular volume deficit.[5] The blood pressure should be assessed immediately upon assuming the erect position, and again after 2 to 3 min (if indicated) to determine whether the pressure drop is sustained. Postural hypotension with dizziness is strongly suggestive of hypovolemia in the absence of autonomic neuropathy or use of medications that are associated with postural hypotension (such as sympatholytic drugs for hypertension).[6] As fluid volume depletion worsens, blood pressure (BP) becomes low in all positions due to loss of compensatory mechanisms. As always, the patient's baseline blood pressure should be used to assess the degree of blood pressure drop (not the commonly accepted "normal" value of 120/80 mmHg). It is interesting to note that BP measured by a sphygmomanometer (with auscultation or palpation) may reflect a lower pressure than is found if arterial pressure is being simultaneously measured with an intraarterial catheter, because peripheral vasoconstriction leads to decreased intensity of Korotkoff sounds. Tachycardia occurs as the heart pumps faster to compensate for the decreased plasma volume.

Changes in Central Venous Pressure

The jugular veins provide a built-in manometer to detect changes in central venous pressure (CVP), and thus fluid volume status, and do not involve an invasive maneuver. Direct measurement of CVP is frequently performed in acutely ill patients and will reveal a reading less than normal in those with FVD (provided cardiopulmonary function is not impaired).

Decreased Capillary Refill

Peripheral blood flow is diminished as a compensatory reaction to FVD. Therefore, measuring the time it takes for capillaries to fill after compression is helpful in detecting the degree of fluid depletion. A study of this phenomenon was done in 30 healthy infants (2–24 months of age) and indicated that normal capillary refilling occurs in 0.81 ± 0.31 sec (as measured in the fingernail bed after applying just the amount of pressure needed to blanch the nail bed).[7] The amount of time it took for capillary refilling to occur in 32 ill infants with diarrhea was also assessed and compared with laboratory indicators of fluid depletion. The investigators found that:

- A refill time <1.5 sec suggested either a normal volume or a deficit of less than 50 mL/kg,
- A refill time of 1.5 to 3.0 sec suggested a deficit between 50 and 100 mL/kg, and
- A refill time of >3.0 sec suggested a deficit greater than 100 mL/kg.

Another group of investigators studied an outpatient sample of 102 children under the age of 4 years and found that increased capillary refill time is a good indicator of fluid depletion (as is decreased skin turgor and increased thirst).[8]

Other Changes

Altered sensorium is the result of decreased cerebral perfusion, secondary to decreased blood volume. Cold extremities reflect peripheral vasoconstriction, which occurs to build up central blood volume. The hematocrit is elevated above baseline due to loss of intravascular fluid and subsequent concentration of the formed elements of blood.

TREATMENT

In planning fluid replacement for the patient with FVD, it is necessary to consider usual maintenance fluid volume requirements and other factors (such as fever) that can influence fluid needs. When the deficit is not severe, the oral route is preferred for replacement, provided the patient is able to drink. However, when fluid losses are acute, the intravenous (IV) route is required. Chapter 10 discusses formulas used in determining maintenance as well as replacement fluid requirements.

Isotonic electrolyte solutions (such as lactated Ringer's or 0.9% NaCl) are frequently used to treat the hypotensive patient with FVD because such fluids expand plasma volume. As soon as the patient becomes normotensive, a hypotonic electrolyte solution (such as 0.45% NaCl) is often used to provide both electrolytes and free water for renal excretion of metabolic wastes. These and additional fluids are discussed in Chapter 10.

If the patient with severe FVD is oliguric, it is necessary to determine whether the depressed renal function is the result of reduced renal blood flow secondary to FVD (prerenal azotemia) or, more seriously, to acute tubular necrosis due to prolonged FVD. The therapeutic test used in this situation is the *fluid challenge test*. One version of the test, as described by Goldberger,[9] is presented below.

1. An initial fluid test volume (200–300 mL in an adult) can be given over a 5- to 10-min period provided the CVP is less than 15 cm water; the patient should be observed for changes in the CVP, BP, and lung sounds. Constant CVP or pulmonary artery wedge monitoring is required to adequately assess the patient's response to the fluid load. A Foley catheter facilitates accurate measurement of urinary output. The type of fluid used for the fluid challenge depends on the clinical situation.
2. If the CVP remains unchanged or does not elevate more than 2 or 3 cm above the initial reading, the BP remains stable (or becomes elevated if hypotension was present initially), and lung sounds remain normal or become no worse, an additional fluid load is given (200 mL over a 10-min period).
3. If the CVP continues below 15 cm, and if vital signs remain unchanged, the infusion is continued at a rate of 500 mL/hr until the urinary output improves and other parameters (such as CVP and BP) return to normal. It is necessary to monitor the CVP, BP, and lung sounds every 15 min. A pulmonary artery catheter is desirable to monitor complex response to fluid loads.
4. If the problem is prerenal azotemia, the urinary output will increase to more than 20 mL/hr within a few hours. Failure to induce an increased urinary output may indicate the presence of acute renal failure or a urinary obstruction.
5. If the patient remains oliguric after the fluid load, and if the CVP and BP have returned to normal, it is necessary to determine whether the oliguria is still prerenal and will respond to further expansion of the blood volume, or whether the volume depletion has led to acute renal failure. If renal failure has occurred, the administration of additional fluids can be dangerous. The physician may elect to use the mannitol infusion test or IV injection of furosemide to evaluate the situation further.

Be aware that prompt treatment of FVD is imperative to prevent the occurrence of renal damage. If

FVD is allowed to progress to acute tubular necrosis, the patient will require strict renal management (see Chapter 17).

NURSING INTERVENTIONS

1. Assess for presence, or worsening, of FVD:
   - Measure and evaluate intake and output (I&O) at least at 8-hr intervals; sometimes hourly measurements are critical. For a valid picture of the patient's fluid balance status, compare the total I&O measurements for 2 or 3 consecutive days (see section on I&O in Chapter 2).
   - Monitor body weight daily. Consider factors necessary to obtain accurate readings (see Chapter 2). Remember that an acute weight loss of 1 lb represents a fluid loss of approximately 500 mL.
   - Monitor for postural hypotension (that is, a drop in the systolic reading >15 mmHg when the patient is moved from a lying to a sitting position).
   - Monitor for tachycardia (pulse increase >15 beats/min) particularly when patient is moved from a lying to a sitting position.
   - Monitor skin and tongue turgor (see Chapter 2).
   - Monitor condition of mucous membranes. Remember that oral membranes will be dry in a mouth breather regardless of fluid status. When in doubt, run a finger over the gum folds to determine whether dryness is present; if it is, FVD is likely present.
   - Monitor concentration of urine; be aware that a low urinary SG in the presence of oliguria is a sign of renal disease. In a volume-depleted patient the urinary SG should be more than 1.020 (indicating healthy renal conservation of fluid).
   - Monitor BUN to creatinine ratio. In FVD, BUN will elevate out of proportion to serum creatinine level (see Table 2-3).
   - Monitor CVP and pulmonary artery wedge pressures if devices are in use. CVP and pulmonary artery wedge pressure monitoring are discussed in Chapter 2.
   - Monitor body temperature; be aware that it will drop below normal when isotonic FVD is moderate or severe, unless infection is present. (Rectal temperatures of 35 °C [95 °F] have been observed in severe FVD.)
   - Monitor level of sensorium; expect that it will decrease as FVD progresses in severity.
2. Give oral fluids if indicated.
   - Consider the patient's "likes" and "dislikes" when offering fluids.
   - Consider the type of fluid the patient has lost. For example, one would select fluids containing sodium and potassium for a patient who has a FVD due to vomiting. See Table 3-1 for the electrolyte content of commonly available beverages. See Table 13-1 for a summary of the electrolyte content of selected body fluids.
   - If the patient is reluctant to drink because of oral discomfort, select fluids that are nonirritating to the mucosa, and provide frequent mouth care (offer saline gargles and apply lubricant to lips).
   - Offer fluids at frequent intervals.
   - Explain to the patient the need for fluid replacement and attempt to gain his or her cooperation.
   - Administer medications as needed if nausea is present to provide relief before fluids are offered.
3. Consider the following interventions for patients with impaired swallowing:
   - Assess gag reflex and ability to swallow water before offering solid foods; have a suction apparatus on hand.
   - Position the patient upright with head and neck flexed slightly forward during feeding (tilting the head backward during swallowing predisposes to aspiration because this position opens the airway).
   - Provide thick fluids or semi-solid foods (such as puddings or gelatin). These are more easily swallowed because of their consistency and weight than are thin liquids.[10]
4. If the patient is unable to eat and drink, discuss the possibility of tube feedings with the physician.
5. Consult with the physician for parenteral fluid directives if the patient is unable to consume fluids by the enteral route. This intervention is important to prevent renal damage related to prolonged FVD. Be aware that the IV route is

TABLE 3–1

Electrolyte Content of Selected Beverages

BEVERAGE	SODIUM (mg)	POTASSIUM (mg)	CALCIUM (mg)	MAGNESIUM (mg)	PHOSPHORUS (mg)
Orange juice, canned 8 fl oz	6	436	21	27	36
Tomato juice, from concentrate, Campbell's, 6 fl oz	589	376	20	—	—
Peach nectar, canned, 8 fl oz	9	33	11	6	7
Dole pineapple juice, canned, 6 fl oz	2	280	28		17
Prune juice, canned, 8 fl oz	11	706	30	36	64
Tea, instant powder, 1 tsp	1	46	0	3	3
Coffee, powdered instant, 1 round tsp	1	64	3	6	5
Pepsi Cola, 12 fl oz	2		0		55
Diet Pepsi Cola, 12 fl oz	2	30	0		29
Diet Coca-Cola, 12 fl oz	8	18	0		28
Sprite, 12 fl oz	46	0	0		
Thirst Quencher, bottled, 8 fl oz	96	26	0	1	22
Kool-aid, from powder, 8 fl oz	14	1	15		7
Tang, orange, from powder, 6 fl oz	1	45	20		18
Milk, 2% fat, 8 fl oz	122	377	297	33	232
Beef broth, 1 cube	1019	27	4	3	19
Chicken broth, 1 cube	1152	18		3	9

Pennington J: Bowes and Church's Food Values of Portions Commonly Used, 16th ed. Philadelphia, JB Lippincott, 1994; with permission.

favored in acute situations and when large volumes of fluid are needed.

6. Be aware that a carefully kept I&O record is necessary to determine the amount and type of fluids to be administered. Usually, abnormally lost fluids are replaced in the volume that has been lost.
7. Be familiar with the usual types of fluids used to treat FVD (review Treatment section above and see Chapter 10).
8. Understand principles of the fluid challenge test and parameters for nursing assessment (see Treatment section above).
9. Monitor response to fluid intake, either orally or parenterally. If therapy is adequate, one should observe the following:
   - Increased urinary volume toward 40 to 60 mL/hr in adults
   - If previously hypotensive, increased BP toward normal
   - Return of pulse rate to baseline
   - Improved sensorium and sense of vitality
   - Improved skin and tongue turgor
   - Decreased dryness of oral mucosa
   - Increased CVP, toward normal
   - Improved wedge pressure readings
   - Normal, or no worse, breath sounds
   - Decreased urinary SG as urinary volume increases
   - Increased body weight, toward preillness level
10. Report inadequate response to fluid therapy to physician and seek appropriate fluid directives before renal damage occurs.
11. Monitor patients with tendency for abnormal fluid retention (such as renal or cardiac problems) for signs of overload during aggressive fluid replacement. A cardiac patient requiring fluid replacement for FVD should be monitored with pulmonary wedge pressures or CVP determinations during fluid replacement.
12. When administering fluids, either orally or parenterally, consider other illnesses that are

Summary of Fluid Volume Deficit

ETIOLOGICAL FACTORS	DEFINING CHARACTERISTICS
Loss of water and electrolytes, as in: • Vomiting • Diarrhea • Excessive laxative use • Fistulas • GI suction • Polyuria • Fever • Excessive sweating • Third-space fluid shifts Decreased intake, as in: • Anorexia • Nausea • Inability to gain access to fluids • Depression	Weight loss over short period (except in third-space losses) • 2% (mild deficit, such as 2.4-lb loss in 120-lb person) • 5% (moderate deficit, such as 6-lb loss in 120-lb person) • ≥8% (severe deficit, such as 10-lb loss or more in 120-lb person) Decreased skin and tongue turgor Dry mucous membranes Urine output < 30 mL/hr in adult Postural hypotension (systolic pressure drops by more than 15 mmHg when patient moves from lying to standing or sitting position) Weak, rapid pulse Slow capillary refill Decreased body temperature, such as 95°–98° F (35°–36.7° C) unless infection is present Central venous pressure less than 4 cm of water in vena cava BUN elevated out of proportion to serum creatinine Urinary specific gravity high Hematocrit elevated Flat neck veins in supine position Marked oliguria, late Altered sensorium Cold extremities, late

occurring concurrently. For example, patients with syndrome of inappropriate antidiuretic hormone secretion (SIADH), potential or actual increased intracranial pressure, renal failure, or preeclampsia require complex management. (These conditions are discussed in later chapters.)

13. Take safety precautions if altered sensorium is present.
14. Turn patient frequently and apply moisturizing agents to skin to avoid skin breakdown.
15. Give frequent oral care.

CASE STUDIES

3-1. An 80-year-old man developed FVD as a result of overzealous diuretic use. After a 13-lb weight loss over 4 days, the CVP dropped to 1 cm of water. Skin turgor over the sternum and medial aspect of the thigh was poor (when skin was pinched, it remained elevated for 6 sec). Urine output was low at 20 mL/hr and the BUN was greatly elevated at 80 mg/dL (normal, 10–20 mg/dL). Body temperature was 36.3 °C (97.4 °F), pulse was 96 and weak in volume, and BP was 140/90 mmHg supine and 122/84 mmHg in a sitting position.

COMMENTARY: This patient had lost 6 L of fluid in a relatively short period; his CVP was far below the normal level of 4 to 11 cm of water. His BUN was elevated; the urine volume was low, particularly for an elderly person. These factors, plus positional hypotension and increased pulse rate, were indicative of FVD. Note that the body temperature was not elevated, probably reflecting the slowed metabolic rate associated with FVD not complicated by infection.

3-2. A 35-year-old woman developed FVD after 4 days of severe diarrhea and poor intake. She weighed 119 lb on admission (preillness weight, 128 lb). Her BUN was 40 mg/dL and serum creatinine was 1.3 mg/dL. Skin turgor was poor and urine output was 15 mL/hr (SG 1.030). Blood pressure was 120/80 mmHg recumbent and fell to 98/60 mmHg when erect. Pulse was 110, weak, and regular.

COMMENTARY: This patient lost 7% of her body weight in 4 days; her BUN was twice normal, whereas her serum creatinine was normal. Postural hypotension, poor turgor, and oliguria all point to FVD.

THIRD-SPACING OF BODY FLUIDS

Third-spacing of body fluids is a unique situation leading to decreased intravascular volume and largely presenting with the same characteristics as those of FVD. However, because it is more difficult to diagnose than direct loss of body fluids, it is given a separate section in this chapter. In addition, third-space fluid losses are discussed in the clinical chapters dealing with specific conditions associated with this phenomenon.

DEFINITION

Third-spacing refers to a shift of fluid from the vascular space into a portion of the body from which it is not easily exchanged with the rest of the ECF. This sequestration of fluid is the result of an alteration in capillary permeability secondary to injury, ischemia, or inflammation.[11] The trapped fluid, although still technically within the body, is essentially unavailable for functional use. Termed *nonfunctional* because it is not able to participate in the normal functions of the ECF compartment, the third-spaced fluid might just as well have been lost externally. Fluid can be sequestered from the intravascular space into potential body spaces (such as the pleural, peritoneal, pericardial, or joint cavities) or it can become trapped in the bowel by obstruction or in the interstitial space as edema after burns or other trauma. Furthermore, it can be trapped in inflamed tissue, as in peritonitis, pancreatitis, or fasciitis.

Major considerations in differentiating the FVD associated with third-spacing from that associated with fluid lost through vomiting or diarrhea are that (1) the latter fluid losses can be observed and measured whereas the former cannot, and (2) decreased body weight does not occur in third-spacing as it does in actual fluid loss. Indeed, patients with third-spacing may *gain* weight as IV fluids are administered to replace the diminished intravascular volume.

PHASES OF THIRD-SPACE FLUID SHIFTS AND ASSOCIATED CLINICAL MANIFESTATIONS

Third-space fluid shifts occur in two phases. The first is described above and involves a shift of fluid from the intravascular space into a nonfunctional fluid space. Clinical manifestations expected with a significant shift of fluid are essentially those of FVD because, although the fluid is in the body, it is functionally unavailable for use. During this period, expect the following:

- Tachycardia and hypotension (effective blood volume is reduced as the fluid shifts out of the vascular space)
- Urine volume less than 30 mL/hr in the adult (decreased plasma volume causes a fall in renal perfusion and, therefore, less urine formation)
- High urinary SG and osmolality (renal attempt to conserve needed water)
- Elevated hematocrit (red blood cells become suspended in a smaller plasma volume as the fluid shifts out of the intravascular space)
- Postural hypotension
- Low CVP
- Poor skin and tongue turgor
- Insignificant body weight changes

During this phase, the body attempts to compensate for the third-space losses of ECF by renal conservation of sodium and water. As with any cause of FVD, it is important to correct the reduced plasma volume before renal perfusion is compromised to the extent that acute tubular necrosis occurs.

After a variable number of days, the fluid shifts back to the vascular space and may impose a temporary hypervolemia. Resolution of the third-space is slower than its accumulation. In some instances the shift of fluid back to the intravascular space occurs within 48 to 72 hrs. In others, it may not occur for 10 days or longer.[12] For example, fluid shifts from major burns or peritonitis are generally reversed within 2 to 3 days, whereas those associated with septic shock may not occur until the underlying cause of the sepsis is addressed.[13] As the extra fluid in the tissues or body spaces shifts back into the intravascular compartment, it is excreted through the kidneys. Excessive fluid administration during the period when fluid is shifting back into the bloodstream may cause circulatory overload, especially in patients with cardiac or renal failure. Assessment is primarily directed at detecting hypervolemia before serious effects occur. For example, observe for polyuria (hourly urine volume may be as high as 200 mL as the excess fluid is excreted), distended neck veins (a sign of fluid overload), moist lung sounds, shortness of breath, elevated CVP, and elevated systolic BP.

PATHOPHYSIOLOGY OF CLINICAL SITUATIONS ASSOCIATED WITH THIRD-SPACE FLUID SHIFTS

Sequestration of fluids (third-spacing) is at least partially the result of altered capillary permeability; therefore, the leaked fluid stems from the vascular space (a compartment of the ECF). Understandably, then, the leaked fluid has the same composition as the ECF. Very large fluid shifts may occur in conditions associated with third-spacing. If there is no oral or IV intake of fluid, the effective circulating volume will decline to a point at which hypotension develops. If fluids are replaced to maintain the vascular volume, the ECF volume will expand and be reflected in weight gain. It is important to note that redistribution of fluid within the body does not appear as a decrease in the patient's weight, nor does it show up on the fluid I&O records; instead, these losses can be detected only by physiological changes in organ function. Not only does weight loss not occur during acute third-spacing, weight may actually be *gained* as fluid is infused to help compensate for the diminished vascular volume.

Because the exact mechanism of third-spacing varies somewhat with the specific cause, it is helpful to consider each separately.

Nonthermal Trauma and Surgery

Traumatic injury results in redistribution of intravascular fluid into the area of injury, thereby reducing the functional ECF volume. The volume of third-spacing varies with the severity of injury. For example, a patient with a fractured hip may lose 1500 to 2000 mL of blood into the tissues surrounding the injury site.[14] Although this fluid will eventually reabsorb (over a period of days or weeks), the deficit can cause an acute reduction in the vascular volume if it is not replaced.

Varying degrees of third-spacing occur in surgical procedures and are related to tissue manipulation and injury. The amount of fluid lost from the extracellular space varies with the extent and nature of the surgical undertaking. Minor operative procedures (such as appendectomy) are associated with considerably less fluid sequestration than are major operative procedures (such as extensive retroperitoneal dissection).[15] For example, a simple laparotomy with a total small bowel exploration can result in 700 mL of ECF distributional loss, whereas an extensive colon resection can cause as much as 2 to 3 L of ECF to sequester into the peritoneal cavity in 2 to 4 hrs.[16] After abdominal surgery, particularly pelvic surgery, fluid accumulates in the peritoneum, bowel wall, and other traumatized tissues. Formation of a third-space after nonthermal traumatic injury occurs immediately and is maximal by 5 to 6 hrs.[17] In the surgical patient, it is difficult to assess fluid loss due to sequestration into the interstitial compartment; for example, the patient with intestinal obstruction may accumulate as much as 6 L of fluid into the bowel wall and lumen.[18] Such unrecognized deficits of ECF during the early postoperative period are manifested primarily as circulatory instability.

Burns

Altered capillary permeability of burned tissue results in an exudation of plasma at the burn site. There is also an increase in fluid flux across capillaries in nonburned tissue that apparently results from hypoproteinemia rather than an alteration in capillary permeability. Formation of edema occurs primarily in the first 24 hrs, with the greatest losses being incurred during the first 8 hrs. For this reason, thermally injured patients should receive 50% of their estimated fluid losses in the first 8 hrs; colloids should be given on the second day to minimize edema formation in the nonburned tissue.[19]

Intestinal Obstruction

Patients suffering from mechanical intestinal obstruction or adynamic ileus may sequester large quantities of ECF equal to many liters. In acute intestinal obstruction, as much as 6 L or more can accumulate within the lumen and wall of the gut.[20] (See Chapter 13 for a more in-depth discussion of intestinal obstruction.)

Inflammation of Intraabdominal Organs

Important third-space fluid losses can occur into the peritoneum, the bowel wall, and other tissues in the presence of inflammatory lesions of the intraabdominal organs. The extent of these losses may not be fully appreciated unless one considers that the total area of the peritoneum is 1.8 m^2 (which is almost equal to the body surface area of the skin).[21] A peritoneal thickness increase of only 1 mm can potentially sequester 18 L of fluid.[22]

Sepsis

Sepsis produces a generalized capillary leak that produces a decrease in the functional ECF volume (while producing interstitial edema). As sepsis persists, protein malnutrition produces hypoproteinemia, which in turn may increase the formation of edema. Other toxic insults to the capillary endothelium (as may occur secondary to snakebites or after the administration of certain drugs, such as interleukin-2) may result in the "capillary leak" syndrome.[23] In these situations, edema forms at the expense of the intravascular volume.

Pancreatitis

In pancreatitis, inflammation and autodigestion by pancreatic enzymes lead to peripancreatic edema as well as fluid loss into the retroperitoneal tissue; a dramatic decrease in plasma volume causes systemic hypovolemia. Clinical signs of fluid loss include hypotension, tachycardia, oliguria, and increased hematocrit due to hemoconcentration. (In the presence of hemorrhagic pancreatitis, the hematocrit may drop rather than elevate.) See Chapter 20 for a more in-depth discussion of fluid and electrolyte problems associated with pancreatitis.

Ascites

The major difference between the fluid shifts described above and the development of ascites in hepatic cirrhosis is the rate of fluid accumulation. Although the above conditions are associated with fluid shifts that typically occur fairly rapidly, cirrhotic ascites develops relatively slowly, allowing time for renal sodium and water retention to replenish the effective circulating blood volume. As a result, patients with cirrhosis typically present with symptoms of edema instead of hypovolemia.[24] An exception could theoretically occur if rapid fluid removal by paracentesis resulted in a quick shift of fluid from the vascular space to the peritoneum (resulting in hypovolemia). Rarely, paracentesis of as little as 1000 mL may lead to circulatory collapse, encephalopathy, and renal failure in patients with hepatic insufficiency.[25] However, recent studies suggest that large-volume paracentesis (4–6 L) can be safely performed in selected patients, provided certain precautions are taken (see discussion of paracentesis in Chapter 21).

FLUID REPLACEMENT

Treatment is directed at correcting the cause of the third-space shift of body fluids. As is the case with any cause of FVD, the reduced plasma volume must be corrected before renal damage occurs.

Although the choice of a replacement fluid depends on the existence of concomitant electrolyte abnormalities, most third-space losses are properly replaced with a balanced salt solution such as lactated Ringer's solution. Attempts to correct the fluid deficit with hypotonic solutions (such as 5% dextrose in water or half-strength saline) may result in clinically significant hyponatremia. Any deficits in red blood cell may require correction by the administration of packed cells to maintain optimal oxygen-carrying capacity of the blood. Large quantities of replacement fluids are often needed to maintain an effective circulating volume. Plasma or plasma substitutes may also be considered for use in addition to replacement electrolyte solutions for patients who have suffered protein loss (as may occur in burns or peritonitis).

Fluid replacement therapy must be tailored to the patient's response. For example, during the first phase, when fluid has shifted from the intravascular space, the aim of fluid therapy is to stabilize BP and pulse and maintain an adequate urine volume (usually 30–50 mL/hr).

FLUID VOLUME EXCESS

Fluid volume excess (FVE) is the result of the abnormal retention of water and sodium in approximately the same proportions in which they normally exist in the ECF (see Fig. 3-2). It is always secondary to an increase in the total body sodium content, which, in turn, leads to an increase in total body water. Because there is isotonic retention of both substances, the serum sodium concentration remains essentially normal.

ETIOLOGICAL FACTORS

This imbalance may be caused by simple overloading with fluids or by diminished function of the homeostatic mechanisms responsible for regulating fluid balance. Etiological factors can include the following:

1. Compromised regulatory mechanisms, as in congestive heart failure, renal failure, cirrhosis of the liver, and steroid excess.
2. Overzealous administration of sodium-containing fluids, particularly to patients with impaired regulatory mechanisms. The commonly used isotonic fluids, 0.9% NaCl and lactated Ringer's solution, contain sizable amounts of sodium and, if used to excess, can easily exceed the tolerance of patients with impaired regulatory mechanisms. Note that 0.9% NaCl contains 154 mEq/L of sodium and that lactated Ringer's has 130 mEq/L.
3. Excessive ingestion of sodium chloride or other sodium salts in the diet. See Table 3-3 for sodium content of compounds used to improve the texture or flavor of food, or to extend freshness. Other "hidden" gains of sodium may result from the use of proprietary drugs such as Alka-Seltzer or the frequent use of hypertonic enemas (such as Fleet enema).

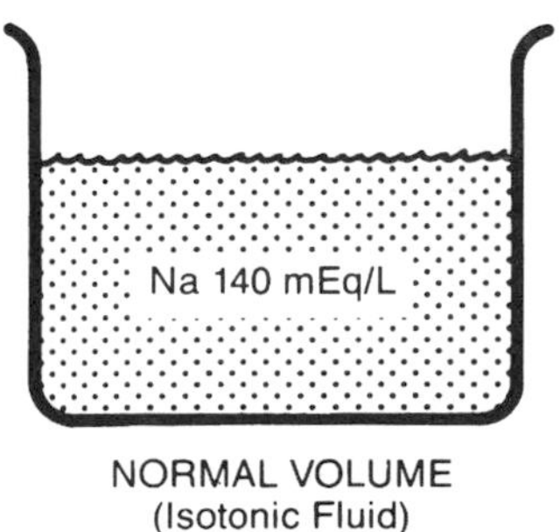

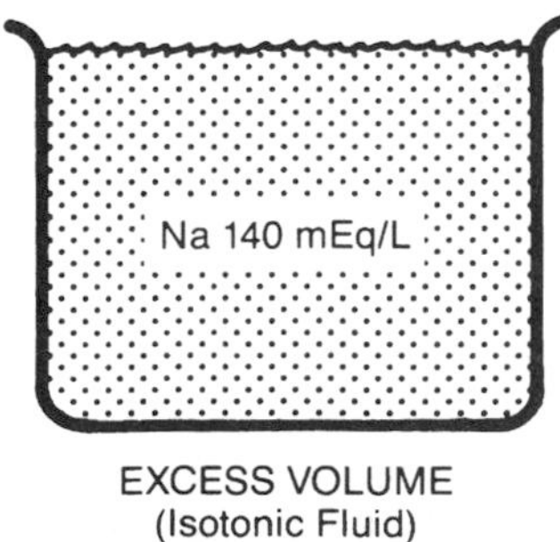

Figure 3–2. Fluid volume excess.

DEFINING CHARACTERISTICS

The defining characteristics of FVE are linked to an excess of fluid in the extracellular compartment and are listed in the Summary of Fluid Volume Excess.

TREATMENT

When reversal of the primary problem is impossible, symptomatic treatment often consists of restriction of sodium and fluids and the administration of diuretics. In some conditions, only one of these therapies is necessary. Sodium-restricted diets and diuretic administration are discussed below, along with the effect of bedrest on mobilization of edematous fluid.

Sodium-Restricted Diets

Sodium content in foods may be expressed as grams of salt, milligrams of sodium, or milliequivalents of sodium. To understand conversions of grams of salt to grams of sodium, recall that sodium represents about 40% of the weight of salt (sodium chloride). Therefore, a gram of sodium chloride is equivalent to 0.4 g of sodium. Dietary prescriptions are more sensibly stated in terms of sodium rather than salt content. According to usual definitions, a mildly restricted diet contains 4 to 5 g of sodium, a moderately restricted one contains 2 g, and a severely restricted diet contains 0.5 g of sodium.[26] To convert milligrams of sodium to milliequivalents, divide the number of milligrams by 23 (the atomic weight of sodium); for example, 1000 mg of sodium is equivalent to 43 mEq of sodium.

The typical American diet contains approximately 10 to 12 grams of salt (NaCl) a day (or 4–4.8 g of sodium).[27] Approximately one third comes from the salt shaker, one-third from processed foods, and one-third from the food itself.[28] Recall that processed foods often have hidden sources of sodium in the form of preservatives, such as monosodium glutamate, baking powder, baking soda, brine, and disodium phosphate. Tables 3-1 and 3-2 list the sodium and potassium contents of some common beverages and foods. Table 3-3 summarizes the sodium content of common food additives. These figures clearly indicate how plentiful sodium is in the average diet.

Sodium-restricted diets are commonly prescribed for patients with fluid excess problems, such as occur with congestive heart failure, hepatic failure with ascites, renal failure, and hypertension. Some patients do well with only mildly restricted diets, whereas others require severe restrictions. A mild sodium-restricted diet requires only light salting of food (about half the usual amount) in cooking and at the table, no addition of salt to foods that are already seasoned (such as canned foods and foods ready to

TABLE 3–2

Sodium, Potassium, and Caloric Content of Selected Fruits and Vegetables

FOOD	SODIUM (mg)	POTASSIUM (mg)	CALORIES
Fruits			
Apple, raw with skin, 1 medium	1	159	81
Apricots, raw, 3 medium	1	313	51
Banana, raw, 1 medium	1	451	105
Raisins, golden seedless, 2/3 cup	12	746	302
Orange, navel, raw, 1 medium	1	250	65
Vegetables			
Carrot, raw, 1 medium	25	233	31
Potato, baked, without skin, 1	8	610	145
Tomato, raw, 1	11	273	26

Pennington J: Bowes and Church's Food Values of Portions Commonly Used, 16th ed. Philadelphia, JB Lippincott, 1994; with permission.

TABLE 3–3

Sodium Content of Common Food Additives

ADDITIVE	SODIUM CONTENT
Salt, Morton	2300 mg/tsp
Baking powder (Calumet)	426 mg/tsp
Baking powder (sodium aluminum silicate)	1205 mg/tbl
Mustard, brown	65 mg/tsp
Catsup, tomato	178 mg/tbl
Horseradish, prepared	14 mg/tbl
Soy sauce, Kikkoman	3074 mg/¼ cup
Worcestershire sauce (Heinz)	234 mg/tbl

Adapted from Pennington J: Bowes and Church's Food Values of Portions Commonly Used, 16th ed. Philadelphia, JB Lippincott, 1994.

cook or eat), and avoidance of foods that are high in sodium. Examples of such foods include salty snack foods, olives, pickles, and luncheon meats.

Patients should be made aware that most canned and ready-to-eat foods already have added salt and thus should be used only as their specific diets allow. Foods that may be used freely include most fresh vegetables and fruits and unprocessed cereals. Cooking from scratch is usually the best way to prepare low-sodium food, and several excellent cookbooks are available for this purpose. Low-sodium baking powder can be found in the dietetic section of many grocery stores, and low-sodium milk, milk products, and bakery goods are available in most large cities. Patients on sodium-restricted diets should also consider the sodium content in "over-the-counter" drugs. For example, one Alka-Seltzer tablet contains 958 mg of sodium bicarbonate.[29]

Because a substantial portion of sodium is ingested in the form of seasoning, use of substitute seasonings plays a major role in cutting sodium intake. Lemon juice, onion, and garlic are excellent substitute flavoring agents, although some patients prefer salt substitutes. Most salt substitutes contain potassium and should be used cautiously by those taking potassium-conserving diuretics (listed in Table 3-4) and by those who have renal impairment. Salt substitutes containing ammonium chloride can be harmful to patients with liver damage. (Salt substitutes are discussed further in Chapter 5 and are listed in Table 5-2).

Diuretics

Diuretics are commonly used drugs that promote increased urine flow. More specifically, they act by inhibiting salt and water reabsorption by the kidney tubules. By inducing a negative fluid balance, these medications are useful in the treatment of conditions associated with FVE.

For the most part, diuretics can be grouped into three major classes:

1. Loop diuretics (such as furosemide, bumetanide, and ethacrynic acid), which act in the thick ascending loop of Henle.
2. Thiazide-type diuretics (such as chlorothiazide and hydrochlorothiazide), which act in the distal tubule and connecting segment.
3. Potassium-sparing diuretics (such as amiloride, spironolactone, and triamterene), which act in the cortical collecting tube.

Examples of other diuretics are acetazolamide, a carbonic anhydrase inhibitor, and mannitol, a nonreabsorbable polysaccharide that acts as an osmotic diuretic.

To achieve excretion of excess fluid, either a single diuretic (such as a thiazide) or a combination of agents may be selected (such as thiazide and spironolactone). The latter combination is particularly helpful in that the two drugs have different sites of action and thus allow more effective control of FVE.

Diuretics may be given orally or parenterally, depending on the particular agent to be administered and the status of the patient. For example, patients with advanced congestive heart failure may have difficulty in absorbing orally administered furosemide (due to decreased intestinal perfusion and perhaps intestinal mucosal edema).[30] In this situation, removal of edema with intravenous furosemide therapy and stabilization of cardiac function may partially correct this absorptive defect, thereby allowing oral therapy to be reinstituted.

Diuretics can have undesirable side effects, such as:

- Extracellular fluid volume depletion
- Hyponatremia
- Alterations in potassium excretion (hypokalemia and hyperkalemia)

TABLE 3–4

Commonly Used Diuretic Agents

DRUG	COMMENTS
Thiazides Examples: chlorothiazide (Diuril), hydrochlorothiazide (Esidrix)	Act by inhibiting sodium reabsorption in the distal tubule and, to a lesser extent, the inner medullary collecting duct Cause loss of sodium, chloride, and potassium Decrease urinary calcium excretion and sometimes result in slightly elevated serum calcium level Potassium supplements or extra dietary potassium may be necessary when these agents are used routinely
Loop diuretics Examples: furosemide (Lasix), ethacrynic acid (Edecrin), bumetanide (Bumex)	Powerful diuretics that act primarily in the thick segment of the medullary and cortical ascending limbs of Henle's loop Cause loss of sodium, chloride, and potassium Potassium supplements or extra dietary K may be necessary when these agents are used routinely
Potassium-conserving diuretics Examples: spironolactone (Aldactone), triamterene (Dyrenium), amiloride	Cause loss of sodium and chloride Conserve potassium Spironoloctone inhibits action of aldosterone (Recall that the hormone aldosterone causes sodium retention and potassium excretion.) Triamterene acts on the distal renal tubule to depress the exchange of sodium Effect of amiloride apparently due to inhibition of sodium entry into the cell from luminal fluid These drugs reduce potassium excretion and may lead to hyperkalemia; thus, potassium supplements are contraindicated, as are salt substitutes containing potassium Often combined with thiazides for effective diuresis; in this case, the hypokalemic tendency of the thiazides may offset the hyperkalemic tendency of triamterene and spironolactone (examples of such combinations are Dyazide and Aldactazide).

- Magnesium wasting
- Alterations in calcium excretion
- Acid–base disturbances

Extracellular Fluid Volume Depletion

Depletion of the ECF volume is a common complication of diuretic use, especially when the potent loop-acting diuretics are used. Although the duration of sodium loss with diuretic use is limited, some patients have a relatively large initial response and develop true volume depletion.[31] This complication is most likely to occur in patients who are concurrently losing fluids from other routes (as in vomiting or diarrhea) or who are unable to take in sufficient amounts of salt and water. Clinical signs of fluid volume depletion include weakness, malaise, muscle cramps, and postural dizziness. Reduction of the effective circulatory volume decreases renal perfusion and can lead to prerenal azotemia, manifested by an increase in the BUN and plasma creatinine concentrations. In general, volume depletion causes a greater rise in the BUN than in the plasma creatinine level. If the patient has an underlying renal insufficiency, the ECF deficit can lead to overt uremia. Most fluid and electrolyte complications associated with use of diuretics occur within the first several weeks of therapy, provided that drug dose, dietary intake, and renal function remain stable.[32]

Hyponatremia

Hyponatremia is seen relatively frequently in patients taking diuretics.[33] Almost all cases of hyponatremia associated with diuretic use are due to a thiazide-type diuretic (as opposed to loop diuretics).[34]

Depression of free water clearance may occur in patients taking routine doses of thiazide diuretics.[35] Excessive water intake is to be discouraged in patients taking these medications.

Hypokalemia

Urinary potassium losses are increased by the thiazide and loop diuretics, often leading to the development of hypokalemia. There is some controversy regarding the seriousness of mild hypokalemia (plasma potassium levels between 3.0 and 3.5 mEq/L). Some physicians view the problem as relatively benign, whereas others believe it increases coronary risk. Although the mechanism for such risk is not known, a possible factor is increased ventricular arrhythmias associated with hypokalemia or hypomagnesemia. Among the potential problems associated with potassium depletion are cardiac muscle irritability (particularly when the patient is also taking digitalis); defects in renal concentrating ability, perhaps leading to interstitial fibrosis; sluggish insulin release, leading to carbohydrate intolerance; and predisposition to rhabdomyolysis (due to decreased striated muscle blood flow).[36] It has been found that urinary potassium loss and potassium depletion are most pronounced in patients who take diuretics and ingest large loads of solute and water; these individuals may need supplemental intake of potassium chloride.[37] However, the most appropriate way to eliminate excessive urinary potassium wasting is through restriction of dietary sodium intake (to about 87 mEq/day).[38] Obviously, the smallest dosage of a diuretic necessary to achieve the desired degree of fluid excretion should be used. Recent studies have indicated that lower dosages of diuretics than are commonly used are capable of achieving the desired effects without producing problems. For example, as little as 12.5 mg of hydrochlorothiazide or 15 mg of chlorthalidone (a thiazide-type agent) produce as large an antihypertensive effect as large doses, with little or no change in plasma potassium concentrations.[39–41]

Hyperkalemia

The potassium-conserving diuretics (such as spironolactone, amiloride, and triamterene) reduce potassium secretion and, as a result, can cause hyperkalemia. To prevent this problem, these drugs should be used with great caution (if at all) in patients with renal failure or in those treated with a potassium supplement or an angiotensin-converting enzyme inhibitor (which also decreases potassium secretion, perhaps by decreasing aldosterone levels).[42,43]

Magnesium Wasting

Magnesium depletion can be induced by thiazide and loop diuretics when they are administered chronically.[44] Oddly, although magnesium depletion is fairly common, most of these losses come from cellular stores as the plasma magnesium concentration often remains within the normal range.[45] A potential problem is cellular magnesium deficit with the increased possibility of cardiac arrhythmias. Magnesium depletion can also contribute to the development of hypocalcemia by reducing parahormone secretion.

Alterations in Calcium Excretion

Thiazide diuretics decrease urinary calcium excretion with both short- and long-term use.[46] Because of decreased calcium excretion in the urine, long-term thiazide administration may lead to overt hypercalcemia.[47] Amiloride also decreases calcium excretion. Conversely, bumetanide, furosemide, and ethacrynic acid increase urinary calcium excretion and therefore, are useful in the treatment of acute hypercalcemic conditions.

Metabolic Acid–Base Disturbances

Hypokalemia occurring with use of thiazide and loop diuretics is often accompanied by metabolic alkalosis. In contrast, the potassium-sparing diuretics can result in both hyperkalemia and metabolic acidosis.

Bedrest

Bedrest alone can induce a diuresis, particularly in cases of heart failure. Mobilization of edematous fluid by the supine position is probably related to diminished peripheral venous pooling and a resultant increase in the effective circulating blood volume, and thus in renal perfusion.[48] Metabolic requirements of peripheral tissues are usually decreased by bedrest so that, in patients with congestive heart failure, there is less demand placed on the weakened myocardium. This action can transfer as much as 400 to 500 mL of interstitial fluid into the central circulation over a few days.[49] Bedrest can cause a 40% increase in glomerular filtration rate and a doubling of urinary sodium excretion in response to diuretics.[50]

NURSING INTERVENTIONS

1. Assess for the presence, or worsening, of FVE:
   - Monitor I&O and evaluate at regular intervals for excessive fluid retention.

Summary of Fluid Volume Excess

ETIOLOGICAL FACTORS

Compromised regulatory mechanisms:
- Renal failure
- Congestive heart failure
- Cirrhosis of liver
- Cushing's syndrome

Overzealous administration of sodium-containing IV fluids

Excessive ingestion of sodium-containing substances in diet or sodium-containing medications

DEFINING CHARACTERISTICS

Weight gain over short period:
- 2% (mild excess, such as 2.4-lb in 120-lb person)
- 5% (moderate excess, such as 6-lb in 120-lb person)
- 8% or greater (severe excess, such as 10-lb gain or greater in 120-lb person)

Peripheral edema (excess of fluid in interstitial space)

Distended neck veins

Distended peripheral veins

Slow-emptying peripheral veins

Central venous pressure > 11 cm of water in vena cava

Moist rales in lungs

Polyuria (if renal function is normal)

Ascites, pleural effusion (when fluid volume excess is severe, fluid transudates into body cavities)

Decreased BUN (due to plasma dilution)

Decreased hematocrit (also due to plasma dilution)

Bounding, full pulse

Pulmonary edema, if severe

- Monitor changes in body weight; be alert for acute weight gain.
- Assess breath sounds at regular intervals for presence, or worsening, of rales.
- Monitor degree of peripheral edema; look for edema in most dependent parts of body (feet and ankles in ambulatory patients, sacral region in bedridden patients). Check for pitting edema (see Fig. 2-3) and measure extent of edema with millimeter tape.
- Monitor degree of distention of peripheral veins.
- Monitor laboratory values (look for low BUN and hematocrit; however, realize that there may well be other causes for abnormalities in these values, such as low protein intake and anemia).

2. Encourage adherence to sodium-restricted diet, if prescribed. Assist dietitian in diet instruction. Review section on sodium-restricted diets under treatment.
3. Instruct patients requiring sodium restriction to avoid over-the-counter drugs without first checking with the health-care adviser.
4. When fluid retention persists despite adherence to dietary sodium intake, consider hidden sources of sodium, such as water supply or use of water softeners.
5. When indicated, encourage rest periods. Lying down favors diuresis of edematous fluid (see the above discussion in section on bedrest).
6. Monitor the patient's response to diuretics. Discuss significant findings with physician.
7. Monitor rate of parenteral fluids and the patient's response. Discuss significant findings with physician.
8. Teach self-monitoring of weight and I&O measurements to patients with chronic fluid retention (such as those with congestive heart failure, renal disease, or cirrhosis of liver).
9. Monitor for worsening of underlying cause of FVE. See Chapters 16, 17, and 21 for specific interventions for patients with cirrhosis and renal and heart failure.
10. If dyspnea and orthopnea are present, position the patient in semi-Fowler's position to favor lung expansion.
11. Turn and position the patient frequently; be aware that edematous tissue is more prone to skin breakdown than is normal tissue.

CASE STUDIES

3-3. A 70-year-old woman with congestive heart failure was admitted to an acute care facility. In addition to distended neck veins and pedal edema, pulmonary edema was present. The CVP was 20 cm of water and the BUN was 8 mg/dL.

COMMENTARY: See Figures 2-3 and 2-1 for examples of pitting edema and distended neck veins. Note in this case study the relatively low BUN, especially for an elderly person (indicating plasma dilution). The CVP was greatly elevated because normal is 4 to 11 cm of water.

3-4. A 10-year-old girl was inadvertently given 3.5 L of isotonic saline (0.9% NaCl) for 3 days postoperatively. A gain of approximately 6 lb over the admission weight was noted. According to laboratory data, the BUN was 6 mg/dL on the third postoperative day.

COMMENTARY: This case is an example of fluid overloading during a period in which the kidneys were less able to excrete the excess. Recall that in the early postoperative period there is a tendency to retain fluids because of increased secretion of adrenal hormones (stress reaction). Fluid overload was reflected by the weight gain and low BUN. A review of the I&O record would also have reflected the problem. Had the staff paid attention to the far greater intake than output, the problem could have been alleviated early.

REFERENCES

1. Condon R, Nyhus L: Manual of Surgical Therapeutics, 8th ed, p 183. Boston, Little, Brown, 1993
2. Ibid
3. Alpers D, Clouse R, Stenson W: Manual of Nutritional Therapeutics, 2nd ed, p 143. Boston, Little, Brown, 1988

4. Gross C, Lindquist R, Woolley A, et al: Clinical indicators of dehydration severity in elderly patients. J Emergency Med 10:267–274,1992
5. Kokko J, Tannen R: Fluids and Electrolytes, 2nd ed, p 72. Philadelphia, WB Saunders, 1990
6. Rose B: Clinical Physiology of Acid-Base and Electrolyte Disorders, 4th ed, p 395. New York, McGraw-Hill, 1994
7. Saavedra J, Harris G, Song L, Finberg L: Capillary refilling in the assessment of dehydration. AJDC 145: 296–298,1991
8. MacKenzie A, Barnes G, Shann F: Clinical signs of dehydration in children. Lancet 2:504–507,1989
9. Goldberger E: A Primer of Water, Electrolytes and Acid-Base Syndromes, 7th ed, p 220. Philadelphia, Lea & Febiger, 1986
10. Gettrust K, Ryan S, Engleman D: Applied Nursing Diagnoses: Guides for Comprehensive Care Planning, p 17. New York, John Wiley & Sons, 1985
11. Schwartz S, Shires T, Spencer F: Principles of Surgery, 6th ed, p 40. New York, McGraw-Hill, 1994
12. Ibid
13. Narins R (ed): Maxwell & Kleeman's Clinical Disorders of Fluid and Electrolyte Metabolism, 5th ed, p 1424. New York, McGraw-Hill, 1994
14. Rose, p 392
15. Schwartz et al, p 41
16. Vannata J, Fogelman M: Moyer's Fluid Balance, 4th ed, p 152. Chicago, Year Book Medical Publishers, 1988
17. Ibid
18. Narins, p 1424
19. Schwartz et al, p 41
20. Narins, p 1424
21. Schwartz et al, p 1452
22. Ibid
23. Szerlip H, Goldfarb S: Workshops in Fluid and Electrolyte Disorders, p 7. New York, Churchill Livingston, 1993
24. Rose, p 392
25. Woodley M, Whelan A (eds): Manual of Medical Therapeutics, 27th ed, p 321. Boston, Little, Brown, 1992
26. Alpers et al, p 325
27. Szerlip, Goldfarb, p 15
28. Ibid
29. Physician's Desk Reference for Nonprescription Drugs, p 1660. Montvale, NJ, Medical Economics, 1995
30. Rose, p 434
31. Ibid, p 427
32. Narins, p 561
33. Rose, p 431
34. Ibid
35. Ashraf N, et al: Thiazide-induced hyponatremia associated with death or neurologic damage in outpatients. Am J Med 70:1163,1981
36. Narins, p 561
37. Ibid, p 562
38. Ibid
39. Johnston G, Wilson R, McDermott B, et al: Low-dose cyclopenthiazide in the treatment of hypertension: A one-year community-based study. Q J Med 78: 135,1991
40. Dahlof B, Hansson L, Acosta J, et al: Controlled trial of enalapril and hydrochlorothiazide in 200 hypertensive patients. Am J Hypertens 1:38,1988
41. McVeigh G, Galloway D, Johnston D: The case for low dose diuretics in hypertension: Comparison of low and conventional doses of cyclopenthiazide. Br Med J 297:95,1988
42. Rose, p 430
43. Narins, p 562
44. Ibid, p 563
45. Rose, p 432
46. Narins, p 563
47. Ibid
48. Ibid, p 548
49. Ring-Larsen H, et al: Diuretic treatment in decompensated cirrhosis and congestive heart failure: Effect of posture. Br Med J 292:1351,1986
50. Szerlip, Goldfarb, p 15

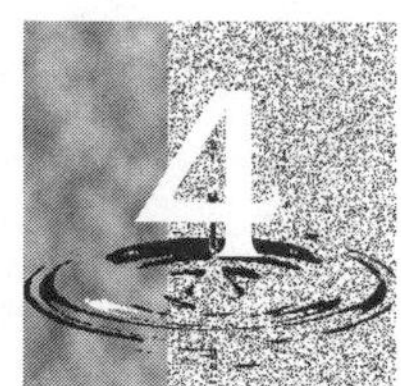

Sodium Imbalances

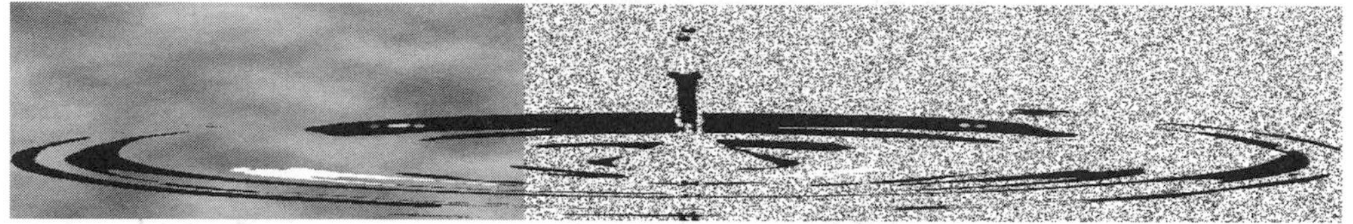

SODIUM BALANCE

Disturbances in sodium balance frequently occur in clinical practice and develop under circumstances varying from the simple to the complex. These imbalances and the nurse's role in their management are discussed in this chapter. First, however, some basic facts about the role of sodium in physiological activities are reviewed.

Sodium is the most plentiful electrolyte in the extracellular fluid (ECF), with a concentration ranging from 135 to 145 mEq/L. More than 95% of the body's physiologically active sodium is in the ECF. In contrast, the intracellular concentration of sodium is small. Maintenance of this asymmetric distribution across cell membranes requires transporting sodium out of the cell against an electrochemical gradient by the adenosine triphosphatase (ATPase) pump.

The fact that sodium does not easily cross the cell wall membrane, in addition to being the dominant electrolyte in quantity, accounts for its primary role in controlling water distribution as well as ECF volume. In general, a loss or gain of sodium is accompanied by a loss or gain of water.

Extracellular sodium concentration has a profound effect on body cells. That is, a low serum sodium level (*hyponatremia*) results in a relatively diluted ECF and allows water to be drawn into the cells. Conversely, a high serum sodium level (*hypernatremia*) results in a relatively concentrated ECF and allows water to be pulled out of cells (Fig. 4-1).

The salt intake per day in the healthy individual varies between 50 and 90 mEq (3–5 g) as sodium chloride.[1] More than this amount is readily available in the diet, in 1 L of lactated Ringer's solution or isotonic saline (0.9% NaCl), or in 2 L of half-strength saline (0.45% NaCl) (see Table 4-1). The sodium balance can be maintained in a healthy individual over a wide range of intakes because the normal kidney can conserve or excrete sodium as needed.[2]

HYPONATREMIA

DEFINITION

Hyponatremia refers to a serum sodium level that is below normal (<135 mEq/L). A low serum concentration does not necessarily mean that the total body sodium is less than normal. In fact, many patients have hyponatremia when there is an excess of total body sodium (as occurs with congestive heart failure or cirrhosis of the liver). When marked hyperlipidemia or hypoproteinemia is present, the serum sodium may appear to be lower than it actually is (pseudohyponatremia).[3] These artifactual readings are less problematic when plasma sodium is measured by ion-specific electrodes, which are now used in many hospital laboratories.[4]

Syndrome of inappropriate antidiuretic hormone secretion (SIADH) produces a special kind of hyponatremia that is associated with excessive water retention. In conditions producing SIADH, there is either too much antidiuretic hormone released or the renal response to the hormone is intensified. Release of antidiuretic hormone (ADH) is termed *inappropriate* because in normal situations a low serum sodium level would depress ADH activity.

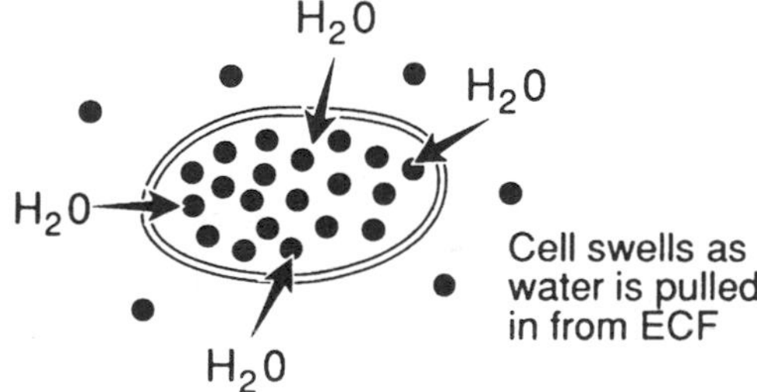

Hyponatremia:
Na less than 130 mEq/L

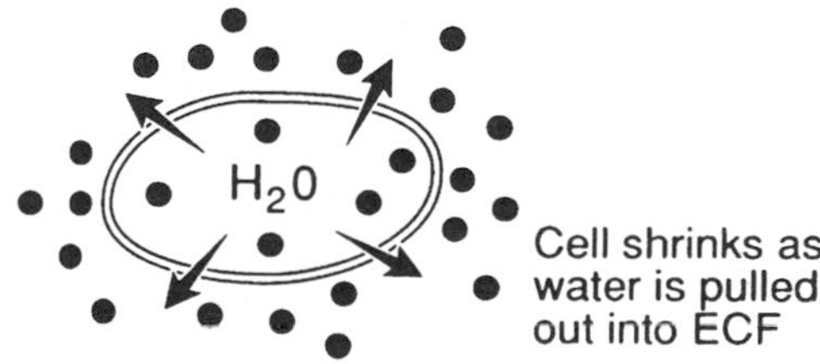

Hypernatremia:
Na greater than 150 mEq/L

Figure 4–1. Effect of extracellular sodium on cell size.

TABLE 4–1

Approximate Sodium Content of Selected Parenteral Fluids

PARENTERAL FLUID	SODIUM (mEq/L)
0.9% NaCl ("Isotonic saline")	154
0.45% NaCl (half-strength saline)	77
0.33% NaCl	56
0.22% NaCl	38
0.11 % NaCl	19
3% NaCl*	513
5% NaCl*	855
Lactated Ringer's solution	130

* Extremely hypertonic fluids.

PATHOPHYSIOLOGY

There are four basic ways in which hyponatremia may occur: (1) loss of sodium, as through the kidney, gastrointestinal (GI) tract, or skin; (2) gain of water, as in high ADH secretion; (3) shift of sodium into the cell, as may occur in potassium deficiency; and (4) shift of water from the cell to the ECF, as may occur in hyperglycemia or mannitol infusion.[5] A common imbalance, hyponatremia can range from mild to severe. When severe, it is often a marker of serious underlying disease. In addition, severe hyponatremia can itself cause major neurological damage and death. As noted in Figure 4-1, a decrease in the serum sodium concentration is expected to cause a shift of water from the ECF to the intracellular space, resulting in generalized cellular edema. Unlike other tissues, the brain's capacity to expand is limited by the bony cranium. Herniation of the brain stem has been found on autopsy in patients who died from severe acute hyponatremia.

As illustrated in Figure 4-2, hyponatremia can be superimposed on a normal fluid volume, on fluid volume deficit (FVD), or on fluid volume excess (FVE). Mechanisms accounting for hyponatremia coupled with ECF volume excess in patients with cirrhosis of the liver and cardiac failure are described in Chapters 21 and 16, respectively. The effect of hyperglycemia on the serum sodium level is discussed in Chapter 18. In general, note that hyperglycemia promotes an osmotic gradient that causes water to move out of the cells into the ECF, thereby diluting the serum sodium level. For every 100 mg/100 mL rise in plasma glucose, the osmotic water shift dilutes the plasma sodium concentration by 1.3 to 1.6 mEq/L.[6]

ETIOLOGICAL FACTORS

Etiological factors associated with hyponatremia are listed in Table 4-2 and are briefly described below.

Diuretics

Hyponatremia is a fairly common and usually mild complication of diuretic therapy. However, severe hyponatremia may develop at times. Diuretic-

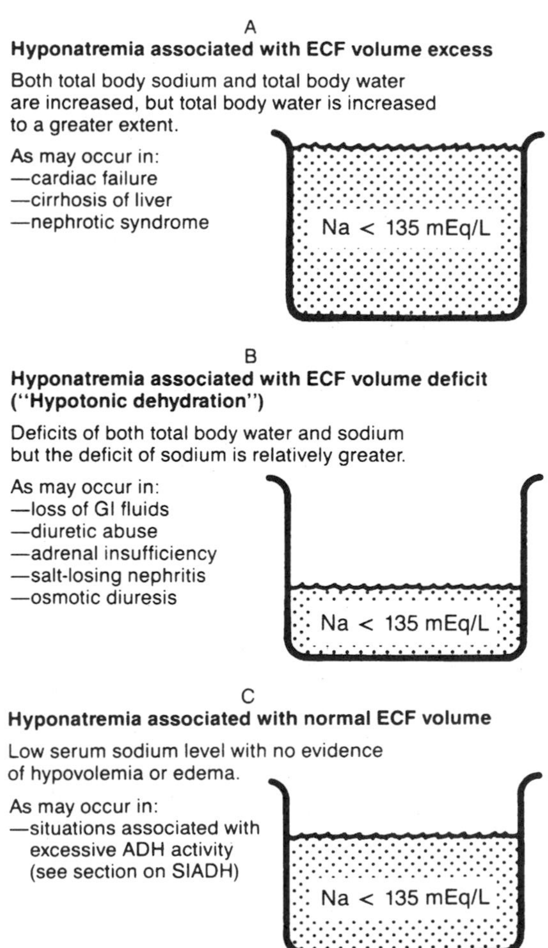

A
Hyponatremia associated with ECF volume excess
Both total body sodium and total body water are increased, but total body water is increased to a greater extent.
As may occur in:
—cardiac failure
—cirrhosis of liver
—nephrotic syndrome
Na < 135 mEq/L
B
Hyponatremia associated with ECF volume deficit ("Hypotonic dehydration")
Deficits of both total body water and sodium but the deficit of sodium is relatively greater.
As may occur in:
—loss of GI fluids
—diuretic abuse
—adrenal insufficiency
—salt-losing nephritis
—osmotic diuresis
Na < 135 mEq/L
C
Hyponatremia associated with normal ECF volume
Low serum sodium level with no evidence of hypovolemia or edema.
As may occur in:
—situations associated with excessive ADH activity (see section on SIADH)
Na < 135 mEq/L

Figure 4–2. Hyponatremic states.

TABLE 4–2

Etiological Factors Associated with Hyponatremia

Loss of sodium

- Use of thiazide diuretics, particularly in combination with low-salt diet, vomiting, diarrhea, or sweating
- Adrenal insufficiency
- Gastrointestinal fluid losses, coupled with excessive water replacement
- Heavy sweating, coupled with excessive water intake
- Salt-losing nephritis

Water gains

- Use of drugs predisposing to SIADH
  - — Intravenous cyclophosphamide (Cytoxan)
  - — Vincristine (Oncovin)
  - — Chlorpropamide (Diabenese)
  - — Tolbutamide (Orinase)
  - — Carbamazepine (Tegretol)
  - — Amitriptyline (Elavil)
  - — Haloperidol (Haldol)
  - — Thioridazine (Mellaril)
  - — Nonsteroidal antiinflammatory drugs
- Presence of tumors predisposing to SIADH
  - — Oat-cell carcinoma of lung
  - — Tumors of pancreas and duodenum
  - — Leukemia
  - — Hodgkin's disease
- Presence of central nervous system disorders predisposing to SIADH
  - — Head injury
  - — Encephalitis
  - — Brain tumor
- Pulmonary disorders
  - — Tuberculosis
  - — Pneumonia
  - — Asthma
  - — Acute respiratory failure
- Release of vasopressin after anesthesia and surgery
- Labor induction with oxytocin
- Irrigation of prostatic bed during transurethral prostatectomy
- Psychotic polydipsia
- Acquired immunodeficiency syndrome (related to multisystem morbidity)
- Excessive administration of dextrose and water solutions (such as 5% dextrose in water), particularly postoperatively

induced severe hyponatremia is primarily a complication of thiazide-type drugs, and most often affects women of small body size who are greater than 60 years of age.[7] In a study of 64 subjects admitted to hospitals for treatment of hyponatremia, it was found that thiazides were either the only cause or a major contributing factor to more than half of the cases of hyponatremia.[8]

Adrenal Insufficiency

Hyponatremia is a common complication of adrenal insufficiency and is due to the effects of aldosterone and cortisol deficiencies. Lack of aldosterone increases renal sodium loss, and cortisol deficiency is associated with increased release of ADH (causing water retention).

Gastrointestinal Fluid Losses

Gastric fluid loss by vomiting or gastric suction can predispose to hyponatremia by the direct loss of sodium. Gains of water (as occurs in the presence of nausea) can further dilute the serum sodium level. Nausea predisposes to water retention and as a result hyponatremia, because it is a potent stimulus for the release of ADH. Despite this effect, however, hyponatremia is not likely to be severe without the intake of free water. When vomiting occurs at home, most patients greatly curtail oral intake and volume depletion usually occurs. In contrast, some vomiting patients may continue to drink while vomiting repeatedly and manage to absorb enough ingested water to develop hyponatremia while maintaining a near-normal plasma volume.[9] In the hospital setting, the erroneous administration of excessive electrolyte-free solutions (such as 5% dextrose in water) can seriously dilute the serum sodium concentration.

Loss of intestinal fluid by diarrhea can also result in an isotonic FVD, leaving the serum sodium within a normal range. The volume depletion induced by diarrhea can also serve as a stimulus for ADH release, leading to renal water retention and hyponatremia. The amount of oral or intravenous (IV) free-water intake frequently determines the severity of hyponatremia. At times, water loss through diarrhea can exceed sodium loss, leading to hypernatremia.

Sweating

Sweat is a hypotonic fluid with a sodium concentration of approximately 30 to 50 mEq/L.[10] Although sweat production is low in the basal state, it may exceed 1 to 2 L/hr in subjects exercising in a dry, hot climate.[11] Hyponatremia can occur when large volumes of sweat are lost and replaced only with water.

Salt-Losing Nephritis

Different kidney conditions can result in renal salt wasting. Among these are chronic interstitial nephropathy, medullary cystic disease, and polycystic kidney disease.[12] The degree of renal sodium wasting can range from mild to severe.

Drugs Predisposing to SIADH

Several drugs (Table 4-2) can impair renal water excretion, thus causing a form of hyponatremia sometimes referred to as SIADH. Some of the major drugs are discussed below.

Chlorpropamide, an oral hypoglycemic agent, can induce SIADH by potentiating the effect of ADH on the kidney.[13] One study reported that 4% of patients in a clinical population receiving chlorpropamide were hyponatremic (suggesting excessive ADH effect).[14] This problem is most likely to occur in patients older than 60 years of age who are also taking a thiazide diuretic.[15]

Cyclophosphamide is an antineoplastic alkylating agent that can increase renal sensitivity to ADH and perhaps its release when given IV in high doses. Because a high fluid intake is generally prescribed to lessen the possibility of hemorrhagic cystitis, severe hyponatremia can result. Use of isotonic saline rather than water to maintain a high urine output can minimize this complication.[16] Vincristine is another antineoplastic drug that can cause hyponatremia, apparently by a neurotoxic effect on the hypothalamus.[17]

Carbamazepine, used as an anticonvulsant, can cause hyponatremia by inducing the release of ADH. Apparently, the hyponatremia caused by this drug is dose-related. Hyponatremia associated with carbamazepine use is particularly common in psychiatric institutions among patients with polydipsia.[18]

Nonsteroidal antiinflammatory drugs (NSAID) decrease renal water excretion because decreased synthesis of prostaglandins potentiates the action of ADH on the kidney. Despite this effect, hyponatremia due solely to these agents is uncommon.[19] Instead, NSAIDs tend to exacerbate the tendency toward hyponatremia in patients with other causes of SIADH.

Tumors Predisposing to SIADH

Probably the most frequent cause of SIADH is oat-cell carcinoma of the lung. Other malignancies associated with this syndrome include carcinomas of the duodenum and pancreas, Hodgkin's disease, leukemia, and lymphoma. In some instances, malignant cells from patients with SIADH have been shown to synthesize and release a substance similar to native ADH ("ectopic ADH production"). In Chapter 22 SIADH in oncology patients is discussed further.

Central Nervous System Disorders Associated With SIADH

Among the central nervous system (CNS) conditions that may be associated with SIADH are psychosis, trauma, neoplasms, and vascular and infectious disorders.[20] For this reason, patients whose symptoms do not improve during correction of the low serum sodium level should be evaluated for CNS pathology.[21] The hyponatremia associated with subarachnoid hemorrhage may not always be caused by inappropriate release of ADH[22]; see Chapter 19 for a more thorough discussion of this topic.

Psychiatric Factors Associated With Hyponatremia

Excessive water intake is relatively common in psychiatric patients and can occasionally cause severe symptomatic hyponatremia. This syndrome is also referred to as "compulsive water drinking" or "self-induced water intoxication." The syndrome of psychosis, intermittent hyponatremia, and polydipsia is a potentially life-threatening problem occurring in approximately 7% of chronically ill psychiatric patients, most of whom are diagnosed with schizophrenia.[23] This dilutional hyponatremia is thought to occur when the rapid ingestion of voluminous quantities of water exceeds the excretory capacity of normally functioning kidneys. Because some of these patients appear to have an increased appetite for salt, they have been observed to self-medicate with table salt.[24]

Hyponatremia in psychiatric patients has been attributed to selected medications used to treat psychoses. For example, carbamazepine is a well-established cause of vasopressin release. (Vasopressin favors water retention.) It has been suggested that patients who smoke may be more likely to be symptomatic because nicotine contributes to transient release of vasopressin, as may the psychosis itself.[25] In a recently reported study of 15 psychiatric patients with severe hyponatremia, all were heavy smokers.[26]

Labor Induction With Oxytocin

Oxytocin, like vasopressin (ADH), is synthesized in the hypothalamus and released by the pituitary gland. Although its primary effects are on uterine function and milk production, it also possesses significant antidiuretic activity. Administration of oxytocin to induce labor, therefore, can cause hyponatremia if improperly used.

In the past, little attention was paid to the water-retentive capacity of oxytocin, and excessive fluid (usually in the form of 5% dextrose in water) was sometimes administered. Severe hyponatremia has developed in some cases after the infusion of less than 3 L of fluid.[27] Intravenous administration of oxytocin in dextrose and water to stimulate labor has resulted in water retention, severe hyponatremia, and seizures in both the mother and the fetus.[28] Safe guidelines for oxytocin administration are discussed in Chapter 23.

Postoperative Hyponatremia

In a recent study of 1088 postoperative patients, Chung et al.[29] reported a 4.4% incidence of hyponatremia (serum $Na^+ < 130$ mEq/L) within 1 week after surgery. Predisposing factors included a temporary increase in vasopressin release after anesthesia and the stress of surgery. Pain enhances the release of vasopressin by direct stimulation of the hypothalamus. Nausea, which is frequently present in postoperative patients, can increase aqueous vasopressin (AVP) release by as much as 1000-fold; the nausea does not have to be associated with vomiting.[30] Because of the tendency for hyponatremia in new postoperative patients, the excessive administration of electrolyte-free solutions during the first 2 to 4 postoperative days should be avoided. In fact, because elevated plasma levels of vasopressin are essentially a universal postoperative occurrence in the first few postoperative days, some researchers state that it may be important to avoid the use of any hypotonic intravenous solution in the immediate postoperative period.[31]

Postoperative Hyponatremia in Menstruant Women

Postoperative hyponatremia is apparently a much more serious problem in menstruant women than in postmenopausal women or men. A recent report has indicated that although women and men are equally likely to develop hyponatremia and hyponatremic encephalopathy after surgery, menstruant women are about 25 times more likely to die or have permanent brain damage (compared with either men or postmenopausal women) if this condition develops.[32] The significantly higher mortality from postoperative hyponatremia in menstruant women may be due, at least in part, to physical factors that affect the ability of the brain to adapt to hyponatremia. Deaths have occurred in young women who have undergone relatively simple surgical procedures, such as endometrial ablation (a relatively new procedure in which the lining of the uterus is ablated by a laser or similar device while an irrigating solution is usually continuously infused into the uterine cavity to facilitate surgical visualization and wash away operative debris) or other elective gynecologic procedures.[33,34] Symptoms that should cause concern in these individuals include nausea and vomiting, headache, and other variable signs. In a study of 40 young women with hyponatremic encephalopathy, all experienced nausea and vomiting, 34 had headache, and some had other symptoms, including weakness, slurred speech, lethargy, confusion, disorientation, bizarre behavior, urinary incontinence, dyspnea, and decorticate posturing. Of the 40 women, 36 sustained an abrupt respiratory arrest postoperatively; at the time of respiratory arrest, the mean plasma sodium level was

113 ± 1 mmol/L (range, 91–128 mmol/L).[35] In summary, it is important to prevent this serious complication by avoiding the excessive use of electrolyte-free or hypotonic fluids in the immediate postoperative period. It is also important to detect developing hyponatremia and institute corrective measures before respiratory insufficiency occurs. Although early symptoms are somewhat nonspecific, the diagnosis can be easily established by measuring the plasma sodium level with virtually no risk to the patient and at minimal cost.[36]

Pulmonary Disorders

Pulmonary disorders associated with SIADH include pneumonia, acute asthma, tuberculosis, acute respiratory failure, pneumothorax, and empyema.[37] The causes are not entirely clear, although increased production of AVP has been suggested. For example, mechanical ventilation, especially when combined with positive expiratory pressure, stimulates AVP release by impeding venous return, thus decreasing cardiac output.[38] Acute hypoxia and hypercapnia also stimulate AVP secretion.[39] Bioassays from tuberculous lung tissue have demonstrated ADH activity.[40]

Postprostatectomy Via Transurethral Resection

During transurethral resection of the prostate (TURP), the urologist must irrigate the prostatic bed with an electrolyte-free solution. If the procedure is prolonged or if the irrigating solution is introduced under pressure, large volumes of the fluid may be absorbed into the circulation. Thus, the fundamental pathology in the TURP syndrome is volume overload and dilutional hyponatremia.[41] In the past, distilled water was used but has been replaced by solutions containing isotonic or slightly hypotonic glycine, mannitol, or sorbitol.[42] Nonetheless, serum sodium concentration can still be lowered by the irrigating solution. Specific side effects vary with the type of irrigant. Profound hyponatremia and a variety of other adverse neurologic and cardiovascular events are reported to follow TURP in 1% to 7% of the cases.[43] The reader is referred to Chapter 14 for further discussion of the TURP syndrome.

Acquired Immunodeficiency Syndrome

Hyponatremia is very common in patients with acquired immunodeficiency syndrome (AIDS).[44] For example, Vitting et al.[45] reported that 56% of the AIDS patients followed prospectively in their study were hyponatremic (mean serum sodium level, 126 ± 4 mEq/L). In another study, Agarwal et al.[46] found that approximately 35% of 103 patients with AIDS admitted for opportunistic infections had serum sodium levels lower than or equal to 130 mEq/L. Although in some patients adrenal insufficiency and volume depletion (as from emesis and/or diarrhea) are responsible for hyponatremia, most patients appear to have SIADH. Conditions that may play a role in hyponatremia are *Pneumocystis carinii* pneumonia, malignancies, and CNS disease.[47] Of course, hyponatremic states are aggravated by the excessive use of hypotonic fluids.

DEFINING CHARACTERISTICS

The defining characteristics of hyponatremia depend on its magnitude, rapidity of onset, and cause. In general, the lower the serum sodium level, the more likely symptoms are to be severe (see Table 4-3). Another major factor is the rapidity of onset. For example, two patients having similar low serum sodium values may have greatly different symptoms if hyponatremia developed slowly in one and quickly in the other. In acute hyponatremia, symptoms develop at a higher rate than they do when hyponatremia is chronic; in the latter case, symptoms may not become evident until the serum sodium is quite low (eg, 110 mEq/L). Severity of symptoms may also vary with the cause. For example, acute water overloading is more likely to cause severe symptoms than is the chronic loss of sodium.

Hyponatremia causes cell hypo-osmolality, which in turn causes all of the clinical manifestations of hyponatremia.[49] Recall that cellular swelling occurs in hyponatremia as the relatively dilute ECF is pulled into the cells. Placing a firm finger pressure over a bony prominence and observing for a fingerprint in the skin is a simple test sometimes done to demonstrate intracellular water excess.[50] Early manifestations of hyponatremia include those involving the GI system, such as nausea and abdominal cramps. However, most of the major manifes-

TABLE 4–3

Clinical Manifestations of Hyponatremia

Rapidity of Drop in Serum Sodium Concentration

Rapidity of development of hyponatremia has a major effect on symptom development. Slowly developing hyponatremia is better tolerated than is acutely developing hyponatremia. For example, patients with chronic hyponatremia may have few if any symptoms with serum sodium levels as low as 115 mEq/L.

Severity of Drop in Serum Sodium Concentration

Patients are often asymptomatic when the serum sodium level is >125 mEq/L. However, when the sodium falls acutely to <125 mEq/L, the following symptoms may occur[48]:

120–125 mEq/L
Nausea
Malaise

115–120 mEq/L
Headache
Lethargy
Obtundation

<110–115 mEq/L
Seizures
Coma

Because there is significant variability in patients, the figures are not necessarily precise. For example, women of childbearing age tend to be at much greater risk of developing severe neurologic symptoms than men or postmenopausal women (presumably because of the effect of female hormones on the ability of the brain to adapt to osmotic changes). There are cases on record in which respiratory arrest has occurred in young women with serum sodium levels at or above 125 mEq/L after acute water overloading in the early postoperative period.

Volume Status

Hyponatremia coupled with ECF volume depletion may produce added symptoms of weakness, fatigue, muscle cramps, and postural dizziness.

Hyponatremia due to SIADH does not produce significant peripheral edema (although water retention has occurred) because about two thirds of the retained water is located inside the cells.

Laboratory Data

By definition, serum sodium level is <135 mEq/L.

Urinary sodium <15 mEq/L indicates renal conservation of sodium and that loss of sodium is from a nonrenal route.

Urinary sodium >20 mEq/L in SIADH

tations of hyponatremia are of a neuropsychiatric nature and are related to cellular swelling. Because the swollen brain has limited room for expansion within the skull, cerebral edema becomes a potentially lethal problem. Brain edema may be so severe that transtentorial herniation (heralded by respiratory arrest) occurs. In general, patients having acute decreases in serum sodium levels have higher mortality rates than do those with more slowly developing hyponatremia. Hyponatremia can reasonably be said to be acute when the serum sodium has fallen by more than 12 mmol/L/day and has been low for less than 48 hrs.[51] Deaths and severe sequelae most commonly occur when the serum sodium level falls below 120 mmol/L and falls by more than 0.5 mmol/L/hr; the complications become even more common when the sodium level drops by more than 1 mmol/L/hr.[52]

Age and Gender Differences

There is a substantial interpatient difference in the susceptibility to symptoms from acute hyponatremia.[53] Perhaps because of differences in cerebral metabolism, women (especially premenopausal women) seem to be at substantially greater risk than men of developing severe neurologic symptoms and irreversible brain damage. It is possible that sex hormones are responsible for this difference as there is no gender difference in the risk of symptomatic hyponatremia in prepubertal children.[54] As described earlier, young women account for most of the reported cases of fatalities secondary to hyponatremia, presumably because their brains are less able to adapt to the effects of hyponatremia than are those of men or postmenopausal women. Because SIADH presents a unique set of circumstances, the clinical manifestations of this disorder are spelled out in Table 4-4.

TABLE 4–4

Clinical Manifestations of SIADH

Water retention

- Intake of fluid greatly exceeds urinary output (as evidenced by I&O records)
- Weight gain (reflecting water retention)
- No significant peripheral edema (water is primarily retained inside the cells, not the interstitium)
- Fingerprint edema over sternum (reflecting cellular edema)
- Signs of cerebral edema (see neurological symptoms below)

Gastrointestinal symptoms

- Anorexia
- Nausea
- Vomiting
- Abdominal cramps

Neurological symptoms

- Lethargy
- Headaches
- Personality changes
- Seizures
- Pupillary changes
- Coma

Laboratory findings

- Hyponatremia
  - — Symptoms usually do not appear unless serum sodium level is <125 mEq/L
  - — Plasma osmolality below normal (reflecting low serum sodium level)
- Low BUN and creatinine
  - — Reflecting state of overhydration
- Urinary signs
  - — Urinary sodium > 20 mEq/L (As opposed to hyponatremia due primarily to sodium loss, where much lower sodium levels are expected due to renal conservation of the needed cation.)
  - — Urinary SG >1.012
  - — Urine osmolality is usually higher than plasma osmolality (urine contains important amounts of sodium and plasma is diluted with water)

SG, specific gravity; SIADH, syndrome of inappropriate antidiuretic hormone secretion.

TREATMENT

The obvious treatment for hyponatremia due to sodium loss is sodium replacement. This may be accomplished orally, by nasogastric tube, or by the parenteral route. For patients able to eat and drink, replacement is easily accomplished because sodium is plentiful in a normal diet. For those unable to take sodium orally or by gastric tube, the parenteral route is necessary. If the plasma volume is below normal, lactated Ringer's solution or isotonic saline (0.9% NaCl) may be prescribed. In the symptomatic patient with normal or excessive plasma volume, it may be necessary to cautiously administer a small volume of 3% or 5% NaCl (extremely dangerous fluids when used incorrectly). (The sodium content of some parenteral fluids is listed in Table 4-1.) In normovolemic patients with chronic asymptomatic hyponatremia, water restriction is generally recommended. If water restriction is unsuccessful in treating chronic hyponatremia, attempts may be made to increase water excretion. This may be achieved by using medications that interfere with urine concentration (such as demeclocycline or lithium). Even more effective is the administration of a loop diuretic (such as furosemide) in conjunction with increased sodium and potassium intake.[55]

Rate of Sodium Replacement in Hyponatremia

The recommended speed and method of treatment of hyponatremia depend on the magnitude of symptoms, how long they have been present, and the status of the ECF volume. The goal of therapy in symptomatic hyponatremia is to reduce brain water and increase the plasma sodium level only to the point necessary to maintain normal respiration and keep the patient seizure-free and alert,[56] and at the same time prevent osmotic demyelination.

Too rapid a correction of hyponatremia, particularly when it has been present more than 48 hrs, can result in an extremely serious condition referred to "osmotic demyelination" or "central pontine myelinolysis." In this situation, it is thought that the rising serum sodium level causes water to be drawn from the brain across the blood–brain barrier, resulting in brain dehydration and injury.

There is disagreement as to what constitutes "too rapid" a correction of hyponatremia. Patients reported to be at greatest risk for osmotic demyelination associated with rapid sodium replacement have been hyponatremic for more than 48 hrs, usually with very low serum sodium concentrations (≤110 mmol/L).[57] In most reported cases, correction of the hyponatremia has exceeded 12 mmol/L during any 24-hr period.[58]

Ayus and Arieff[59] argue that the judicious rapid correction of acute hyponatremia (that developing within 24–48 hrs) is warranted to prevent seizures, cerebral herniation, respiratory arrest, and death.[60] They caution, however, that too rapid correction (defined as >25 mEq/L during the first 48 hrs of treatment) may result in cerebral demyelination.[61]

It appears that a definitive recommendation for the treatment of severe hyponatremia cannot be made with certainty.[62] Rose[63] states that it seems advisable to raise the plasma sodium concentration in asymptomatic patients at a maximum average rate of 0.5 mEq/L/hr or 12 mEq/L/day. In contrast, for patients who already have severe neurologic symptoms associated with hyponatremia, the risk of untreated hyponatremia and associated cerebral edema is greater than the potential harm of too rapid correction. In this situation, Rose states that hypertonic saline should be given to elevate the serum sodium level more quickly (1.5–2 mEq/L/hr for 3–4 hrs or until the severe neurologic symptoms abate); even then, the elevation in the plasma sodium concentration should not exceed 12 to 15 mEq/L/day.[64]

Syndrome of Inappropriate Antidiuretic Hormone Secretion

If the problem is SIADH, treatment is directed at eliminating the underlying cause if possible (eg, radiation therapy for a tumor secreting ectopic ADH-like substances, or discontinuing a drug that increases ADH secretion). If this is not possible, alleviation of water overload by fluid restriction is indicated. Fluid is restricted to the extent that urinary and insensible losses induce a negative water balance (ie, fluid loss exceeds intake). Laboratory values and clinical status are used as guides for fluid restriction. The most important parameters are serum and urine electrolytes and osmolality, fluid intake and output, and body weight records.

For patients with mild hyponatremia, fluid restriction may be all that is needed. More severe cases may require the IV administration of a small amount of hypertonic saline (3% or 5% NaCl), in addition to fluid restriction, to provide sodium in a minimal fluid volume. Furosemide is often used in conjunction with hypertonic saline to promote water excretion and decrease the risk of FVE and its dangerous sequelae (such as pulmonary edema). Use of hypertonic saline alone elevates the serum sodium level only transiently because most of the administered sodium is rapidly lost in the urine. In contrast, furosemide causes loss of both water and sodium; but when the sodium is given back as hypertonic saline, the result is a net removal of water.[65]

If the underlying cause of SIADH is chronic, as in patients with inoperable tumors producing ectopic ADH, other therapeutic measures must be considered. Although the mainstay of therapy in this setting is water restriction, it is not well tolerated by some patients over a prolonged period. For such patients, the administration of a variety of medications has been recommended. Among these are loop diuretics in conjunction with increased salt intake, or other medications such as urea, demeclocycline, and lithium. In some patients, loop diuretics (such as furosemide) have been administered concomitantly with salt tablets to increase the serum sodium level when SIADH is present. Other patients have been placed on a high-salt, high-protein diet (the unused protein is excreted as urea) to increase renal solute load and thus increase urinary output.[66] Urea can also be given as a medication, usually in a dose ranging from 30 to 60 g/day.[67] Possible drawbacks to the use of urea are unpalatability and some GI discomfort. Demeclocycline and lithium carbonate are medications that block the action of ADH on the renal collecting duct, thereby causing increased urinary output (nephrogenic diabetes insipidus). Lithium's side effects limit its usefulness. In contrast, demeclocycline in a dose of 600 to 1200 mg/day is usually well tolerated.[68] However, it has several disadvantages, including nephrotoxicity when hepatic function is impaired, delayed onset of action for several days, and persistent effect for several days after treatment has been discontinued.[69] The choice of agents in chronic SIADH depends partly on the urine osmolality of the individual patient.[70]

NURSING INTERVENTIONS

1. Identify patients at risk for hyponatremia. As noted in Table 4-2, many common conditions can lower the serum sodium concentration.
   - Being aware of patients at risk for hyponatremia is crucial to monitoring for the occurrence of subtle early changes associated with this imbalance. As explained earlier in the chapter, a profound hyponatremia can be fatal if not detected early and treated appropriately.
2. Review medications the patient is receiving, noting those that predispose to hyponatremia (such as thiazides or the drugs listed in Table 4-2 associated with SIADH).
3. Monitor fluid losses and gains for all patients at risk for hyponatremia. Look for loss of sodium-containing fluids (such as GI secretions or sweat), particularly in conjunction with a low-sodium diet or excessive water intake either orally or IV.
4. Monitor laboratory data for serum sodium levels lower than normal.
5. Monitor for presence of GI symptoms, such as anorexia, nausea, vomiting, and abdominal cramping, as these may be early signs of hyponatremia. Of course, these symptoms must be evaluated in relation to other findings, such as fluid gains and losses, amount of sodium intake, and laboratory data.
6. Monitor for CNS changes, such as lethargy, confusion, muscular twitching, convulsions, and coma. Be aware that more severe neurological signs are associated with very low sodium levels that have fallen rapidly due to water overloading.
7. For patients able to consume a normal diet, encourage foods and fluids with a high sodium content. For example, broth made with one beef cube contains approximately 900 mg (39 mEq) of sodium; 8 oz of canned tomato juice contains approximately 700 mg (30 mEq) of sodium.[71] Sodium content of additional fluids can be found in Table 3-1.
8. When administering sodium-containing IV fluids to patients with cardiovascular disease, monitor especially closely for signs of circulatory overload. These include moist rales in the lungs (the greater the sodium concentration, the greater the risk). Sodium content of some of the major IV fluids is listed in Table 4-1.
9. Avoid giving large water supplements to patients receiving isotonic tube feedings, particularly if routes of abnormal sodium loss are present or water is being retained abnormally (as in SIADH) (see Chapter 12).
10. Use extreme caution when administering hypertonic saline solutions (3% or 5% NaCl). Be aware that these fluids can be lethal if infused carelessly (see Clinical Tip: Nursing Considerations in Administration of Hypertonic Saline Solutions).
11. Be aware of the effect a low serum sodium level can have on patients receiving lithium. A low serum sodium level causes a relative increase in lithium retention and predisposes to toxicity. Because of this, decreased tolerance to lithium occurs in patients with protracted sweating and diarrhea. In such instances, supplemental salt and fluid should be administered. Because diuretics promote sodium loss, patients taking lithium should not use diuretics unless they are under close medical supervision. For all patients on lithium therapy, an adequate salt intake should be assured. The patient's food intake should be checked and the physician informed of anorexia. (Seek a dietary consultation if indicated.)
12. To avoid serious sodium deficiency, instruct patients with adrenal insufficiency to do the following:
    - Take steroid-replacement medications as prescribed.
    - Keep several days' dosage on their person when traveling.

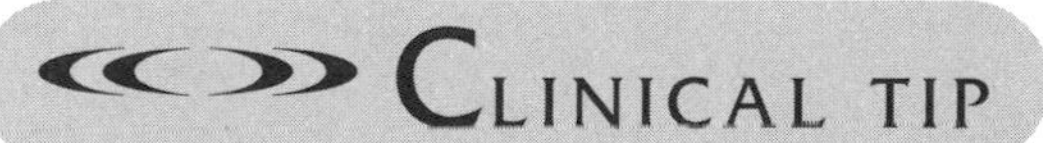

Nursing Considerations in Administration of Hypertonic Saline Solutions (3% and 5% NaCl)

Check the serum sodium level before administering these solutions and frequently thereafter

Administer these solutions only in settings where the patient can be closely monitored:

Watch for signs of pulmonary edema and worsening of neurological signs. (Furosemide may be prescribed to promote water loss and prevent pulmonary edema.)

Use a volume-controlled apparatus to administer the fluid; maintain close vigilance on the device as none is foolproof

Be aware that a definitive recommendation for the treatment of severe hyponatremia cannot be made with certainty. However, consider that factors affecting the rate of administration include (1) length of time the hyponatremia has been present, and (2) severity of symptoms.

For example, sodium replacement should occur more slowly in patients who have had hyponatremia for greater than 48 hrs (as opposed to <48 hrs); this is because these individuals are at increased risk for osmotic demyelination (also referred to as central pontine myelinolysis).

It appears that sodium replacement should occur more rapidly in patients with severe neurological symptoms and *acute* hyponatremia (hyponatremia present for <48 hours); this is because the risk of untreated hyponatremia and associated cerebral edema is greater than the potential harm of too rapid correction of the plasma sodium level.[72]

It seems advisable to raise the plasma sodium concentration in *asymptomatic* hyponatremic patients at a maximum rate of 0.5 mEq/L/hr or 12 mEq/L/day.[73]

According to Ayus and Arieff,[74] the judicious rapid correction of *acute* hyponatremia (that developing within 24 to 48 hours) is warranted to prevent seizures, cerebral herniation, respiratory arrest, and death. They caution, however, that too rapid correction (defined as more than 25 mEq/L during the first 48 hours of treatment) may result in cerebral demyelination.

According to Rose,[75] for patients who have severe neurological symptoms, hypertonic saline should be given to elevate the serum sodium level by 1.5 to 2 mEq/L/hour for 3 to 4 hours or until the severe neurological symptoms abate; even then, however, the elevation in the plasma sodium concentration should not exceed 12 to 15 mEq/L/day.

- Wear an identification bracelet stating need for steroids in case of emergency.
- Seek consultation with a health-care provider in times of excessive stress.
- Monitor their weight and fluid intake and output (I&O) changes and report significant findings to the health care provider.
- Increase dietary salt intake as indicated during presence of excessive sweating or diarrhea (or other causes of sodium loss).

13. Monitor patients with decreased adrenal function for signs of acute adrenocortical insufficiency (adrenal crisis) when they are exposed to severe stress (such as surgery, trauma, emotional upset, excessive heat, or prolonged medical illness). Look for extreme weakness, acute onset of nausea and vomiting, hypotension, confusion, and even shock.

Because SIADH requires special nursing management, an assessment for this condition is provided in Table 4-5 and nursing interventions during therapy for SIADH are described in Table 4-6. Recovery from this dilutional state is usually rapid if the condition is recognized early and appropriate measures are initiated. The nurse plays a vital role in preventing serious consequences of this disorder.

TABLE 4–5

Nursing Assessment for SIADH

1. Identify patients at risk (see Table 4-2).
2. Maintain accurate I&O.
   - Look for fluid intake greatly exceeding output; I&O should be totaled and the overall picture observed for several consecutive days.
3. Maintain daily body weight records.
   - Look for sudden weight gain (recall that 1 L of fluid weighs approximately 2.2 lb).
   - Although there will be an acute weight gain, do not expect to detect significant peripheral edema because most (approximately two thirds) of the excess fluid will be retained inside the cells, not in the interstitial space.
4. Monitor serum sodium concentrations.
5. Observe for gastrointestinal symptoms, which usually occur early.
   - Be alert for anorexia, nausea, vomiting, and abdominal cramping.
6. Observe the neurologic status carefully.
   - Be particularly alert for personality changes, headache, lethargy, seizures, and coma.

TABLE 4–6

Nursing Interventions Related to Therapy for SIADH

1. Restrict fluids to the prescribed level.
   - Consider all routes of intake (eg, oral fluids, "keep-open" IV, piggyback medications).
   - Gain the patient's cooperation, if he or she is rational, by explaining the need for fluid restriction.
   - Place "fluid restriction" signs at the bedside.
   - Remove the water pitcher.
   - Explain the need for fluid restriction to visitors.
   - Space the allotted fluid allowance over the 24-hour period.
   - Minimize the risk of accidental overadministration of IV fluids by using a volume-controlled device.
2. Maintain an accurate I&O record and study its pattern.
   - A greater urinary output than fluid intake is desired because it indicates a negative water balance. (Remember, the excessive water load must be excreted before significant improvement occurs.)
3. Maintain an accurate body-weight record.
   - With proper therapy, expect to see an acute decline in body weight due to excretion of excess water. Recall that a liter of fluid is equivalent to 2.2 lb; for example, a weight loss of 6.6 lb over a period of 1 to 2 days indicates a loss of approximately 3 L.
4. Assess neurologic signs.
   - With appropriate therapy, an increased level of consciousness and increased muscle strength is hoped for. Unfortunately, neurological damage induced by SIADH is not always reversible, particularly if treatment is delayed.
5. Initiate safety precautions.
   - Elevate siderails for the patient with a decreased level of consciousness; be prepared for seizure activity; modify other aspects of the patient's environment as indicated.
6. Monitor serum sodium levels.
   - With appropriate therapy, the sodium concentration should elevate slowly toward normal. It is important that the correction not take place too rapidly.
7. Administer hypertonic saline, when prescribed, with great caution.
   - Review the facts regarding administration of hypertonic saline (Clinical Tip, p 75).

SIADH, syndrome of inappropriate antidiuretic hormone secretion.

Nursing interventions related to SIADH in part involve monitoring to detect the disturbance before it becomes severe, and to determine if the response to therapeutic interventions is adequate. Change interventions involve restricting fluids (step 1 in Table 4-6) and initiating safety precautions when indicated (step 5 in Table 4-6) (see Summary of Hyponatremia).

Summary of Hyponatremia

ETIOLOGICAL FACTORS	DEFINING CHARACTERISTICS
Loss of sodium • Use of diuretics • Loss of GI fluids • Adrenal insufficiency • Osmotic diuresis • Salt-losing nephritis *Gains of water* • Excessive administration of D_5W • Psychogenic polydipsia • Excessive water administration with isotonic or hypotonic tube feedings *Disease states associated with SIADH* • Oat-cell carcinoma of lung • Carcinoma of duodenum or pancreas • Head trauma • Stroke • Pulmonary disorders (tuberculosis, pneumonia, asthma, respiratory failure) *Pharmacologic agents that may impair renal water excretion* • Chlorpropamide (Diabenese) • Cyclophosphamide (Cytoxan) • Vincristine (Oncovin) • Thioridazine (Mellaril) • Fluphenazine (Prolixin) • Carbamazepine (Tegretol) • Oxytocin (Pitocin)	Anorexia Nausea Vomiting Lethargy Confusion Muscular twitching Seizures Coma Respiratory arrest Serum Na <135 mEq/L Serum osmolality <285 mOsm/kg Urinary Na level varies with cause of hyponatremia

CASE STUDIES

4-1. A 50-year-old man was started on hydrochlorothiazide and a low-sodium diet for the treatment of hypertension. After 2 weeks, he began to complain of weakness, abdominal cramping, leg cramps, and postural dizziness. On examination he was found to have decreased skin turgor and flat neck veins in the supine position. Laboratory data included the following:

Na = 118 mEq/L
K = 2.2 mEq/L
Cl = 66 mEq/L
Plasma osmolality = 240 mOsm/kg

COMMENTARY: This patient was obviously hyponatremic, as indicated by the low plasma sodium level and osmolality. In this instance, the hyponatremia was accompanied by decreased fluid volume (as evidenced by the decreased skin turgor and flat neck veins). In addition, the plasma potassium and chloride levels were quite low. Thiazide diuretics promote both sodium and potassium excretion and predispose to hypochloremic alkalosis (metabolic alkalosis). Sodium loss, coupled with a low sodium intake, caused hyponatremia.

4-2. A 40-year-old man with polycystic kidney disease developed nausea, vomiting, and diarrhea. He stopped eating but drank large quantities of water. Over a period of 4 days, he developed progressive lethargy and had a grand mal seizure. Laboratory data included:

Na = 108 mEq/L
Cl = 72 mEq/L
BUN = 142 mg/dL
Creatinine = 12 mg/dL

COMMENTARY: This patient lost sodium through vomiting and diarrhea and replaced only water. He continued to lose sodium through the kidneys because of his renal disease. The neurological symptoms were due to dilution of the already low serum sodium level by excessive water intake, resulting in brain swelling.

4-3. A 58-year-old man with a history of inoperable oat-cell carcinoma of the lung was admitted to the hospital; according to his family, he had a 2-week history of progressive lethargy. Laboratory data included the following:

Plasma Na = 105 mEq/L
Urinary Na = 76 mEq/L
Cl = 72 mEq/L
Urinary osmolality = 800 mOsm/kg

COMMENTARY:The history of an oat-cell lung tumor strongly suggests the presence of ectopic ADH production. Lethargy is a prominent symptom of hyponatremia due to water excess. Laboratory data revealed an extremely low plasma sodium level. In contrast, note the relatively high urinary sodium level indicative of the "salt-wasting" of SIADH.

4-4. After an automobile accident, a 30-year-old woman was admitted to the emergency department of a small suburban hospital. She had sustained facial fractures and a possible head injury (evidenced by temporary loss of consciousness at the accident scene). During the first 3 days of her hospitalization, she received an average of 4 L of fluid daily (despite persistent low urinary output). She became increasingly lethargic and complained of headache and nausea. On the 4th day she had a grand mal seizure and was noted to have papilledema and Babinski's sign. At that time, her serum sodium level was 110 mEq/L. Despite intensive treatment, she died within a week. On autopsy, her brain was found to be swollen, and she weighed 10 pounds more than when admitted (despite almost no caloric intake during her hospitalization).

COMMENTARY: Patients with head injuries (especially when facial injuries are also present) are at risk for SIADH and should be monitored closely for it. Care should be taken to avoid fluid-overloading head-injured individuals (see Chapter 19). Note that this patient did not have any concomitant injuries that necessitated large fluid volume replacement. Weight on autopsy was greater than on admission because water was abnormally retained in cells throughout her body. No peripheral edema was present because the excess water was retained *intracellularly*, not in the interstitial space. This patient's death could have been prevented had those providing care looked at the I&O record and paid attention to the obvious warning signs of SIADH. For example, despite the 4000 mL/day intake, she excreted less than 600 mL on most days. Nurses' notes made frequent mention of the presence of lethargy, nausea, abdominal cramping, and headache.

4-5. A 23-year-old healthy woman (mother of two children) underwent an elective vaginal hysterectomy. Postoperatively, this 110-lb woman received 5% dextrose in 0.45% NaCl at a rate of 175 mL/hr for a period of approximately 20 hrs, even though her urinary output was less than 500 mL each shift. No abnormal routes of fluid loss were present. On the evening of her surgery, she complained of nausea and headache. In the early morning of the first postoperative day she was combative and disoriented. Two hours later, blood work revealed a serum sodium level of 126 mEq/L (no baseline sodium level was available as preoperative values were not obtained). One-half hour later, she was unresponsive to verbal stimuli. At this time, her serum sodium level was 122 mEq/L. Despite resuscitative efforts, she progressed on a downhill course and subsequently died several weeks later without regaining consciousness.

COMMENTARY: Cerebral edema was apparent on autopsy. Apparently this patient suffered hyponatremic encephalopathy, resulting in respiratory arrest and her subsequent death. (See the section on Postoperative Hyponatremia in Menstruant Women in this chapter.) The cause of the hyponatremia was the greatly excessive administration of hypotonic fluid during a period when her ability to excrete fluid was limited (due to the effects of increased ADH activity in the postoperative period). Recall that ADH activity is increased for the first 2 to 4 postoperative days due to the stress of surgery, as well as the presence of pain and nausea. The I&O record showed a disproportionately large fluid intake to output ratio for all three shifts. In fact, from the time of her return from surgery to the catastrophic neurologic event, this patient received approximately 3.5 L of hypotonic fluid and excreted less than 1.5 L of urine. The excess hypotonic fluid caused her serum sodium level to drop quickly, accounting for the severe neurologic symptoms despite a serum sodium level of more than 120 mEq/L. This patient's death could have been easily prevented by the administration of an isotonic fluid (or at least by avoiding the greatly excessive rate of the hypotonic electrolyte fluid). Had her symptoms been recognized earlier, and the appropriate treatment instituted, the condition could likely have been safely reversed.

HYPERNATREMIA

DEFINITION

Hypernatremia refers to a greater-than-normal serum sodium level, that is, a serum level greater than 145 mEq/L.

PATHOPHYSIOLOGY

Normally, the body defends itself against the development of hypernatremia by both increasing the release of ADH and stimulating thirst by the osmoreceptors in the hypothalamus.[76] Thus, when the serum sodium level begins to increase, the resultant retention of water and increased water intake lower the sodium concentration. Naturally, failure of these responses can lead to hypernatremia. Hypernatremia is virtually never seen in an alert patient with a normal thirst mechanism and access to water.

Causes of hypernatremia include a gain of sodium in excess of water, or a loss of water in excess of sodium. Disease states capable of causing a significant acute alteration in the serum sodium level frequently produce a concomitant change in the ECF volume. Thus, hypernatremia often occurs with either FVD or FVE. See Figure 4-3 for further explanations.

Hypernatremia associated with a near normal ECF volume

Loss of water causes elevation of serum sodium level; does not lead to volume contraction unless water losses are massive.

As may occur in:
—increased insensible water loss (as in hyperventilation)

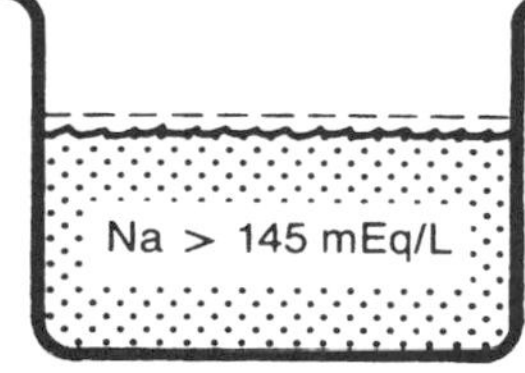

Hypernatremia associated with ECF volume deficit ("Hypertonic dehydration")

Losses of both sodium and water but relatively greater loss of water.

As may occur in:
—profuse sweating
—diarrhea, particularly in children
—aged individuals with poor water intake (recall that the aged kidney loses part of its ability to concentrate urine and thus cannot conserve water as it should)

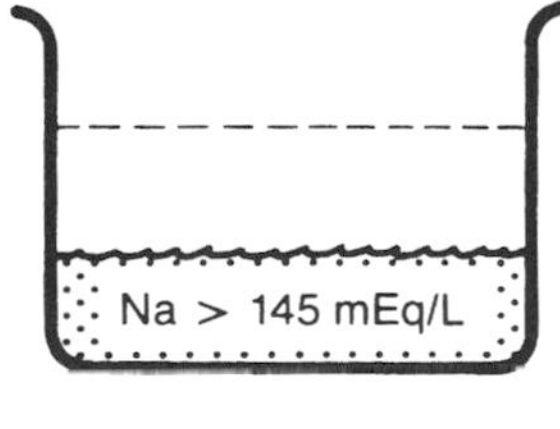

Hypernatremia associated with fluid volume excess

Gains of both sodium and water, but relatively greater gain of sodium.

As may occur:
—administration of hypertonic sodium solutions or substances (such as sodium bicarbonate in cardiac arrest)

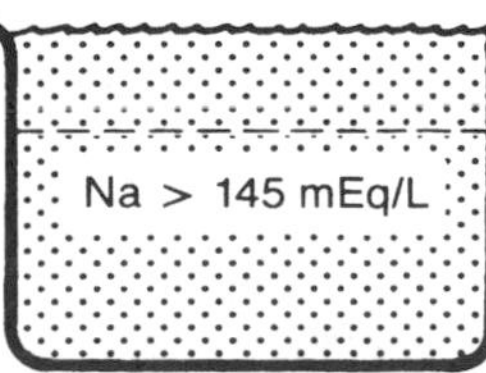

Figure 4-3. Hypernatremic states.

As noted in Figure 4-1, initially hypernatremia favors the shrinkage of cells as fluid is pulled away from them into the hypertonic ECF. It is this cellular dehydration in the brain that produces its contraction and is largely responsible for the neurologic symptoms of hypernatremia. Contraction of the brain may cause mechanical traction on delicate cerebral vessels and produce vascular trauma. Autopsies on patients who died from hypernatremia have shown widespread cerebral vascular bleeding.

The cerebral shrinking caused by hypernatremia is transient. Usually within a few hours, by means of complex mechanisms, the brain begins to adapt to the extracellular hyperosmolality by raising the amount of intracellular solutes and thereby minimizing its water loss. With increased intracellular solute, water movement back into the brain is initiated and the brain volume moves toward normal. This adaptation accounts for the relative absence of symptoms in patients with slow-developing high serum sodium levels (sometimes up to levels of 170–180 mEq/L).[77] Conversely, severe hypernatremia that develops over a period of less than 24 hrs is often fatal.

ETIOLOGICAL FACTORS

Etiological factors associated with hypernatremia are listed in Table 4-7 and are briefly described below. In general, it should be noted that the etiology of hypernatremia is quite different in children and in adults. For example, in infants the most common cause is diarrhea, whereas in the elderly, it is infirmity with inability to obtain sufficient free-water intake.

Water Deprivation

Hypernatremia may occur in any patient with a diminished mental status because the ability to perceive and respond to thirst is impaired. In adults, hypernatremia is most often seen in patients older than 60 years.[78] Not only are older persons at increased risk for illness and diminished mental status, increasing age is associated with lowered osmotic stimulation of thirst and decreased ability of the kidneys to conserve water in times of need. Infants, because they are unable to ask for water, are also at increased risk.

TABLE 4–7

Etiological Factors Associated With Hypernatremia

Deprivation of water, most common in unconscious or debilitated patients unable to perceive or respond to thirst (such as the elderly stroke patient)

Deprivation of water in infants, very young children, or retarded individuals unable to communicate thirst

Hypertonic tube feedings without adequate water supplements (see Chapter 12)

Greatly increased insensible water loss (as in hyperventilation or in extensive denuding effects of uncovered second- or third-degree burns)

Watery diarrhea

Ingestion of salt in unusual amounts (as in faulty preparation of oral electrolyte-replacement solutions)

Excessive parenteral administration of sodium-containing fluids
- Hypertonic saline (3% or 5% NaCl)
- Sodium bicarbonate ($NaHCO_3$) in cardiac arrest or treatment of lactic acidosis
- 0.9% NaCl (when primary fluid loss is water)

Diabetes insipidus if the patient does not experience, or cannot respond to, thirst; or if fluids are excessively restricted

Less common are heatstroke, near drowning in sea water (which contains a sodium concentration of approximately 500 mEq/L), accidental introduction of hypertonic saline into maternal circulation during therapeutic abortion, and malfunction of either hemodialysis or peritoneal dialysis systems

Insensible Water Loss

A typical adult with a normal body temperature will lose approximately 1000 mL of water per day through respiration and evaporation from the skin (insensible water loss). When any condition is present that increases this insensible water loss (such as fever, hyperventilation, pulmonary infections, tracheostomy, exposure to hot environmental temperatures, or massive burns), hypernatremia may result.

Watery Diarrhea

Gastrointestinal fluid losses are a major cause of hypernatremia in children, and apparently result from a combination of hypotonic fluid loss in diarrheal stools, increased insensible water loss associated with concomitant fever, and excessive sodium administration in formulas or IV fluids. Fortunately, the incidence of this imbalance has decreased in recent years because more appropriate lower-solute replacement fluids are used (providing adequate amounts of free water). Loss of hypotonic fluid in the stool of end-stage liver disease patients treated with lactulose may also result in severe hypernatremia.[79]

Excessive Sodium Intake

Ingestion or IV infusion of too much salt can induce hypernatremia. Acute or fatal hypernatremia due to excessive sodium intake has been reported after the accidental substitution of sodium chloride for sugar in infant formulas. It can also result from improperly prepared oral electrolyte solutions (addition of too much NaCl or $NaHCO_3$). Fatalities have resulted from the administration of 5% sodium chloride solution instead of the intended 5% dextrose solution because parenteral fluid containers were not checked carefully. Other causes of hypernatremia include excessive administration of $NaHCO_3$ during cardiac arrest or in the treatment of lactic acidosis. Elevated serum sodium levels can even occur from the administration of an isotonic sodium chloride solution (0.9% NaCl) if the patient's fluid deficit is primarily water.

Ingestion of sea water (which has a sodium concentration of 450–500 mEq/L) can lead to severe hypernatremia.[80] Also, fatalities have been reported with the accidental administration of hypertonic salt solutions into the maternal circulation instead of the amniotic cavity during therapeutic abortion attempts.[81]

Diabetes Insipidus

Diabetes insipidus (DI) is a water balance disorder that is associated either with a lack of ADH or with an end-organ (kidney) resistance to the effects of ADH, leading to water diuresis. Hypernatremia will result if insufficient water is replaced either orally or IV. As a rule, however, the serum sodium level remains normal because the individual with DI experiences thirst and drinks sufficient fluid to replace the lost urine volume. There are two types of DI, central and nephrogenic. Central DI (CDI) is sometimes referred to as neurogenic, and nephrogenic DI (NDI) is sometimes referred to as renal.

Central DI is due to a relative lack of ADH and is sometimes called vasopressin-sensitive DI because it responds favorably to vasopressin (ADH) administration. This form of DI may occur after head trauma (particularly caused by fractures at the base of the skull or surgical procedures near the pituitary) or as a result of infection, primary tumor, or metastatic tumor. It may also be idiopathic; approximately 50% of the patients with CDI have no known underlying pathology.

Nephrogenic DI is due to failure of the kidney to respond to ADH, not to a deficit of the hormone. This condition is sometimes referred to as vasopressin-resistant DI because the administration of vasopressin does not relieve the disorder. It may occur as a rare genetic disorder or may be acquired. Acquired NDI is much more common and may be the result of electrolyte disorders (such as hypokalemia or hypercalcemia), chronic renal failure, or drugs such as lithium, demeclocycline, and methoxyflurane (a halogenated anesthetic).[82] Fortunately, the NDI caused by hypercalcemia and hypokalemia is usually reversible within 1 to 12 weeks after correction of the imbalance.[83]

DEFINING CHARACTERISTICS

Defining characteristics of hypernatremia are given in Table 4-8. When the patient is awake, thirst is the usual early sign of developing hypernatremia.

TABLE 4–8
Defining Characteristics of Hypernatremia

Thirst (Note that thirst is so strong a defender of serum sodium in normal individuals that hypernatremia never occurs unless the person is rendered unconscious or is denied access to water; ill persons may have an impaired thirst mechanism.)

Elevated body temperature

Dry and sticky mucous membranes

Restlessness and weakness in moderate hypernatremia

Disorientation, delusions, and hallucinations in severe hypernatremia; or, patient may be lethargic when undisturbed and irritable and hyperreactive when stimulated

Lethargy, stupor, or coma (The level of consciousness depends not only on actual sodium levels, but on the rate of development of hypernatremia. For example, a patient may have a serum sodium level of 170 mEq/L and remain conscious if the imbalance developed slowly.)

Muscle irritability and convulsions

Signs of irritability and high-pitched cry in infants

Laboratory data:

- Serum sodium >145 mEq/L
- Serum osmolality >295 mOsm/kg
- Urinary SG > 1.015 as the kidneys attempt to conserve needed water, provided water loss is from a route *other* than the kidney (such as the GI tract, skin, or lungs). If the physiological defect involves water loss from the kidney (as occurs in complete diabetes insipidus), the urinary SG will be very low.

It should be noted that thirst, by stimulating water intake, normally protects against hypernatremia. Thus, hypernatremia generally occurs in individuals either unable to perceive or unable to respond to thirst (eg, adults with an altered mental status or infants). An awake, alert patient with hypernatremia can be assumed to have a hypothalamic lesion affecting the thirst center.[84]

Like hyponatremia, the primary manifestations of hypernatremia are neurological in nature. The earliest signs are lethargy, weakness, and irritability. These symptoms can progress to twitching, seizures, coma, and death if the hypernatremia is severe. Although convulsions may occur from an acute, rapid increase of plasma sodium by 15 to 20 mEq/L within 24 hrs or less, they usually occur with a sodium concentration greater than 160 mEq/L.[85] Presumably these symptoms are the consequence of cellular dehydration (resulting from pulling of fluid from the cells into the hyperosmotic ECF). If hypernatremia is severe, permanent brain damage can occur, especially in children. Brain damage is apparently due to subarachnoid hemorrhages that result from tearing of vessels during brain contraction. Because of rupture of cerebral vessels, a lumbar puncture may reveal blood in the cerebrospinal fluid. Symptoms in infants often include marked irritability and a high-pitched cry, with a depressed sensorium ranging from lethargy to frank coma. In adults, the symptoms of hypernatremia are often difficult to separate from those of the underlying pathology, which is often of a catastrophic nature.

As is the case with hyponatremia, the rapidity of onset is an important determinant of the severity of symptoms as well as the eventual outcome of hypernatremia. A high plasma sodium level that evolves over days to weeks is associated with minimal to mild neurologic symptoms because the CNS cells have time to adapt to hyperosmolar changes.[86]

If the hypernatremia is accompanied by FVD, other symptoms such as postural hypotension may occur. Other physical signs of water deficit are dry, hot skin with decreased sweating; thick, rubbery-feeling skin; and fever of CNS origin.[87] Hypernatremia is the only state in which dry, sticky mucous membranes are characteristic.[88]

TABLE 4–9

Clinical Manifestations of Diabetes Insipidus

Excessive urinary output regardless of fluid intake:
- Urinary output usually ranges between 3 to 20 liters per 24 hr (depending on the severity of the pathologic process)
- Urinary output often exceeds 200 mL/hr
- In complete DI, urinary specific gravity <1.010, urine osmolality <300 mOsm/L
- In partial DI, urinary specific gravity and urinary osmolality are somewhat higher (such as 1.010 to 1.023 and 300 to 800 mOsm/L, respectively)
- Inability of kidneys to concentrate urine by fluid restriction (a common test for this disorder)

Intense thirst in the alert patient, resulting in an intake that corresponds to the urinary volume

Serum osmolality and sodium levels greater than normal if water intake does not match urinary losses (severe hypovolemia may occur with inadequate fluid intake)

Diabetes Insipidus

The most prevalent signs of DI are polyuria and polydipsia. Depending on the severity of the disease, the degree of polyuria in DI can range from 3 to 20 L in 24 hrs. In complete CDI and NDI, the urinary specific gravity and osmolality are quite low (<1.010 and 300 mOsm/L, respectively). In partial CDI and NDI, the urinary specific gravity and osmolality are somewhat higher (1.010–1.023 and 300–800 mOsm/L, respectively). This is because the patient has some remaining ability to concentrate urine. Clinical manifestations of DI are summarized in Table 4-9.

As a rule, the patient with an intact thirst mechanism will drink sufficient fluids to maintain the sodium balance (ie, an essentially normal serum sodium and serum osmolality). Unfortunately, the frequency of urination and drinking often interferes with other activities when the condition is severe.

If the patient is not able to perceive or respond to thirst or if parenteral fluid replacement is inadequate, polyuria will lead to severe dehydration (hypernatremia and hyperosmolality of plasma) with weight loss, tachycardia, and even shock.

TREATMENT

Hypernatremia is treated either by the addition of water or by the removal of sodium, depending on the cause of the imbalance. If water loss is the cause, water needs to be added; if sodium excess is the cause, sodium needs to be removed. Too rapid a correction of hypernatremia can result in cerebral edema, seizures, permanent neurological damage, and death. The reasons for this is as follows: Hypernatremia initially pulls water from brain cells and produces brain contraction; however, after a few hours the brain begins to adapt by increasing the intracellular solute level.[89] Rapid lowering of the plasma sodium can render the plasma relatively hypoosmotic to the brain cells and allow water to be pulled into the cells, producing cerebral edema. (Note that the blood–brain barrier prevents the intracellular solutes from being diluted at the same rate as the solute in the plasma.) To minimize the risk of complications, it is currently recommended that the plasma sodium concentration be gradually lowered to normal unless the patient has symptomatic hypernatremia.[90] In both children and adults, fluid therapy is administered such that normonatremia is achieved over a period of approximately 48 hrs.[91] Because chronic hypernatremia is well tolerated, rapid correction offers no advantage and may be harmful because of the potential for causing brain edema. According to one group of investigators, chronic hypernatremia (defined as hypernatremia that has been present for >2 days) should not be corrected faster than 0.7 mEq/L/hr or approximately 10% of the serum sodium concentration per day.[92] In contrast, acute hypernatremia (present for <12 hrs) may be treated more rapidly.[93] In acute symptomatic hypernatremia, the serum sodium concentration may be reduced by 6 to 8 mEq/L in the first 3 to 4 hrs, but thereafter the rate of decline should not be more than 1 mEq/L/hr.[94]

Standard formulas exist for calculating the degree of free-water deficit in hypernatremic patients. Generally, sufficient free water is given in the form of hypotonic fluids (ranging from 5% dextrose in water to 0.45% sodium chloride solution) to lower the plasma sodium level gradually over a period of approximately 48 hrs.[95] Plasma electrolytes should be monitored at frequent intervals, such as every 2 hrs.[96] Disease states that cause hypernatremia also often cause a decrease in the extracellular fluid volume. In most cases, it may be safer to correct hypernatremia concomitantly with repletion of the volume deficit with half-strength saline (0.45% NaCl) or half-strength lactated Ringer's solution; this is because too rapid correction of the hyperosmolar ECF by 5% dextrose in water may cause convulsions and coma.[97] Patients who have sustained both water and sodium losses and who show evidence of circulatory insufficiency may need to receive isotonic saline (0.9% NaCl) until they become hemodynamically stable; after stabilization, 0.45% NaCl may be infused.[98]

Diabetes Insipidus

The standard treatment of patients with complete CDI has been ADH replacement by means of vasopressin administration. Vasopressin may be administered in different forms, depending on the clinical situation.

Vasopressin (8-arginine vasopressin) is a short-acting aqueous ADH replacement possessing antidiuretic and pressor effects, which can be given subcutaneously, intramuscularly, or intranasally. This preparation is useful when a rapidly acting, short-duration ADH replacement is indicated, particularly after cranial surgery.[99] When a longer-acting preparation is desirable, desmopressin (a synthetic analogue of vasopressin), may be used; this agent has a stronger antidiuretic effect than arginine vasopressin but has negligible pressor activity.[100]

Until the polyuria is controlled by vasopressin therapy, careful attention must be paid to replacement of fluid (particularly if the patient has a decreased level of consciousness or other disturbances interfering with the perception of thirst or the ability to drink). However, it is important to recall that a potential complication of vasopressin therapy is water intoxication (excessive retention of water).

If the patient with CDI has some residual capacity to secrete ADH, drugs that increase the release of ADH or enhance its action on the kidney may be used instead of hormonal replacement therapy. Such drugs include chlorpropamide (Diabinese), an oral hypoglycemia agent, and carbamazepine (Tegretol), an anticonvulsant.

Paradoxically, thiazide diuretic agents are sometimes used to decrease the polyuria associated with both CDI and NDI.[101] It is believed that the thiazides act by decreasing the amount of sodium ions that reach the distal tubules of the kidneys. Patients taking thiazides for treatment of DI should be instructed to avoid liberal use of salt because it decreases the effectiveness of the drug.

NURSING INTERVENTIONS

1. Identify patients at risk for hypernatremia (review Table 4-7).
2. Monitor fluid losses and gains. Look for abnormal losses of water or low water intake, and for large gains of sodium as may occur with prescription drugs having a high sodium content. For example, 24 g of carbenicillin disodium (a possible daily dose) contain 142 mEq of sodium.[102] Fleet enema solution also has a high sodium content.
3. Monitor for symptoms of hypernatremia (see Table 4-8). Evaluate these in relation to other factors in the patient's history.
4. Monitor serum sodium levels as frequently as indicated.
5. Prevent hypernatremia in debilitated patients unable to perceive or respond to thirst by offering them fluids at regular intervals. If fluid intake remains inadequate, consult with the physician to plan an alternate route for intake, either by tube feedings or by the parenteral route.
6. If tube feedings are used, give sufficient water to keep the serum sodium and the blood urea nitrogen (BUN) levels within normal limits (see Chapter 12).
7. Monitor the patient's response to corrective parenteral fluids by reviewing serial sodium levels and observing any changes in neurological signs. With gradual decrease in the serum sodium level, the neurological signs should improve, not worsen. Be aware that the serum sodium

level should be decreased gradually (see Treatment section above and Case Study 4-2).

8. For patients with DI:
   A. Monitor parameters outlined in Table 4-10.
   B. Ensure that the alert DI patient with intact thirst mechanism is allowed to drink at will; also, ensure that this individual is near a bathroom as frequent voiding is anticipated until the condition is brought under control.
   C. Ensure that the patient with a decreased level of consciousness or other disability interfering with drinking is given adequate fluid; if the patient is unable to take fluids orally, consult with the physician to obtain parenteral fluid orders. Anticipate performing this intervention in neurological patients, particularly in the early postoperative period.
   D. Administer medications for DI with an understanding of their actions.
   E. Be aware that a potential complication of vasopressin administration is water intoxication (excessive retention of water causing a low serum sodium level). This is particularly important because it is difficult to regulate vasopressin dosage in patients with rapidly fluctuating clinical states.
   F. Educate patients regarding the proper use of prescribed medications and how to monitor and record fluctuations in their fluid input and output (I&O) and body weight (see Summary of Hypernatremia).

TABLE 4–10

Assessment for Diabetes Insipidus

1. Be aware of patients at risk for DI
   Central DI
   - Head trauma (particularly with fractures at the base of the skull or surgical procedures near the pituitary)
   - Cerebral infections
   - Brain tumors

   Nephrogenic DI
   - Hypokalemia
   - Hypercalcemia
   - Certain drugs (such as lithium and demeclocycline)
2. Maintain an accurate I&O record for at-risk patients.
   - Look for a significantly greater output than intake (a danger signal of impending hypernatremia). Fortunately, many patients keep themselves "in balance" by drinking approximately as much as they urinate. It is helpful to calculate and record cumulative amounts for several days to obtain a more accurate account of the patient's fluid balance status, particularly if onset of polyuria was insidious.
3. Be alert for polyuria in at-risk patients.
   - It is frequently necessary to measure hourly urine volumes in such individuals to foster early detection. For example, a frequent directive in the care of postoperative neurosurgical patients is to report a urine volume greater than 200 mL in each of 2 consecutive hours or more than 500 mL in a 2-hr period.
4. Monitor urinary SG in at-risk patients.
   - A persistently dilute urine is a hallmark of DI. (The SG may be as low as 1.005.)
5. Monitor serum sodium levels at least once a day (more often as indicated) in at-risk patients.
   - Look for hypernatremia (serum sodium >145 mEq/L). Once vasopressin therapy has been initiated, look for hyponatremia (a possible rebound effect).
6. Monitor body weights.
   - Look for weight loss paralleling polyuria. Maintaining a weight chart helps detect excessive fluid loss, particularly when I&O records are in doubt (as may occur in incontinent patients).

DI, diabetes insipidus; SG, specific gravity.

SUMMARY OF HYPERNATREMIA

ETIOLOGICAL FACTORS	DEFINING CHARACTERISTICS
Deprivation of water (most common in those unable to perceive or respond to thirst)	Thirst usually occurs early
Increased insensible water loss (as in hyperventilation)	Dry, sticky mucous membranes
Watery diarrhea	Fever may be present
Ingestion of salt in unusual amounts	Severe hypernatremia • Disorientation • Hallucinations • Lethargy when undisturbed • Irritability when stimulated • Focal or grand mal seizures • Coma
Excessive parenteral administration of sodium-containing solutions • Hypertonic saline (3% or 5% NaCl) • Sodium bicarbonate • Isotonic saline	Serum sodium >145 mEq/L
Near drowning in sea water	Serum osmolality >295 mOsm/kg
Heatstroke	Urinary SG >1.015, provided water loss is from nonrenal route
Diabetes insipidus if water intake is inadequate	For diabetes insipidus, see Table 4-10

CASE STUDIES

4-6. An 80-year-old woman living in a nursing home had a stroke and developed aphasia and hemiplegia. Because of her neurological deficits, she required a great deal of assistance to eat and drink. Due to lack of attention from the staff, she ingested insufficient water and developed a serum sodium of 188 mEq/L.

COMMENTARY: A serum sodium concentration greater than 150 mEq/L is virtually never seen in an alert patient with a normal thirst mechanism and access to water.[103] This hypernatremic patient represents a common problem in patients with decreased awareness and inability to drink. One researcher stated that hypernatremic dehydration constitutes a "sentinel health event" in patients without documented rapid free-water loss. A *sentinel health event* is defined as an illness or death that should be preventable, given adequate care, or at least should cause those caring for the patient to ask why the event occurred.[104] In the absence of free-water loss, hypernatremic dehydration probably indicates fluid deprivation (a form of neglect).

4-7. A 60-year old woman with a serum sodium level of 185 mEq/L was transferred from a nursing home to an acute care facility. Aggressive IV therapy with large volumes of 5% dextrose in water was instituted and her serum sodium dropped to 145 mEq/L in 5 hrs. She became unresponsive; a lumbar puncture revealed an opening pressure of 32 cm of water (normal is 10–20 cm of water).

COMMENTARY: This patient had been hypernatremic for some time, allowing her brain to adapt to the hyperosmolal state by increasing brain osmolality. (In hypernatremia, brain volume initially declines and then begins to adapt toward normal within several hours.)[105] Once this cerebral adaptation has occurred, any rapid lowering of the serum sodium level creates an osmotic gradient, allowing water to move into the brain, increasing brain size, and causing cerebral edema. This is precisely what happened in this patient; had the serum sodium been decreased gradually, the cerebral edema would not have occurred.

4-8. Over a 16-hr period, a young child was inadvertently given 800 mL of 5% NaCl solution (containing 855 mEq/L of sodium) instead of the prescribed 5% dextrose in half-strength saline (containing 77 mEq/L of sodium). She developed lethargy, convulsions, and coma before the error was discovered. Despite resuscitative efforts, the child died.

COMMENTARY: Instead of a hypotonic sodium fluid, this child received a grossly hypertonic sodium solution, causing fatal brain damage. This terrible event would never have occurred had the fluid been checked properly before being administered.

4-9. A 55-year-old comatose woman with a basal skull fracture was transferred to a medical center from a small suburban hospital. Her urine output was noted to be 200 mL/hr and her serum sodium was 170 mEq/L. Urine osmolality was 80 mOsm/kg (extremely dilute, reflecting excessive water loss in the urine) and the serum osmolality was 360 mOsm/kg (reflecting hypernatremia). A diagnosis of central DI was made and vasopressin was administered. In 3 days the serum sodium level had fallen to 130 mEq/L.

COMMENTARY: This patient was not hydrated adequately at the onset and thus developed hypernatremia. The staff should have been alert for CDI because of the nature of the injury (basal skull fracture). Excessive use of vasopressin caused the development of hyponatremia.

4-10. For the past 6 months a 65-year-old man had received diuretics to manage his hypertension. During a visit to his physician, he reported that he was more thirsty than usual and frequently had to get up at night to urinate (nocturia). Laboratory analysis found his serum potassium to be 2.4 mEq/L. He was hospitalized for evaluation; it was found that he could concentrate his urine to only 300 mOsm/kg on fluid restriction (instead of the expected 1200–1400 mOsm/kg in normal renal function). After correction of the hypokalemia, his renal concentrating ability and urine volume eventually returned to normal.

COMMENTARY: This patient had acquired nephrogenic DI due to hypokalemia. Many patients with potassium depletion complain of polyuria; it is caused by a reduced ability to concentrate the urine due to decreased responsiveness to ADH. This resistance to ADH may be due to an interference with the generation and action of cyclic adenosine monophosphate (AMP).[106] Although the nephrogenic DI associated with hypokalemia is usually reversible, recall that more severe changes are possible with prolonged hypokalemia. The serum sodium level was not elevated because the patient managed to drink sufficient fluids to match the increased output of dilute urine.

4-11. A physician prescribed 20 mL of 0.9% sodium chloride to be administered over 30 min to a hypotensive newborn; instead of a vial of 0.9% NaCl, the nurse inadvertently obtained a vial of 14.6% NaCl.[107] (Unfortunately, the vial's label did not clearly warn that the solution was highly concentrated and required dilution.) Two doses were administered from the vial and the infant developed apnea and required intubation. Blood was drawn and showed a serum sodium level of 195 mEq/L.

COMMENTARY: The greatly elevated serum sodium level resulted in severe, permanent brain damage, requiring that the child be institutionalized. An important lesson to learn from the tragic event reported here is the need to carefully check all vials before administering any solution.

SODIUM AND HEAT STRESS

Physiological disturbances related to heat stress range from mild to severe. This discussion describes the relationship between sodium and the major types of heat-related disorders.

HEAT SYNCOPE

Heat syncope is associated with postural hypotension, which occurs when blood is diverted to peripheral tissues for cooling. Diminished venous return to the heart and reduction of cardiac output lead to cerebral ischemia, which accounts for the syncope. This condition is most likely to occur in persons deficient in salt and water, particularly if cardiovascular disease is present. Thus, patients receiving diuretics are at increased risk. Treatment other than rest in a cool environment generally is not needed.

HEAT EDEMA

Shortly after entering a hot climate, slight swelling of the hands and feet is very common among unacclimatized individuals (those not accustomed to the heat). Most often occurring in women, the edema disappears as heat tolerance is gained. Likely causes are salt and water retention from salt supplementation, increased aldosterone production, and oliguria after heat-induced vasodilation.[108] Fortunately, this is a self-limiting condition that does not require treatment.

HEAT CRAMPS

As the name implies, *heat cramps* are characterized by painful muscle contractions in persons exposed to heat stress. More specifically, heat cramps are painful, intermittent contractions of skeletal muscles after strenuous activity in a hot environment. (Of interest, they most often occur in individuals in excellent physical condition who are accustomed to working in a hot environment. Such individuals are able to produce large quantities of sweat in response to strenuous exercise and heat stress.)

Precipitating factors are strenuous exercise, hemodilution (due to large water intake with no salt), and cooling of the muscle. Because individuals with heat cramps are hyponatremic, it is believed that the mechanism for heat cramp production is sodium depletion in the muscle. Typically, heat cramps occur toward the end of a strenuous period, after bathing in cool water.[109]

Ingestion of salt before or during exercise is usually an effective prophylaxis for heat cramps. To replace salt lost in sweat, salt can be added to foods as a seasoning or can be consumed in liquids having salt as a component. Once heat cramps have occurred, treatment involves salt ingestion, either orally or IV. For severe, unrelenting cramps, oral or IV salt solutions quickly relieve all signs.[110]

HEAT EXHAUSTION

Heat exhaustion is a common yet vague clinical entity. Although pure forms are uncommon, heat exhaustion can be divided into two major forms: (1) associated primarily with sodium depletion (hyponatremia) and (2) associated with dehydration (water deficit with hypernatremia).

Heat Exhaustion Due Primarily to Salt Depletion

Heat exhaustion due to salt depletion occurs when large volumes of sweat from heat-stressed individuals are replaced by adequate volumes of water but too little salt. This condition differs from heat cramps in two ways: (1) it tends to occur in individuals who are *not* accustomed to heat stress, and (2) it involves systemic effects beyond skeletal muscle cramps. Among these are fatigue, weakness, giddiness, frontal headache, anorexia, nausea, vomiting, and diarrhea.[111] Because water is consumed to replace the lost sweat, marked weight loss may not occur. Treatment consists of administering salted liquids by mouth. If necessary, isotonic saline (0.9% NaCl) may be given IV.

Heat Exhaustion Due to Water Depletion

This form of heat exhaustion is caused when sweat losses are not replaced by the individual working under heat stress, resulting in a negative water balance. As a rule, this set of circumstances is experienced by individuals for whom the water supply is limited (eg, soldiers or laborers who are unable to gain access to water). Clinically, there is intense thirst, fatigue, weakness, discomfort, and impaired judgment.[112] Body temperature is almost always elevated, although not to the level associated with heatstroke. The person with *heat exhaustion due to water depletion* usually has a temperature that is normal or lower than 39 °C (102 °F), whereas the person with heatstroke usually has a much higher temperature. Left untreated, heat exhaustion condition may terminate in heatstroke.[113]

Treatment consists of water replacement. However, as discussed earlier in the chapter, rapid correction of severe hypernatremia must be guarded against to avoid initiating convulsive seizures. It has been recommended that the serum osmolality be decreased at a rate no faster than 2 to 4 mOsm/hr.[114] If possible, water should be given orally. However, if the patient is vomiting or unconscious, the solution of choice is 5% dextrose in water; when the serum sodium has fallen to 150 mEq/L, hypotonic saline (0.45% NaCl) can be substituted for water.[115]

HEATSTROKE

Heatstroke is likely with elevation of body temperature beyond a critical point (in the range of 106 ° to 108 °F).[116] Symptoms include delirium, dizziness, abdominal distress, and eventually loss of consciousness. Symptoms are related in part to reduced circulatory volume brought about by excessive sweating. Others are directly related to the effects of hyperthermia on the brain and other body tissues. Autopsies on individuals who died from heatstroke have shown hemorrhages and parenchymatous cellular degeneration throughout the body.

Two forms of heatstroke are often described, classic and exercise-induced. Classic heatstroke occurs primarily in invalids or in the elderly during a sustained heat wave. In contrast, exertion-induced heatstroke usually occurs in well-conditioned athletes or workers whose physical means to dissipate heat are exceeded by endogenous heat production. Examples include football players, marathon runners, and military recruits.

Most important in the treatment of heatstroke is lowering body temperature to a safe level. Among the methods used are cold water immersion with skin massage,[117] compressed air/warm water sprays,[118] and strategically placed ice packs.[119] It has been suggested that effective body cooling may occur with water having a temperature of 15 ° to 16 °C (59 ° to 61 °F).[120]

Placement of IV lines and tracheal intubation are necessary, as is placement of a rectal thermistor to measure core temperature. Hypotension is likely to be present as blood is shunted to the periphery for cooling. Excessive fluid replacement should be guarded against because pulmonary edema could result as cooling promotes return of peripheral blood to the central circulation. Sodium levels are variable and often depend on conditions leading to heatstroke. The most important laboratory measurements at time of admission are arterial blood gases, serum electrolyte concentrations, and complete blood count. Treatment is based on results and other clinical findings.

PREVENTIVE MEASURES AND RATIONALES

Heat disorders can often be prevented, or at least minimized, by some relatively simple measures.

1. Before engaging in sustained strenuous activity, undergo acclimatization to a hot environment.
   - Exposure to heat for several hours each day while performing a reasonably heavy workload will increase tolerance to heat in 1 to 3 weeks.[121] Acclimatized individuals attain an increased maximum rate of sweating, increased plasma volume, and decreased loss of salt in the sweat and urine. The latter two effects are related to an increased production of aldosterone. (Although the sodium content of sweat in these individuals is less than that in nonacclimatized persons, it can still be the source of significant sodium loss.)
2. To offset the body's loss of water and salt in sweat, drink cool liquids at regular intervals while undergoing heat stress.
   - First, consider fluids that are inappropriate for replacing losses. Alcohol is certainly contraindicated because it has diuretic effects but, more important, because it can alter judgment about heat exposure. Furthermore, a brief period of moderate or heavy alcohol intake often appears to cause loss of acclimatization.[122] Coffee and tea are not recommended for sole use in fluid replacement as these beverages

have diuretic properties and predispose to further fluid loss.

- Depending on individual need, fluid replacement can be in the form of water, a sodium chloride solution, or a balanced electrolyte solution. *Water is often sufficient* when the subject has taken in a normal diet supplying ample sodium, potassium, and other electrolytes. However, sustained losses of sweat over prolonged periods may necessitate electrolyte replacement in addition to water. A solution of sodium chloride (4 tsp of salt to a gallon of water) for oral consumption may suffice to prevent heat cramps.[123] Care must be taken to avoid excessive salt and insufficient water intake because this practice predisposes to water-depletion heat exhaustion that can culminate in heatstroke.[124]
- A few oral electrolyte-rehydrating fluids are available commercially and usually contain varying quantities of carbohydrates in the form of simple sugars or glucose polymers. Advantages of carbohydrates in replacement fluids are improved endurance during strenuous exertion (due to muscle glycogen sparing) and pleasant taste (perhaps ensuring that they will be consumed in greater quantity than plain water or electrolyte solutions). However, a potential difficulty with carbohydrates is their effect on gastric emptying time, that is, the higher the solution's carbohydrate content or osmolality, the more likely gastric emptying is to be inhibited, thereby reducing the rate of fluid absorption into the system. Some researchers believe that fluids with a high carbohydrate concentration slow gastric emptying and produce satiety, thus discouraging further intake of needed fluids.[125]

To compare the effects of drinking distilled water versus drinking a carbohydrate–electrolyte solution* on physiological disturbances during prolonged strenuous exercise in the heat, Carter and Gisolfi[126] studied seven men during and after vigorous bouts of cycle exercise. They concluded that the carbohydrate–electrolyte beverage used in their study maintained plasma volume at a level higher than water during exercise, supplied an energy source, and rehydrated subjects faster than water during recovery.

- The number of people participating in marathons and triathlons has greatly increased over the past decade. Electrolyte disturbances are more likely to occur during events that last a prolonged period in the heat. During triathlon events in high environmental temperatures, volume depletion and hyponatremia are likely if the athlete replaces sweat losses with water (although in inadequate amounts) but no salt. As Hiller[127] reported, it is common for endurance athletes to be both volume-depleted and hyponatremic after races, such as triathlons, lasting longer than 8 hrs. In these situations, the exercise-induced hyponatremia is a combination of massive unreplaced sodium losses associated with partially replaced massive water losses. Hiller[128] recommends that endurance athletes practice programmed replacement of hourly fluid losses (such as 500 mL of fluid for each 1-lb weight loss), and that they use some form of sodium replacement during events lasting longer than 4 hrs. He further recommends that they prepare by increasing their salt intake during the period before the event during which they become acclimatized. If sodium-containing fluids are needed to treat athletes after the events, 5% dextrose in normal saline may be used for races lasting longer than 4 hrs and 5% dextrose in either normal or half-normal saline for events lasting less than 4 hrs.[129]

3. Strenuous activity on hot days should be curtailed as much as possible.
   - Periods of prolonged exercise, such as training programs or athletic events, should take place during the cooler parts of the day (before 8 AM and after 5 PM). Care should be taken to avoid direct solar heat radiation during the hottest hours of the day (11 AM to 2 PM).
4. When possible, loose, porous clothing should be worn to allow for heat dissipation.
   - A hat and light-colored clothing are helpful in decreasing the amount of heat absorbed from direct sunlight, although workers in specific jobs may need different types of

---

*Composed of 4.85% polycose, 2.65% fructose, 9.2 mM Na, 5.0 mM K, 2.1 mM Ca, 2.1 mM Mg, 9.6 mM Cl, 250 mOsm/L.

clothing. For example, those working with radiant heat should wear reflective garments. Unfortunately, the nature of some work requires that special protective clothing be worn, further predisposing to heat injury. For example, welders and others exposed to sparks should wear self-extinguishing materials like "green cotton," that is, cotton treated with flame retardant.[130]

- Firefighters must wear heavy protective clothing (often rubberized) that predisposes them to increased heat stress. Engaging in strenuous activity while dressed in impervious plastic sweat clothing is potentially disastrous. The belief that this activity can safely result in weight loss in overweight athletes is erroneous.

5. During extreme high temperatures, individuals without air conditioners or fans should make use of "cooling centers" that are usually available in most communities.
   - Unfortunately, many elderly inner-city residents are hesitant to leave their homes for cooling centers during heat waves because of a fear of burglaries or vandalism.
6. Adequate fluids should be provided for confused or otherwise debilitated patients unable to respond to thirst.
7. Coaches and trainers in athletic programs and supervisors in the workplace should be aware of the warning signs of heat disorders and the measures to deal with them.
8. Participants and planners of competitive sports events should consider the following points:
   A. Competitors should train in the heat before the big event to promote acclimatization.
   B. Competitors should avoid fluid restriction before the start of the event. Pre-event dehydration results in a reduction of the body's sweating and, therefore, cooling abilities.
   C. Fluid stations should be readily available at strategic locations to allow the competitors to replace needed fluids.
   D. Competitors and race officials should be aware that events lasting longer than 4 hrs are more likely to produce fluid and electrolyte problems than are those lasting less than 4 hrs.
   E. Trained spotters should be placed at regular intervals during the event to identify competitors with early signs of heat injury. Cooling and fluid replacement should be initiated on the spot. Athletes should use the "buddy system" and assume mutual responsibility for each other's well-being during the event.
9. Because children are less efficient thermoregulators than adults, they are at increased risk for heat illness. Like adults, children should undergo a period of acclimatization before indulging in heavy exercise in hot temperatures and should modify their physical activity in the face of high ambient temperature and humidity. Although they may benefit from drinking carbohydrate–electrolyte-containing solutions, for the majority of young athletes, cold water remains the preferred choice for fluid replacement during exercise.[131]

REFERENCES

1. Schwartz S (ed): Principles of Surgery, 6th ed, p 64. New York, McGraw-Hill, 1994
2. Narins R (ed): Clinical Disorders of Fluid and Electrolyte Metabolism, 5th ed, p 1196. New York, McGraw-Hill, 1994
3. Ibid, p 591
4. Kovacs L, Robertson G: Disorders of water balance—hyponatremia and hypernatremia. Baillier's Clinical Endocrinology and Metabolism 6(1):107–127,1992
5. Oh M, Carroll H: Disorders of sodium metabolism: Hypernatremia and hyponatremia. Crit Care Med 20(1):94–103,1992
6. Narins, p 592
7. Szerlip H, Goldfarb S: Workshops in Fluid and Electrolyte Disorders. New York, Churchill Livingstone, 1993
8. Sterns R: Severe symptomatic hyponatremia, treatment and outcome: A study of 64 cases. Ann Intern Med 107:656,1987
9. Narins, p 595
10. Rose B: Clinical Physiology of Acid-Base and Electrolyte Disorders, 4th ed, p 391. New York, McGraw-Hill, 1994
11. Ibid
12. Narins, p 595
13. Rose, p 662
14. Weissman P, Shenkman L, Gregerman R: Chlorpropamide hyponatremia: Drug-induced inappropriate antidiuretic hormone activity. N Engl J Med 284:65–71, 1971
15. Kadowaki T, Hagura R, Kajinuma H, et al: Chlorpropamide-induced hyponatremia; Incidence and risk factors. Diabetes Care 6:468,1983

16. Rose, p 662
17. Kokko J, Tannen R: Fluids and Electrolytes, 2nd ed, p 1000. Philadelphia, WB Saunders, 1990
18. Narins, p 598
19. Rose, p 662
20. Narins, p 588
21. Ibid, p 599
22. Wijdicks et al: Atrial natriuretic factor and salt-wasting after aneurysmal subarachnoid hemorrhage. Stroke 22:1519,1991; 17:137,1985
23. Shutty M, Leadbetter R: Salt appetite with psychosis, intermittent hyponatremia and polydipsia. Am J Psychiatry 150:4,1993
24. Ibid
25. Kokko, Tannen, p 165
26. Ellinas P, Rosner F, Jauma J: Symptomatic hyponatremia associated with psychoses, medications, and smoking. J Nat Med Assoc 85:135–140,1993
27. Narins, p 597
28. Rose, p 663
29. Chung et al: Postoperative hyponatremia. Arch Intern Med 146:333,1986
30. Narins, p 599
31. Ayus J, Wheeler J, Arieff A: Postoperative hyponatremic encephalopathy in menstruant women. Ann Intern Med 117:891–897,1992
32. Ibid
33. Arieff A, Ayus J: Endometrial ablation complicated by fatal hyponatremic encephalopathy. JAMA 270:1230–1232,1993
34. Ayus J, Wheeler J, Arieff A: Postoperative hyponatremic encephalopathy in menstruant women. Ann Intern Med 117:891–897,1992
35. Ibid
36. Ibid
37. Rose, p 662
38. Narins, p 599
39. Brown R: Disorders of water and sodium balance. Postgraduate Med 93(4):227–246,1993
40. Narins, p 598
41. Ellis R, Carmichael J: Hyponatremia and volume overload as a complication of transurethral resection of the prostate. J Family Pract 33(1):89–91,1991
42. Narins, p 1419
43. Ibid
44. Glassock R, et al: Human immunodeficiency virus (HIV) and the kidney. Ann Intern Med 112:35,1990
45. Vitting et al: Frequency of hyponatremia and nonosmolar vasopressin release in the acquired immunodeficiency syndrome. JAMA 263:973,1990
46. Agarwal et al: Hyponatremia in patients with the acquired immunodeficiency syndrome. Nephron 53:317,1989
47. Rose, p 661
48. Rose, p 671
49. Oh, Carroll, p 94
50. Pemberton L, Pemberton D: Treatment of Water, Electrolyte, and Acid–Base Disorders in the Surgical Patient, p 77. New York, McGraw-Hill, 1994
51. Narins, p 599
52. Ibid
53. Rose, p 671
54. Arieff A, Ayus J, Fraser C: Hyponatremia and death or permanent brain damage in children. Br Med J 304:1218,1992
55. Chernow B (ed): The Pharmacologic Approach to the Critically Ill Patient, 3rd ed, p 560. Baltimore, Williams & Wilkins, 1994
56. Ayus J, Arieff A: Symptomatic hyponatremia: Correcting sodium deficits safely. J Crit Illness 5(9):905–918,1990
57. Brunner J, et al: Central pontine myelinolysis and pontine lesions after rapid correction of hyponatremia: A prospective magnetic resonance imaging study. Ann Neurol 27:61,1990
58. Narins, p 601
59. Ayus J, Arieff A: Symptomatic hyponatremia: Making the diagnosis rapidly. J Crit Illness 5(8):846–856,1990
60. Ayus J, Arieff A: Symptomatic hyponatremia: Correcting sodium deficits safely. J Crit Illness 5(9):905–918,1990
61. Ibid
62. Rose, p 678
63. Ibid
64. Ibid
65. Chernow, p 959
66. Rose, p 684
67. Ibid
68. Narins, p 606
69. Ibid
70. Rose, p 684
71. Pennington J: Bowes & Church's Food Values of Portions Commonly Used, 15th ed, p 177. Philadelphia, J B Lippincott, 1989
72. Rose, p 678
73. Ibid
74. Ayus J, Arieff A: Symptomatic hyponatremia: Correcting sodium deficits safely. J Crit Illness 5(9): 905–918,1990
75. Rose, p 678
76. Ibid, p 263
77. Ibid, p 711
78. Ibid, p 697
79. Narins, p 1525
80. Ibid, p 1526
81. Ibid, p 1525
82. Ibid, p 636
83. Rose, p 704
84. Ibid, p 712
85. Pemberton, p 101
86. Ibid
87. Ibid, p 102
88. Schwartz, p 66
89. Rose, p 710
90. Ibid, p 721

91. Narins, p 1529
92. Oh, p 94
93. Ibid
94. Chernow, p 960
95. Narins, p 1529
96. Ibid
97. Schwartz, p 76
98. Votey S, Peters A, Hoffman J: Disorders of water metabolism: Hyponatremia and hypernatremia. Emerg Med Clin North Am 7:749,1989
99. Bell T: Diabetes insipidus. In: Endocrine and Metabolic Disturbances in the Critically Ill. Crit Care Nurs Clin N Am December:682,1994
100. Ibid
101. Oh, p 94
102. Goldberger E: A Primer of Water, Electrolyte and Acid-Base Syndromes, 7th ed, p 35. Philadelphia, Lea & Febiger, 1986
103. Rose, p 697
104. Himmelstein D, Jones A, Woolhander S: Hypernatremic dehydration in nursing home patients: An indicator of neglect. J Am Geriatr Soc 31:466,1983
105. Rose, p 710
106. Ibid, p 704
107. Cohen M: Sodium chloride vial concentrations above 0.9% should make you nervous. Intravenous Nurses Society Newsline 15(5):8,10,1994
108. Ibid
109. Ibid, p 1559
110. Ibid, p 1560
111. Ibid
112. Ibid
113. Ibid
114. Narins, p 1561
115. Ibid
116. Guyton A: Textbook of Medical Physiology, 8th ed, p 807. Philadelphia, WB Saunders, 1991
117. Costrini A: Emergency treatment of exertional heatstroke and comparison of whole body cooling techniques. Med Sci Sports Exerc 22(1):15,1990
118. Wyndham C, Strydom B, Cooke H: Methods of cooling subjects with hyperpyrexia. J App Physiol 14:771,1959
119. Kielblock A, VanRensberg J, Franz R: Body cooling as a method for reducing hyperpyrexia. South African Med J 69:378,1986
120. Magazinik A, et al: Tap water, an efficient method for cooling heatstroke victims—A model in dogs. Aviat Space Environ Med 5:864,1980
121. Guyton, p 807
122. Narins, p 1526
123. LaDou J: Occupational Medicine, p 111. Norwalk, Appleton & Lange, 1990
124. Narins, p 1567
125. Goldberger, p 35
126. Carter J, Gisolfi C: Fluid replacement during and after exercise in the heat. Med Sci Sports Exerc 21:532,1989
127. Hiller W: Dehydration and hyponatremia during triathlons. Med Sci Sports Exerc 21:S219,1989
128. Ibid
129. Ibid
130. Eisma T: Cool under fire: Wearers of heat-protective clothing must avoid heat stress. Occup Health Saf November:26,1989
131. Squire D: Heat illness: Fluid and electrolyte issues for pediatric and adolescent athletes. Pediatr Clin N Am 37(5):1085–1090,1990

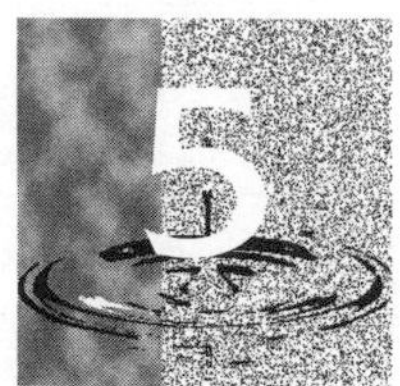

Potassium Imbalances

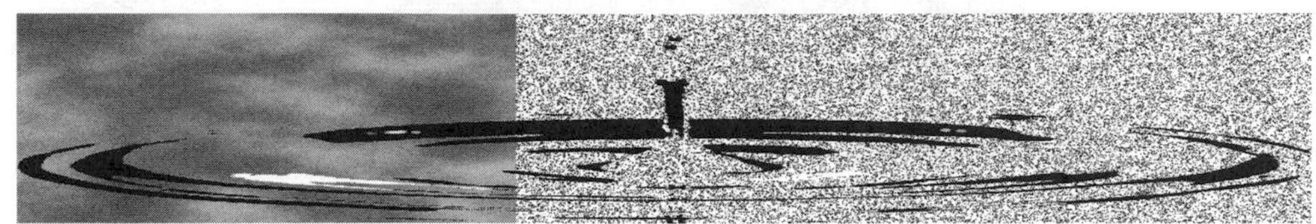

Disturbances in potassium balance are common because they are associated with a number of disease and injury states. Unfortunately, they may also be induced by the administration of a variety of medications as well as by therapies such as hyperalimentation and chemotherapy.

It is important to review some pertinent facts about potassium before proceeding to discussions of hypokalemia and hyperkalemia.

POTASSIUM BALANCE

Potassium is the major *intracellular* electrolyte; in fact, 98% of the body's potassium is inside the cells. The remaining 2% is in the extracellular fluid (ECF): this 2% is all-important in neuromuscular function. For example, alterations in plasma potassium concentrations can significantly affect myocardial irritability and rhythm. Electrocardiogram (ECG) changes associated with serum potassium level variations are illustrated in Figure 5-1.

Normal renal function is necessary for maintenance of potassium balance as 80% of the potassium excreted daily from the body is by way of the kidneys. The other 20% is lost through the bowel and sweat glands.

Potassium must be replaced daily, either enterally or parenterally; approximately 40 to 60 mEq/day suffice in the adult if there are no abnormal losses occurring. Dietary intake in the average adult is 50 to 100 mEq/day.[1] Because potassium is plentiful in the normal diet (in meat, fruits, and some vegetables), poor dietary intake rarely causes hypokalemia; however, it contributes to other causes of hypokalemia.

Potassium is constantly moving in and out of cells according to the body's needs, under the influence of the sodium–potassium pump. For example, alterations in acid–base balance can have a significant effect on potassium distribution: potassium ions move into the cells when alkalosis is present and out of the cells when acidosis occurs. In the presence of acid–base disturbances, the plasma potassium level may not reflect the true status of total body potassium stores. The reader is referred to Chapter 9 for a more thorough discussion of the effect of acidemia and alkalemia on plasma potassium concentration.

HYPOKALEMIA

Most laboratories list the normal plasma potassium range as 3.5 to 5.0 mEq/L. *Hypokalemia* refers to a below-normal serum potassium concentration. Mild hypokalemia is arbitrarily defined as ranging between 3.0 and 3.5 mEq/L. This degree of potassium depletion is usually well tolerated in the absence of digitalis therapy or severe hepatic disease.[2] Moderate hypokalemia is arbitrarily said to range between 2.5 and 3.0 mEq/L, whereas severe hypokalemia is generally defined as $<$2.5 mEq/L.[3] Hypokalemia usually indicates a real deficit in total potassium stores; however, it may occur in patients having normal potassium stores when alkalosis is present (because alkalosis causes a temporary shift of serum potassium into the cells). Hypokalemia is a common disturbance with a number of etiologies. Frequently, a combination of factors predisposes to hypokalemia.

ETIOLOGICAL FACTORS

Gastrointestinal Losses

Gastrointestinal (GI) losses of potassium are probably the most common cause of potassium depletion. Vomiting and gastric suction frequently lead to hypokalemia, partly because of actual potassium loss in gastric fluid, but largely because of increased renal potassium loss associated with metabolic alkalosis. (Recall that loss of acidic gastric fluid causes metabolic alkalosis; then, the kidneys attempt to conserve hydrogen ions to correct the pH disturbances. In this process, potassium ions are lost in greater amounts.)

Relatively large amounts of potassium are contained in intestinal fluids; for example, diarrheal fluid may contain as much as 30 mEq/L. Therefore, potassium deficit occurs frequently with diarrhea, prolonged intestinal suction, recent ileostomy, and villous adenoma. A dramatic cause of diarrheal potassium loss occurs with villous adenomas, with which up to 1 to 3 L of potassium-rich fluid (as high as 80 mEq/L) may be lost.[4]

Renal Losses

Hyperaldosteronism increases renal potassium wasting and can lead to severe potassium depletion. Primary hyperaldosteronism is relatively rare, occur-

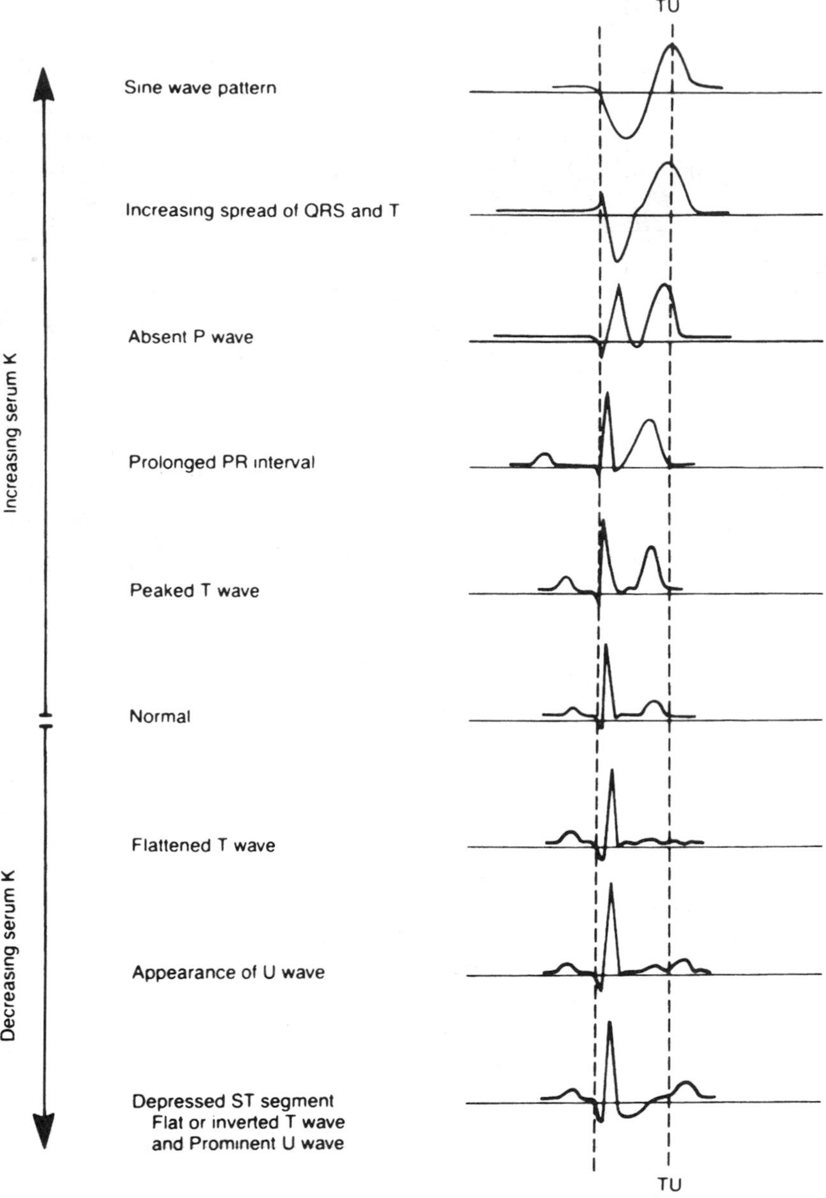

Figure 5–1. ECG manifestations of hypokalemia and hyperkalemia. Either extreme in the serum potassium level may lead to ventricular fibrillation; ventricular standstill or complete heart block is more common in hyperkalemia. From Zull D: Disorders of potassium metabolism. Emerg Med Clin North Am 7(4):783, 1989.

ring in patients with adrenal adenomas and adrenal hyperplasia. Secondary hyperaldosteronism is a common occurrence in patients with cirrhosis, nephrotic syndrome, congestive heart failure, and malignant hypertension.

Potassium-losing diuretics, such as the thiazides, furosemide, and ethacrynic acid, can certainly induce hypokalemia, particularly when given in high doses to patients with poor potassium intake. Approximately 20% to 30% of patients taking 50 mg of hydrochlorothiazide (HCTZ) daily develop hypokalemia.[5] Combined use of thiazides and furosemide greatly increases the likelihood of serious hypokalemia. Surreptitious use of diuretics to control weight is an increasing problem in these days of easy drug availability.

Renal potassium wasting may also be caused by certain medications, such as amphotericin B, gentamicin, cisplatin, and levodopa (L-dopa).[6] In fact, hypokalemia due to increased urinary losses occurs in up to half of patients receiving amphotericin B.[7] Also implicated as potential causes of hypokalemia are some of the penicillin derivatives (including sodium penicillin, ampicillin, carbenicillin, oxacillin, nafcillin, and ticarcillin).[8]

High serum glucocorticoid levels, as occur in Cushing's syndrome, or excessive steroid administration, for conditions such as arthritis or asthma, can cause potassium depletion.

European licorice contains glycyrrhizinic acid, a substance that has a pharmacological action similar to mineralocorticoid; thus, excessive intake of this substance can cause hypokalemia.

The osmotic diuresis associated with glucosuria causes real potassium wasting, which is presumably associated with increased fluid delivery to the distal tubular potassium secretory site.

Shift Into Cells

In alkalosis, hydrogen ions shift out of the cells to help correct the pH defect; potassium ions from the ECF move into the cells to maintain electroneutrality. (See Chapter 9 for a more thorough discussion of the effects of alkalemia on plasma potassium concentration.)

Entry of potassium into skeletal muscle and hepatic cells is promoted by insulin. Thus, patients with persistent insulin hypersecretion may experience hypokalemia. This is often seen in individuals receiving high-carbohydrate parenteral fluids (as in hyperalimentation). Later in the chapter insulin administration is discussed as a therapeutic measure for temporary relief of life-threatening hyperkalemia.

Catecholamines promote potassium entry into the cells. Therefore, transient hypokalemia can be induced when epinephrine release is enhanced by the stress of an acute illness, such as an episode of coronary ischemia, acute head trauma, and post-cardiopulmonary resuscitation. Similarly, the plasma potassium concentration can fall by 0.5 to 1 mEq/L after the administration of a beta-adrenergic agonist (such as albuterol or dobutamine) to treat asthma or heart failure.[9]

Hypothermia stimulates the cellular uptake of extracellular potassium; this hypokalemic effect is reversible upon rewarming.[10] If the hypokalemia is treated with vigorous potassium replacement, "overshoot" hyperkalemia may occur. If irreversible tissue necrosis occurs during a period of profound hypothermia (as in patients who are essentially dead after accidental hypothermia), a plasma potassium concentration of more than 10 to 20 mEq/L may be found.[11]

Sweat Losses

Potassium deficit related to heavy perspiration is most likely to occur in persons who are acclimated to heat as sweat glands in these individuals tend to excrete more potassium than in those who are not acclimated to heat stress. The mechanism involved is presumably the result of an aldosterone-related effect attempting to conserve sodium (the primary electrolyte in sweat). Sweat losses exceeding 10 L/day have been reported in individuals exercising in a hot climate.

Poor Intake

Patients unable or unwilling to eat a normal diet for a prolonged period are candidates for hypokalemia. However, strict fasting usually induces only a moderate depletion of total body potassium if normal homeostatic mechanisms are present. Usually poor intake is coupled with other problems in individuals with low serum potassium levels. For example, in addition to poor intake, individuals with anorexia nervosa frequently abuse diuretics and laxatives and induce vomiting to maintain a low body weight. Also, alcoholics frequently have other factors predisposing to hypokalemia (such as vomiting, diarrhea, and magnesium deficiency). Refeeding a malnourished patient can lead to serious hypokalemia if inadequate potassium is supplied because insulin release is stimulated by the feeding and promotes anabolism with entry of potassium into the cells.

DEFINING CHARACTERISTICS

Because potassium is the major cation in intracellular fluid (ICF), it is understandable that potassium deficit can result in widespread derangements in normal physiological functioning. Some of the more common changes are discussed below. It must be remembered that severe hypokalemia can result in death from cardiac or respiratory arrest. Clinical signs are usually not present until the potassium level falls below 3.0 mEq/L. Among the exceptions are patients with even mild hypokalemia who are receiving digitalis (predisposing them to a greater chance for dysrhythmias) and patients with hepatic failure (who are more prone to hepatic encephalopathy because of increased ammonia production).

Cardiac Changes

The major cardiac effects of hypokalemia include abnormalities of electrophysiology and contractility. The most important cardiac derangement associated with hypokalemia is the potential for a variety of atrial and ventricular arrhythmias, particularly in patients with ischemic myocardial disease and those receiving digitalis preparations. Because hypokalemia is associated with increased binding of digitalis to Na^+-K^+-ATPase, cardiac sensitivity to digitalis preparations is heightened by hypokalemia.[12] In many instances, hypokalemia and hypomagnesemia occur together; the most serious consequence of this combination of imbalances is increased cardiac irritability and risk for arrhythmias.

Neuromuscular Changes

Potassium levels less than 3.0 mEq/L may be associated with muscular weakness and adynamic ileus. At least two mechanisms are involved; the first involves changes in the resting membrane potential and the other has to do with altered operation of intracellular enzymes. Muscle weakness does not usually start until the plasma potassium concentration is less than 2.5 mEq/L; the lower extremities are usually involved first (particularly the quadriceps).[13] Later, in severe cases, the muscles of the trunk and upper extremities are involved, eventually causing death from respiratory failure if the condition is not corrected. Symptoms, such as anorexia, nausea, vomiting, prolonged gastric emptying, gaseous distention, and paralytic ileus, are due to weakness of the smooth muscles of the GI tract and impairment of the response to parasympathetic stimulation.

Renal Changes

Prolonged potassium depletion can lead to inability to maximally concentrate urine. This, in turn, results in dilute urine, polyuria, nocturia, and polydipsia. The reduced ability to concentrate urine is the result of a decreased responsiveness to antidiuretic hormone (ADH).[14] The resistance to ADH appears to be due to interference with the generation and action of cyclic adenosine monophosphate (cAMP).[15]

Rhabdomyolysis

A condition called *rhabdomyolysis* (disintegration of striated muscle fibers with excretion of myoglobin in the urine) can occur with potassium depletion. Rhabdomyolysis is usually only seen when the plasma potassium level is less than 2.5 mEq/L.[16] Possible causes of this condition are muscle ischemia due to direct effects of hypokalemia on muscle cell metabolism; it is made worse by exercising because hypokalemia blocks the vasodilation that normally occurs during exercise.[17]

TREATMENT

The best treatment for hypokalemia is prevention. For patients at risk, a diet with ample potassium content should be provided. Table 5-1 lists some foods with high potassium content. However, once hypokalemia has developed, dietary potassium intake may be ineffective replacement because most potassium in foods is complexed to anions that metabolize into bicarbonate.[18] For example, potassium-rich foods such as orange juice or bananas contain phosphate and citrate rather than chloride and therefore are less likely to correct hypokalemia associated with metabolic alkalosis. Therefore, patients with significant hypokalemia associated with metabolic alkalosis should be given potassium chloride (KCl).[19] Because KCl is efficiently absorbed through the GI tract, no more solution should be given orally than would be given intravenously (IV) over 2 to 3 hrs.[20]

When dietary intake is inadequate, the physician may prescribe one of the commercially prepared potassium substitutes (available in liquids, effervescent tablets, capsules, or slow-release tablets) (see Clinical Tip: Nursing Considerations in Administering Oral Potassium Supplements). Also available for potassium supplementation are potassium-containing salt substitutes (which usually contain

TABLE 5–1

Some Foods with High Potassium Content

FOOD	POTASSIUM (mg)	POTASSIUM (mEq APPROXIMATE)
Fruits		
Apricots, raw, 3 medium	313	8.0
Bananas, raw, 1 medium	451	11.6
Cantaloupe, raw, 1 cup pieces	494	12.7
Dates, dried, 10	541	13.9
Orange, 1 medium	250	6.4
Raisins, dried, seedless, 2/3 cup	751	19.3
Vegetables		
Avocado, raw, Florida, 1 medium	1484	38.1
Carrot, raw, 1 medium	233	6.0
Potato, baked, without skin, 1 medium	610	15.6
Tomato, red, raw, 1	273	7.0
Beverages		
Apricot nectar, canned, 8 fl oz	286	7.3
Orange juice, canned, 8 fl oz	436	11.2
Milk, 1% fat, 8 fl oz	381	9.8

Pennington J: Bowes and Church's Food Values of Portions Commonly Used, 16th ed. Philadelphia, JB Lippincott, 1994.

between 50 and 65 mEq of potassium per level teaspoon)(see Table 5-2).[21] When possible, treatment of hypokalemia by oral replacement is favored because this route allows the serum potassium to rise slowly in equilibration with the intracellular compartment.

Usual maintenance requirements for potassium are 40 to 60 mEq/day in patients with no abnormal routes of potassium loss or other above-average needs for replacement (such as hyperalimentation). When potassium cannot be consumed in adequate amounts in the diet, and when oral potassium supplements are not feasible, the IV route is indicated for replacement. The IV route is mandatory for patients with severe hypokalemia (such as <2.5 mEq/L)(see Clinical Tip: Nursing Considerations in Administering Potassium Intravenously).

Although KCl is usually used to replace potassium deficits, the physician may prescribe potassium acetate or potassium phosphate. Potassium acetate can be used to treat patients with potassium loss associated with metabolic acidosis (as in renal tubular acidosis and potassium-losing nephritis); the acetate is metabolized to bicarbonate and thus helps correct the acidosis. Potassium phosphate is used when the patient has deficits of both potassium and phosphate.

Factors such as shifting of potassium in and out of the cells make it difficult to precisely identify the amount of potassium needed to correct potassium deficit by assessing plasma potassium levels. However, in general, when the plasma potassium level falls from 4.0 to 3.0 mEq/L, there is apparently a deficit of 200 to 400 mEq of potassium.[39] An additional 200 to 400 mEq potassium deficit will lower the plasma potassium concentration to 2.0 mEq/L.[40]

As with other imbalances, the aim of treatment in hypokalemia is to get the patient out of danger, not to immediately correct the entire potassium deficit. A case described by Rose[41] dramatically makes this point: a patient with profound hypokalemia had flaccid paralysis; when 80 mEq of potassium was administered over 15 min, the ECG changed from one typical of hypokalemia to one characteristic of severe hyperkalemia. It must be remembered that the administered potassium needs

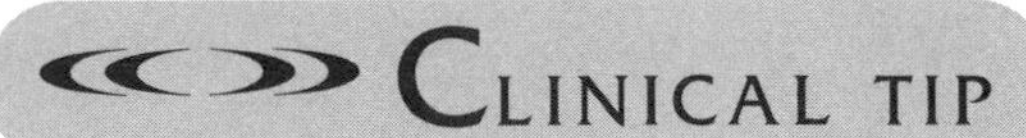

Nursing Considerations in Administering Oral Potassium Supplements

1. The most common adverse reactions to oral potassium salts are nausea, vomiting, abdominal discomfort, and diarrhea. To help minimize GI irritation, administer potassium supplements immediately after meals or with food.

2. Hyperkalemia can result from oral overdosage, just as it can from intravenous overdosage. Therefore, care should be taken to administer the intended dose. Because there are numerous forms of potassium supplements available commercially, with highly variable concentrations, it is important to check the physician's order carefully against the preparation's label (some trade names are quite similar).

3. A single oral dose of potassium should probably not exceed the hourly intravenous dose (used in more life-threatening situations).[22] The ingestion of more than 160 mEq can produce a potentially fatal increase in the serum potassium concentration to >8.0 mEq/L, even when normal renal function is present.[23]

4. Potassium supplements are contraindicated in patients receiving potassium-sparing diuretics (ie, spironolactone [Aldactone], triameterene [Dyrenium], and amiloride [Midamor]).

5. Dosages of potassium supplements need to be decreased (or perhaps even discontinued) if the patient begins to use generous portions of potassium-containing salt substitutes.

6. Slow-release tablets should be administered with a full glass of water to help them dissolve in the GI tract. Observe patients taking slow-release KCl tablets for GI bleeding as these tablets may cause intestinal and gastric ulceration. Do not crush potassium tablets unless the manufacturer's directions specifically state that it is appropriate.

7. Effervescent potassium supplements should be dissolved in 3 to 8 oz cold water, juice, or suitable beverage and consumed slowly.[24]

8. The majority of patients with hypokalemia have mild to moderate decreases in serum potassium levels (such as 3.0–3.5 mEq/L); this range is usually well tolerated in the absence of digitalis therapy or severe hepatic disease. Provided they can swallow, these patients can usually be treated with oral potassium supplements in the range of 60–80 mEq/day.[25]

time to equilibrate with cellular stores; it may take days to totally correct the entire potassium deficit.

NURSING INTERVENTIONS

1. Be aware of patients at risk for hypokalemia and monitor for its occurrence (see Summary of Hypokalemia.) Because hypokalemia can be life-threatening, it is important to detect it early.
2. Assess digitalized patients at risk for hypokalemia especially closely for symptoms of digitalis toxicity because hypokalemia potentiates the action of digitalis. Be aware that the physician usually prefers to keep the serum potassium level in the high normal range in digitalized patients.

(text continues on page 104)

TABLE 5–2

Potassium and Sodium Content of Some Salt Substitutes

FOOD	POTASSIUM (mg/tsp)	SODIUM (mg/tsp)
Morton Lite salt	1500 (38 mEq)	1100
Morton salt substitute	2800 (72 mEq)	—
Morton seasoned salt substitute	2100 (54 mEq)	—
No Salt salt alternative	2500 (64 mEq)	5
No Salt salt alternative, seasoned	1330 (34 mEq)	2
Nu-Salt	528 (13.5 mEq)	0
Table salt (reference)	—	2300

Pennington J: Bowes and Church's Food Values of Portions Commonly Used, 16th ed, p 286. Philadelphia, JB Lippincott, 1994.

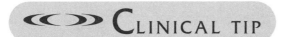

Nursing Considerations in Administering Potassium Intravenously

1. Concentrated potassium solutions from ampules should never be administered without first being diluted appropriately.

   Because of reports of deaths caused by the accidental injection of undiluted potassium chloride injections, the United States Pharmacopeia (USP) recently renamed the drug "potassium chloride for injection concentrate." To decrease the likelihood of mistaking the concentrate for a ready-to-use solution, the caps and overseals bear the words "must be diluted" and black bands with the words "must be diluted" appear on ampules (effective January 15, 1993).[26] Furthermore, in order to minimize errors, many hospitals have removed potassium chloride for injection concentrate from nursing units and replaced it with minibags of potassium chloride injection 20 mEq/100 ml.[27] The rationale is that if that form of the drug is administered in error, it is not likely to seriously harm anyone.

2. The appropriate dilution of potassium chloride solutions depends on (a) the amount of fluid the patient can tolerate, (b) the site of administration (peripheral or central vein), and (c) the patient's tolerance for pain at the infusion site.

   Fluid Tolerance

   It is safer to dilute potassium to the maximal point allowed without exceeding the patient's tolerance for fluid. For example, if a patient requires 80 mEq of KCl in 24 hr, and the fluid intake for that period is 2000 mL, the 80 mEq of KCl should be divided equally between the 2 L of allowable fluid (that is, 40 mEq/L). However, if a patient requires more potassium than can be administered at "typical" dilutions, it becomes necessary to administer more concentrated solutions. See below.

(continued)

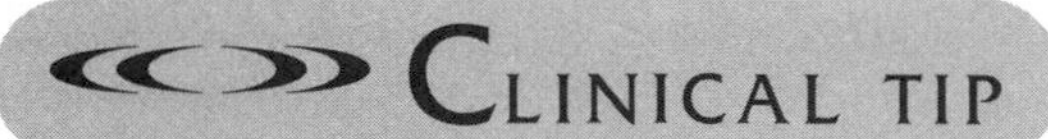

Nursing Considerations in Administering Potassium Intravenously (cont.)

Site

Peripheral Vein. A typical concentration of potassium for peripheral veins is 20 to 40 mEq/L.[28] The most frequently recommended maximal concentration of KCl in a peripheral vein is 60 mEq/L because higher concentrations are very irritating, resulting in pain and sclerosis of veins.[29,30]

Central Vein. The maximal recommended concentration in a central vein is variably defined as 140 mEq/L (14 mEq/100 mL) [31] to 200 mEq/L (20 mEq/100 mL).[31] Unlike peripheral veins, central veins have a large blood flow, thereby allowing dilution of the irritating potassium solution. Although some authors have expressed concern that administering concentrated potassium solutions through central veins near the myocardium could cause dysrhythmias, this was not shown to be a problem in a study of 495 sets of KCl infusions administered to a population in a medical intensive care unit.[33]

Tolerance for Pain at Infusion Site

Administration of KCl in a peripheral vein at a concentration >40 mEq/L is often associated with discomfort that increases as the concentration of KCl increases. Pain is more likely if the patient already has phlebitis associated with prolonged intravenous cannulation at the site and other irritating medications are also administered. The following steps are helpful in minimizing pain associated with the administration of KCl solutions:

(A) Dilute the KCl as much as possible.
(B) If a central line is in place, consider using this site for the infusion because rapid blood flow will dilute the KCl solution.
(C) If necessary, discuss with the physician the use of a small volume of lidocaine (either as a bolus through the IV device before the infusion or added to the solution) to minimize pain. Several studies have indicated that this method is of some benefit in alleviating pain associated with concentrated KCl solutions in peripheral veins:

> In a double-blind study of 28 subjects, researchers evaluated the effectiveness of a pretreatment IV bolus dose of 3 mL of lignocaine (versus a placebo bolus dose of 3 mL of 0.9% NaCl) at the infusion site in alleviating pain associated with the administration of concentrated KCl solutions (20 mEq/100 mL) over a 2-hr period. They concluded that pain at the IV site was signficantly reduced in the group that received the lignocaine bolus dose.[34]
>
> In an earlier study, the effect of lidocaine in alleviating pain induced by intravenous KCl administration was evaluated in six healthy volunteers.[35] Each subject received KCl in a concentration of 200 mEq/L (10 mEq of KCl in 50 mL D_5W) in both arms. One of the infusions had 10 mg of lidocaine added (although the subject was not told which infusion contained the lidocaine). The solutions were infused over 1 hr and each person was asked to rate the degree of pain in each arm on a 7-point scale (1 = mild, 7 = severe). It was found that pain was significantly less in the arm with the lidocaine (mean, 3.17) than in the arm without lidocaine (mean, 6.17). It is worth noting, however, that pain was still at least moderate in the group receiving the lidocaine.

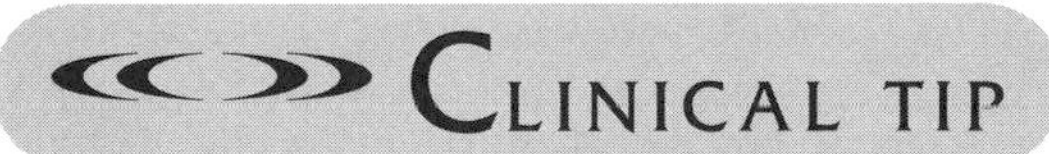

Nursing Considerations in Administering Potassium Intravenously (cont.)

Tolerance for Pain at Infusion Site (cont.)

3. Rate of administration is dependent on the urgency for potassium replacement:

   In usual situations, potassium is administered at a rate not exceeding 10 mEq/hr. In the presence of mild to moderate hypokalemia, it is safer to administer potassium at a rate no faster than 10–20 mEq/hr. Rates greater than 40 mEq/hr are not recommended because of the possibility of producing transient hyperkalemia and arrhythmias.[36] However, as much as 40–100 mEq/hr have reportedly been given to patients with paralysis or life-threatening arrhythmias.[37] Rapid potassium administration is potentially dangerous even in severely potassium-depleted patients and should be used only in life-threatening situations—ECG monitoring is essential in this setting.

4. Because potassium is primarily eliminated through the kidneys, it is important to monitor carefully the rate of urinary output. When giving potassium, a urine output >30 mL/hr is recommended to avoid producing transient hyperkalemia.[38] If potassium replacement is needed in oliguric patients, the amount is reduced according to the level of renal function.

5. Because dextrose administered concurrently with potassium can cause a transient shift of potassium into the cells, urgent potassium replacement for severely hypokalemic patients is usually accomplished with a nondextrose solution (such as 0.9% sodium chloride solution).

6. Protocols for the safe administration of potassium solutions in specific institutions/agencies should be jointly written by nurses, physicians, and pharmacists. Such protocols are immensely helpful in preventing problems with potassium infusions. General precautions include:

   (A) Limit the amount of potassium available in a single container (such as 20 mEq in 100 mL of solution) to avoid accidental overinfusion
   (B) Use an infusion pump to control the flow rate, and carefully monitor the rate to be sure that the pump doesn't malfunction. (Also, remember that KCl inadvertently administered into subcutaneous tissue is extremely injurious and needs to be detected early; pumps will continue to infuse KCl, regardless of whether the cannula is in the vein or subcutaneous tissue).
   (C) Mix KCl solutions with great care. Preferably, KCl solutions should be mixed in the pharmacy. If required to mix these solutions on a nursing unit, squeeze the medicine ports of plastic containers while they are in the upright position and then mix by inversion and agitation. Never add KCl to a hanging container (this can result in a high concentration bolus of the drug being administered). Commercially available premixed potassium-containing solutions are available in commonly prescribed concentrations for routine infusions.

3. Take measures to prevent hypokalemia when possible.
   A. Prevention may take the form of encouraging extra potassium intake for at-risk patients (when the diet allows). Some foods high in potassium (and relatively low in sodium) are listed in Table 5-1. Of course, one must always consider dietary restrictions imposed by other conditions (such as diabetes mellitus or obesity).
   B. When hypokalemia is due to abuse of laxatives or diuretics, education of the patient may help alleviate the problem. Part of the nursing history and assessment should be directed at identifying problems amenable to prevention through education.

Summary of Hypokalemia

ETIOLOGICAL FACTORS

Gastrointestinal Loss
- Diarrhea
- Laxative abuse
- Prolonged gastric suction
- Villous adenoma

Renal Loss
- Potassium-losing diuretics
- Hyperaldosteronism
- Sodium penicillin, carbenicillin, or amphotericin B
- Steroid administration
- Osmotic diuresis

Shift into Cells
- Alkalosis
- Excessive secretion or administration of insulin
- Hyperalimentation

Poor Intake
- Anorexia nervosa
- Alcoholism
- Debilitation

DEFINING CHARACTERISTICS

Skeletal Muscle
- Fatigue
- Weakness (initially most prominent in legs, especially the quadriceps, and then extending to the arms; involvement of respiratory muscles soon follows)
- Cramps
- Rhabdomyolysis

Cardiovascular System
- Increased sensitivity to digitalis
- ST segment depression
- Flattened T waves
- Ventricular arrhythmias
- Cardiac arrest

Gastrointestinal System
- Decreased bowel motility (intestinal ileus)

Renal System
- Impaired urinary concentrating ability when hypokalemia is prolonged, causing dilute urine, polyuria, nocturia, and polydipsia
- Increased ammonia production and H^+ excretion

Lab Data
- Serum potassium <3.5 mEq/L
- Often associated with alkalosis

4. Keep in mind the points summarized in Clinical Tip: Nursing Considerations in Administering Oral Potassium Supplements when administering potassium supplements.
5. Educate patients regarding the use of salt substitutes, keeping the following facts in mind:
   A. Salt substitutes may contain from 50 to 60 mEq of potassium per teaspoon. Although they are often viewed as helpful for those taking potassium-losing diuretics (such as furosemide or thiazides), they can be dangerous for patients taking potassium-conserving diuretics (such as spironolactone, triamterene, and amiloride).
   B. As with any potassium-containing substance, there is a danger of hyperkalemia with excessive use, particularly if renal function is impaired and/or the patient is taking pharmacologic potassium supplements.
6. Be thoroughly familiar with the nursing considerations involved with administering potassium intravenously (see Clinical Tip: Nursing Considerations in Administering Potassium Intravenously).

CASE STUDIES

5-1. A 40-year-old woman was admitted to the hospital with complaints of progressive muscle weakness. She had been taking a thiazide diuretic for several weeks and had recently developed vomiting and diarrhea. Postural hypotension was noted to be present (110/70 mmHg when supine and 90/60 mmHg when upright). Skin turgor was reduced. Laboratory data included the following:

Plasma K = 2 mEq/L
HCO_3 = 40 mEq/L
Cl = 70 mEq/L

COMMENTARY: This patient had increased losses of potassium from the GI tract as well as in the urine. Her major presenting symptom, diffuse progressive muscle weakness, is common in hypokalemia. In addition to hypokalemia, signs of FVD were present (reduced skin turgor and postural hypotension). Recall that postural hypotension can also be a sign of hypokalemia. On questioning, it was found that she was taking a friend's diuretic to induce weight loss. Note the presence of hypochloremic alkalosis (below-normal chloride and greatly elevated bicarbonate).

5-2. A 65-year-old man with a draining intestinal fistula was receiving a total parenteral nutrition (TPN) solution at the rate of 120 mL/hr. The total potassium intake was 100 mEq/day. On a routine ECG, flattened T waves, ST segment depression, and arrhythmias were detected. A blood sample was then drawn that revealed a plasma potassium level of 2.5 mEq/L. The rate of TPN infusion was tapered promptly, the serum glucose levels were monitored closely, and an IV infusion of KCl was initiated in a peripheral vein at the rate of 10 mEq/hr. After alleviation of the signs of hypokalemia, the TPN infusion was slowly reinstituted with adequate potassium added.

COMMENTARY: Potassium requirements in the patient receiving TPN are variable, ranging between 18 and 80 mEq/L of solution administered.[42] Most often there is greater than usual potassium need as, during nutritional repletion, potassium will be deposited in the newly synthesized cells, causing serum levels to fall abruptly if potassium is not supplied in sufficient amounts. This patient's needs were even greater than usual because intestinal fistulas result in significant potassium loss.

5-3. A 31-year-old woman with a history of acute leukemia was admitted to an acute care facility with fever. On admission, her serum potassium level was 4.1 mEq/L. To deal with the infection, she was started on ticarcillin disodium, 3 g intravenous piggyback (IVPB) every 4 hrs, and tobramycin, 90 mg, IVPB, every 8 hrs. Isotonic saline was administered at a rate of 40 mL/hr. On the third day of hospitalization, her serum potassium was noted to have fallen to 2.8 mEq/L. She complained of weakness, fatigue, anorexia, and constipation. Potassium was replaced by the parenteral route until oral supplements could be tolerated.

COMMENTARY: As noted earlier in this chapter, sodium penicillin is associated with increased renal losses of potassium, particularly when volume depletion is present.

HYPERKALEMIA

Hyperkalemia refers to a greater-than-normal serum potassium concentration. It seldom occurs in patients with normal renal function. Apparently the incidence of hyperkalemia is twice as high in hospitalized adults older than 60 years of age than in younger hospitalized adults.[43] Like hypokalemia, hyperkalemia is often due to iatrogenic (treatment-induced) causes. Although less common than hypokalemia, it is often more dangerous because cardiac arrest is more frequently associated with high serum potassium levels.

ETIOLOGICAL FACTORS

Some of the causes of hyperkalemia are simple and straightforward (such as direct gain exceeding the kidney's excretory rate). Others are related to shifts of potassium out of the cells into the plasma, or to decreased production of aldosterone, which causes potassium retention. Note the potassium-elevating influence exerted by several commonly used drugs, particularly when there are preexisting abnormalities in potassium metabolism. (See pp. 107–108.)

Pseudohyperkalemia

A number of causes of factitious ("pseudo") hyperkalemia exist. When the blood sample is allowed to hemolyze, potassium leaks from ruptured erythrocytes into the serum. In a recent study, 61 (19.8%) of 308 patients were found to have single elevated serum potassium measurements on samples that were noted to be grossly hemolyzed.[44] Other causes of pseudohyperkalemia include marked leukocytosis or thrombocytosis, drawing blood above a site where potassium is being infused, and obtaining a sample from an extremity in which repeated clenching and unclenching of the fist has been performed. Pseudohyperkalemia should be suspected when there is no apparent cause for elevated plasma potassium and there are no changes in muscle strength or on ECG tracings.[45]

Although the effect of fist clenching has been recognized for many years,[46] it continues to be a problem. Don et al.[47] reported a case in which a man was admitted for evaluation of hyperkalemia. Blood drawn from this individual in an outpatient setting (using a tourniquet with repeated fist clenching and unclenching) had a serum potassium concentration of 6.9 mmol/L. In the hospital, blood drawn from an indwelling catheter (without use of a tourniquet and fist clenching) had a normal value of 4.1 mmol/L. (It increased to 5.1 mmol/L within 1 min after application of a tourniquet and repeated fist clenching.) The researchers concluded that it is advisable to avoid fist clenching altogether when obtaining samples for potassium testing and to rely on venous stasis alone, if needed, as an aid in performing phlebotomy.

Failure to be aware of factitious causes of hyperkalemia can result in aggressive treatment of the nonexistent hyperkalemia with serious lowering of serum potassium levels. Some clinicians favor obtaining an ECG when the reported value exceeds 6.0 mEq/L. Absence of ECG evidence for hyperkalemia is usually consistent with a factitious reading because higher levels of hyperkalemia, 7 to 10 mEq/L, are almost always accompanied by ECG abnormalities.[48] However, on rare occasions, severe hyperkalemia can present without typical ECG manifestations. Moderate levels of hyperkalemia are more difficult to detect by ECG. A recent study of 220 ECGs performed on patients at risk for hyperkalemia indicated that ECG interpretations made by two separate physicians were not especially good predictors of hyperkalemia; this caused the researchers to caution that it is prudent to delay treatment for hyperkalemia in stable patients until confirmatory serum values can be obtained to confirm the presence of hyperkalemia.[49]

Decreased Renal Excretion

A major cause of hyperkalemia is decreased renal excretion of potassium. This is understandable when one considers that the kidney is the major route of potassium excretion. Significant hyperkalemia, therefore, is commonly seen in untreated patients with renal failure, particularly when potassium is being liberated from cells during infectious processes or exogenous sources of potassium are excessive (as in diet or medications).

A deficiency of adrenal steroids causes sodium loss and potassium retention; thus, hypoaldosteronism and Addison's disease predispose to hyperkalemia. Between 40% and 65% of patients with chronic adrenal insufficiency manifest hyperkalemia on initial diagnosis.[50] Hyporeninemic hypoaldosteronism (type IV renal tubular acidosis) is a common renal cause of hyperkalemia. This condition is usually seen in elderly persons with mild renal insufficiency, many of whom are diabetic as well.[51]

Potassium-conserving diuretics, such as spironolactone (Aldactone), triamterene (Dyrenium), and amiloride (Midamor), are commonly implicated as causes of hyperkalemia (particularly when there is renal dysfunction, potassium supplementation, or concomitant use of other drugs predisposing to potassium retention). Serious and even fatal complications have been associated with these drugs.[52]

Trimethoprim (an antimicrobial) can impair renal excretion of potassium; therefore, when given in high doses to AIDS patients with *Pneumocystis carinii* pneumonia, it can produce hyperkalemia.[53] In a recent study, it was reported that hyperkalemia occurred in 20% to 53% of patients with AIDS while they were receiving high doses of trimethoprim in combination with sulfamethoxazole or dapsone for the treatment of *Pneumocystis carinii* pneumonia.[54]

Hyperkalemia occurs with a variety of nonsteroidal antiinflammatory drugs (NSAID) in association with renal insufficiency. However, only indomethacin (Indocin) and piroxican (Feldene) have been reported to produce clinically significant hyperkalemia in patients without underlying renal disease.[55] It appears that hyperkalemia is related to reduced plasma and urinary aldosterone levels.[56]

High Potassium Intake

Although sustained hyperkalemia is rarely observed after potassium ingestion in individuals with normal renal function, it can occur with massive oral potassium ingestion or by rapid IV potassium administration.

A case was reported in which a young physician took potassium in the form of a potassium-containing salt substitute to ward off hypokalemia after diuretic use and a bout of diarrhea.[57] On admission to a hospital, her plasma potassium concentration was 8.4 mmol/L. An ECG revealed signs of severe hyperkalemia (peaked T waves, absent P wave, and a broadened QRS complex). She experienced cardiorespiratory arrest and was resuscitated. After treatment, the hyperkalemia resolved; however, posthypoxic brain damage occurred.

Although excessive potassium intake by the oral route is less dangerous than the IV route (because GI absorption may be limited by either vomiting or diarrhea from the large potassium load), the above case illustrates that care is required with potassium administration in all situations. Cases are on record in which both intentional and accidental oral potassium overdosages have resulted in fatalities.[58,59]

Although potassium-containing salt substitutes are often recommended for patients requiring sodium restriction, they are contraindicated for patients on potassium-restricted diets or those with renal disease who have diminished capacity to excrete potassium. Note in Table 5-2 that the potassium content in most salt substitutes is quite high.

Because it is possible to exceed the renal tolerance of any patient with rapid IV potassium administration, extreme caution is required when administering potassium solutions (see Clinical Tip: Nursing Considerations in Administering Potassium Intravenously). The serum concentration of potassium increases as storage time of blood increases; therefore, aged blood should not be given to patients with impaired renal function (see Chapter 10). Even the potassium content of high-protein oral nutrient supplements can be a problem in some patients.

Shift of Potassium out of Cells

Shifting of potassium out of the cells into the extracellular fluid is influenced by many factors, such as tissue injury, lysis of malignant cells during chemotherapy, catabolism, and acidemia. For example, an elevated plasma potassium concentration should be anticipated when extensive tissue trauma has occurred, as can happen in crushing injuries or severe infections. Similarly, it can occur with lysis of malignant cells after administration of chemotherapy, particularly in lymphomas, leukemia, and myeloma. Starvation also causes cellular breakdown and release of potassium into the extracellular space.

Potassium leaks out of the cells in acidosis as hydrogen ions enter the cells to help correct the acidic extracellular pH. However, there is evidence that the extent of potassium shifting from the cells that occurs in acidemia is greatly influenced by the *cause* of the acidemia. That is, more shifting is associated with metabolic acidosis due to the accumulation of nonorganic acids (as occurs in diarrhea and renal failure) than in metabolic acidosis due to organic acids (such as lactic acidosis or ketoacidosis). Respiratory acidosis has less effect on potassium shifting than does metabolic acidosis. (The reader is referred to Chapter 9 for a more thorough discussion of this topic.)

Beta-adrenergic blockers (such as propranolol) increase the risk of hyperkalemia by interfering with entry of potassium into the cells. The increase in plasma potassium concentration is usually modest (0.2–0.5 mEq/L) and corrects on discontinuation of the drug.[60] Dangerous hyperkalemia is rarely due to beta-blockers alone,[61] but these blockers can exacerbate hyperkalemia in patients with other risk factors.[62] For example, dialysis patients treated with propranolol (Inderal) exhibit an approximately 1.0 mEq/L increase in predialysis serum potassium levels.[63] Digoxin has produced fatal hyperkalemia when taken in large amounts.[64] Although digitalis toxicity is aggravated by hypokalemia, severe digitalis intoxication poisons the Na^+-K^+-ATPase pump, resulting in potassium release from the cells and hyperkalemia.[65]

Other Causes

One study found captopril (an angiotensin-converting enzyme inhibitor) to be one of the drugs most frequently implicated in producing hyperkalemia.[66] Significant hyperkalemia has been reported in association with captopril in patients with renal insufficiency, presumably due to captopril's inhibitory effect on aldosterone secretion.[67]

Cyclosporin can cause hyperkalemia through a combination of mechanisms. For example, it can decrease potassium excretion, decrease prostaglandin production, and lower plasma renin and aldosterone levels.[68] Cyclosporin-induced hyperkalemia does not seem to be related either to dosage or duration of therapy.[69]

Because chronic heparin administration blocks a step in aldosterone synthesis, occasionally it can cause hyperkalemia.[70] Elevated serum potassium levels have been produced with heparin doses of 20,000 units/day.[71] Yet there are infrequent reports of heparin-induced hyperkalemia, despite widespread use of this drug.[72] However, in one study, heparin usage was present in a substantial percentage of patients having other conditions favoring hyperkalemia.[73]

DEFINING CHARACTERISTICS

Cardiac Effects

As the plasma potassium concentration is increased, disturbances in cardiac conduction occur. The earliest changes, often appearing at a serum potassium level greater than 6 mEq/L, are peaked narrow T waves and a shortened QT interval. If the serum potassium level continues to rise, the PR interval becomes prolonged and is followed by disappearance of the P waves. Finally, there is decomposition and prolongation of the QRS complex. Ventricular arrhythmias and cardiac arrest may occur at any point in this progression (see Fig. 5-1).

Hyperkalemia slows the heart rate, may cause atrioventricular (AV) block, and prolongs depolarization.[74] Factors exaggerating ECG changes of hyperkalemia are low serum sodium and calcium levels, as well as acidosis and a high serum magnesium concentration. These changes are counteracted by an increased serum calcium level, explaining why calcium infusion is an emergency treatment for serious hyperkalemia. Medications that may aggravate hyperkalemia include procainamide, propranolol, and heparin.[75]

In profound hyperkalemia, the heart becomes dilated and flaccid due to decreased strength of contraction (related to a decreased number of active muscle units). Detrimental myocardial effects of hyperkalemia are more pronounced when the serum potassium level elevates rapidly.

Neuromuscular Effects

Severe hyperkalemia causes muscle weakness and even paralysis related to a depolarization block in muscle. Typically, muscle weakness does not occur until the plasma potassium concentration is more than 8 mEq/L.[76] Usually muscle weakness and paralysis first affect the large muscles of the legs, followed by trunk and upper extremity muscles. Fortunately, the muscles controlled by the cranial nerves are spared, as are the muscles of respiration.[77] Cardiac muscle is also weakened by hyperkalemia; the ultimate cause of death may be cardiac failure in diastole.

Gastrointestinal Changes

Gastrointestinal symptoms, such as nausea, intermittent intestinal colic, or diarrhea, can occur in hyperkalemic patients.[78] These changes have been attributed to smooth-muscle hyperactivity.

TREATMENT

Restriction of Potassium Intake and Drugs Potentiating Hyperkalemia

In nonacute situations, adequate treatment may be limited to restriction of dietary potassium and discontinuance of agents predisposing to hyperkalemia (including potassium-sparing diuretics, potassium supplements, and potassium-containing salt substitutes). Other drugs that have a predisposing effect to hyperkalemia include nonsteroidal antiinflammatory agents, captopril, and beta-adrenergic blockers. (See previous discussion of possible etiological factors for hyperkalemia.)

Methods to Promote Potassium Excretion

Sodium Polystyrene Sulfonate

Sodium polystyrene sulfonate is a cation exchange resin that can be given orally or rectally to remove potassium from the body by exchanging sodium for potassium in the intestinal tract. Because it exchanges about 1.5 mEq Na^+ for each 1 mEq K^+ removed, the patient's tolerance for sodium must be considered.[79] For example, severe congestive heart failure limits the amount of resin that can be safely administered. Although it is an effective method for managing developing hyperkalemia because of its relatively slow onset, it should not be the sole treatment for severe hyperkalemia.

When given orally, it is usually administered with an osmotic agent (such as sorbitol) to prevent constipation. If the oral route cannot be used, the drug can be given by enema and retained for a period of at least 30 to 60 min. Each enema can lower the plasma potassium concentration by as much as 0.5 to 1.0 mEq/L.[80]

Dialysis

Dialysis can remove potassium effectively but should be reserved for situations in which more conservative methods do not suffice. Although peritoneal dialysis can be started relatively quickly, it is not as effective as hemodialysis. (For example, using 2-L exchanges cycled every 45 min, peritoneal dialysis can remove approximately 10–15 mEq/hr of potassium, as compared to 25–30 mEq/hr for hemodialysis.)[81] A major limitation of hemodialysis is the time needed to prepare the patient for the procedure.

Diuretics

In patients with normal renal function, diuretics (such as furosemide, 40–80 mg IV, or ethacrynic acid, 50–100 mg IV) have been shown to be effective in promoting potassium excretion and decreasing the total body potassium level.[82] These agents are most likely to be used in patients with chronic hyperkalemia due to hypoaldosteronism or heart failure.[83] Loop diuretics are of limited value in patients with severely impaired glomerular filtration rates.

Emergency Measures

Three generally accepted stop-gap measures for treating severe hyperkalemia include IV administration of (1) calcium gluconate, (2) sodium bicarbonate, and (3) insulin and hypertonic dextrose. These methods, and a relatively new treatment (use of a selective $beta_2$-adrenergic agonist) are briefly described below.

Calcium Gluconate

The intravenous administration of calcium gluconate immediately antagonizes the effects of hyperkalemia on the heart, even when the plasma calcium level is normal.[84] This protective effect begins within 1 or 2 min but lasts only about 30 to 60 min. However, this action allows time for one of the measures described below (administration of either insulin and hypertonic dextrose or sodium bicarbonate) to force serum potassium into the cells. The usual dose is 10 mL of a 10% calcium gluconate solution administered slowly over 2 to 3 min under electrocardiographic monitoring.[85] Calcium should be used only when absolutely necessary in patients taking digitalis, as hypercalcemia potentiates the toxic effects of digitalis on the myocardium. If calcium must be given to patients receiving digitalis, it should be added to 100 mL of 5% aqueous dextrose solution (D_5W) and infused slowly over 20 to 30 min.[86]

Sodium Bicarbonate

Sodium bicarbonate infusion temporarily shifts potassium into the cells, and is especially helpful if the patient has metabolic acidosis. The typical dose is a 50-mEq bolus of $NaHCO_3$ infused slowly over a 5-min period.[87] The onset of action is about 5 to 10 min and the effect lasts for about 2 hrs.[88] Possible problems associated with this treatment include expansion of the extracellular fluid and precipitation of congestive heart failure in patients with cardiac disease, as well as precipitation of tetany in patients with preexisting hypocalcemia.

Insulin and Glucose

Intravenous insulin stimulates potassium uptake by the cells, thereby reducing the plasma potassium concentration. A usual prescription is 10 units of regular insulin with 50 g of glucose given over 60 min.[89] (For example, this could be accomplished by adding 10 units of regular insulin to 500 mL of a 10% glucose solution.) The typical onset of insulin's hypokalemic action is about 30 min, and the effects may last for up to 4 to 6 hrs.

Beta$_2$-Adrenergic Agonists

Similar to insulin, the beta$_2$-adrenergic agonists temporarily force potassium into the cells.[90] The most frequently used agents for this purpose are salbutamol and albuterol; as a rule, the doses for lowering the plasma potassium concentration are significantly greater than the doses used for treating asthma.[91] In the nebulized form, albuterol (10–20 mg) has been shown to lower the plasma potassium concentration for up to 2 hrs.[92] Because of reports of ventricular arrhythmias with the use of beta$_2$-agonists, it has been suggested that these agents be used only when other approaches to control hyperkalemia have been unsuccessful.[93] Beta$_2$-adrenergic agonists should not be used in patients with active coronary disease.[94]

NURSING INTERVENTIONS

1. Be aware of patients at risk for hyperkalemia and monitor for its occurrence (see Summary of Hyperkalemia). Because hyperkalemia is life-threatening, it is imperative to detect it early.
2. Take measures to prevent hyperkalemia when possible by following guidelines for administering potassium safely, both orally and IV (see Clinical Tip: Nursing Considerations in Administering Oral Potassium Supplements and Clinical Tip: Nursing Considerations in Administering Potassium Intravenously).
3. Avoid administration of potassium-conserving diuretics, potassium supplements, or salt substitutes to patients with poor renal function.
4. Caution patients to use salt substitutes sparingly if they are taking other supplementary forms of potassium or are taking potassium-conserving diuretics (such as spironolactone, triamterene, and amiloride).
5. Caution hyperkalemic patients to avoid foods high in potassium content. These include chocolate, coffee, cocoa, tea, dried fruits, dried beans, whole-grain breads, and milk desserts.[95] Meat and eggs also contain substantial amounts of potassium (review Table 5-1). (Foods with minimal potassium content include butter, margarine, cranberry juice or sauce, ginger ale, gumdrops or jellybeans, lollipops, root beer, sugar, or honey.)[96]
6. To avoid false reports of hyperkalemia, take the following precautions:
   A. Avoid prolonged use of tourniquet while drawing blood sample.
   B. Do not allow patient to exercise extremity immediately before drawing blood sample.
   C. Take blood sample to the laboratory as soon as possible (serum must be separated from cells within 1 hr after collection).
   D. Avoid drawing blood specimen from a site above an infusion of potassium solution (or any solution for that matter). See section on obtaining blood samples in Chapter 2.
7. Be familiar with usual treatment regimens for hyperkalemia.

SUMMARY OF HYPERKALEMIA

ETIOLOGICAL FACTORS

Pseudohyperkalemia
- Prolonged tight application of tourniquet; fist clenching and unclenching immediately before or during blood drawing
- Hemolysis of blood sample
- Leukocytosis
- Thrombocytosis

Decreased Potassium Excretion
- Oliguric renal failure
- Potassium-conserving diuretics
- Hypoaldosteronism

High Potassium Intake
- Improper use of oral potassium supplements
- Excessive use of salt substitutes
- Rapid intravenous potassium administration
- Rapid transfusion of aged blood

Shift of Potassium out of Cells
- Acidosis
- Tissue damage, as in crushing injuries
- Malignant cell lysis after chemotherapy

DEFINING CHARACTERISTICS

Neuromuscular Effects
- Vague muscular weakness
- Flaccid muscle paralysis (first noticed in legs, later in arms and trunk; respiratory muscles and muscles supplied by cranial nerves are usually spared)
- Paresthesias of face, tongue, feet, and hands

Cardiovascular System
- Tall, peaked T waves
- Widened QRS complex progressing to sine waves
- Ventricular arrhythmias
- Cardiac arrest

Gastrointestinal System
- Nausea
- Intermittent intestinal colic or diarrhea

Laboratory Data
- Serum potassium >5.0 mEq/L
- Often associated with acidosis

CASE STUDIES

5-4. A 60-year-old man visited his family physician complaining of chronic tiredness and increased skin pigmentation. On examination, his blood pressure was found to be low (98/60 mmHg). Blood tests revealed a plasma potassium level of 6.8 mEq/L and a plasma sodium level of 132 mEq/L. The BUN was 20 mg/dL and the serum creatinine was 1.2 mg/dL.

COMMENTARY: This patient was diagnosed as having adrenal insufficiency. Recall that aldosterone regulates sodium and potassium balance by causing sodium retention and potassium excretion. Thus, a deficit of aldosterone results in potassium retention and elevation of the plasma potassium level. Note that the patient has normal renal function, as evidenced by the BUN and creatinine levels. Increased skin pigmentation is common in adrenal insufficiency.

5-5. A 30-year-old man with chronic renal failure developed vomiting and diarrhea. Because he became very weak, his family brought him to the emergency room. In addition to severe muscle weakness, he was noted to have decreased skin turgor. An ECG revealed tall, peaked T waves and widening of the QRS complex. Blood tests revealed a plasma potassium level of 9.4 mEq/L and a creatinine level of 2.9 mg/dL.

COMMENTARY: Due to fluid volume depletion after the bout of vomiting and diarrhea, this patient developed decreased renal perfusion and a reduced ability to excrete potassium. Because of the life-threatening situation (evidenced by the high plasma potassium level and the ECG changes), he was treated with calcium gluconate and sodium bicarbonate. A dextrose and saline solution was administered to achieve volume replacement. After volume repletion, kidney perfusion improved and the patient was again able to excrete potassium. Remember that patients with chronic renal failure can become seriously ill when volume depletion and thus decreased renal perfusion occur.

5-6. A 65-year-old woman was admitted to the emergency room complaining of abdominal cramping and numbness in her extremities. Laboratory data revealed a BUN of 96 mg/dL and a creatinine of 3.9 mg/dL. The serum potassium was 8.6 mEq/L. She was given a retention enema of Kayexalate (sodium polystyrene sulfonate) in 20% sorbitol. Fifty milliliters of 50% dextrose and 10 units of regular insulin were given intravenously. An infusion of 5% dextrose and 0.45% NaCl containing two ampules of sodium bicarbonate was started at a rate of 25 mL/hr. By the next day, the serum potassium was reduced to 5.0 mEq/L.

COMMENTARY: Kayexalate is an ion-exchange resin that causes sodium to be exchanged for potassium in the intestine, resulting in potassium excretion by this route. Hypertonic dextrose and insulin favor cellular uptake of potassium, and sodium bicarbonate, by alkalinizing the plasma, also causes potassium to shift temporarily into the cells.

REFERENCES

1. Schwartz S (ed): Principles of Surgery, 6th ed, p 71. New York, McGraw-Hill, 1994
2. Rose B: Clinical Physiology of Acid-Base and Electrolyte Disorders, 4th ed, p 811. New York, McGraw-Hill, 1994
3. Latta K, et al: Perturbations in potassium balance. Clin Lab Med 13(1):149–156, 1993
4. Zull D: Disorders of potassium metabolism. Emerg Med Clin North Am 7(4):771, 1989
5. Ibid
6. Narins R (ed): Clinical Disorders of Fluid and Electrolyte Metabolism, 5th ed, p 671. New York, McGraw-Hill, 1994
7. Rose, p 797
8. Narins, p 671
9. Rose, p 779
10. Pemberton L, Pemberton D: Treatment of Water, Electrolyte, and Acid-Base Disorders in the Surgical Patient, p 178. New York, McGraw-Hill, 1994
11. Rose, p 782
12. Chernow B (ed): The Pharmacologic Approach to the Critically Ill Patient, 3rd ed, p 989. Baltimore, Williams & Wilkins, 1994
13. Rose, p 800
14. Ibid, p 803
15. Ibid
16. Ibid, p 802
17. Ibid
18. Zull, p 785
19. Ibid
20. Ibid
21. Rose, p 810
22. Szerlip H, Goldfarb S: Workshops in Fluid and Electrolyte Disorders, p 93. New York, Churchill Livingstone, 1993
23. Rose, p 826
24. Lacey R, et al: Drug Information Handbook, 2nd ed, p 769. Hudson (Cleveland), Lexi-Comp, Inc., American Pharmaceutical Association, 1994
25. Rose, p 811
26. Eng J: USP institutes new mandates for potassium chloride for injection concentrate (Letter). Oncol Nurs Forum 20(1):11,1993
27. Davis N: Med Errors: Potassium perils. Am J Nurs 95(3):14,1995
28. Pemberton, Pemberton, p 187
29. Rose, p 811
30. Woodley M, Whelan M: Manual of Medical Therapeutics, 27th ed, p 52. Boston, Little, Brown, 1992
31. Pemberton, Pemberton, p 187
32. Kruse J, Carlson R: Rapid correction of hypokalemia using concentrated intravenous potassium chloride infusions. Arch Intern Med 150:613–617,1990
33. Ibid
34. Lim E, et al: Efficacy of lignocaine in alleviating potassium chloride infusion pain. Anesth Intensive Care 20(2):196–198,1992
35. Morrill G, Katz M: The use of lidocaine to reduce the pain induced by potassium chloride infusion. J Intravenous Nurs 11(2):105–108,1988
36. Pemberton, Pemberton, p 187

37. Rose, p 811
38. Pemberton, Pemberton, p 183
39. Narins, p 682
40. Rose, p 809
41. Ibid
42. Zaloga G (ed): Nutrition in Critical Care, p 387. St. Louis, Mosby, 1994
43. Kleinfeld M, Corcoran A: Hyperkalemia in the elderly. Comprehensive Therapy 16(9):49–53,1990
44. Rimmer J, Horn J, Gennari J: Hyperkalemia as a complication of drug therapy. Arch Intern Med 147:867,1987
45. Rose, p 817
46. Skinner S: A cause of erroneous potassium levels. Lancet 1:478,1961
47. Don et al: Pseudohyperkalemia caused fist clenching during phlebotomy. N Engl J Med 322:1290,1990
48. Kokko J, Tannen R: Fluids and Electrolytes, 2nd ed, p 251. Philadelphia, WB Saunders, 1990
49. Wrenn K, et al: The ability of physicians to predict hyperkalemia from the ECG. Ann Emerg Med 20:1229–1232,1991
50. Kokko, Tannen, p 262
51. Zull, p 788
52. Schwartz A, Cannon-Babb M: Hyperkalemia due to drugs in diabetic patients. Am Fam Pract 39(1):225,1989
53. Choi M, et al: Trimethoprim-induced hyperkalemia in a patient with AIDS. N Engl J Med 328(10): 703–706,1993
54. Medina I, et al: Oral therapy for *Pneumocystis carinii* pneumonia in the acquired immunodeficiency syndrome—a controlled trial of trimethoprim-sulfamethoxazole versus trimethoprim-dapson. N Engl J Med 323:776–782,1990
55. Rimmer et al, p 869
56. Schwartz, Cannon-Bobb, p 225
57. van der Loeff H, van Schijndel S, Thijs L: Cardiac arrest due to oral potassium intake. Intensive Care Med 15:58,1988
58. Illingsworth R, Proudfoot A: Rapid poisoning with slow-release potassium. Br Med J 281:485,1980
59. Wetli C, Davis J: Fatal hyperkalemia from accidental overdose of potassium chloride. JAMA 240:1339,1978
60. Schwartz, Cannon-Bobb, p 227
61. Zull, p 788
62. Rimmer et al, p 869
63. Kokko, Tannen, p 268
64. Schwartz, Cannon-Bobb, p 228
65. Zull, p 788
66. Rimmer et al, p 869
67. Ibid
68. Kokko, Tannen, p 268
69. Schwartz, Cannon-Bobb, p 229
70. Zull, p 789
71. Kokko, Tannen, p 268
72. Ibid
73. Rimmer et al, p 869
74. Huerta B, Lemberg L: Potassium imbalances in the coronary unit. Heart Lung 14:193,1985
75. Ibid
76. Rose, p 845
77. Pemberton, Pemberton, p 170
78. Rimmer et al, p 869
79. Woodley M, Whelan M, p 53
80. Rose, p 851
81. Kokko, Tannen, p 256
82. Narins, p 738
83. Rose, p 851
84. Narins, p 736
85. Rose, p 849
86. Narins, p 736
87. Ibid
88. Ibid
89. Ibid, p 737
90. Rose, p 850
91. Kupin W, Narins R: The hyperkalemia of renal failure: Pathophysiology, diagnosis and therapy. In Bourke E, et al (eds): Moving Points in Nephrology, vol 102, pp 1–22. Contrib. Nephrol. Basel, Karger, 1993
92. Narins, p 738
93. Ibid
94. Rose, p 851
95. Goldberger E: A Primer of Water, Electrolytes and Acid-Base Syndromes, 7th ed, p 256. Philadelphia, Lea & Febiger, 1986
96. Ibid

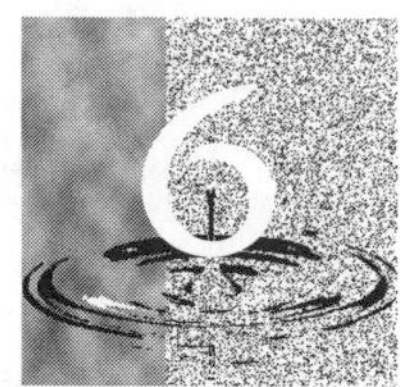

Calcium Imbalances

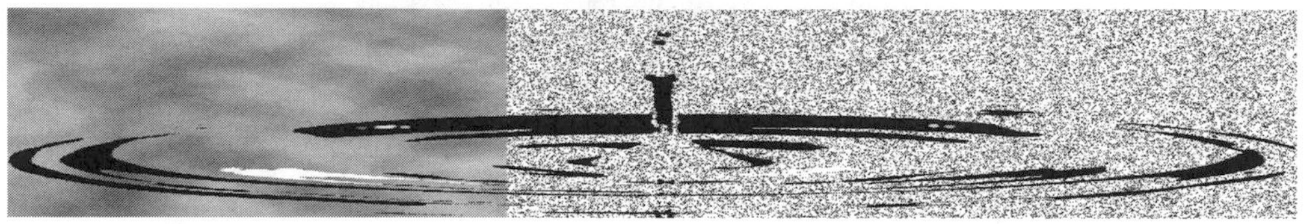

Because many factors affect calcium regulation, there are a multitude of causes of altered calcium balance. Both hypocalcemia and hypercalcemia are relatively common imbalances, particularly in the acutely ill patient. For example, in one study, 64% of the patients in the intensive care unit were found to be hypocalcemic.[1] The opposite imbalance, hypercalcemia, is often seen in patients with malignant disease. To facilitate understanding of calcium disturbances, a review of factors affecting calcium balance follows.

CALCIUM BALANCE

DISTRIBUTION AND FUNCTION

Over 99% of the body's calcium is concentrated in the skeletal system, where it is a major component of strong, durable bones and teeth. About 1% of skeletal calcium is rapidly exchangeable with blood calcium; the rest is more stable and only slowly exchanged. The small amount of calcium located outside the bone circulates in the serum partly bound to protein and partly ionized. Calcium exerts a sedative action on nerve cells and plays a major role in the transmission of nerve impulses. It helps regulate muscle contraction and relaxation, including normal heart beat. Calcium plays a vital role in the cardiac action potential and is essential for cardiac pacemaker automaticity.[2] It is also involved in blood clotting and hormone secretion.

SERUM CONCENTRATION

The test most frequently performed in clinical settings to measure serum calcium is "total calcium," with results normally ranging from 8.5 to 10.5 mg/dL. The total calcium in serum is the sum of the ionized (47%) and nonionized (53%) calcium components. The nonionized portion consists of calcium bound to albumin (40%) and the portion chelated to anions (13%), which include citrate and phosphate.

Most laboratories have the capability to directly measure the ionized calcium level (normal range, 4.0–5.0 mg/dL). This is highly desirable, especially in critically ill patients, because it is the ionized calcium that is physiologically active and clinically important. It has been recommended that blood obtained for ionized calcium be drawn anaerobically with minimal use of heparin, placed on ice, and measured immediately (in a manner similar to that used for measurement of arterial blood gases).[3]

When only the total serum calcium level is available, the reading must be evaluated in relation to the serum albumin concentration. In the noncritically ill patient, it is estimated that a decrease in the serum albumin of 1.0 g/dL will decrease the total calcium by 0.8 mg/dL.[4] For example, if the patient's serum albumin level is below normal by 1 g/dL (eg, 2.5 g/dL rather than 3.5 g/dL), the measured total serum calcium concentration of 8.0 mg/dL should be adjusted upward to 8.8 mg/dL. In this situation, the ionized calcium level would be estimated at about half of the adjusted value (4.4 mg/dL). The direct relationship between albumin and total calcium often leads clinicians to ignore a low total serum calcium level in the presence of a similarly low serum albumin level.

The above estimation is not valid when situations are present that affect pH (and thus the percentage of ionized calcium). When the arterial pH increases (alkalosis), more calcium becomes bound to protein. Although the total serum calcium remains unchanged, the ionized portion decreases. Therefore, symptoms of hypocalcemia often occur in the presence of alkalosis. Acidosis (low pH) has the opposite effect; that is, less calcium is bound to protein and therefore, more exists in the ionized form. Signs of hypocalcemia will develop only rarely in the presence of acidosis, even when the total serum calcium level is lower than normal. The estimation described above is also not valid when situations are present that increase the quantity of plasma anions available to bind with calcium (such as citrate, lactate, and phosphate), thus reducing the ionized calcium level.

REGULATION

Many biochemical and hormonal factors act to maintain a normal calcium balance. Among the most important are parathyroid hormone, calcitonin, and calcitriol (an active metabolite of vitamin D). Parathyroid hormone (PTH) promotes a transfer of calcium from the bone to plasma (raising the plasma calcium level). The bones and teeth are ready sources for replenishment of low plasma calcium levels. Parathyroid hormone also augments the intestinal absorption of calcium and enhances the net renal calcium reabsorption.

Calcitonin (produced by C cells in the thyroid as well as several other tissues) is a physiological antagonist of PTH. Calcitonin secretion is directly stimulated by a high serum calcium concentration. At high levels, calcitonin inhibits bone resorption; the resultant reduced flux of calcium from bone causes a reduction in the serum calcium level. Because high levels of calcitonin have a hypocalcemic effect, calcitonin is thought to play a role in protecting against acute hypercalcemia.[5] However, its effect is thought to be minor when compared to that of PTH and calcitriol.[6]

Calcitriol (1,25-dihydroxyvitamin D_3) is a hormone that increases the extracellular calcium concentration by three main actions: (1) it promotes calcium absorption from the intestine; (2) it enhances bone resorption of calcium; and (3) it stimulates renal tubular reabsorption of calcium.

The daily recommended oral dietary intake of calcium is 1000 to 1500 mg.[7] Approximately one-third to one-half of the ingested calcium is absorbed, primarily through the small intestine. Calcium is excreted by both the gastrointestinal (GI) and urinary tracts.

CALCIUM DEFICIENCY-ASSOCIATED DISEASES

OSTEOPOROSIS

Osteoporosis is associated with prolonged low intake of calcium. It is characterized by loss of bone mass causing bones to become porous, brittle, and therefore susceptible to fracture. This disease causes 1.5 million fractures and costs $10 billion in the United States each year.[8] Although serum calcium levels are usually normal in these individuals, *total* body calcium stores are greatly diminished. Bone loss begins at an earlier age in women than in men and is accelerated by menopause. However, men also develop negative calcium balance in later years. A dual process is involved in osteoporosis: increased bone resorption and inadequate bone formation. Menopause leads to rapid bone loss in women because estrogen deficiency reduces calcium absorption and increases excretion; as a result, bone loss far outpaces bone deposition.

Risk of developing serious bone problems is greater in postmenopausal, physically inactive women who are elderly, white or Asian, thin and small-framed, smokers, and have a diet deficient in calcium.[9] Inactivity predisposes to bone loss by reducing the efficiency of calcium use. Conversely, regular physical exercise (such as running, walking, or bicycling) slows the rate of bone loss and improves calcium balance.

Considering the magnitude of the problems associated with osteoporosis, prevention is the only cost-effective approach. If dietary calcium intake is low, it should be increased to at least the recommended daily allowance of 800 mg/day for adults and 1200 mg/day for adolescents and young adults.[10] Increased physical activity should be encouraged, and bone toxins (such as cigarettes and heavy alcohol ingestion) should be eliminated. Also, estrogen replacement therapy may be beneficial in preventing osteoporosis when it is started at or within a few years after menopause and continued for at least 15 to 20 years.[11] See Chapter 25 for further discussion of osteoporosis.

HYPERTENSION

Several studies indicate support for the concept that ingesting a high-calcium diet reduces blood pressure, at least in some individuals. However, the mechanisms by which dietary calcium can modify blood pressure are not clearly understood.

HYPOCALCEMIA

Hypocalcemia is defined as a total serum calcium level of less than 8.5 mg/dL, and an ionized calcium concentration of less than 4.0 mg/dL. As described earlier, hypoalbuminemia is a common cause of a reduced total serum calcium concentration; however, this is sometimes referred to as "pseudohypocalcemia" because the ionized calcium remains normal despite a low total calcium level.[12] In this situation, the patient is asymptomatic and does not require treatment. On the other hand, an alkalotic patient often has a decreased ionized calcium level (and therefore is symptomatic) although the total serum calcium level is normal. Thus, when total serum calcium measurements are performed to assess calcium balance, the need to consider the results in relation to the serum albumin level as well as acid–base status is obvious. Conditions associated with hypocalcemia are briefly discussed below.

ETIOLOGICAL FACTORS

Surgical Hypoparathyroidism

Primary hypoparathyroidism causes hypocalcemia, as does surgical hypoparathyroidism; however, the latter is a more common cause. Hypocalcemia is usually seen when the operation involves removal of a parathyroid adenoma, total or near-total thyroidectomy, or bilateral neck surgery for cancer.[13] Hypocalcemia reportedly occurs in up to 70% of patients undergoing parathyroidectomy, particularly when a severe hyperparathyroid state was present before surgery.[14] Transient hypocalcemia reportedly occurs in 5% to 10% of patients undergoing thyroidectomy.[15] The hypocalcemia may occur immediately or 1 to 2 days postoperatively and usually lasts less than 5 days.[16]

The most likely mechanism for hypocalcemia after radical neck dissection is ischemia to the parathyroid tissue after dissection and hemostatic maneuvers. Intraoperative release of calcitonin has been suggested as a possible mechanism for hypocalcemia that complicates thyroid surgery.[17] It is also possible that trauma to the parathyroid glands does not allow PTH to increase as needed to elevate the low serum calcium level, thus contributing to the hypocalcemia. If permanent parathyroid damage has not occurred, parathyroid insufficiency resolves as edema at the surgical site lessens and revascularization occurs, allowing reestablishment of parathyroid gland integrity.

Permanent hypocalcemia associated with thyroid surgery (which may be defined as a hypocalcemia lasting 2 months or longer) is due to accidental removal of the parathyroid glands or to vascular necrosis.[18] Fortunately, permanent post-surgical hypoparathyroidism occurs in only a small percentage of patients; the frequency of this complication is partially dependent on the technical skill of the surgeon.[19] Surgeons performing thyroidectomies and parathyroidectomies strive to preserve the blood supply to the parathyroid glands.[20] Extensive neck surgery (as in radical neck dissection for cancer) is more likely to be associated with permanent hypoparathyroidism than are less involved surgical maneuvers.

Most patients who develop hypocalcemia after neck surgery are asymptomatic; however, some may develop paresthesias, laryngeal spasm, or tetany.[21] It has been recommended that the serum ionized calcium level be checked every 12 hrs after neck surgery (and more frequently if symptoms of hypocalcemia are present) until the serum ionized concentration begins to elevate, indicating recovery of the parathyroid glands.[22] Of course, symptomatic patients should receive supplemental calcium to increase the serum calcium level to the low normal range.

It is possible that postoperative hypoparathyroidism may manifest itself months to years after neck surgery; therefore, in at-risk patients serum ionized calcium levels should be monitored serially. It is also possible that stress can induce hypocalcemia in these individuals; therefore, critically ill patients with a history of neck surgery should have a serum calcium test performed.[23]

Acute Pancreatitis

Inflammation of the pancreas causes release of proteolytic and lipolytic enzymes; it is believed that calcium ions combine with the fatty acids released by lipolysis, forming soaps, and thus decreasing the serum calcium concentration. Some investigators have found that there is an inadequate PTH response to the hypocalcemia caused by acute pancreatitis.[24] In any event, hypocalcemia is a common problem, occurring in as many as 40% to 75% of patients with acute pancreatitis.[25] See Chapter 20 for a more extensive discussion of this topic.

Magnesium Abnormalities

The serum magnesium level influences both PTH secretion and action, and thus the serum calcium level. Severe hypomagnesemia (<1 mg/dL) inhibits PTH secretion. One study reported that 22% of the hypocalcemia patients in their sample also had hypomagnesemia.[26] Chronic hypomagnesemia associated with impaired PTH secretion and hypocalcemia can occur in malnourished alcoholics and in the renal magnesium-wasting associated with cisplatin therapy.[27] Hypomagnesemic hypocalcemia responds poorly to calcium therapy alone but does respond to magnesium replacement.[28]

Hyperphosphatemia

Progressive hyperphosphatemia that develops rapidly is associated with hypocalcemia and the deposition of amorphous calcium phosphate salts in the organs and tissues.[29] Although severe hypocalcemia usually results from hyperphosphatemia, it is possible that the serum phosphorus and calcium concentrations may rise together if rapid bone breakdown is the basic cause.[30]

Alkalosis

Blood pH alters Ca^{2+} binding to serum proteins. As described earlier, alkalosis can induce a decreased ionized serum calcium concentration as a result of increased binding of Ca^{2+} to albumin. Although the total calcium concentration remains normal in this situation, tetany (presumably caused by the fall in ionized calcium) can occur if the blood pH rises above 7.6.[31]

Inadequate Vitamin D

Inadequate consumption of vitamin D or insufficient exposure to the sun (ultraviolet radiation) can cause reduced calcium absorption and thus lead to hypocalcemia. Deficiency of vitamin D occurs in malabsorptive states, as described below.

Malabsorption Syndromes

Intestinal malabsorptive disorders are likely to lead to hypocalcemia by decreasing the absorption of vitamin D, bile salts, and calcium.[32] Hypocalcemia has been found in 7% of patients who have undergone partial gastrectomy with gastrojejunostomy.[33] It may also occur after ileal bypass in obese persons,[34] Crohn's disease, pancreatic insufficiency, and hepatobiliary disease.[35]

Infusion of Citrated Blood

Decreases in ionized Ca^{2+} values during blood transfusion correlate with speed of transfusion and circulating citrate levels.[36] Citrate is present in bank blood to act as an anticoagulant and to preserve the life of the blood. Usually the citrate in blood is rapidly metabolized by the liver and presents no problem for calcium balance. However, when blood is transfused faster than the excess citrate can be metabolized, hypocalcemia results. Recall that citrate is negatively charged and calcium is positively charged, resulting in an attraction between these ions. Therefore, transient hypocalcemia can occur with massive administration of citrated blood (as in exchange transfusions in neonates), as citrate combines with ionized calcium and temporarily removes it from the circulation (also referred to as "chelation"). Citrate metabolism is hindered in the presence of liver disease, shock, and hypothermia. Also at increased risk for citrate-induced ionized calcium deficit during massive transfusion are small children, elderly or osteoporotic patients, and those who have been bedridden for extended periods; all of these individuals tend to have inadequate stores of bone calcium and therefore are less able to compensate for declined ionized calcium levels. When citrate intoxication occurs, it may be manifested as circumoral paresthesias, muscle tremors, or tetany; it does not affect coagulation.[37] Hypocalcemia has also been observed during plasmapheresis.[38]

The infusion of packed red blood cells (instead of whole blood) lowers the amount of citrate infused, and thus decreases the already low risk for hypocalcemia after transfusions. However, there is sufficient citrate even in packed red blood cells to affect calcium balance. For example, Chernow et al.[39] reported a significant fall in total serum calcium (from 9.49 ± 0.11 to 7.6 ± 0.11 mg/dL) in 21 patients after transfusion with packed red blood cells.

Current recommendations suggest the administration of calcium only when patients develop symptomatic hypocalcemia; this is because calcium infusion can be associated with ventricular dysrhythmias and thus should not be used indiscriminately.[40]

Drugs

Many medications can predispose to hypocalcemia. Some are listed in Table 6-1 with a brief description of the underlying mechanisms.

Alcoholism

The hypocalcemia associated with chronic alcoholism has numerous causes. Among these are the direct effect of ethanol, intestinal malabsorption,

TABLE 6–1

Drugs With Calcium-Lowering Effects

DRUG	MECHANISM
Loop diuretics (such as furosemide)	Increases renal excretion of calcium
Anticonvulsants (especially Dilantin and phenobarbital)	Inhibits gastrointestinal calcium absorption and causes faulty vitamin D metabolism
Citrate-buffered blood and blood products	Presumably binds ionized Ca^{2+} with citrate
Phosphates (orally, IV, or enema)	Phosphate combines with calcium
Mithramycin	Decreases calcium mobilization from bone
Calcitonin	Decreases calcium mobilization from bone
Drugs that lower serum Mg level (such as cisplatin and gentamycin)	By inducing hypomagnesemia, may decrease calcium mobilization from bone
EDTA (disodium edetate)	Physically combines with calcium for excretion
Alcohol (chronic abuse)	Multiple factors (see text)
Certain radiographic contrast media	Those containing chelating agents combine with calcium

low levels of 25-(OH)-D_3, hypomagnesemia, hypoalbuminemia, respiratory and metabolic alkalosis, and pancreatitis.[41] The most significant of these is probably hypomagnesemia. Magnesium replacement increases responsiveness to PTH and correction of the hypocalcemia.

Neonatal Hypocalcemia

There are two types of hypocalcemia in newborn infants. The first occurs early after birth, during the first 3 days of life. This type is attributed to parathyroid immaturity and/or maternal hyperparathyroidism (resulting in neonatal parathyroid gland suppression) and most often resolves within the first week of life.[42] Among the predisposing factors for this condition are prematurity, maternal insulin-dependent diabetes mellitus, and asphyxia at birth. A second type of neonatal hypocalcemia occurs about 1 week after birth and is associated with hyperphosphatemia and hypomagnesemia. Hypocalcemia in infants with this "late-onset" condition can be caused by feeding milk with a high phosphorus level, leading to hyperphosphatemia and then to hypocalcemia. Low serum calcium levels can persist until the parathyroid glands function well enough to respond.[43]

Sepsis

The underlying basis for hypocalcemia in septic patients is unclear. It is postulated that calcium moves from the extracellular compartment into the cells and that the hormonal response to hypocalcemia is inadequate.[44] Possible causes for hypocalcemia in a group of Gram-negative sepsis patients described by Zaloga and Chernow[45] are acquired parathyroid gland insufficiency, dietary vitamin D deficiency, or renal hydroxylase insufficiency. Treatment of ionized hypocalcemia in sepsis is not recommended unless the patient is symptomatic because calcium administration appears to increase organ dysfunction.[46]

Other Factors

Medullary thyroid carcinoma may produce hypocalcemia if calcitonin (a calcium-lowering hormone) is secreted by the tumor. And, as discussed earlier, conditions associated with low serum albumin levels (such as cirrhosis of the liver and the nephrotic syndrome) are frequently associated with a low total serum calcium concentration. Often, the ionized calcium concentration is normal and there are no symptoms of hypocalcemia.

In a recent study, hypocalcemia was reported in 17.9% of 66 patients with acquired immunodeficiency syndrome (AIDS).[47] The researchers postulated that intestinal malabsorption of vitamin D is the most likely cause of hypocalcemia in this patient population.

DEFINING CHARACTERISTICS

Clinical manifestations of hypocalcemia vary widely among patients and depend on severity, duration, and rate of development. The concurrent presence of hypomagnesemia and hypokalemia can potentiate the neurological and cardiac abnormalities associated with hypocalcemia.

Neuromuscular Manifestations

Tetany, the most characteristic manifestation of hypocalcemia, refers to the entire symptom complex induced by increased neural excitability. Findings may include sensations of tingling around the mouth (circumoral paresthesia) and in the hands and feet, as well as spasms of the muscles of the extremities and face. The increase in nerve membrane excitability causes fibers to discharge spontaneously, eliciting tetanic contractions. Although laryngeal spasms may occur, they only rarely result in asphyxia.[48]

When hypocalcemic patients lack overt signs of tetany, neuromuscular excitability (latent tetany) can be elicited in two ways. One involves placing a blood pressure cuff on the upper arm and inflating to above systolic pressure for about 3 min and observing for carpal spasm (Trousseau's sign, see Fig. 2-4). Trousseau's sign is not specific for hypocalcemia as it is negative in about 30% of individuals with latent tetany and positive for a small percentage of healthy individuals.[49] Another test involves tapping over the facial nerve just anterior to the ear and observing for ipsilateral facial muscle contraction (Chvostek's sign). This sign is also not specific for hypocalcemia as it may occur in some healthy adults.

Cardiovascular Manifestations

In some patients altered cardiovascular hemodynamics may be the most significant effect of hypocalcemia. This is understandable when considering the important role calcium ions play in the contraction of cardiac muscle. The cardiovascular effects of hypocalcemia include decreased myocardial contractility leading to a reduced cardiac output, hypotension which is refractory to fluids and vasoconstrictive agents, and decreased responsiveness to digitalis.[50] Dysrhythmias associated with hypocalcemia can range from bradycardia to ventricular tachycardia and asystole. Hypocalcemia prolongs the QT interval, predisposing the patient to life-threatening ventricular dysrhythmia. Often cardiac patients are already predisposed to both hypocalcemia and hypomagnesemia because they are taking potent loop diuretics.

Central Nervous System Manifestations

Severe hypocalcemia can cause convulsions and, in fact, these may be the initial manifestation.[51] Hypocalcemia may also cause impaired higher cerebral function. For example, anxiety, depression, confusion, and frank psychoses may occur.

Other Changes

There are indications that hypocalcemia can affect respiratory function. When hypocalcemia was induced in dogs by the administration of a chelating agent, transdiaphragmatic pressures were found to be reduced.[52] The decreased diaphragmatic strength in these experimental animals was apparently not related to changes in cardiac output.[53]

In chronic hypocalcemia, the skin may be dry and scaling, the nails brittle, and the hair dry and easily shed; cataracts are common. Chronic hypocalcemia in children can retard growth and lower the IQ.

TREATMENT

As noted above, there are numerous etiological factors associated with hypocalcemia. Ideally, treatment is directed at alleviating the cause. If this is impractical or ineffective, the following general measures should be considered.

Acute Hypocalcemia

Acute symptomatic hypocalcemia is a medical emergency, requiring prompt administration of intravenous (IV) calcium. Parenteral calcium salts include calcium gluconate, calcium chloride, and calcium gluceptate. Although calcium chloride produces a significantly higher ionized calcium than an equimolar amount of calcium gluconate, it is not used as often because it is more irritating to the vein and can cause tissue sloughing if allowed to infiltrate. Because calcium is very irritating, it is advisable to administer calcium through a central line whenever possible.[54] For symptoms of severe hypocalcemia in adults, 10 to 20 mL of 10% calcium gluconate (90 mg elemental calcium/10 mL), administered at a rate not exceeding 2 mL/min, may be prescribed.[55,56] This may be followed by the infusion of 30 to 40 mL of 10% calcium gluconate in 500 mL or 1000 mL of 5% aqueous dextrose (D_5W) or 0.9% NaCl over a 4-hr period.[57] (Calcium should not be mixed with any solution containing bicarbonate because of the possibility of precipitation.) Patients receiving digitalis should be monitored electrocardiographically during the infusion as calcium administration may produce fatal arrhythmias if the infusion is given rapidly.[58] The serum calcium level should be monitored every 4 to 6 hrs and the infusion rate adjusted to avoid recurrent symptomatic hypocalcemia.[59]

An infusion of calcium gluconate may be needed to correct postoperative symptomatic hypocalcemia in the first 24 to 48 hr after neck surgery (such as thyroidectomy, radical neck dissection, or parathyroidectomy). The flow rate is titrated according to clinical signs and serum calcium levels.

Chronic Hypocalcemia

When oral calcium supplements can be tolerated, the oral route is preferred over the IV route because it is safer. Oral calcium intake can be provided as either carbonate, gluconate, or lactate salts. In general, 1 or 2 g of elemental calcium daily, in four divided doses, is sufficient.[60] In some cases, long-term management may require the use of vitamin D preparations. These should be used with caution if severe hyperphosphatemia is present, because of the danger of calcium phosphate precipitation in the soft tissues. If hyperphosphatemia is present, oral phosphate-binding medications (such as aluminum hydroxide) may be indicated.

NURSING INTERVENTIONS

1. Be aware of patients at risk for hypocalcemia and monitor for its occurrence (see Summary of Hypocalcemia). Also, review previous sections for explanations of etiological factors and defining characteristics.
2. Be prepared to adopt seizure precautions when hypocalcemia is severe.
3. Monitor condition of airway closely as laryngeal stridor can occur.
4. Take safety precautions if confusion is present.
5. Be aware of factors related to the safe administration of calcium replacement salts (see Clinical Tip: Nursing Considerations in the Administration of IV Calcium).
6. Educate individuals in high-risk groups for osteoporosis (especially postmenopausal women not on estrogen therapy) about the need for adequate dietary calcium intake.
   A. Most sources recommend that the calcium intake for older persons be 1000 to 1500 mg each day. The best way for healthy individuals to ensure an adequate calcium intake is to eat a wide variety of foods from the four food groups daily.
   B. Calcium supplements may be necessary for individuals unable to consume sufficient calcium in their diets, such as those who do not tolerate milk or dairy products.
   C. Individuals with a tendency to form renal stones should be encouraged to consult their physicians before greatly increasing their calcium intake. For such individuals, the physician must determine a safe calcium dosage range; this is usually determined by studying urinary calcium levels. Also, these individuals should drink no less than 2 to 3 quarts of fluid a day to protect against stone formation.
7. Inform individuals at risk for osteoporosis about the value of regular physical exercise in decreasing bone loss. Walking is tolerated well by all age groups and is an excellent form of exercise, as is bicycling. (See Chapter 25 for further discussion of exercise and osteoporosis.
8. To prevent osteoporosis in later years, educate young women about the need for a normal diet ensuring adequate calcium intake. Also, discuss the calcium loss associated with alcohol and nicotine use. Smoking lowers estrogen levels and interferes with the body's absorption of calcium; women who smoke are at greater risk of developing osteoporosis.

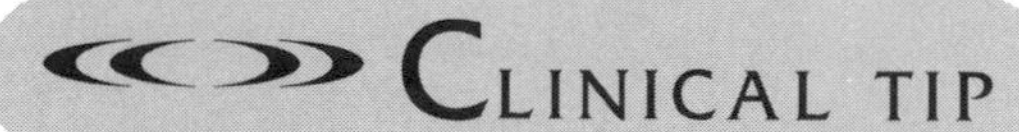

Nursing Considerations in the Administration of IV Calcium

1. The dosage of calcium prescribed for a specific hypocalcemic patient depends on the severity of hypocalcemia, as well as its cause.
2. The most commonly prescribed calcium preparations for IV use are:
   Calcium Gluconate: 10 mL of a 10% solution contains 90 mg (4.5 mEq) of elemental Ca^{2+} (suitable for either IV or IM use)
   Calcium Chloride: 10 mL of a 10% solution contains 270 mg (13.5 mEq) of elemental Ca^{2+} (suitable only for IV use)
3. Calcium preparations may be given by slow IV push (if indicated) or may be added to compatible parenteral fluids (such as 500 mL to 1000 mL of 0.9% NaCl, lactated Ringer's solution, or D_5W) for slow infusion.
4. Calcium preparations are irritating to veins. While they may be given undiluted via IV push, it is preferable to dilute them first with an equal volume of distilled water or isotonic saline.[61]
5. Calcium chloride is especially irritating to veins and may cause venous sclerosis; for this reason, administration through a central vein is recommended.[62] Because calcium gluconate is less irritating to veins, it is more frequently prescribed (although it contains only one third as much elemental calcium as calcium chloride). If a peripheral administration site is necessary, the largest available vein should be used. Do not use small hand veins.[63] Great care should be taken to avoid extravasation of calcium solutions (especially calcium chloride) because they can cause severe soft tissue damage.
6. Calcium preparations should not be administered with bicarbonate or phosphate because a precipitate will form.[64]
7. Calcium should be administered cautiously (with ECG monitoring) to patients taking digitalis because accidental hypercalcemia induced by too rapid infusion of calcium could precipitate digitalis toxicity.
8. Frequent monitoring of the patient's response to calcium replacement therapy is indicated. Serum calcium levels should be checked frequently (such as every 1–4 hours) and the dosage adjusted accordingly.[65] Adequacy of treatment can also be monitored by following Chvostek's and Trousseau's signs, the ECG, and hemodynamic parameters.[66]

CASE STUDIES

6-1. A 46-year-old woman with end-stage renal disease was admitted with a secondary diagnosis of seizure activity and multi-infarct dementia. She required dialysis twice a week. On admission, laboratory data from a venous blood sample revealed the following:

Na	=	138 mEq/L
BUN	=	41 mg/dL
K	=	5.8 mEq/L
Creatinine	=	8.2 mg/dL
Total Ca	=	7.0 mg/dL
Albumin	=	3.0 g
PO_4	=	7.1 mEq/L
HCO_3	=	13.5 mEq/L

SUMMARY OF HYPOCALCEMIA

ETIOLOGICAL FACTORS

Surgical hypoparathyroidism (may follow thyroid surgery or radical neck surgery for cancer)

Primary hypoparathyroidism

Malabsorption

Acute pancreatitis

Excessive administration of citrated blood

Alkalotic states (causing decreased calcium ionization)

Hyperphosphatemia

Sepsis

Hypomagnesemia

Medullary carcinoma of thyroid

Hypoalbuminemia (as in cirrhosis, nephrotic syndrome, and starvation)

DEFINING CHARACTERISTICS

Neuromuscular

- Numbness, tingling of fingers, circumoral region, and toes
- Muscle cramps, which can progress to muscle spasms, tremor, and twitching
- Hyperactive deep-tendon reflexes
- Trousseau's sign
- Chvostek's sign
- Convulsions (usually generalized but may be focal)
- Spasm of laryngeal muscles

Cardiovascular

- Decreased myocardial contractility with a reduction in cardiac output
- ECG: Prolonged QT interval
- Arrhythmias, ranging from bradycardia to ventricular tachycardia and asystole

Mental

- Impaired higher cerebral functioning, such as depression, emotional instability, anxiety, or frank psychoses

Gastrointestinal

- Diarrhea

Total serum calcium level below 8.5 mg/dL or ionized calcium level below 4 mg/dL

COMMENTARY: Note the low total calcium level and the presence of hypoalbuminemia. With correction for the low serum albumin level, the serum calcium would be nearer to normal. (Recall that for every gram the serum albumin is below the normal level of 4–5 g, 0.8 mg must be added to the reported calcium level; because the albumin level is 1 or 2 g below normal, 0.8 or 1.6 mg must be added to the reported calcium level, making it 7.8–8.6 mg/dL.) Although the total calcium level was below normal, the ionized fraction of the calcium was normal; thus, symptoms of hypocalcemia were not present. Note that this patient has metabolic acidosis (evidenced by the low serum bicarbonate level); both hypoalbuminemia and acidosis favor increased calcium ionization. Rapid correction, or overcorrection, of acidosis in a renal patient predisposes to precipitation of hypocalcemic symptoms. Hyperphosphatemia was present, a major factor in explaining the hypocalcemia. Among the medications prescribed for this patient were Basaljel (to bind the excess phosphate) and Os-Cal (a calcium supplement). Seizure activity was managed by the administration of Dilantin and phenobarbital (seizures were related to the cerebral infarcts, not to hypocalcemia).

6-2. A hysterical young woman was admitted to the emergency department after an automobile accident in which she fractured her arm. She complained of circumoral paresthesia and then fainted. Arterial blood gas findings included a pH of 7.55 (alkalosis) and an arterial carbon dioxide pressure ($PaCO_2$) of 20 mmHg (normal, 40 mmHg).

COMMENTARY: Hyperventilation secondary to hysteria is a common cause of tetany in the hospital emergency department. In this situation, the tetany resulted from a reduction in the plasma ionized calcium level consequent to respiratory alkalosis. Fainting was due to cerebral ischemia caused by the low $PaCO_2$ (recall that a low $PaCO_2$ causes cerebral vasoconstriction). The total serum calcium level was probably normal, although the ionized fraction decreased. Correction of the hyperventilation (and thus of respiratory alkalosis) will restore the ionized calcium level to normal and alleviate symptoms.

HYPERCALCEMIA

The prevalence of hypercalcemia in the hospital inpatient population ranges from 0.6% to 3.6%.[67] If allowed to become severe, hypercalcemia is associated with significant morbidity and mortality; therefore, it is important to detect this imbalance early.

ETIOLOGICAL FACTORS

Malignancy and primary hyperparathyroidism account for most of the cases of hypercalcemia. In contrast, causes such as thiazide diuretics, immobilization, lithium use, and vitamin D and A intoxication account for only a small percentage of the cases.[68]

Malignancies

Malignancies most often associated with hypercalcemia include breast and lung cancers and multiple myeloma.[69] See Chapter 22 for a more thorough discussion of tumors associated with hypercalcemia.

Primary Hyperparathyroidism

Hypercalcemia caused by primary hyperparathyroidism results from increased PTH production, and about 75% of the cases are caused by single adenomas.[70] Due to increased PTH, hyperparathyroidism causes increased bony release of calcium, augmented intestinal calcium absorption, and renal reabsorption of calcium. Hypercalcemia also occurs in some hyperthyroid patients. When total serum calcium is measured, approximately 10% to 20% of hyperthyroid patients have elevated values; the percentage is even higher when ionized calcium is measured.[71]

Immobilization

Bone mineral is lost during immobilization, sometimes causing elevation of total calcium in the bloodstream. The hypercalcemia associated with immobilization is the result of an imbalance between the rates of bone formation and bone resorption. This process is more conspicuous in patients with Paget's disease or in those in whom bone turnover is increased (such as adolescents during a growth spurt). Factors leading to hypercalcemia during immobilization are still largely unexplained.

Drugs

A variety of drugs have calcium-elevating effects; some of these are listed in Table 6-2. Thiazide-induced hypercalcemia may be partially mediated by volume contraction that increases renal reabsorption of calcium; also, it is thought that thiazides have a direct effect on distal tubular calcium reabsorption.

Use of lithium to treat manic-depressive patients has been reported to cause hypercalcemia and high circulating iPTH levels.[72] Too aggressive treatment of hypoparathyroidism, rickets, or osteomalacia with vitamin D is the most common cause of vitamin D intoxication and its associated hypercalcemia. Excessive vitamin A intake can increase bone resorption and lead to hypercalcemia; it appears that large doses of vitamin A increase bone resorption. The widespread use of vitamin A analogues to treat acne and other skin conditions has occasionally been associated with hypercalcemia.[73]

Milk-alkali syndrome can occur in peptic ulcer patients treated for a prolonged period with milk and alkaline antacids, particularly calcium carbonate. This condition only develops when both calcium and alkali are ingested together.[74] Patients who

TABLE 6–2
Drugs with Calcium-Elevating Effects

DRUG	MECHANISM
Thiazide diuretics	Decrease renal calcium excretion
Lithium	Decreases renal calcium excretion
Prolonged megadoses of vitamins A and D	Vitamin A likely increases calcium mobilization from bone; vitamin D increases GI calcium absorption and mobilization of calcium from bone
Theophylline	Perhaps increases effect of endogenous parathyroid hormone
Milk with soluble alkali (especially calcium carbonate)	Multiple mechanisms

take large quantities of calcium-containing antacids may present with marked hypercalcemia.[75]

Renal Transplantation

Hypercalcemia may occur after successful renal transplantation as a result of increased PTH production by hyperplastic parathyroid glands. As a rule, it disappears within 6 months after transplantation as the glands undergo involution, although it may persist for up to 24 months. If the serum calcium is persistently greater than 12 mg/dL, parathyroidectomy may be considered.

DEFINING CHARACTERISTICS

The magnitude of the serum calcium elevation and the length of time during which it developed have a major significance for clinical findings, as does the underlying cause of hypercalcemia. For example, acute hypercalcemia is more symptomatic than chronic hypercalcemia. Also, malignancies can present with severe hypercalcemia (>15 mg/dL) more commonly than other conditions.[76]

In some patients mild hypercalcemia is found on routine examinations; others may present in hypercalcemic crisis. As a rule, symptoms of hypercalcemia are proportional to the serum calcium level, although this is not always the case.

Neuromuscular Changes

Hypercalcemia reduces neuromuscular excitability because it acts as a sedative at the myoneural junction. Symptoms such as muscular weakness and depressed deep tendon reflexes may occur.

Gastrointestinal Symptoms

Constipation, anorexia, nausea, and vomiting are common symptoms of hypercalcemia. Constipation results from decreased GI motility caused by calcium's action on smooth muscle and nerve conduction, as well as from dehydration.[77] Delayed gastric emptying, nausea, and vomiting are also related to altered GI motility. Patients with hypercalcemia are predisposed to duodenal ulcer disease because of the increased gastric acid secretion, promoted by calcium on the parietal cells of the stomach. Pancreatitis is another potential GI complication of severe hypercalcemia and is probably related to calcium deposits in the pancreatic ducts.

Behavior Changes

Behavior changes may range from subtle alterations in personality to acute psychosis, and may include confusion, impairment of memory, and bizarre behavior. Although the cause of these symptoms is not known, it has been suggested that increased calcium in the cerebrospinal fluid is involved.[78] The more severe symptoms tend to occur when the serum calcium level is approximately 16 mg/dL or higher. In a study of eight hypercalcemic cancer inpatients during a period of 66 patient-days, Mahon[79] found that the most evident changes were those affecting mental status. For example, many subjects could not remember their home telephone numbers or perform simple mathematical computations. Some displayed inappropriate behaviors, such as pulling out a Foley catheter while the balloon was inflated. When serum calcium levels decreased toward normal values, the mental symptoms subsided.

Renal Changes

Disturbed renal tubular function produced by the hypercalcemia can cause polyuria and polydipsia. More specifically, this disturbed function is a form of nephrogenic diabetes insipidus that is usually reversible within 1 to 12 weeks after correction of the imbalance. The concentrating defect may become clinically apparent when the plasma calcium concentration exceeds 11 mg/dL.[80] Renal colic may occur as a result of kidney stones, which may form from the excess calcium presented to the kidneys for excretion. Calcium salts deposited in the kidney can cause renal failure.

Cardiovascular Changes

Calcium is important in cardiac function; it exerts a positive inotropic effect on the heart and reduces heart rate in a way similar to the effect of cardiac glycosides. As described earlier, calcium administration to patients receiving digitalis must be done with extreme care because it can precipitate severe arrhythmias (with shortening of the QT interval on ECG).

Hypercalcemia cause alterations in myocardial muscle function and rhythm disturbances. Bradycardia, first-, second-, and third-degree heart block, and bundle branch block may occur.[81] Hypercalcemia can also affect the systemic vasculature, perhaps leading to hypertension. The mechanism for the increase in blood pressure may be multifactorial. For example, serum levels of epinephrine and norepinephrine are higher in hypercalcemic patients than in those with normocalcemia, and elevated renin activity has been reported in patients with primary hyperparathyroidism.[82]

TREATMENT

Treatment for hypercalcemia is directed at reducing the serum calcium level by increasing urinary calcium excretion, inhibiting bone resorption, blocking intestinal calcium absorption, or enhancing formation of calcium complexes. Treatment should also be directed at correcting the underlying cause of hypercalcemia when possible.

General Conservative Measures

When hypercalcemia is not life-threatening, treatment may be limited to simple actions such as ensuring an adequate fluid intake to avoid volume depletion and eliminating drugs that can contribute to hypercalcemia (such as thiazide diuretics, vitamin D preparations, or calcium-containing antacids). Whenever possible, the patient should be encouraged to be active (as immobility predisposes to hypercalcemia).

Fluid Replacement

Because most patients with severe hypercalcemia are volume-depleted, isotonic saline (0.9% NaCl) may be ordered initially at a rate of 300 to 500 mL/hr until the intravascular volume has been restored.[83] Volume expansion with isotonic saline dilutes the plasma calcium, increases the glomerular filtration rate, and increases renal calcium excretion. A dose of 4 to 5 L of saline over 24 hrs, or more if tolerated, may be given; the serum calcium level may fall by 2 to 3 mEq/L over 8 to 24 hrs.[84] A slowed saline infusion is maintained to promote renal calcium excretion after volume replacement has been achieved.

Cardiovascular and renal function should be assessed before rapid saline infusion because fluid overload and congestive heart failure are potential complications. Furosemide should be used as necessary after the plasma volume has been expanded to prevent volume overload and to enhance calcium excretion. It may be necessary to monitor the central venous pressure (CVP) to detect fluid overload, particularly in the elderly or those with marginal cardiac reserve; at least, breath sounds should be monitored at regular intervals. Hourly intake and output (I&O) records should be maintained. Losses of potassium and magnesium will result from the large urinary output, which must be corrected as indicated by laboratory data.

When the use of saline and furosemide, as described above, is ineffective or contraindicated, different measures may be instituted. Among these are the administration of biphosphonates, mithramycin, calcitonin, glucocorticoids, and phosphate salts. In some situations, either peritoneal or hemodialysis may be indicated.

Biphosphonates

The biphosphonates are a relatively new group of compounds that retard bone turnover and therefore are helpful in the management of hypercalcemia. These agents act mainly by inhibiting the activity and number of osteoclasts and are usually effective in normalizing serum calcium only in cases where hypercalcemia is due to a bone-resorbing mechanism (such as breast cancer and certain hematologic malignancies).[85] Etidronate and other biphosphonates, such as pamidronate, are becoming the agents of choice for treating hypercalcemia.[86] These agents provide a significant decrease in serum calcium while having few side effects.

Mithramycin

Mithramycin (an antineoplastic agent) lowers serum calcium by inhibiting osteoclastic bone resorption and by decreasing bone turnover. This drug is usually effective in hypercalcemia caused primarily by increased bone resorption (such as occurs with many malignancies and hyperparathyroidism). Because mithramycin is potentially nephrotoxic, it should be used cautiously in patients with impaired renal function. Due to the potential for nephrotoxicity and hepatotoxicity, the long-term use of mithramycin is limited. Liver enzymes and renal function should be monitored during therapy with this drug. Side effects can include anorexia, nausea, vomiting, bone marrow suppression, and thrombocytopenia.

Calcitonin

By inhibiting bone resorption, salmon calcitonin may temporarily lower the serum calcium level by 1 to 3 mg/dL within hours.[87] Calcitonin is a safe drug but its hypocalcemic effect is mild and many individuals become unresponsive to it after 6 to 10 days of treatment.[88] Side effects include nausea, vomiting, diarrhea, facial flushing, and rarely, allergic reactions.

Glucocorticoids

Glucocorticoids can reduce the serum calcium level by inhibiting calcium absorption in the intestine and by inhibiting osteoclastic bone resorption. They are effective in reducing serum calcium in hypercalcemia due to hypervitaminosis A or sarcoidosis as well as hematolic malignancies.[89] Steroid therapy may be initiated with hydrocortisone, 5 mg/kg body weight per day for 2 to 3 days; later, the dose is reduced to a maintenance level.[90] A drawback of glucocorticoids is that clinically significant reductions in serum calcium may not occur for 5 to 10 days after therapy is initiated.[91] Due to the slow onset of action, glucocorticoids are combined with other therapeutic measures when used to treat patients with severe hypercalcemia. Possible complications associated with glucocorticoids include hyperglycemia and sodium and water retention.

Phosphate Salts

Phosphate salts reduce serum calcium concentration by several mechanisms. For example, phosphate inhibits bone resorption. Also, oral phosphate therapy inhibits intestinal calcium absorption by forming poorly soluble calcium salts. However, the following point should be considered. Increasing the serum phosphate concentration alters the extracellular calcium–phosphate equilibrium to promote calcium deposition into bone and soft tissue (metastatic calcification). Due to the risk of soft-tissue calcification, phosphate therapy should be limited primarily to patients with low serum phosphate levels (<3.0 mg/dL) and adequate renal function. Phosphate salts may be administered orally as Phospho-Soda or Neutra-Phos. Intravenous phosphate therapy should be used with extreme caution in the treatment of hypercalcemia because it can cause severe calcification in various tissues, including the vein in which it is given.

NURSING INTERVENTIONS

1. Be aware of patients at risk for hypercalcemia and monitor for its presence. See Summary of Hypercalcemia and review above sections on etiological factors and defining characteristics.
2. Increase patient mobilization when feasible; recall that immobilization favors hypercalcemia. Hospitalized patients at risk for hypercalcemia should be ambulated as soon as possible; outpatients should be told the importance of frequently moving about.

Summary of Hypercalcemia

ETIOLOGICAL FACTORS

Hyperparathyroidism

Malignant neoplastic disease (lung tumors, breast tumors, and multiple myeloma account for more than 50% of the cases)

Drugs
- Thiazide diuretics
- Excessive vitamin A or D
- Overuse of calcium supplements
- Overuse of calcium-containing antacids
- Lithium
- Theophylline

Prolonged immobilization

DEFINING CHARACTERISTICS

Neuromuscular
- Muscle weakness
- Decreased deep-tendon reflexes

Renal
- Polyuria (nephrogenic diabetes insipidus)
- Hypercalciuria, perhaps leading to renal stones

Gastrointestinal
- Anorexia
- Nausea
- Vomiting
- Constipation

Cardiovascular
- Arrhythmias
- Heart block
- ECG: Shortened Q-T interval
- Increased digitalis sensitivity
- Hypertension

Mental
- Impaired higher cerebral functioning, such as confusion, emotional instability, anxiety, frank psychoses, lethargy or coma

3. Encourage the oral intake of sufficient fluids to keep the patient well hydrated. Sodium-containing fluids should be given, unless contraindicated by other conditions, as sodium favors calcium excretion. One should always consider the patient's "likes" and "dislikes" when encouraging oral fluids. Patients at home should be instructed to drink 3 to 4 quarts of fluid per day, if possible.
4. Discourage excessive consumption of milk products and other high-calcium foods. Depending on the cause of hypercalcemia, dietary restrictions do not necessarily need to be stringent. Consult with physician and dietitian as indicated.
5. Encourage adequate bulk in the diet to offset the tendency to constipation.
6. Take safety precautions if confusion or other mental symptoms of hypercalcemia are present. Explain to the patient and family that the mental changes associated with hypercalcemia are reversible with treatment (see Case Study 6-3 and 6-4).
7. Be aware that cardiac arrest can occur in patients with severe hypercalcemia; be prepared

to deal with this emergency situation.

8. Be aware that bones may fracture more easily in patients with chronic hypercalcemia as bone resorption has been excessive, weakening the bony structure. Transfer patients cautiously.
9. Educate home-bound oncology patients with a predisposition for hypercalcemia, as well as their families, regarding symptoms that occur with this condition. Instruct them to report symptoms to the health care providers before they become severe. In a study reported by Mahon,[92] constipation, confusion, anorexia, increasing bone pain, weight loss, and weakness were the symptoms that most frequently caused readmission of cancer patients. In a study of 22 hospitalized and 18 ambulatory cancer patients, Coward[93] reported that 90% were unaware that hypercalcemia might be a complication of their cancer. Furthermore, only one of the patients knew the symptoms of cancer-induced hypercalcemia. Almost 70% of the patients did not recall being told of measures that might prevent hypercalcemia.
10. Be alert for signs of digitalis toxicity when hypercalcemia occurs in digitalized patients.
11. Be familiar with the treatment modalities for hypercalcemia and associated nursing functions (see Treatment section in this chapter and in Chapter 22).
12. Help prevent formation of calcium renal stones in patients with long-standing hypercalcemia or immobilization by:
    A. Forcing fluids to maintain a dilute urine, thus avoiding supersaturation of precipitates.
    B. Encouraging fluids that yield an acid ash (such as prune or cranberry juice) as a urinary pH of less than 6.5 favors calcium solubility. (Be aware that dietary modifications do not usually alter urinary pH significantly; therefore, pharmacological acidifying agents [such as ascorbic acid, potassium acid phosphate, or methionine] may be prescribed by the physician to ensure a uniformly low pH.)
    C. Preventing urinary stasis by frequently turning the immobilized patient, elevating the head of the bed, and having the patient sit up if this can be tolerated.
    D. Encouraging weight-bearing and ambulation as soon as possible.

CASE STUDIES

6-3. A 76-year-old woman, described as poorly nourished, was admitted through the emergency department. According to her family, she had become progressively confused and weaker over the past 2 to 3 weeks and was incontinent of large amounts of urine; also, she had vomited frequently and was constipated. On assessment she was found to be responsive only to painful stimuli. Skin turgor was poor. A fracture in her left hip was confirmed by film. Bowel sounds were hypoactive. The blood pressure was 96/50 mmHg, pulse 136 beats/min, and respirations 28 breaths/min. While in the emergency department, the patient suffered cardiac arrest three times and was successfully resuscitated. The serum calcium was found to be 18.6 mg/dL. A solution of 0.45% NaCl containing KCl was infused at a rate of 200 mL/hr. Lasix, 20 mg, was given as an IV push every 6 hrs. By the 36th hour, her serum calcium was 16.1 mg/dL. However, rales were heard at the bases of both lungs and periods of shortness of breath developed. Also, she was noted to have 2+ pitting peripheral edema. The IV fluids were cut back to 75 mL/hr. Mithramycin was administered. By the fifth day, the serum calcium was 13.4 mg/dL and the patient was more alert, although responding inappropriately. She remained incontinent of urine and complained of pain. Constipation was relieved by enemas. On the sixth day, mithramycin was repeated and she was begun on Neutra-Phos, 500 mg four times daily. On the seventh day, she was alert and oriented most of the time. Her lungs were clear and there was no edema. When encouraged, she took oral fluids and foods. Also, she was able to void in the bedpan and was only occasionally incontinent. Active bowel sounds were heard in all four quadrants. The serum calcium was 8.1 mg/dL. She was diagnosed as having carcinoma of the ovary with metastases to the bone; radiation therapy and chemotherapy were administered. She was discharged on Neutra-Phos, 500 mg four times daily.

COMMENTARY: This patient displayed classic symptoms of hypercalcemia; they included weakness, confusion, vomiting, constipation, polyuria, and, worst of all, cardiac arrest. The treatment regimen was also close to a textbook picture in that saline fluids were given rapidly in conjunction with IV Lasix. Because of her advanced age, she had difficulty tolerating fluids at a rate of 200 mL/hr, as evidenced by the rales and shortness of breath. Mithramycin was needed to help correct the hypercalcemia, as was Neutra-Phos. Over a period of days, the hypercalcemia was slowly corrected; note that her mental status improved as the serum calcium level diminished.

6-4. A 40-year-old woman with cancer of the cervix and vulva had documented bone and lung metastases and was cared for at home. However, when she became lethargic and developed inappropriate behavior, her family brought her to the emergency room. Other symptoms included severe weakness, nausea, and vomiting, no bowel movement for 5 days, inability to eat and drink for 2 days, and poor skin turgor. Bowel sounds were hypoactive in all four quadrants. Abnormalities noted on laboratory data included a serum calcium level of 16.4 mg/dL and a serum potassium of 2.8 mEq/L. Initial orders (first 24 hrs) included the following:

1. Add 40 mEq of KCl to a liter of 0.9% NaCl solution and infuse at a rate of 250 mL/hr; alternate with a solution of 0.45% NaCl with 40 mEq of KCl at a rate of 250 mL/hr.
2. Lasix, 20 mg, IV push every 6 hrs
3. Neutra-Phos, 500 mg, by mouth four times daily

COMMENTARY: After 3 days, the serum calcium was 12.2 mg/dL and the serum potassium was 3.7 mEq/L. The patient remained confused. On the 6th day, mithramycin was administered. Saline infusions and furosemide were continued. By the 7th day, the serum calcium was down to 9.5 mg/dL. On the 9th day, she was discharged home on Neutra-Phos, 500 mg three times daily, with a serum calcium level of 8.9 mg/dL. At the time of discharge, she was responding appropriately and was oriented to her surroundings.

REFERENCES

1. Chernow et al: Hypocalcemia in critically ill patients. Crit Care Med 10:848,1982
2. Chernow B (ed): The Pharmacologic Approach to the Critically Ill Patient, 3rd ed, p 777. Baltimore, Williams & Wilkins, 1994
3. Yucha C, Toto K: Calcium and phosphorus derangements. In Endocrine and Metabolic Disturbances in the Critically Ill. Crit Care Nurs Clin North Am December:749,1994
4. Rose B: Clinical Physiology of Acid-Base and Electrolyte Disorders, 4th ed, p 891. New York, McGraw-Hill, 1994
5. Narins R (ed): Clinical Disorders of Fluid and Electrolyte Metabolism, 5th ed, p 282. New York, McGraw Hill, 1994
6. Yucha, Toto, p 750
7. Chernow, p 779
8. Wyngaarden J, Smith L, Bennet J (eds): Cecil Textbook of Medicine, 19th ed, p 1426. Philadelphia, WB Saunders, 1992
9. Wyngaarden et al, p 1506
10. Ibid, p 1430
11. Ibid
12. Yucha, Toto, p 751
13. Chernow, p 780
14. Condon R, Nyhus L: Manual of Surgical Therapeutics, 8th ed, p 251. Boston, Little, Brown, 1993
15. Ibid
16. Chernow, p 780
17. Narins, p 1025
18. Bourrel C, et al: Transient hypocalcemia after thyroidectomy. Ann Otol Laryngol 102:496,1993
19. Narins, p 1025
20. Pemberton L, Pemberton D: Treatment of Water, Electrolyte, and Acid-Base Disorders in the Surgical Patient, p 216. New York, McGraw-Hill, 1994
21. Chernow, p 780
22. Ibid
23. Ibid
24. Narins, p 1484
25. Ibid, p 1026
26. Whong S: Predictors of clinical hypomagnesemia. Arch Intern Med 144:1794,1984
27. Narins, p 277
28. Chernow, p 781
29. Narins, p 1084
30. Ibid, p 1085
31. Kokko J, Tannen R: Fluids and Electrolytes, 2nd ed, p 357. Philadelphia, WB Saunders, 1990
32. Narins, p 1028
33. Merideth S, Rosenberg I: Gastrointestinal-hepatic disorders and osteomalacia. Clin Endocrinol Metab 9:131,1980
34. Pemberton, Pemberton, p 173
35. Narins, p 1028
36. Chernow, p 778
37. Condon, Nyhus, p 241

38. Narins, p 1029
39. Chernow et al, p 851
40. Condon, Nyhus, p 240
41. Narins, p 1029
42. Chernow, p 781
43. Narins, p 1026
44. Narins, p 1483
45. Zaloga G, Chernow B: Pathogen mechanisms for hypocalcemia during gram negative sepsis (Abstr). Crit Care Med 14(4):405,1986
46. Lawler D: Hormonal response in sepsis. In Sepsis. Crit Care Nurs Clin North Am September:272,1994
47. Peter S: Disorders of serum calcium in acquired immunodeficiency syndrome. J Natl Med Assoc 84(7):626–628,1992
48. Olinger M: Disorders of calcium and magnesium. Emerg Med Clin North Am 7(4):800,1989
49. Narins, p 1030
50. Yucha, Koko, p 753
51. Olinger, p 800
52. Aubier M et al: Effect of hypocalcemia on diaphragmatic strength generation. J Appl Physiol 58:2054–2061,1985
53. Zaloga G: Nutrition in Critical Care, p 649. St. Louis, CV Mosby, 1994
54. Yucha, Koko, p 753
55. Narins, p 1030
56. Woodley M, Whelan A: Manual of Medical Therapeutics, 27th ed, p 432. Boston, Little, Brown, 1992
57. Narins, p 1031
58. Ibid
59. Woodley, Whelan, p 432
60. Kokko, Tannen, p 617
61. Gahart B: A Handbook of Intravenous Medications, 9th ed, p 85. St. Louis, CV Mosby, 1993
62. Szerlip H, Goldfarb H: Workshops in Fluid and Electrolyte Disorders, p 188. New York, Churchill Livingstone, 1993
63. Lacy C, Armstrong L, Lipsy R, Lance L: Drug Information Handbook, 2nd ed, p 142. Hudson (Cleveland) Lexi-Comp, Inc. American Pharmaceutical Association, 1994–1995
64. Yucko, Koko, p 753
65. Ibid, p 754
66. Zaloga, Chernow, p 784
67. Narins, p 1011
68. Yucha, Toto, p 756
69. Goni M, Tolis G: Hypercalcemia of cancer: An update. Anticancer Res 13:1155–1160,1993
70. Narins, p 1014
71. Ibid, p 1015
72. Ibid, p 1019
73. Ibid, p 1015
74. Ibid, p 1017
75. Olinger, p 805
76. Narins, p 1020
77. Ibid, p 1021
78. Ibid, p 1020
79. Mahon S: Symptoms as clues to calcium levels. Am J Nurs 87(3):354,1987
80. Rose, p 704
81. Yucha, Toto, p 756
82. Narins, p 1020
83. Woodley, Whelan, p 429
84. Szerlip H, Goldfarb H: Workshops in Fluid and Electrolyte Disorders, p 171. New York, Churchill Livingstone, 1993
85. Goni, Tolis, p 1158
86. Ibid, p 172
87. Woodley, Whelan, p 430
88. Olinger, p 830
89. Szerlip, Goldfarb, p 172
90. Narins, p 1031
91. Woodley, Whelan, p 430
92. Mahon, p 354
93. Coward D: Hypercalcemia knowledge assessment in patients at risk of developing cancer-induced hypercalcemia. Oncology Nurs Forum 15(4):471,1988

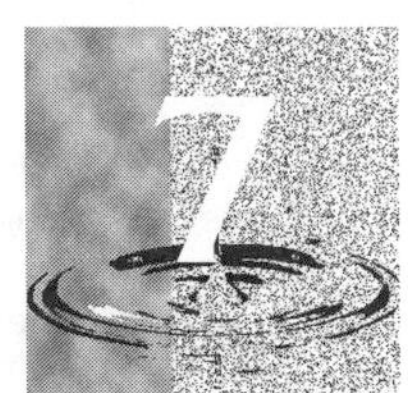

Magnesium Imbalances

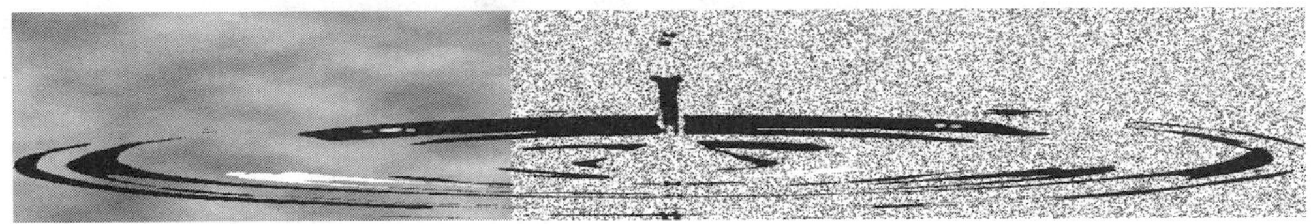

MAGNESIUM BALANCE

Approximately two-thirds of the body's magnesium is located in the skeleton and one-third is in the intracellular fluid; only about 1% is in the extracellular fluid (0.3% in the serum).[1] The normal serum magnesium level can be expressed in mEq/L, mmol/L, or mg/dL (see Table 7-1). (For comparison of these measures, 1 mEq of magnesium is synonymous with 0.5 mmol or 12 mg.) About one-third of the magnesium in serum is bound to proteins; the rest is ionized.

FUNCTIONS

Magnesium has a critical role in intracellular metabolism. It participates in more than 300 enzymatic reactions, especially those processes involving the production and utilization of adenosine triphosphate (ATP).[2] Extracellular magnesium is implicated in neuronal control, neuromuscular transmission, and cardiovascular tone.[3]. Its high concentration in bone relates magnesium closely to calcium and phosphorus. However, because it is a major intracellular ion, it is also closely related to potassium.

HOMEOSTASIS

The recommended daily allowance for magnesium is 300 mg for women and 350 mg for men; the average American dietary magnesium intake is about 500 mg/day.[4] Magnesium is plentiful in green vegetables, grains, nuts, meats, and seafood.

Dietary magnesium is absorbed primarily in the jejunum and ileum. Although little is known about the control of intestinal magnesium absorption, it is thought that it may be increased by parathyroid hormone and growth hormone.[5]

The kidneys are the primary route of magnesium excretion. Fortunately, the kidneys are capable of conserving magnesium efficiently in times of need and excreting it when it is not needed. For example, when magnesium deficiency is present, urinary excretion may fall to less than 1 mEq (0.5 mmol) per day.[6] Also, the kidneys are capable of excreting excess magnesium; therefore, sustained hypermagnesemia is difficult to maintain when normal renal function exists because renal magnesium excretion increases in proportion to the load presented to the kidney.[7]

LABORATORY ASSESSMENT

Assessment of magnesium status is problematic. Although the serum concentration of magnesium is the test most available for clinical use, it is a relatively insensitive measure. This is because only a fraction (0.3%) of the body's total magnesium content is located in the serum. Whereas a less than normal serum magnesium level is most often indicative of total body magnesium deficiency, normal serum magnesium concentrations may exist in some individuals with magnesium deficiency. A high index of suspicion should be used for patients whose clinical condition suggest magnesium depletion but whose serum magnesium is normal or only slightly reduced.[8] The serum magnesium may not fall until several hours after the onset of an acute illness (such as myocardial infarction).[9]

Other more involved methods exist for evaluating magnesium status. Among these are measuring intracellular magnesium in red blood cells and white blood cells and measuring skeletal muscle magnesium. One group of investigators found that 47% of patients admitted to a respiratory intensive care unit had magnesium content in quadriceps muscle

TABLE 7–1

Normal Serum Magnesium Values

EXPRESSION OF MEASUREMENT	NORMAL RANGE
Milliequivalents per 1000 mL (mEq/L)	1.3–2.1
Millimoles per 1000 mL (mmol/L)	0.65–1.1
Milligrams per 100 mL (mg/10 dL)	1.6–2.5

below the lower limit of normal; only 9.4% of the same population had subnormal serum magnesium concentrations.[10] Another group of researchers found that 53% of 104 patients admitted to a coronary care unit had low magnesium content in blood mononuclear cells, but only 7.7% had below normal serum magnesium concentrations.[11] Another type of test involves measuring 24-hr urinary magnesium excretion. This is helpful because patients with magnesium deficiency can be expected to conserve magnesium, excreting less magnesium in the urine per day than individuals with a normal magnesium balance. Under normal circumstances, given average magnesium intake and total body stores, 24-hr urinary magnesium excretion ranges from 120 to 140 mg.[12] In the absence of agents or conditions that promote magnesium excretion, a 24-hr urinary magnesium excretion of less than 25 mg suggests magnesium deficiency.[13] A more elaborate test is the magnesium load test; this involves obtaining a 24-hr baseline urine magnesium determination, followed by the administration of 30 mmol of magnesium sulfate in 500 mL of 5% aqueous dextrose (D_5W) over 12 hrs; urine is collected for 24 hrs from the beginning of the infusion.[14] Patients with normal total magnesium stores are expected to excrete 60% to 80% of the administered magnesium, whereas patients with magnesium deficiency will excrete less than 50%.

A curious relationship exists between magnesium and calcium; although low serum levels of these electrolytes produce similar effects (that is, increased neuromuscular irritability), their actions sometimes antagonize each other. For example, magnesium narcosis can be antagonized by parenteral calcium administration.

HYPOMAGNESEMIA

Hypomagnesemia (and possibly magnesium depletion) is a common clinical problem, both in ambulatory and hospitalized patients. For example, hypomagnesemia was found to be present in 10.2% of 5100 consecutive ambulatory and hospitalized patients in one study.[15] Much higher rates are observed in critically ill patients. A recent study found that 61% of patients admitted to two postoperative intensive care units had lower than normal serum magnesium levels.[16] Similarly, 65% of patients with normal renal function in a medical intensive care unit population were found to have lower than normal serum magnesium levels.[17]

ETIOLOGICAL FACTORS

Gastrointestinal Losses

An important route for magnesium loss is the gastrointestinal (GI) tract. Losses may take the form of drainage from nasogastric suction, diarrhea, or fistulas. Because fluid from the lower GI tract is richer in magnesium (10–14 mEq/L) than is fluid from the upper tract (1–2 mEq/L), losses from diarrhea and intestinal fistulas are more likely to induce magnesium deficit than are those from gastric suction.[18] However, hypomagnesemia will occur in patients with prolonged nasogastric suction, especially if parenteral fluids are magnesium free.

Because the distal small bowel is the major site of magnesium absorption, any disruption in small bowel function (as occurs in intestinal resection or inflammatory bowel disease) can lead to hypomagnesemia. One study reported that 15 of 42 patients with malabsorption syndromes had subnormal serum magnesium levels[19]; the degree of hypomagnesemia showed a rough correlation with the degree of steatorrhea. In the presence of steatorrhea, it is believed that magnesium ions are excreted in the stool in the form of magnesium soaps. In another study, 50% of 191 patients developed hypomagnesemia in the first postoperative year after bowel resection for the treatment of morbid obesity.[20]

Alcoholism

Chronic alcoholism is the most common cause of hypomagnesemia in the United States. One study found that 30% of all alcoholics and 86% of patients with delirium tremens had hypomagnesemia during the first 1 to 2 days of hospitalization.[21] Although there are no convincing data to indicate that hypomagnesemia causes delirium tremens, it is likely that magnesium deficiency aggravates alcohol withdrawal.[22] For this reason, it is recommended that the serum magnesium level be measured every 2 or 3 days in hospitalized alcoholic patients undergoing withdrawal.[23] Although the serum magnesium level may be normal on admission, it can fall as a result of metabolic changes associated with therapy (such as the intracellular shift of magnesium associated with intravenous [IV] glucose administration).

Decreased dietary intake of magnesium is a major factor in the development of hypomagnesemia in alcoholics. Other factors include increased GI losses (due to episodic emesis and diarrhea) and intestinal malabsorption. In addition, alcohol ingestion is believed to increase magnesium excretion in the urine.

Refeeding After Starvation

In the catabolic state, the protein structure of cells is metabolized as energy sources; as a result, intracellular ions are lost and total body concentrations of these ions (magnesium, potassium, and phosphate) are decreased.[24] Conversely, during nutritional repletion, these electrolytes are taken from the serum and deposited into newly synthesized cells. Thus, if the enteral or parenteral feeding formula is deficient in magnesium content, serious hypomagnesemia will occur. Serum levels of these primarily intracellular ions should be measured at regular intervals during the administration of IV total parenteral nutrition and even during enteral feedings, especially in patients who have undergone a period of starvation. See Chapters 11 and 12 for further discussions of this topic.

Drugs Disrupting Magnesium Homeostasis

The loop diuretics (furosemide, bumetanide, and ethacrynic acid) increase urinary magnesium excretion. Although the loop diuretics are the most potent magnesuric diuretics, long-term use of thiazide diuretics may also lead to mild hypomagnesemia.[25]

Although the exact mechanism is not clear, it has been demonstrated that aminoglycosides (such as gentamycin, tobramycin, and kanamycin) are associated with urinary magnesium wasting. For example, one study found that of 55 patients receiving aminoglycoside antibiotics, 38% developed hypomagnesemia associated with renal magnesium wasting.[26] Amphotericin B (an antifungal agent) can also cause hypomagnesemia.[27]

Cis-platinum (cisplatin) administration is associated with hypomagnesemia secondary to increased urinary excretion of magnesium; this potentially nephrotoxic chemotherapeutic agent causes hypomagnesemia in a dose-related manner.[28] Cyclosporin usage in renal transplant patients may produce a significant drop in the serum magnesium concentration, presumably by increasing renal magnesium wasting.[29]

Recall that citrate is a preservative added to collected blood to prolong its longevity. Rapid administration of citrated blood (eg, faster than 1.5 mL/kg/min) can temporarily drop the ionized magnesium level because citrate chelates circulating magnesium ions (and calcium ions).[30] This is most likely to occur when citrate clearance is diminished by renal or hepatic disease or by hypothermia.[31]

Other Factors

Magnesium deficiency is often seen in patients with diabetic ketoacidosis. It is primarily the result of increased renal excretion of magnesium during osmotic diuresis (caused by the high glucose load) and of the shifting of magnesium into cells that occurs with insulin therapy (see Chapter 18).

Some causes of renal disease, such as glomerulonephritis, pyelonephritis, and renal tubular acidosis, may produce hypomagnesemia by impairing renal magnesium reabsorption. However, remember that with *advanced* renal disease (glomerular filtration rate [GFR] $<$10–25 mL/hr), *hyper*magnesemia usually results from impaired renal magnesium excretion.[32]

Pancreatitis may cause hypomagnesemia in much the same way that it causes hypocalcemia (see Chapter 20 for a discussion of this topic). In addition, any condition associated with hypercalcemia, such as excessive doses of vitamin D or calcium supplements, may result in renal magnesium loss.[33] It should be noted that magnesium and calcium share a common route of absorption in the intestinal tract and appear to have a mutually suppressive effect; thus, if calcium intake is unusually high, calcium will be absorbed in preference to magnesium, and vice versa.

Magnesium deficiency has also been described in burn patients and is possibly related to loss of magnesium during débridement and bathing of denuded skin. Other conditions believed to predispose to hypomagnesemia are sepsis and hypothermia.[34] Also, postoperative patients may have increased magnesium loss in the urine due to increased aldosterone release associated with stress from the operative procedure.[35]

Administration of magnesium-free, sodium-rich IV fluids to induce extracellular fluid expansion can cause hypomagnesemia. In fact, any condition predisposing to excessive calcium or sodium in the urine can augment renal excretion of magnesium as magnesium is normally reabsorbed in the kidney with calcium and sodium.[36]

DEFINING CHARACTERISTICS

Some of the effects of hypomagnesemia are directly caused by the low serum magnesium level, whereas others are due to secondary changes in potassium and calcium metabolism. Manifestations of magnesium deficiency do not usually occur until the serum magnesium level is less than 1 mEq/L. However, because the serum magnesium concentration may underestimate intracellular magnesium depletion, a high index of suspicion for magnesium deficiency is warranted.[37]

Neuromuscular Changes

Neuromuscular hyperexcitability with muscular weakness, tremors, and athetoid movements may be seen. Other manifestations may include tetany, generalized tonic-clonic or focal seizures, laryngeal stridor, and positive Chvostek's and Trousseau's signs. The neuromuscular symptoms of hypomagnesemia are similar to those occurring in hypocalcemia and result mainly from increased neuronal excitability. Because severe hypomagnesemia may ultimately result in hypocalcemia and hypokalemia, it is possible that the symptoms may be partly due to these disturbances. Vague but nonspecific GI symptoms have been described; for example, dysphagia may develop.

Cardiovascular Effects

Magnesium deficiency predisposes to cardiac arrhythmias, such as premature ventricular contractions, supraventricular tachycardia, and ventricular fibrillation. In fact, tachyarrhythmias are a well-documented complication of magnesium depletion. Because standard antiarrhythmic drugs and defibrillation may be ineffective in controlling ventricular arrhythmias associated with magnesium deficiency, refractory arrhythmias should be treated with IV magnesium salts. Intracellular magnesium depletion in the myocardium is even more likely to predispose to arrhythmias if hypokalemia is also present.[38] Electrocardiographic (ECG) changes observed in hypomagnesemia include PR and QT interval prolongation, widened QRS complex, ST segment depression, and T wave inversion.[39]

Increased susceptibility to digitalis toxicity is associated with low serum magnesium levels. An experiment with animals found that the uptake of digoxin by myocardial cells was enhanced by magnesium depletion.[40] One report found that hypomagnesemia was present twice as often in digitalis-toxic patients (21%) as in nontoxic patients (10%).[41] This is important because patients receiving digoxin are also likely to be on diuretic therapy, which predisposes to renal loss of magnesium.

Central Nervous System Changes

Because decreased serum magnesium increases irritability of nerve tissue, convulsions may occur. Disorientation is common. Other changes may include ataxia, vertigo, depression, and psychosis.

Metabolic Effects

Associated Imbalances

Imbalances commonly associated with hypomagnesemia include hypokalemia, hypocalcemia, and hypophosphatemia. In a recent study of hypomagnesmic patients, 43% had hypokalemia, 29% had hypophosphatemia, and 22% had hypocalcemia.[42] It is likely that the latter two accompany hypomagnesemia because severe magnesium depletion interferes with the secretion of parathyroid hormone (PTH), which is needed to return calcium and phosphorus to normal ranges. Hypokalemia is a relatively common finding in hypomagnesemic patients because the kidneys are not able to conserve potassium when magnesium deficiency exists. This hypokalemia accompanying hypomagnesemia is often refractory to potassium replacement alone, requiring the replacement of both potassium and magnesium before correction of the imbalance can occur. The plasma magnesium concentration should always be measured in patients with otherwise unexplained hypokalemia.[43]

Insulin Resistance

Magnesium has been found to influence peripheral tissue responsiveness to insulin and also to affect insulin secretion by the pancreas.[44] Hypomagnesemia has been reported in a variety of settings involving insulin resistance.[45] However, the relationship between hypomagnesemia and insulin resistance is not clear.

TREATMENT

Magnesium replacement may be indicated even when the serum magnesium concentration is normal; this is because total body magnesium stores may be decreased despite normomagnesemia. Magnesium deficiency is treated by correcting the cause of the imbalance (when possible) and supplying magnesium to correct the deficit. Serum magnesium levels may normalize rather quickly, but sustained magnesium replacement for several days is usually needed to replace cellular magnesium deficits. Provided the patient is able to eat, mild magnesium deficiency can be corrected by diet alone; principal dietary sources of magnesium are green vegetables, meat, seafood, dairy products, and cereals.[46] When symptoms of hypomagnesemia are absent, it is best to administer magnesium orally to avoid causing abrupt increases in the plasma magnesium level.[47] Magnesium salts in tablet form (such as magnesium oxide) can be given orally to replace continuous excessive losses. Unfortunately, diarrhea is a side effect that can interfere with the usefulness of oral magnesium preparations.

Magnesium may be given IV or by deep intramuscular injection (although painful) when indicated. Parenteral magnesium is especially helpful in individuals with symptomatic hypomagnesemia or malabsorption. Before magnesium administration, renal function should be assessed as the kidneys are primarily responsible for the elimination of magnesium. When renal function is impaired in those receiving magnesium, blood levels should be closely monitored. During parenteral magnesium replacement, serum magnesium levels should be monitored, as should deep tendon reflexes. Marked depression of deep tendon reflexes signals too high a serum magnesium level and is an indication that no further magnesium should be administered.[48] Reports of serum levels at which loss of the patellar reflex occurs are variable; some studies state that it is decreased at 4 to 7 mEq/L and is lost at 10 to 15 mEq/L.[49] Other studies state that it is lost when serum magnesium levels are more than 6 mEq/L.[50] In any event, deep tendon reflexes disappear before respiratory paralysis and heart block occur.

Patients with severe hypomagnesemia (defined as <1 mg/dL) should receive special attention. For example, in the treatment of life-threatening arrhythmias, Zaloga and Chernow[51] recommend 1 to 2 g (8–16 mEq) of magnesium sulfate intravenously over 5 min (while ECG monitoring is continuously performed). They further recommend that this bolus dose be followed by an infusion of 1 to 2 g/hr of magnesium sulfate for the next few hours and then the dose be reduced to 0.5 to 1 g/hr as a maintenance infusion (provided renal function is normal).

Magnesium sulfate is available in 10%, 20%, and 50% solutions; 1 g of magnesium sulfate is equivalent to 2 mL of a 50% solution, 5 mL of a 20% solution, and 10 mL of a 10% solution.[52] A report of severe hypermagnesemia resulting from improperly written or executed orders for IV magnesium sulfate pointed out the need for extreme caution in administering magnesium.[53] Three cases of severe hypermagnesemia were attributed to the inadvertent use of 50-mL vials of 50% magnesium sulfate. In two cases, the orders called for "one amp" of 50% magnesium sulfate by slow IV infusion. Although the prescriber intended that a 2-mL ampule be given, a 50-mL ampule was substituted. In the third case, the order was for a 50-mL vial of 50% dextrose. Instead, a 50-mL vial of magnesium sulfate was mistakenly used. The author emphasizes the need to recognize the potency of currently available electrolyte solutions and the importance of physicians writing precise orders pertaining to their use. Certainly orders containing terms such as "amp" or "vial" without further specification should not be written by physicians or accepted by nurses. The third case emphasizes the need to read product labels carefully before use. Never rely solely on the size, shape, or label design of the container for product identification. General nursing considerations related to administering of magnesium salts are listed in Clinical Tip: Nursing Considerations in Administering IV Magnesium.

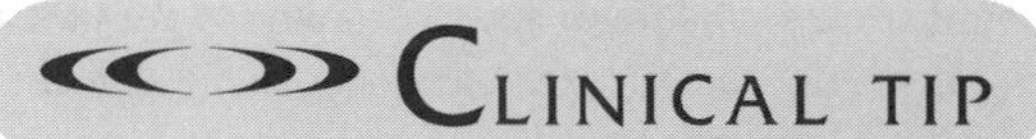

Nursing Considerations in Administering IV Magnesium

1. The extent of magnesium replacement needed for specific hypomagnesemic patients may vary widely according to (a) the severity of the magnesium deficiency, and (b) the current level of renal function. Generally, the more severe the symptoms, the more aggressive the therapy must be.
2. Carefully check the order for IV magnesium. Be sure that it stipulates one of the following:
   A. Concentration of the solution to be administered (as well as the number of milliliters), fluid in which it is to be diluted, and the time frame over which it is to be given. For example: "Give 2 mL of 50% $MgSO_4$, diluted in 100 mL of 0.9% sodium chloride, over one hr."
   B. Number of grams of magnesium sulfate to be administered, along with the required dilution, and time frame over which it is to be administered. For example: "Give 1 g of $MgSO_4$, diluted in 100 mL of 0.9% sodium chloride, over one hr."

   Recall that magnesium sulfate ($MgSO_4$) is available in concentrations of 10%, 20%, and 50%. One gram of magnesium sulfate is contained in 10 mL of a 10% solution, 5 mL of a 20% solution, and 2 mL of a 50% solution. Obviously, serious errors can occur if the wrong concentration is used.
3. Never accept order for "amps" or "vials" without further specifications.
4. Use IV magnesium with great caution in patients with impaired renal function (as evidenced by an elevated serum creatinine level). Recall that the primary route of magnesium excretion is via the kidneys; thus, it is easy to induce hypermagnesemia when renal impairment is present. If magnesium replacement is required in a patient with renal impairment, the physician will probably reduce the dose to be administered by 25% to 50% of that needed for a patient with normal renal function.
5. Monitor urine output at regular intervals throughout the magnesium infusion. It should be maintained at a level of at least 100 mL every 4 hr.[54] An output less than this amount raises the question of adequate urinary elimination of magnesium.
6. Check deep tendon reflexes (such as patellar "knee jerk") before each dose of magnesium, or periodically during continuous infusion of the drug. If reflexes are absent, do not give additional magnesium, and notify the physician. (Because deep tendon reflexes are decreased before adverse respiratory and cardiac effects occur, the presence of knee jerks can usually be relied on to indicate that life-threatening hypermagnesemia is not present.)
7. Therapeutic doses of magnesium can produce flushing and sweating because magnesium acts peripherally to produce vasodilation. Inform the patient that this might occur to minimize concern.
8. Check blood pressure, pulse, and respirations every 15 minutes and monitor the serum magnesium level at regular intervals. Look for a sharp fall in blood pressure or respiratory distress; both are signs of hypermagnesemia. (This can be induced rather easily with improper doses of magnesium.) Patients receiving very aggressive magnesium therapy should receive close cardiac monitoring.
9. If the patient displays signs of severe hypermagnesemia, stop IV administration of magnesium and run in the IV solution from the primary line (as appropriate) to keep the vein open. Notify the physician and be prepared to administer artificial ventilation and IV calcium (if prescribed).
10. Because magnesium is primarily an intracellular ion, it may take several days to completely correct cellular deficits. Therefore, normal serum magnesium values do not necessarily imply that the magnesium depletion has been corrected.

OTHER CONDITIONS THAT MAY BENEFIT FROM MAGNESIUM ADMINISTRATION

Briefly described in Table 7-2 are the possible rationales for using magnesium in the treatment of patients with eclampsia, myocardial infarction, angina, and acute asthma. The use of magnesium in patients with diabetes mellitus is discussed below.

Although a strong association between magnesium deficiency and insulin resistance has been shown, no study has demonstrated a causal relationship between the two.[61] Hypomagnesemia has been demonstrated in both insulin-dependent and non-insulin-dependent diabetics. Probably the magnesium deficiency in these patients is caused by increased urinary magnesium losses due to chronic glycosuria. Although there are data relating magnesium deficiency to insulin resistance, the exact physiologic role of magnesium deficiency in diabetes is not clear. Therefore, a consensus statement published by the American Diabetic Association in 1992

TABLE 7–2

Conditions That May Benefit from Magnesium Administration

Severe Preeclampsia/Eclampsia	Prevent or control convulsions Lower blood pressure Inhibit uterine contractions (See Chapter 23 for a more thorough discussion of magnesium administration in this disorder.)
Myocardial Infarction	Postulated that magnesium infusion decreases some arrhythmias and decreases the size of ischemic injury after an acute myocardial infarction (presumably by acting as a coronary artery vasodilator, potential antithrombotic agent, and a calcium competitor). Several large studies have shown conflicting results regarding the value of magnesium in reducing mortality following acute myocardial infarction (MI). A 1992 study (the LIMIT-2 trial) of over 2000 patients with acute MIs showed a mortality decrease of 24% when magnesium was administered.[55] However, findings from a study of over 50,000 patients presented in late 1993 from the ISIS-4 Collaborative Group suggest there is no benefit from the routine use of magnesium in acute MI.[56] The 1994 ACLS Guidelines recommend magnesium administration in acute MI when there is known or suspected magnesium deficiency; the recommended dose for acute MI prophylaxis is 1–2 g (2–4 mL of 50% magnesium sulfate) diluted in 100 mL of normal saline over 5–60 min (followed with 0.5–1.0 g/hr up to 24 hrs).[57]
Coronary Artery Spasm and Angina	Magnesium has been likened to "nature's physiologic calcium channel blocker" because it promotes vascular effects similar to those seen with calcium channel blockers (vasodilation and prevention of vasospasm). (There are insufficient data at present to recommend that magnesium be given as routine treatment for angina.[58])
Acute Asthma	Postulated that magnesium relaxes bronchial smooth muscle and produces dilatation of the airways.[59] (Some authorities believe that more systematic, controlled studies should be conducted before this therapy is recommended since hypermagnesemia can depress neuromuscular and cardiovascular function.[60])

Summary of Hypomagnesemia

ETIOLOGICAL FACTORS

Inadequate Intake
Prolonged administration of magnesium-free fluids
Starvation
TPN without adequate magnesium supplementation
Chronic alcoholism

Increased Gastrointestinal Losses
Diarrhea
Laxative abuse
Fistulas
Prolonged nasogastric suction
Vomiting
Malabsorption syndromes

Increased Renal Losses
Drugs
- Loop and thiazide diuretics
- Mannitol
- Cisplatin
- Cyclosporine
- Aminoglycosides
- Carbenicillin
- Amphotericin B
- Digitalis
- Pentamidine

Diuresis
- Uncontrolled diabetes mellitus
- Hyperaldosteronism

SIADH

Changes in Magnesium Distribution
Pancreatitis
Thermal injury
Drugs causing shift into cells
- Insulin
- Glucose
- Catecholamines

Citrate Chelation
- Citrated blood products
- Plasmapheresis

Hungry bone syndrome

DEFINING CHARACTERISTICS

Neuromuscular
Muscle weakness
Muscle twitching, cramps
Paresthesias
Chvostek's sign
Trousseau's sign

Cardiovascular
Increased sensitivity to digitalis
Hypertension
Arrhythmias—
- Premature ventricular contractions, ventricular fibrillation, torsades de pointes, atrial fibrillation, paroxysmal supraventricular tachycardia

Increased sensitivity to ischemic heart disease arrhythmias
Coronary artery spasm

ECG changes—
- Prolonged QT and PR intervals, widened QRS complex, depressed ST segment

Metabolic
Hypocalcemia
Hypokalemia
Hypophosphatemia
Insulin resistance

Central Nervous System
Depression
Agitation
Confusion
Psychosis

suggests that only patients who have documented hypomagnesemia with diabetes mellitus receive magnesium supplements.[62] The group stated that in the absence of prospective studies, it is possible that decreased magnesium levels may represent a marker rather than a cause of disease. They further stated that it is appropriate to measure the serum magnesium concentration in patients especially at risk of magnesium deficiency (namely, those with acute myocardial infarction, ketoacidosis, ethanol abuse, long-term parenteral nutrition, use of magnesium-losing drugs, and congestive heart failure).

Magnesium given to patients with non-insulin-dependent diabetes has been reported to decrease the hyperaggregability of platelets typically seen in these individuals.[63] It has been suggested that magnesium might play a protective role against thrombotic cerebrovascular and myocardial infarction, and that magnesium deficiency might accelerate their progression.[64]

NURSING INTERVENTIONS

1. Be aware of patients at risk for hypomagnesemia and monitor for its presence. See Summary of Hypomagnesemia and review above sections for a discussion of etiological factors and defining characteristics.
2. Assess digitalized patients at risk for hypomagnesemia especially closely for symptoms of digitalis toxicity as a deficit of magnesium predisposes to toxicity.
3. Be prepared to take seizure precautions when hypomagnesemia is severe.
4. Monitor condition of airway as laryngeal stridor can occur.
5. Take safety precautions if confusion is present.
6. Be familiar with magnesium replacement salts and factors related to their safe administration. Review Treatment section above and Clinical Tip: Nursing Considerations in Administering IV Magnesium.
7. Be aware that magnesium-depleted patients may experience difficulty in swallowing. (Dysphagia is probably related to the athetoid or choreiform movements associated with magnesium deficit.) If difficulty in swallowing is suspected, test the ability to swallow with water before offering oral medications.
8. When magnesium deficit is due to abuse of diuretics or laxatives, educating the patient may help alleviate the problem. Part of the nursing assessment should be directed toward identifying problems amenable to prevention through education.
9. Be aware that most commonly used IV fluids have either no magnesium or a relatively small amount. For example, D_5W, isotonic saline, and lactated Ringer's solution have no magnesium. Prolonged use of magnesium-free parenteral fluids with no oral intake of magnesium and abnormal losses of magnesium by the GI or renal route will eventually lead to hypomagnesemia. When indicated, discuss need for magnesium replacement with physician.
10. For patients experiencing abnormal magnesium losses who are able to consume a general diet, encourage the intake of magnesium-rich foods (such as green vegetables, meat, seafood, dairy products, and cereal).

CASE STUDIES

7-1. A 65-year-old emaciated woman with carcinoma of the stomach was started on a total parenteral nutrition (TPN) protocol because she was unable to eat or tolerate enteral tube feedings. On the seventh day, when electrolytes were checked for the first time, the serum magnesium was found to be 0.8 mEq/L. She was lethargic and had coarse tremors, most notable in the arms. Total parenteral nutrition was stopped and 12 mL of 50% magnesium sulfate was added to 1 L of 10% glucose in water and infused over 3 hrs. Additional magnesium was administered over the next 2 days. Total parenteral nutrition was slowly restarted with adequate magnesium supplementation.

COMMENTARY: Serum electrolytes should be measured regularly during TPN. In fact, they should be measured daily for the first 5 days. The purpose is to detect abnormalities before they become severe. Requirements for the intracellular ions potassium, magnesium, and phosphate vary with calorie and nitrogen intake and the nutritional state of the patient. As the anabolic state is achieved with TPN, these ions are incorporated into the newly synthesized cells. In this way, extracellular deficits will develop if inadequate amounts are provided in the nutrient solution.

7-2. A 50-year-old man with a history of chronic alcoholism was admitted for treatment. He had been on a diet of only alcoholic beverages for a week and then stopped drinking for a few days. Because of nausea, he ate very little. On examination, he was noted to have hyperactive knee jerks. Laboratory findings included a serum magnesium level of 0.7 mEq/L.

COMMENTARY: Hypomagnesemia is a frequent occurrence in alcoholic patients. Contributing to poor dietary intake of magnesium as a major cause of magnesium deficiency is the increased renal loss of this electrolyte associated with excessive alcohol intake.

7-3. A 40-year-old man developed a high-output intestinal fistula after treatment for an intestinal obstruction. For 2 weeks he received only isotonic saline (0.9% NaCl) and 5% dextrose in water with added KCl. He developed choreiform movements of the arms and muscle twitching. In addition, he was noted to be confused. Laboratory findings included:

Serum Na = 140 mEq/L
K = 3.3 mEq/L
Mg = 0.7 mEq/L

COMMENTARY: Although the serum sodium level is normal, the magnesium is far below normal and there is some degree of hypokalemia, despite addition of KCl to the IV fluids. Recall that intestinal fluid contains approximately 10 to 12 mEq/L of magnesium. These losses were not replaced as the IV fluids were magnesium-free. With a negative magnesium balance, there is often a below-normal serum potassium, even with adequate intake.

HYPERMAGNESEMIA

Although hypermagnesemia is much less common than hypomagnesemia, it may occur more frequently than previously thought. In one study, as many as 86% of hypermagnesemic patients were not clinically identified.[65] Serum magnesium concentrations tend to be good predictors of magnesium excess. Most causes of hypermagnesemia are iatrogenic.

ETIOLOGICAL FACTORS

Renal Failure

Hypermagnesemia is most likely to occur in patients with renal insufficiency (especially if creatinine clearance is <30 mL/min).[66] This is understandable because magnesium is primarily excreted by the kidneys and, therefore, diminished renal function results in abnormal renal magnesium retention. The predisposition of patients with renal failure to hypermagnesemia is aggravated if they are given magnesium to control convulsions or if they inadvertently receive one of the many commercial antacids or laxatives containing variable amounts of magnesium salts (see Table 7-3). Despite its relatively low prevalence (as compared to that of hypomagnesemia), hypermagnesemia probably occurs more frequently than it should because clinicians are often unaware of the magnesium content of various preparations.[67]

Renal patients may also receive an exogenous magnesium load during hemodialysis, because of either an inadvertent use of hard water or an error in manufacture of the concentrate used for preparing the dialysate.

Elderly persons are at greater risk for hypermagnesemia because they have age-related reduced renal function and tend to consume more magnesium-containing preparations (such as antacids or

TABLE 7–3

Some Commonly Used Medications Containing Magnesium

ANTACIDS	LAXATIVES
Aludrox	Citrate of Magnesia
Camalox	Milk of Magnesia
Creamalin	Haley's M-O
Delcid	
Di-Gel	
Gelusil	
Maalox	
Mylanta	
Riopan	
Silain-Gel	
Simeco	
Trisagel	

mineral supplements) than younger individuals. Also, the elderly may have GI disorders (eg, gastritis and colitis) that alter the GI mucosal barrier and thus increase absorption of magnesium.[68]

Other Factors

Overly vigorous treatment with magnesium salts can cause hypermagnesemia in patients with normal renal function, as can conventional doses in those with renal impairment. Magnesium sulfate is sometimes administered to treat eclampsia or to delay delivery. In either case, excessive magnesium administration can cause both maternal and fetal hypermagnesemia. In a recent study of the use of magnesium sulfate as a tocolytic agent on 111 women, investigators reported that side effects were common but were rarely severe enough to cause cessation of therapy.[69] They cautioned that because 90% of parenterally administered magnesium sulfate is cleared by the maternal kidneys, the drug should be administered with extreme caution in women with impaired renal function. It is possible to exceed the renal tolerance of patients with normal renal function if excessive magnesium is accidentally administered during treatment of symptomatic hypomagnesemia or when too much magnesium is added to parenteral nutrition fluids.

Transient elevations in serum magnesium levels can occur during periods of extracellular fluid volume depletion, as in adrenal insufficiency or after diuretic abuse. Hypermagnesemia can also be related to untreated diabetic ketoacidosis when catabolism causes release of cellular magnesium that cannot be excreted due to the oliguria associated with fluid volume depletion.

An elevated magnesium level can be artifactual (false-positive) when blood specimens are drawn with an excessively tight tourniquet or allowed to hemolyze.

DEFINING CHARACTERISTICS

Because magnesium is not routinely measured with other electrolytes, one must maintain a high index of suspicion for hypermagnesemia in at-risk patients. The clinical manifestations of hypermagnesemia largely reflect the ion's action on the nervous and cardiovascular systems.

Hypermagnesemia diminishes neuromuscular transmission and can depress skeletal muscle function and cause neuromuscular blockade.[70] Hypocalcemia may accompany hypermagnesemia because the latter suppresses PTH secretion.

Cardiovascular effects of hypermagnesemia are related to its "calcium channel blocker" effect on cardiac conduction and smooth muscle of blood vessels.[71] Arrhythmias occurring with hypermagnesemia may include bradycardia, atrioventricular (AV) block, and asystole. Changes seen on ECG tracings may include shortening of the QT interval as well as T wave abnormalities and prolongation of the QRS and PR intervals. Hypotension tends to occur early in hypermagnesemia and is related to vasodilatation.

The reader is referred to the Summary of Hypermagnesemia for a list of some rough relationships between the serum levels of magnesium and expected symptoms. However, it should be emphasized that authorities do not agree on precise serum magnesium levels and correlation with clinical signs and symptoms. In fact, quite variable results may be found in the literature. For example, some researchers indicate that deep tendon reflexes are usually lost when the serum magnesium concentration exceeds 6 mEq/L[72]; others describe this as occurring at a level of 10 to 15 mEq/L.[73] Most investigators seem to agree that deep tendon reflexes become hypoactive before respiratory depression occurs, making this an important area for assessment. Despite the wide variations in reports of levels at which symptoms occur, it is clear that the patients at risk for hypermagnesemia (especially those receiving magnesium infusions) must be closely monitored for potential problems. Rizzo et al.[74] reported a case in which a 27-year-old diabetic woman was inadvertently given two 25-g bottles of magnesium sulfate over a 6-hr period for treatment of hypomagnesemia. (This occurred after an order was placed for "2 amps of magnesium sulfate" to be administered in 1 L of intravenous fluids.) Profound hypermagnesemia (9.85 mmol/L) resulted and caused total neuromuscular blockade and a pseudocoma state that mimicked a midbrain syndrome. Fortunately, the patient eventually recovered although she received a greatly larger dose of magnesium than intended. (*One* gram of magnesium sulfate provides 97.6 mg, 4 mmol, or 8 mEq of elemental magnesium.)[75]

Summary of Hypermagnesemia

ETIOLOGICAL FACTORS

Acute and chronic renal failure (particularly when magnesium-containing medications are used)

Excessive magnesium administration during treatment of eclampsia or to delay labor (affects both mother and fetus)

Excessive doses of magnesium during treatment of hypomagnesemia

Excessive use of magnesium-containing antacids or laxatives by elderly persons (who have age-related decreased renal function)

Adrenal insufficiency

Hemodialysis with excessively hard water or with a dialysate high in magnesium content

CLINICAL INDICATORS

Serum Magnesium Level (mEq/L)*	
3–5	Peripheral vasodilatation with facial flushing, sense of warmth, and tendency for hypotension; nausea and vomiting
4–7	Drowsiness; decreased deep tendon reflexes; muscle weakness
5–10	More severe hypotension and bradycardia
7–10	Loss of patellar reflex
10	Respiratory depression
10–15	Respiratory paralysis; coma
15–20	Cardiac arrest

*These are only general ranges; precise levels at which signs and symptoms are expected to develop are not uniformly defined. Reports in the literature vary widely in regard to symptoms and the level at which they appear (see text).

TREATMENT

The best treatment for hypermagnesemia is prevention. This can be accomplished by avoiding administration of magnesium to patients with renal failure and by carefully administering magnesium salts to seriously ill patients.

In the presence of hypermagnesemia, any parenteral or oral magnesium salt should be discontinued. This may be all that is needed if the deep tendon reflexes are still present. Neuromuscular and cardiac toxicity of hypermagnesemia can be antagonized transiently by the intravenous administration of 10 to 20 mL of 10% calcium gluconate over 10 min.[76] (Recall that calcium acts as a direct antagonist to magnesium.) Mechanical ventilation may be needed for patients with compromised respiratory function. A temporary pacemaker may be needed for bradyarrhythmias.[77] Dialysis (either peritoneal or hemodialysis) may be needed for treating hypermagnesemic renal failure patients.

NURSING INTERVENTIONS

1. Be aware of patients at risk for hypermagnesemia and assess for its presence. See Summary of Hypermagnesemia and preceding sections explaining etiological factors and defining characteristics.

   When hypermagnesemia is suspected, assess the following parameters:
   - Vital signs: Look for low blood pressure and shallow respirations with periods of apnea.
   - Patellar reflexes: If absent, notify physician as this usually implies a serum magnesium level greater than 6 mEq/L. If allowed to progress, cardiac or respiratory arrest could occur.

- Level of consciousness: Look for drowsiness, lethargy, and coma.

2. Do not give magnesium-containing medications to patients with renal failure or compromised renal function. (Be particularly careful in following "standing orders" for bowel preparation for radiography because some of these include the use of magnesium citrate.)
3. Caution patients with renal disease to check with their health care providers before taking over-the-counter medications. See Table 7-3 for a list of some commonly used medications containing magnesium.
4. Be aware of factors related to safe parenteral administration of magnesium salts. Review Clinical Tip: Nursing Considerations in Administering IV Magnesium.

CASE STUDIES

7-4. A 43-year-old woman was awaiting a kidney transplant when an order was written for a barium enema. Routine orders for bowel preparation in the institution included the administration of magnesium citrate as a laxative. Without considering the need to modify directives for a renal patient, the preparation was administered. Shortly after administration of magnesium citrate, the patient became very lethargic and developed muscular weakness.

COMMENTARY: Magnesium salts should never be given to patients with acute or chronic renal disease because diseased kidneys are incapable of eliminating magnesium. Blindly following standing orders caused serious problems for this patient. Hemodialysis was performed on an emergency basis.

7-5. A 62-year-old woman with chronic glomerulonephritis took Maalox (a magnesium-containing antacid) to alleviate gastric discomfort. She developed lethargy and difficulty in breathing. On admission to an acute care facility, her serum magnesium level was found to be 7.8 mEq/L (normal, 1.5–2.5 mEq/L). Ten mEq of calcium gluconate were administered to alleviate respiratory depression. Hemodialysis was initiated.

COMMENTARY: As above, magnesium-containing medications are contraindicated in patients with acute or chronic renal disease. Part of patient education should be directed at the need to avoid such preparations.

REFERENCES

1. Matz R: Magnesium deficiencies and therapeutic uses. Hosp Pract April 30:79–92,1993
2. Reinhart R: Magnesium deficiency: Recognition and treatment in the emergency medicine setting. Am J Emerg Med 10:78–83,1992
3. Narins R (ed): Maxwell & Kleeman's Clinical Disorders of Fluid and Electrolyte Metabolism, 5th ed, p 373. New York, McGraw-Hill, 1994
4. Matz, p 80
5. Ibid
6. Ibid
7. Reinhart, p 78
8. Narins, p 1100
9. Reinhart, p 79
10. Fiaccadori E, et al: Muscle and serum magnesium in pulmonary intensive care unit patients. Crit Care Med 16:751–759,1988
11. Ryzen E, et al: Low blood mononuclear cell magnesium in intensive cardiac care unit patients. Am Heart J 111:475–480,1986
12. White J, Campbell K: Magnesium and diabetes: A review. Ann Pharmacother 27:775–780,1993
13. Matz, p 80
14. Zaloga G, Chernow B: Divalent ions: Calcium, magnesium, and phosphorus. In Chernow B (ed): The Pharmacologic Approach to the Critically Ill Patient, Chapter 46, 3rd ed, p 794. Baltimore, Williams & Wilkins, 1994
15. Jackson C, Meier D: Routine serum magnesium analysis: Correlation with clinical state in 5100 patients. Ann Intern Med 69:743,1968
16. Chernow B, et al: Hypomagnesemia in patients in postoperative intensive care. Chest 95(2):391,1989
17. Ryzen et al: Magnesium deficiency in a medical intensive care unit population. Crit Care Med 13(1):19,1985
18. Chernow et al: Hypomagnesemia: Implications for the critical care specialist. Crit Care Med 10:193,1982
19. Booth et al: Incidence of hypomagnesemia in intestinal malabsorption. Br Med J 2:141,1963
20. Hallberg D: Magnesium problems in gastroenterology. Acta Med Scand 662:62,1981
21. Sullivan et al: Magnesium metabolism in alcoholism. Am J Clin Nutr 63:297,1963
22. Zaloga G, Chernow B: Magnesium metabolism in critical illness. Crit Care Q 6:24,1983
23. Ibid
24. Silberman H, Eisenberg D: Parenteral and Enteral Nutrition for the Hospitalized Patient, 2nd ed, p 309. E. Norwalk, CT, Appleton & Lange, 1989

25. Rose B: Clinical Physiology of Acid-Base and Electrolyte Disorders, 4th ed, p 431. New York, McGraw-Hill, 1994
26. Zaloga et al: Hypomagnesemia is a common complication of aminoglycoside therapy. Clin Res 31: 261A,1983
27. Narins, p 679
28. Kokko H, Tannen R: Fluids and Electrolytes, 2nd ed, p 641. Philadelphia, WB Saunders, 1990
29. Narins, p 1391
30. Zaloga, Chernow, p 24
31. Ibid
32. Ibid
33. Chernow et al, 1982, p 193
34. Ibid
35. Pemberton L, Pemberton D: Treatment of Water, Electrolyte, and Acid-Base Disorders in the Surgical Patient, p 244. New York, McGraw-Hill, 1994
36. Chernow et al, 1982, p 193
37. Olerich M, Rude R: Should we supplement magnesium in critically ill patients? New Horizons 2(2):186–192,1994
38. Rose, p 432
39. Chernow et al, 1982, p 194
40. Goldman et al: The effect on myocardial ^{3}H-digoxin of magnesium deficiency. Proc Soc Exp Biol Med 136:747,1971
41. Beller et al: Correlation of serum magnesium levels and cardiac digitalis intoxication. Am J Cardiol 33:225,1974
42. Pemberton, Pemberton, p 244
43. Szerlip H, Goldfarb S: Workshops in Fluid and Electrolyte Disorders, p 92. New York, Churchill Livingstone, 1994
44. White, Campbell, p 777
45. Matz, p 81
46. Kokko, Tannen, p 638
47. Narins, p 1110
48. Toto K, Yucha C: Magnesium. In Endocrine and Metabolic Disturbances in the Critically Ill. Crit Care Nurs Clin North Am 6(4):767–783,1994
49. Kokko, Tannen, p 642
50. Narins, p 1111
51. Zaloga, Chernow, 1994, p 794
52. Toto, Yucha, p 775
53. Hoffman et al: An amp by any other name: The hazards of intravenous magnesium dosing (Letter). JAMA 261:557,1989
54. Gahart B: Handbook of Intravenous Medications, 9th ed, p 403. St. Louis, CV Mosby, 1993
55. Woods K, Fletcher S, Roffe C, Haider Y: Intravenous magnesium sulphate in suspected acute myocardial infarction: results of the second Leicester Intravenous Magnesium Intervention Trial (LIMIT-2). Lancet 339:1553–1558, 1992
56. ISIS Collaborative Group. ISIS-4: A randomised study of intravenous magnesium in over 50,000 patients with suspected acute myocardial infarction. Circulation 88(suppl):1–292, Abstract, 1993
57. Cummis R (ed): Textbook of Advanced Cardiac Life Support, pp 1–55. Dallas, American Heart Association, 1994
58. Ibid, p 779
59. Okayama et al: Bronchodilating effect of intravenous magnesium sulfate in bronchial asthma. JAMA 257:1076–1078,1987
60. Zaloga, Chernow, 1994, p 796
61. American Diabetes Association: Magnesium supplementation in the treatment of diabetes. Diabetes Care 15(8):1065–1067,1992
62. Ibid
63. Matz, p 82
64. Ibid
65. Rude R: Magnesium metabolism and deficiency. Endocrinol Metab Clin North Am 22:377–394,1993
66. Toto, Yucha, p 779
67. Kokko, Tannen, p 970
68. Clark B, Brown R: Unsuspected morbid hypermagnesemia in elderly patients. Am J Nephrology 12:336–343,1992
69. Dudley D, Gagnon D, Varner M: Long-term tocolysis with intravenous magnesium sulfate. Obstet Gynecol 73:373,1989
70. Zaloga, Chernow, 1994, p 796
71. Toto, Yucha, p 779
72. Narins, p 1111
73. Kokko, Tannen, p 642
74. Rizzo M, et al: Hypermagnesemic pseudocoma. Arch Intern Med 153:1130–1132,1993
75. Narins, p 1110
76. Woodley M, Whelan A: Manual of Medical Therapeutics, 27th ed, p 436. Boston, Little, Brown, 1992
77. Ibid

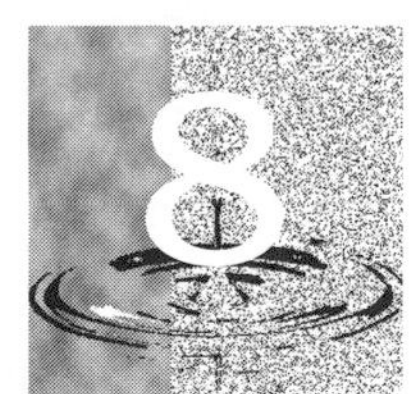

Phosphorus Imbalances

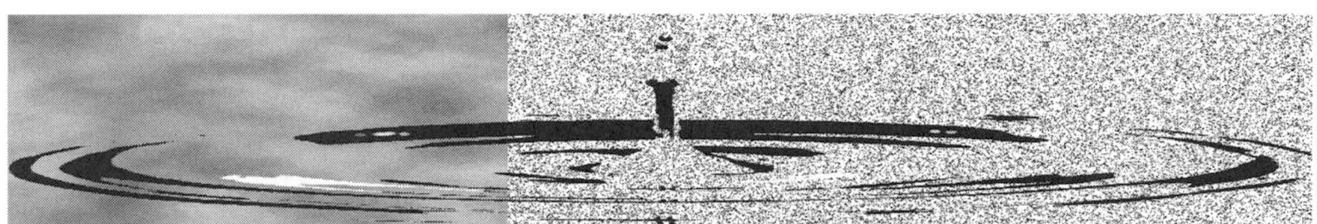

The increased recognition of the frequency of phosphorus disturbances and the increased use of therapeutic interventions that profoundly affect overall phosphorus balance have roused a greater interest in phosphorus metabolism.

PHOSPHORUS BALANCE

Phosphorus is a critical constituent of all tissues of the human body. It is essential to the function of muscle, red blood cells, and the nervous system, and to the intermediary metabolism of carbohydrate, protein, and fat.

The normal serum phosphorus level in adults ranges from 2.5 to 4.5 mg/dL (0.81–1.45 mmol/L). Levels are greater in children, presumably because of the higher rate of skeletal growth. Serum levels may fluctuate throughout the day; for example, glucose intake, insulin administration, or hyperventilation can lower the serum phosphorus concentration by increasing cellular uptake. Because phosphorus is primarily an intracellular ion, serum levels may not always reflect the total body stores. Phosphorus circulates in the bloodstream in three major forms: protein bound (12%), complexed (33%), and ionized (55%); it is the ionized form that is physiologically active.[1] Most laboratories measure total phosphorus.

The usual dietary intake of phosphate ranges between 800 and 1200 mg/day.[2] Adequate dietary intake is ensured by a normal diet as phosphorus is plentiful in many foods, including red meat, fish, poultry, eggs, milk products, and legumes. Most ingested phosphate is absorbed in the jejunum. However, absorption can be impaired by certain medications (such as phosphate-binding antacids) or by malabsorptive disorders. Maintenance of normal phosphate balance requires an efficient renal conservation mechanism because the kidneys are the major route of excretion of phosphorus, being responsible for approximately 90% of the phosphorus excreted daily. During times of low phosphate intake, the kidneys retain more phosphorus.

HYPOPHOSPHATEMIA

Hypophosphatemia refers to a serum phosphorus concentration below the lower limit of normal (<2.5 mg/dL); it is considered to be severe at a concentration of less than 1.0 mg/dL.[3] It may occur in the presence of total body phosphorus deficit or merely reflect a temporary shift of phosphorus into the cells. When doubt exists about the presence of phosphorus depletion, it is helpful to measure the urinary excretion of phosphorus. In patients with phosphorus depletion, the urinary phosphorus drops markedly to less than 100 mg and often less than 50 mg/day.[4]

ETIOLOGICAL FACTORS

A wide variety of clinical disorders and therapeutic interventions can cause hypophosphatemia. These etiological factors are listed in the Summary of Hypophosphatemia and are discussed briefly below. Essentially, these factors fall into one of three categories: (1) shift of phosphate from the extracellular fluid (ECF) into the cells; (2) decreased absorption of phosphate from the gastrointestinal (GI) tract; and (3) increased renal phosphate losses.[5] Usually at least two, and often all three, of these mechanisms are present in a given situation.[6] Many of the precipitating causes are treatment-related. For example, Halevy and Bulvik[7] reported that medications contributed to hypophosphatemia in 82% of the patients in their study; among the implicated medications were intravenous (IV) glucose, antacids, anabolic steroids, and diuretics.

Glucose Administration

Glucose administration causes endogenous release of insulin, which in turn promotes the transport of both glucose and phosphorus into the cells (primarily of the skeletal muscle and liver). Normally the decline in serum phosphorus does not exceed 0.5 mg/dL,[8] although the response is more severe in starving patients. A survey of 100 patients with hypophosphatemia showed that parenteral administration of glucose was the cause in 45% of the cases.[9] A lesser effect is associated with oral glucose intake.

Hyperalimentation

Development of severe hypophosphatemia in malnourished patients receiving total parenteral nutrition (TPN) without adequate phosphorus replacement has been well documented and may occur within the first 24 hrs, although it often becomes evident only after 2 to 3 days of treatment. It is caused by a rapid influx of phosphorus into the body's muscle mass at the initiation of anabolism (tissue building) after a period of catabolism.

Respiratory Alkalosis

Prolonged, intense hyperventilation can depress serum phosphorus to values in the vicinity of 0.5 mg/dL, presumably by inducing respiratory alkalosis. Clinical situations associated with respiratory alkalosis include Gram-negative bacteremia, withdrawal from chronic alcoholism, heat stroke, acute salicylate poisoning, primary hyperventilation, and thyrotoxicosis.

Hypophosphatemia associated with alkalosis is secondary to increased cellular phosphate uptake. Although the underlying mechanism is unknown, it is likely that alkalosis stimulates glycolysis, increasing the formation of phosphorylated intermediates and thereby pulling more phosphorus into the cells.[10] This process causes a precipitous fall in the serum phosphorus concentration.

Alcoholism

A common cause of severe hypophosphatemia is alcoholism. In one study, hypophosphatemia was found in 30.4% of alcoholic patients admitted to medical services (as compared to only 1.8% of matched nonalcoholic patients).[11] Factors contributing to phosphate depletion in alcoholics include poor intake, vomiting, use of antacids, and diarrhea. The fact that some alcoholics develop phosphate depletion in the absence of these factors suggests the presence of other mechanisms, perhaps the effects of ethanol per se, magnesium deficiency, ketoacidosis, and hypocalcemia.[12]

Excessive Pharmacological Phosphate Binding

Antacids are used in uremic patients to bind with dietary phosphorus and prevent its absorption, thus normalizing serum phosphorus concentrations. However, excessive phosphorus binding by aluminum hydroxide, magnesium hydroxide, or aluminum carbonate gels may cause severe hypophosphatemia, particularly when there is poor dietary intake of phosphorus. Phosphate-binding antacids are more likely to produce hypophosphatemia when other conditions associated with this imbalance are present, such as diuretic therapy, renal tubular defects, or hyperparathyroidism.

Diabetic Ketoacidosis

Patients with poorly controlled diabetes who have glycosuria, ketonuria, and polyuria lose phosphate excessively into the urine. Although patients with untreated ketoacidosis may have normal or slightly elevated serum phosphorus levels, administration of insulin and parenteral fluids quickly causes serum phosphorus levels to drop below normal (see Chapter 18).

Insulin Administration

Because insulin promotes glycolysis, it causes a shift of phosphorus into the cells. In a study reported by Van Landingham et al.[13] hypophosphatemia was found in 30% of tube-fed patients. This usually occurred in patients who were treated with insulin for hyperglycemia and the condition was assumed to be secondary to intracellular transport of phosphate.

Nutritional Recovery Syndrome

The nutritional recovery syndrome is sometimes referred to as the "refeeding syndrome." Hypophosphatemia may occur during the administration of calories in normally required amounts to patients with severe protein-calorie malnutrition (such as those with anorexia nervosa, elderly debilitated patients who are unable to eat, or alcoholics). The nutritional recovery syndrome occurs most commonly with overzealous refeeding of simple carbohydrates. A prerequisite for the syndrome is that the cells be capable of anabolism; during the anabolic phase there is an influx of phosphorus into the cells (primarily the body's muscle mass).

Excessive Catecholamine Secretion

Epinephrine may be a key mediator of hypophosphatemia and may explain partially the hypophosphatemia of sepsis, myocardial infarction, and other conditions associated with epinephrine release.[14]

Thermal Burns

Hypophosphatemia is common in patients with extensive burns and usually appears within several days after injury. The mechanism by which it develops is not clear. Because burn patients often hyperventilate, it is possible that respiratory alkalosis occurs and results in acceleration of glycolysis causing hypophosphatemia. It has also been postulated that urinary loss of phosphate may occur during the diuresis of salt and water, or that phosphorus may be taken up by the cells as the burned patient becomes anabolic.

Other Factors

A survey of 100 hypophosphatemic patients suggested that diuretics were the cause in 7%.[15] Other possible causes include GI malabsorption syndrome, vitamin D deficiency, acute gout (presumably due to pain-induced hyperventilation), hypokalemia, hypomagnesemia, and hypocalcemia. Hypomagnesemia fosters hypophosphatemia through increased urinary losses of phosphate. Hypocalcemia can cause phosphaturia through stimulation of parathyroid hormone release.[16]

Reversal of hypothermia causes a shift of phosphate into the cells and may cause hypophosphatemia.[17] Patients with panic disorders may have a significant incidence of hypophosphatemia, at least partly due to respiratory alkalosis.[18] Moderate (usually well tolerated) hypophosphatemia is also common after kidney transplant and is the result of renal phosphaturia, glucocorticoid therapy, persistent hyperparathyroidism, and use of antacids.[19] Low birth weight infants may develop hypophosphatemia when fed human milk rather than cow's milk.[20]

DEFINING CHARACTERISTICS

Most signs and symptoms of phosphorus deficiency apparently result from deficiency of adenosine triphosphate (ATP), 2,3-diphosphoglycerate (2,3-DPG), or both. Cellular energy resources are impaired by ATP deficiency and oxygen delivery to tissues by 2,3-DPG deficiency.

Central Nervous System Changes

Cellular deficiencies of ATP and 2,3-DPG can produce a wide range of neurological symptoms, which may include irritability, apprehension, weakness, numbness, paresthesias, ataxia, lack of coordination, confusion, unequal pupils, nystagmus, convulsive seizures, and coma.[21] The basic cause of these central nervous system disturbances is not clear; possibly it is related to a decreased availability of phosphate that in turn causes reduced ATP synthesis in the brain.[22]

Hematological Changes

Hypophosphatemia affects all the blood cells, but changes in the red cells are most pronounced. As stated above, a decline in 2,3-DPG levels in erythrocytes occurs in hypophosphatemia. Recall that 2,3-DPG is an enzyme in red blood cells that normally interacts with hemoglobin to promote the release of oxygen. Thus, low levels of 2,3-DPG may reduce the delivery of oxygen to peripheral tissues, resulting in tissue hypoxia. Hemolytic anemia may occur because the red cells are more fragile and easily destroyed as a result of low ATP levels. This circumstance is particularly significant in critically ill patients who cannot tolerate even modest decreases in oxygen delivery.

In laboratory animals, hypophosphatemia has been noted to produce depression of the chemotactic and phagocytic activity of granulocytes. These abnormalities are apparently reversible with correction of the hypophosphatemia. It is thought that hypophosphatemia impairs granulocytic function by interfering with ATP synthesis. Obviously, patients with impaired leukocyte function are at greater risk of infection.

Skeletal Muscle Changes

Muscle damage may develop as the ATP level in the muscles declines. This is manifested clinically by muscle weakness, release of creatinine phosphokinase (CPK), and, at times, acute rhabdomyolysis (disintegration of striated muscle). Profound muscular weakness has been described in severely hypophosphatemic patients, as has muscular pain. Elevations in CPK levels have been reported in patients with serum phosphate concentrations less than 1 mg/dL for 1 to 2 days.[23] It is possible that muscle cell injury could be the result of disrupted functioning of chemical processes important in maintaining cellular membrane integrity.

Ventilatory Changes

Several investigators have reported weakness of the chest muscle in hypophosphatemic patients.[24,25] Ventilatory muscle fatigue may arise from cellular depletion of ATP, impaired cellular oxygenation, and central respiratory depression. Respiratory failure is most likely to occur in patients with underlying lung disease. Varsano et al.[26] recommended that the possibility of hypophosphatemia be considered for each patient who develops acute ventilatory failure or presents a problem of respiratory weaning. In some cases, patients can be removed from the ventilator soon after phosphate repletion has been achieved.[27]

Cardiac Changes

There are indications that severe hypophosphatemic patients have decreased cardiac contractility that can be corrected with phosphorus replacement.[28] A reversible congestive cardiomyopathy may occur.[29] Phosphate depletion may also be associated with a decreased sensitivity to inotropic and vasoconstrictive medications.[30] And, there may be an increased incidence of arrhythmias in hypophosphatemic patients.[31]

Other Factors

There are indications that phosphorus deficiency may produce an insulin-resistant state, resulting in hyperglycemia.[32] Prolonged and severe hypophosphatemia may also be accompanied by severe metabolic acidosis.

TREATMENT

Mild-to-Moderate Hypophosphatemia

Treatment of hypophosphatemia varies with the cause and severity of the imbalance. If mild and asymptomatic, it may be managed adequately by treatment of the primary disorder.[33] Because phosphorus is plentiful in the diet, improved nutrition may suffice. However, if hypophosphatemia is likely to persist, therapy may require oral supplementation. Often, milk is recommended for the treatment of chronic phosphate deficiency because it is high in phosphate; it is also an excellent source of calcium and potassium. Of course, if calcium is contraindicated, milk is not recommended. If milk is not tolerated, Neutra-Phos capsules (250 mg of elemental phosphorus and 7 mEq each of sodium and potassium per capsule) or Neutra-Phos K (250 mg of elemental phosphorus and 14 mEq of potassium), or Fleet Phospho-Soda (815 mg of elemental phosphorus and 33 mEq of sodium per 5 mL) may be prescribed as needed.[34] Nausea and diarrhea are side effects that may limit dosage of these agents.

Severe Hypophosphatemia

Severe hypophosphatemia (<1 mg/dL) is dangerous and requires intravenous replacement, because oral phosphate preparations, when given in large amounts, usually cause diarrhea. Two intravenous preparations are available (sodium phosphate and potassium phosphate).[35] If the patient is oliguric, sodium salts rather than potassium salts should be administered.[36] Dosage is guided by serial determinations of serum phosphate levels (such as every 6 hrs) and clinical response. Zaloga and Chernow[37] recommend giving 0.6 mg/kg/hr if phosphate depletion is recent and uncomplicated; if it is prolonged and multifactorial, 0.9 mg/kg/hr is recommended. After the serum level rises above 2 mg/dL, enteral replacement should be started and carried out over 5 to 7 days to replace cellular phosphate deficits.[38] Possible dangers of IV phosphorus administration include hyperphosphatemia and hypocalcemia. Another consideration is that calcium and phosphate should not be administered in the same IV infusion because of the risk of precipitation.

Phosphorus replacement in patients receiving TPN is discussed in Chapter 11; replacement in patients with diabetic ketoacidosis is discussed in Chapter 18.

NURSING INTERVENTIONS

1. Identify patients at risk for hypophosphatemia. See the Summary of Hypophosphatemia and discussion of etiological factors.
   - Extremely malnourished patients being started on TPN or large caloric intake by tube feeding (refeeding syndrome in starving patients) are particularly at risk.
   - Also at great risk are alcoholic patients undergoing withdrawal therapy and initial treatment with IV glucose fluids.

Summary of Hypophosphatemia

ETIOLOGICAL FACTORS	DEFINING CHARACTERISTICS
Glucose administration	Paresthesias
Refeeding after starvation	Muscle weakness (perhaps manifested as decreased strength of hand grasp and difficulty speaking)
Hyperalimentation	Muscle pain and tenderness
Alcohol withdrawal	Mental changes, such as apprehension, confusion, delirium, and coma
Diabetic ketoacidosis	Decreased cardiac contractility
Respiratory alkalosis	Acute respiratory failure (related to chest muscle weakness)
Phosphate-binding antacids	Seizures
Recovery phase after severe burns	Decreased tissue oxygenation
	Serum phosphate <2.5 mg/dL

- Similarly at great risk are patients with diabetic ketoacidosis during the early treatment period with insulin and IV fluids. This is particularly true if serum phosphate levels were low on admission. Fortunately, low-dose insulin therapy has decreased the incidence of rapid phosphate cellular shifts during early treatment (see Chapter 18).

2. Monitor patients at risk for hypophosphatemia. See Summary of Hypophosphatemia and discussion of defining characteristics.
   - Monitor serum phosphate levels in patients at high risk. Notify physician when levels are low. Hypophosphatemia is profound when serum levels are less than 1.0 mg/dL.
   - Be alert for paresthesias, particularly about the mouth.
   - Be alert for muscle weakness and pain. Test hand grasp strength on a serial basis to monitor for muscle weakness. Monitor for changes in speech that may reflect muscular weakness.
   - Be alert for mental changes associated with hypophosphatemia, such as apprehension, confusion, delirium, and decreased level of consciousness.
   - Be alert for signs of cardiac and ventilatory failure in patients with severe hypophosphatemia.
3. Be aware that severely hypophosphatemic patients are thought to be at greater risk for infection because of changes in white blood cells. As always, take precautions to prevent infections (as in meticulous care of central lines for TPN patients).
4. Administer IV phosphate products cautiously and monitor clinical response as well as serum phosphate levels. Because it is possible to give too much phosphorus, monitor for signs of hyperphosphatemia and of the salt in which it is administered. For example, excessive administration of potassium phosphate could cause paresthesias of the extremities, flaccid paralysis, listlessness, confusion, weakness, arrhythmias, heart block, and ECG abnor-

malities. Serum potassium or sodium levels (depending on the replacement salt) should be monitored in addition to the serum phosphorus levels.

5. Be aware that sudden increase in the serum phosphorus level during treatment can cause hypocalcemia. For this reason, serum calcium levels should be monitored. Watch for twitching around the mouth, laryngospasm, positive Chvostek's sign, and paresthesias.
6. Be aware of the need to introduce hyperalimentation *gradually* in patients who are malnourished. Gradual introduction of the feeding solution is less apt to be associated with rapid shifts of phosphate into the cells. Frequently monitor rates of TPN flow.
7. Monitor for diarrhea in patients taking oral phosphorus supplements; consult with physician if it persists or becomes severe.
8. Mix powdered oral phosphorus supplements with chilled or iced water to make them more palatable. Also, palatability may be increased by refrigerating the solution made from the powder. (Any palatable juice or beverage may be used in place of water.)

CASE STUDY

8-1. A 40-year-old woman with a prolonged history of severe diarrhea, nausea, and anorexia was admitted. Two months earlier she had undergone a bilateral salpingo-oophorectomy for ovarian cancer and a radium implant. A 30-lb weight loss was sustained over the previous 4 months. Weight on admission was 88 pounds. A retroperitoneal small-bowel fistula was found and surgical repair of the fistula and a colostomy were performed. After she suffered a multitude of postoperative complications, TPN was begun. At this time, serum electrolytes were found to be:

Na^+ = 136 mEq/L
PO_4 = 3.4 mg/dL
Cl^- = 93 mEq/L
CO_2 content = 31 mEq/L
K^+ = 3.6 mEq/L
Glucose = 128 mg/dL
Ca^{2+} = 8.7 mg/dL
BUN = 8 mg/dL

Eight days later, her condition had markedly deteriorated. A glucose intolerance (blood glucose, 270 mg/dL) required the administration of regular insulin, 20 units, every 6 hrs. Inflammation was noted at the central line insertion site. At this time, her serum phosphate level was 0.4 mg/dL (normal, 2.5–4.5 mg/dL). Assessment revealed slurred speech and drooping of the mouth and tongue. The patient appeared restless and anxious and complained of numbness all over.

The next day, muscle twitching and gross abnormal movements were noted. The patient was unable to grasp objects with her hands and was too weak to raise her arms. She complained of pain whenever anything touched her skin. At this time, her serum phosphate level was 0.2 mg/dL. A nutritional consultation was made and IV phosphate administration was started.

Two days later her speech remained slurred, spastic movements continued, and intense sensitivity to touch remained. However, her glucose intolerance had improved. Spot checks decreased from 2% to 0.10% glucose. Slowly, over a period of days, her hand grasps became perceptibly stronger and the muscle pain diminished. Numbness eventually disappeared. Three weeks later, the patient was discharged with a serum phosphate level of 4.5 mg/dL.

COMMENTARY: The fact that this patient had essentially been starving caused her to suffer the nutritional recovery syndrome when overzealous refeeding was initiated with inadequate phosphorus in the TPN solution. Note that the serum phosphorus concentration reached extremely low levels before it was noticed and treated. Typical signs of hypophosphatemia were present. Even after the serum phosphorus concentration was raised to normal levels, it took days for the clinical manifestations to resolve (indicating sustained cellular deficits). This patient was allowed to become critically ill before the cause of her problem was diagnosed and treated.

HYPERPHOSPHATEMIA

Moderate hyperphosphatemia is said to be present when the serum level is 4.6 to 6.0 mg/dL; severe hyperphosphatemia exists at a phosphorus level of more than 6.0 mg/dL.

ETIOLOGICAL FACTORS

Three basic mechanisms can lead to hyperphosphatemia; these include: (1) reduced renal phosphate excretion; (2) shift of phosphorus from the intracellular space into the extracellular fluid; and (3) increased phosphate intake or absorption.

Decreased Renal Excretion of Phosphorus

An increase in the serum phosphorus concentration is observed in patients with chronic renal failure when the glomerular filtration rate (GFR) is 25 mL/min or less. Also, hyperphosphatemia is common in acute renal failure.

Shift of Intracellular Phosphate to Extracellular Fluid

Large quantities of phosphates may be released into the circulation when chemotherapy is administered for neoplastic conditions (particularly acute lymphoblastic leukemia and lymphoma) and are the result of cell destruction and liberation of intracellular phosphates ("tumor lysis"). Shift from the cellular space to the extracellular space can also occur when sepsis, severe hypothermia, and rhabdomyolysis are present.[39] Recall that muscle tissue contains the bulk of soft-tissue phosphate. Therefore, necrosis of muscle is a potent cause of hyperphosphatemia. Situations associated with rhabdomyolysis include direct trauma, viral infections, and heat stroke.

High Phosphate Intake

It is possible to impose an excess phosphorus load if phosphate substances are administered incorrectly, whether IV, orally, or in the form of phosphate-containing enemas. Even when renal function is normal, it is possible to cause hyperphosphatemia when phosphate-containing solutions are administered too rapidly. Substantial absorption of phosphorus can occur from the large bowel when Fleet Phospho-Soda is given as an enema. This is especially problematic for patients who have slowed colonic motility or defects in the bowel mucosa. A case was recently reported in which a constipated geriatric patient received multiple Fleet's enemas (six over a 12-hr period), resulting in life-threatening hyperphosphatemia (22 mg/dL).[40] Use of laxatives containing sodium phosphate may also result in accidental phosphate poisoning. Fatal hyperphosphatemia (59.6 mg/dL), secondary to enteral administration of Fleet Phospho-Soda, was recently reported in a 64-year-old man with colonic ileus.[41] Blood transfusions can be a source of exogenous phosphorus because of leakage from the blood cells during storage.

Large intake of vitamin D, either therapeutic or self-administered, causes increased phosphorus absorption that, together with impaired renal function, can result in hyperphosphatemia.

Hyperphosphatemia may develop in infants fed cow's milk, which contains more phosphate than human milk. Patients taking large quantities of milk for peptic ulcer management may develop increased serum phosphorus levels.

DEFINING CHARACTERISTICS

The clinical signs of hyperphosphatemia are primarily the ones of hypocalcemia as it is induced as the elevated serum phosphate combines with ionized calcium. Insoluble calcium phosphate is formed when the calcium–phosphate product exceeds 75.[42]

Hypocalcemia and Tetany

Because of the reciprocal relationship between phosphorus and calcium, a high serum phosphorus level tends to cause a low calcium concentration in the serum. Tetany can result and present as sensations of tingling in the tips of the fingers and around the mouth. These sensations may increase in severity and spread proximally along the limbs and to the face and be followed by numbness. Muscle spasms and pain may occur. Symptoms of tetany are most likely to occur in patients who are hyperphosphatemic because of a high

Summary of Hyperphosphatemia

ETIOLOGICAL FACTORS	DEFINING CHARACTERISTICS
Renal failure Chemotherapy, particularly for acute lymphoblastic leukemia and lymphoma Large intake of milk, as in treatment of peptic ulcer Use of cow's milk in infants Overzealous administration of phosphorus supplements, orally or IV Excessive use of Fleet's phosphosoda as enema solution or laxative, particularly in children and individuals with slow bowel elimination Large vitamin D intake (increases phosphorus absorption)	Short-term consequences: symptoms of tetany, such as tingling of fingertips and around mouth, numbness, and muscle spasms Long-term consequences: precipitation of calcium phosphate in nonosseous sites, such as the kidney, heart, arteries, skin, or cornea Serum phosphate >4.5 mg/dL

phosphate load, either exogenous or endogenous. Because patients with renal disease often have some degree of acidosis, they are less prone to develop symptoms of hypocalcemia because acidosis favors increased calcium ionization.

Soft-Tissue Calcification

High levels of serum inorganic phosphate are harmful because they promote precipitation of calcium phosphate in nonosseous sites. One such site is the kidney, where precipitation of calcium phosphate can result in progressive renal impairment. Other sites include heart, lungs, skin, and cornea. Soft-tissue calcification is seen primarily in patients with chronic renal failure and long-term serum phosphate elevation. An attempt is made to control the hyperphosphatemia and thus keep the calcium and phosphate product below 70 mg/dL. Recall that normal serum levels of calcium (8.5–10.5 mg/dL) and phosphate (2.5–4.5 mg/dL) have a product of approximately 30 to 40 mg/dL.

Other Effects

One effect of hyperphosphatemia is an increase in red blood cell 2,3-DPG levels. In patients with chronic renal failure, hyperphosphatemia helps protect against the adverse effects of anemia on tissue oxygenation.

TREATMENT

When possible, treatment is directed at the underlying disorder. If due to excessive phosphate administration in drugs or in milk, the disorder is rather easily remedied by eliminating the products. Dietary restriction of phosphorus intake is also indicated.

Phosphate-binding agents, such as aluminum hydroxide (Amphogel) and aluminum carbonate (Basaljel), are frequently used to decrease the serum phosphate level in patients with renal disorders.

In acute hyperphosphatemia, IV saline infusions may promote renal phosphate excretion, provided the patient has functional kidneys. It may be necessary to administer hypertonic dextrose in conjunction with regular insulin to temporarily drive phosphorus into the cells. Either hemodialysis or peritoneal dialysis may be needed for patients with compromised renal function.

NURSING INTERVENTIONS

1. Administer prescribed enteral and IV phosphate supplements cautiously and monitor serum phosphate levels periodically during their use.
2. Identify patients at risk for hyperphosphatemia and monitor for signs of tetany, such as tingling sensations in the fingertips and around the mouth, and presence of muscle cramps or positive Chvostek's and Trousseau's signs.
3. Instruct patients that improper use of phosphate-containing laxatives may result in acute phosphate poisoning.
4. Be aware that phosphate-containing enemas can result in hyperphosphatemia if not used judiciously, particularly in individuals with slow bowel emptying and mucosal defects that hasten absorption. Instruct patients accordingly. See Summary of Hyperphosphatemia.

CASE STUDY

8-2. An elderly woman was admitted to the hospital with abdominal pain and constipation that had been present for 5 days. Abdominal x-ray revealed multiple fecal impactions. Over a period of 12 hrs, six Fleet Phospho-Soda enemas were administered to attempt to correct the constipation; however, no relief was obtained. The patient's condition deteriorated and she was noted to have positive Chvostek's and Trousseau's signs. Blood tests revealed a serum phosphorus level of 22 mg/dL (normal, 2.5–4.5 mg/dL) and a total serum calcium level of 5.4 mg/dL (normal, 8.5–10.5 mg/dL). Intravenous fluids were maintained using central venous monitoring and calcium gluconate was administered by continuous infusion. In the first 24 hrs, 6.7 L of fluids were administered. Within 24 hrs, serum electrolyte levels returned to near normal values (phosphorus, 4.7 mg/dL; calcium, 9.3 mg/dL). The paralytic ileus resolved slowly, after the fecal impactions were manually removed, with the assistance of isotonic enemas. The patient was discharged to an extended care facility in 2 weeks.[43]

COMMENTARY: Most cases of hyperphosphatemia due to phosphate enemas have occurred in young children. However, severe electrolyte abnormalities can also occur in adults, particularly when conditions are present that cause prolonged retention of the enema solution. In this case, paralytic ileus and fecal impaction promoted retention of the phosphate solution and precipitated the extreme hyperphosphatemia and hypocalcemia described. Both of these imbalances were directly caused by the retained hypertonic phosphate solution. The high phosphorus content of the enema, which was absorbed through the colon, caused a rise in the serum phosphorus level; the elevated serum phosphorus level caused a reciprocal drop in the serum calcium level. Elderly patients with atonic colons and poor renal function are particularly at risk. In these patients, use of enemas should be carefully supervised, and whenever possible, isotonic enemas should be used.

REFERENCES

1. Zaloga G, Chernow B: Divalent ions: Calcium, magnesium, and phosphorus. In Chernow B (ed): The Pharmacologic Approach to the Critically Ill Patient, 3rd ed, Chapter 46, p 796. Baltimore, Williams & Wilkins, 1994
2. Ibid, p 796
3. Narins R (ed): Clinical Disorders of Fluid and Electrolyte Metabolism, 5th ed, p 1046. New York, McGraw-Hill, 1994
4. Pemberton L, Pemberton D: Treatment of Water, Electrolyte, and Acid-Base Disorders in the Surgical Patient, p 228. New York, McGraw-Hill, 1994
5. Zaloga, Chernow, p 798
6. Narins, p 1055
7. Halevy J, Bulvik S: Severe hypophosphatemia in hospitalized patients. Arch Intern Med 148:153,1988
8. Knochel J: The pathophysiology and clinical characteristics of severe hypophosphatemia. Ann Intern Med 137:205,1977
9. Juan D, Elrazak M: Hypophosphatemia in hospitalized patients. JAMA 242:163,1979
10. Narins, p 1051
11. Ryback R, et al: Clinical relationship between serum phosphorus and other blood chemistry values in alcoholics. Arch Intern Med 140:673,1980
12. Knochel, p 205

13. Van Landingham et al: Metabolic abnormalities in patients supported with enteral tube feeding. J Parenteral Enteral Nutrition 5(4):322,1981
14. Narins, p 1053
15. Juan, p 163
16. Tucker S, Schimmel E: Postoperative hypophosphatemia: A multifactorial problem. Nutr Rev 47(4):111,1989
17. Zaloga, Chernow, p 797
18. Balon J, et al: Relative hypophosphatemia in patients with panic disorders. Arch Gen Psychiatry 45:294,1988
19. Zaloga, Chernow, p 798
20. Narins, p 1051
21. Narins, p 1070
22. Narins, p 1070
23. Knochel, p 213
24. Newman J: Acute respiratory failure associated with hypophosphatemia. N Engl J Med 297:1101,1977
25. Gravelyn T, et al: Hypophosphatemia-associated respiratory muscle weakness in a general inpatient population. Am J Med 84:870,1988
26. Varsano et al: Hypophosphatemia as a reversible cause of refractory ventilatory failure. Crit Care Med 11:908,1983
27. Narins, p 1068
28. O'Connor L, et al: Effect of hypophosphatemia in myocardial function in man. N Engl J Med 291:901, 1977
29. Peppers M, et al: Hypophosphatemia and hyperphosphatemia. Crit Care Clin North Am 7:201,1991
30. Narins, p 1068
31. Venditti F, et al: Hypophosphatemia and cardiac arrhythmias. Miner Electrolyte Metab 13:19,1987
32. DeFronzo R, Lang R: Hypophosphatemia and glucose intolerance: Evidence for tissue insensitivity to insulin. N Engl J Med 303:1259–1263,1980
33. Woodley M, Whelan A: Manual of Medical Therapeutics, 27th ed, p 435. Boston, Little, Brown, 1992
34. Ibid
35. Yucha C, Toto K: Calcium and phosphorus derangements. In Endocrine and Metabolic Disturbances in the Critically Ill, p 763. Crit Care Nurs Clin North Am December, 1994
36. Narins, p 1078
37. Zaloga, Chernow, p 800
38. Ibid
39. Ibid
40. Korzets A, et al: Life-threatening hyperphosphatemia and hypocalcemic tetany following the use of Fleet enemas. J Am Geriatr Soc 40:620–621,1992
41. Fass R, et al: Fatal hyperphosphatemia following Fleet phospho-soda in a patient with colonic ileus. Am J Gastroenterol 88(6):929–932,1993
42. Zaloga, Chernow, p 801
43. Korzets et al, p 620

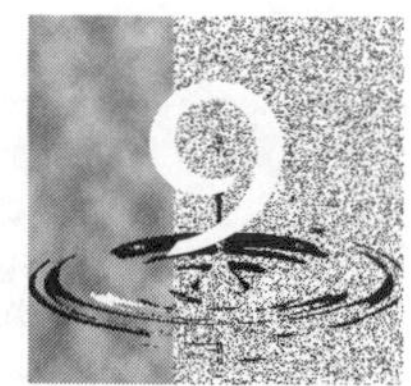

Acid–Base Imbalances

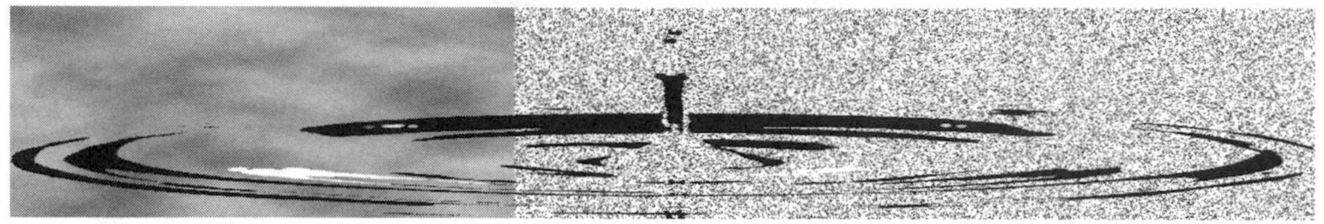

This chapter provides a basic explanation of acid–base imbalances. Etiological factors and defining characteristics of each of the four imbalances are presented, followed by brief discussions of their treatment. For the nursing interventions used to deal with these disturbances, the reader should see the later chapters concerning specific situations associated with acid–base imbalances.

Before turning to the four acid–base disturbances, it is helpful to review how the body regulates the acid–base balance.

REGULATION OF ACID–BASE BALANCE

The body has the remarkable ability to maintain plasma pH within the narrow normal range of 7.35 to 7.45. It does so by means of chemical buffering mechanisms, by the kidneys, and by the lungs. pH is defined as hydrogen ion concentration; the more hydrogen ions, the more acidic the solution. The pH range that is compatible with life (6.8–7.8) represents a tenfold difference in hydrogen ion concentration in plasma.

It has been estimated that metabolism normally produces 13,000 mEq/day of hydrogen ions; less than 1% of this amount is excreted by the kidneys. Therefore, renal shutdown can be present for hours or days before life-threatening acid–base imbalance occurs, yet cessation of breathing for minutes produces critical acid–base changes.

CHEMICAL BUFFERING MECHANISMS

Chemical buffers are substances that prevent major changes in the pH of body fluids by removing or releasing hydrogen ions; they can act within a fraction of a second to prevent excessive changes in hydrogen ion concentration.

The body's major buffer system is the bicarbonate (HCO_3)–carbonic acid (H_2CO_3) buffer system. Normally, there are 20 parts of bicarbonate to 1 part of carbonic acid. If this ratio is upset, the pH will change. It is the ratio that is important in maintaining pH, not absolute values.

Example: In a healthy individual:
HCO_3, 24 mEq/L [20 parts]
(pH = 7.4)
H_2CO_3, 1.2 mEq/L [1 part]

In an individual with chronic obstructive lung disease, one might see:

HCO_3, 48 mEq/L [20 parts]
(pH = 7.4)
H_2CO_3, 2.4 mEq/L [1 part]

Carbon dioxide (CO_2) is a potential acid. When CO_2 is dissolved in water, it becomes carbonic acid: $CO_2 + H_2O = H_2CO_3$. Thus, when CO_2 is increased, the carbonic acid content is also increased, and vice versa.

If either bicarbonate or carbonic acid is increased or decreased so that the 20:1 ratio is no longer valid, acid–base imbalance results. Figure 9-1 demonstrates changes in plasma pH when the bicarbonate:carbonic acid ratio is altered.

Other less important buffer systems in the extracellular fluid (ECF) include the inorganic phosphates

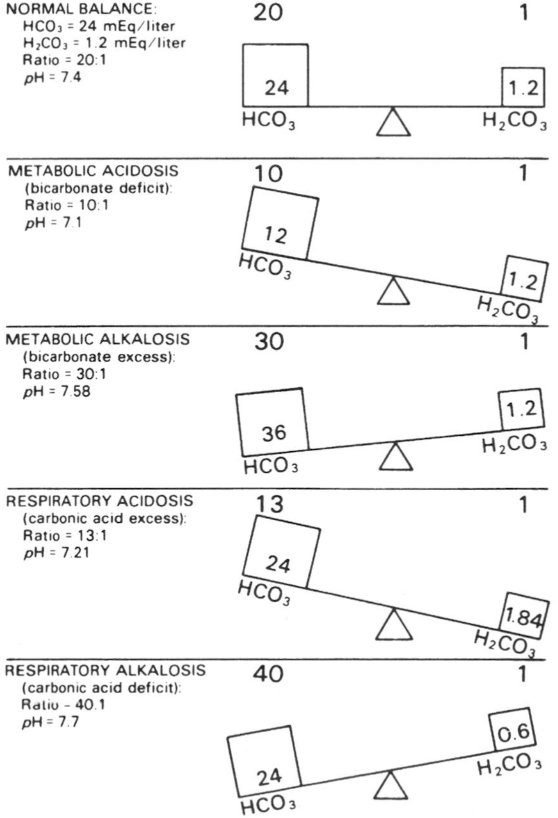

Figure 9-1. Examples of pH changes with alterations in the bicarbonate:carbonic acid ratio.

and the plasma proteins. Intracellular buffers include proteins, organic and inorganic phosphates, and, in red blood cells, hemoglobin.

KIDNEYS

The kidneys regulate the bicarbonate level in ECF; they are able to regenerate bicarbonate ions as well as reabsorb them from the renal tubular cells.

In the presence of respiratory acidosis, and most cases of metabolic acidosis, the kidneys excrete hydrogen ions and conserve bicarbonate ions to help restore balance. (The kidneys obviously cannot compensate for the metabolic acidosis created by renal failure.)

In the presence of respiratory and metabolic alkalosis, the kidneys retain hydrogen ions and excrete bicarbonate ions to help restore balance.

As stated earlier, renal compensation for imbalances is slow (a matter of hours or days).

LUNGS

Under the influence of the respiratory center, the lungs control the CO_2 (and thus carbonic acid) content of ECF by adjusting ventilation in response to the amount of CO_2 and, to a lesser extent, oxygen in the blood.

An acute rise in the partial pressure of CO_2 in arterial blood ($PaCO_2$) is a powerful stimulant to respiration. The stimulatory effect of increased CO_2 reaches its peak within a few minutes; however, it gradually declines for the next 1 or 2 days to as little as 20% of the initial effect.[1] Therefore, after several days, elevation of blood CO_2 has only a weak effect as a respiratory stimulant.

Partial pressure of O_2 in arterial blood (PaO_2) influences respiration; however, decreased PaO_2 normally will not stimulate alveolar ventilation significantly until it falls to very low levels. For example, ventilation approximately doubles when the PaO_2 falls to 60 mmHg and increases almost sixfold when it falls to 20 mmHg.[2]

Also, the lungs compensate for metabolic disturbances by either conserving or retaining CO_2.

1. In the presence of metabolic acidosis, respiration is increased, causing greater elimination of CO_2 (to lighten the acid load).
2. In the presence of metabolic alkalosis, respiration is decreased, causing CO_2 to be retained (increasing the acid load).

Faulty pulmonary function disrupts the acid–base balance. For example, hypoventilation due to chronic obstructive pulmonary disease (COPD) causes excessive CO_2 retention and respiratory acidosis; hyperventilation due to hysteria causes excessive elimination of CO_2 and respiratory alkalosis. Of course, the lungs are unable to compensate for metabolic pH disturbances when there is severe pulmonary dysfunction; in these instances, compensation must be accomplished solely by the kidneys.

MEASUREMENT OF ACID–BASE BALANCE

Before discussing acid–base measurement, it is useful to review the definition of "acid" and "base." Simply stated, an acid is a substance that can donate hydrogen ions. For example, H_2CO_3 (carbonic acid) $\rightarrow H^+$ (hydrogen ion) + HCO_3^- (bicarbonate). A base is a substance that can accept hydrogen ions (H^+). For example, $HCO_3^- + H^+ \rightarrow H_2CO_3$.

The best way to evaluate acid–base balance is by measuring arterial blood gases (Table 9-1). Arterial blood gases (ABG) sample blood that has come from various parts of the body (not just one extremity as is the case with venous blood). Also, arterial blood gives information on how well the lungs are oxygenating the blood.

Note in Table 9-1 that only two of the listed measures are actually of gases ($PaCO_2$ and PaO_2). However, reporting the nonrespiratory component (bicarbonate) is essential to understanding the respiratory measures. In review, the $PaCO_2$ is controlled by the lungs and refers to the pressure exerted by dissolved CO_2 gas in blood. CO_2 should be considered as an acid substance because, when dissolved in water, it forms carbonic acid (H_2CO_3). Also, PaO_2 refers to the pressure exerted by dissolved oxygen in the blood.

In the evaluation of acid–base status, the reporting of CO_2 content is often confusing. This measure is usually included with electrolyte determinations. Although listed on the laboratory sheet as "CO_2,"

TABLE 9–1

Arterial Blood Gases

TERM	NORMAL VALUE	DEFINITION-IMPLICATIONS
pH	7.35–7.45	Reflects H^+ concentration; acidity increases as H^+ concentration increases (pH value decreases as acidity increases) • pH <7.35 (acidosis) • pH >7.45 (alkalosis)
$PaCO_2$	35–45 mmHg	Partial pressure of CO_2 in arterial blood • When <35 mmHg, hypocapnia is said to be present (respiratory alkalosis) • When >45 mmHg, hypercapnia is said to be present (respiratory acidosis)
PaO_2	80–100 mmHg	Partial pressure of O_2 in arterial blood
Standard HCO_3	22–26 mEq/L	HCO_3 concentration in plasma of blood that has been equilibrated at a $PaCO_2$ of 40 mmHg, and with O_2 to fully saturate the hemoglobin

it is actually a measure of the sum of bicarbonate (24 mEq/L) and dissolved CO_2 gas (1.2 mEq/L). Note the normal ratio of 20 parts of HCO_3 to 1 part of dissolved CO_2 gas. Thus, in normal situations, the CO_2 content should be 25.2 mEq/L.[3] Because CO_2 content primarily reflects the concentration of bicarbonate, it is largely a measure of the nonrespiratory (or metabolic) component of acid–base balance. Instead of merely using CO_2 as a term, it is important to clarify whether it refers to the gas ($PaCO_2$) or the CO_2 content.

To assure patient safety and accuracy, only clinicians specially instructed in drawing blood gas samples should perform this maneuver. Listed at the end of the chapter, after discussion of the four primary acid–base imbalances, are guidelines for interpreting blood gases (Clinical Tip) and information regarding the calculation of expected compensatory changes (Table 9-8).

EFFECT OF pH ON POTASSIUM BALANCE

Acid–base changes can produce concurrent changes in potassium distribution between cellular and extracellular fluid. Generally, acidemia causes potassium to shift from the cells and thus elevates plasma potassium concentration. Just the opposite occurs with alkalemia; that is, potassium shifts into the cells, thus lowering the plasma potassium concentration. In the past, it was thought that the inverse relationship between pH and plasma potassium concentration was so precise that it could be expressed in mathematical terms. However, the relationship between pH and plasma potassium concentration is more complex than was originally assumed.[3]

ALKALEMIA

A shift of potassium into the cells can occur in alkalemia, either metabolic or respiratory.[4] In alkalemic states, hydrogen ions (H^+) are released from the cellular buffers and move into the ECF to help correct the elevated pH. In turn, to preserve electroneutrality, extracellular potassium enters the cells. Generally, the degree of hypokalemia caused by alkalemia is relatively mild (plasma potassium falls <0.4 mEq/L for each 0.1 unit increase in pH).[5] Although the effect of alkalemia itself is relatively small, hypokalemia is commonly present in patients with metabolic alkalosis. Partly this is because common causes of hypokalemia (such as potassium-losing diuretics and vomiting) also cause loss of hydrogen ions (thereby inducing alkalosis).[6] Apparently there is little change in plasma potassium concentration with respiratory alkalosis.[7]

ACIDEMIA

A shift of potassium out of the cells can occur in acidemia, either metabolic or respiratory. However, respiratory acidosis is a weaker stimulus for potassium shifting than is metabolic acidosis. In acidemic states, hydrogen ions shift into the cells to help correct the low plasma pH; in turn, to preserve electroneutrality, cellular potassium moves from the cells into the ECF.

The cause of metabolic acidosis apparently has an effect on the extent to which the plasma potassium concentration will elevate. For reasons that are not clearly understood, hyperkalemia is *less* marked when the acidosis is due to organic acids (such as lactic acidosis or ketoacidosis) than when it is due to nonorganic acids (as seen in acidosis due to renal failure or diarrhea).[8,9] In fact, lactic acidosis typically does *not* cause hyperkalemia.[10] Hyperkalemia *does* occur in untreated diabetic ketoacidosis, but it is due more to insulin lack and hyperosmolality than it is to acidemia.[11] The shift of cellular potassium to the bloodstream in a patient with diarrhea becomes clinically important because it may result in normokalemia (masking the true state of potassium deficit, perhaps leading to inadequate potassium replacement therapy). It has been stated that highly variable increases in plasma potassium levels (ranging between 0.2 and 1.7 mEq/L for every 0.1 unit reduction in arterial pH) may occur when the cause of metabolic acidosis is nonorganic acid accumulation.[12] However, other investigators state that no clear quantitative relationship exists.[13]

In summary, it is helpful to remember the following points when considering potassium balance in relation to pH:

1. Potassium shifts are generally more pronounced in acidemia than they are in alkalemia.[14]
2. Metabolic pH disturbances have a greater effect on plasma potassium concentrations than do respiratory pH disturbances.[15–17]
3. Metabolic acidosis due to the accumulation of nonorganic acids (as occurs in diarrhea and renal failure) has a greater effect on plasma potassium elevation than does metabolic acidosis due to the accumulation organic acids (as occurs in lactic acidosis and ketoacidosis).

METABOLIC ACIDOSIS

Metabolic acidosis (HCO_3 deficit) is a clinical disturbance characterized by a low pH (increased hydrogen concentration) and a low plasma bicarbonate concentration. It can be produced by a gain of hydrogen ion or a loss of bicarbonate. In compensation, the lungs hyperventilate to decrease the $PaCO_2$ concentration (movement in the same direction as the primary bicarbonate disturbance).

ANION GAP

Metabolic acidosis can be divided into two forms, depending on the values of the serum anion gap:

$$\text{Anion gap (AG)} = Na^+ - (Cl^- + HCO_3^-) \\ = 12 \pm 2 \text{ mEq/L.}$$

As the equation demonstrates, sodium represents the major cation in body fluids, and chloride and bicarbonate represent the two major anions. There are other anions in body fluid that are not accounted for in the equation, including anionic proteins, phosphates, sulfates, and organic anions (such as ketones and lactic acid). Normally the sum of these unmeasured anions should be no greater than 12 ± 2 mEq/L.[18] However, in some situations, these anions are markedly increased and the AG is greater than expected. These situations are referred to as high AG metabolic acidosis. On the other hand, if the primary problem is direct loss of bicarbonate, gain of chloride, or decreased renal ammonia production, the AG will be within normal limits (12 ± 2 mEq/L). Table 9-2 lists causes of metabolic acidosis classified as either high or normal AG. (Normal values for AG may vary according to the laboratory performing the assays.)

High Anion Gap Acidosis

Lactic Acidosis

Lactic acidosis is most commonly seen in patients with significant cardiopulmonary problems and sepsis.[19] When intracellular oxygen is not available, energy is produced by the anaerobic metabolic pathways, producing lactate and hydrogen ions (which in turn form lactic acid in the bloodstream). Accumulation of lactic acid produces

TABLE 9–2

Causes of Metabolic Acidosis Classified as High Anion Gap or Normal Anion Gap

HIGH ANION GAP (GAIN OF UNMEASURED ANIONS)	NORMAL ANION GAP
Diabetic ketoacidosis	Diarrhea
Starvational ketoacidosis	Biliary or pancreatic fistulas
Alcoholic ketoacidosis	
Lactic acidosis	Excessive administration of isotonic saline or ammonium chloride
Renal failure	
Poisonings:	
• Salicylate	Ureteroenterostomies
• Ethylene glycol	Renal tubular acidosis
• Methyl alcohol	Acetazolamide (Diamox)

a profound decrease in pH. Correlation of elevated lactate levels with mortality in critically ill patients is well established; for example, an arterial lactate level of $\geq$10 mmol/L is associated with a 95% mortality rate.[20] The normal arterial lactate level is $\leq$2.5 mmol/L. Lactate is a credible clinical indicator of tissue hypoxia because it reflects anaerobic metabolism.[21]

Example: The high AG in a patient with lactic acidosis:

$$\begin{aligned} Na^+ &= 131 \text{ mEq/L} \\ HCO_3^- &= 9 \text{ mEq/L} \\ Cl^- &= 86 \text{ mEq/L} \\ AG &= Na^+ - (HCO_3^- + Cl^-) \end{aligned}$$

$$131 - (9 + 86) = 36 \text{ mEq/L}$$

(normal, 12 ± 2 mEq/L)

Although it is commonly accepted that high lactate levels should be accompanied by high AG acidosis, recent studies suggest that more than half of critically ill patients with high lactate levels show normal AG acidosis.[22,23] Probably this is because of the high incidence of preexisting hypoalbuminemia, hyperchloremia, and mixed acid–base disorders in patients in intensive care units.[24]

Ketoacidosis

Both glucose and oxygen are required for energy production in normal cellular metabolism, and insulin is required for transporting glucose across the cell wall. Lack of insulin leads to utilization of metabolic pathways that produce ketones (strong acids) rather than CO_2.[25] More specifically, diabetic ketoacidosis occurs in diabetic patients with a severe insulin deficiency coupled with excessive secretion of counterregulatory hormones. Due to insulin deficiency, lipolysis is increased, releasing free fatty acids that are delivered to the liver where they are converted to ketones. Accumulation of ketones (anions) causes a reciprocal decrease in bicarbonate and an increase in the AG.

Hepatic ketone production is a normal consequence of starvation; yet, the excess ketones are rarely a cause of severe acidosis in healthy nondiabetic persons. However, alcoholics who have gone on a recent drinking binge and are eating poorly may suffer significant ketoacidosis. Although ketosis is initiated by starvation, alcohol itself stimulates ketoacid production. Thus, alcoholic ketoacidosis can produce concentrations of ketones in the blood that are similar to those seen in severe diabetic ketoacidosis. Alcoholic ketoacidosis is reported to occur in two vastly different populations: chronic alcoholics and young children. In children, alcoholic ketoacidosis typically occurs when a small child who has fasted overnight awakens and samples an alcoholic drink left out by the parents the previous evening.[26]

Toxic Substances

Ingestion of toxic substances such as salicylates, ethylene glycol, and methanol produces metabolites that cause metabolic acidosis with a high AG. Excessive salicylate ingestion alters peripheral metabolism, causing overproduction of organic acids. Ethylene glycol is metabolized to glycolic acid and oxalic acids, and methanol is transformed to formaldehyde and formic acid.[27] Abnormal increases in these anions cause a reciprocal decrease in bicarbonate and elevation of the AG.

Renal Failure

Recall that the kidneys are responsible for regulating the serum bicarbonate concentration. During renal failure with uremia this capability is compromised, resulting in bicarbonate's replacement with sulfate, phosphate, or various organic acids. Uremic acidosis usually occurs when the glomerular filtration rate (GFR) is reduced to less than 20 to 30 mL/min.[26]

Example: The normal AG in a patient with ureterosigmoidostomy:

Na^+ = 134 mEq/L
HCO_3^- = 10 mEq/L
Cl^- = 115 mEq/L
AG = $Na^+ - (HCO_3^- + Cl^-)$
134 − (10 + 115) = 9 mEq/L

Normal Anion Gap Acidosis

Diarrhea

Diarrhea causes direct loss of bicarbonate in the stool, ECF volume depletion, and concentration of the remaining serum chloride, resulting in hyperchloremic acidosis. Because no change is caused in the "unmeasured" anions, the AG remains within normal limits. The same mechanism is seen in pancreatic and biliary fistulas, through which bicarbonate-rich fluid is lost in external drainage.

Hyperchloremic acidosis often develops in patients with urinary diversion into the sigmoid colon. Apparently it is associated with bicarbonate secretion into the colon in exchange for the reabsorption of urinary chloride. The same changes may occur with urinary diversion to an ileal segment.

Excessive Chloride

Excessive infusion of chloride-containing fluids, such as isotonic sodium chloride (0.9% NaCl) or ammonium chloride, can cause hyperchloremic acidosis. Other causes include renal tubular acidosis and carbonic anhydrase inhibitors. Renal tubular acidosis exists in various forms and can be characterized by either bicarbonate loss in the urine or inability to generate new bicarbonate. As the plasma bicarbonate level decreases, the chloride level increases. Carbonic anhydrase inhibitors (such as acetazolamide) cause renal bicarbonate wasting.

Decreased Anion Gap

Most often, a decreased AG is due to either severe dilution or hypoalbuminemia. Hypoalbuminemia is not a surprising cause since albumin accounts for most of the nonchloride or nonbicarbonate anions in the blood. A decreased AG may also be due to an increase in unmeasured *cations* (as in lithium intoxication).

Metabolic acidosis can be acute or chronic. Expected blood gas changes for uncompensated, partly compensated, and completely compensated metabolic acidosis are presented in Table 9-3.

DEFINING CHARACTERISTICS

Both etiological factors and defining characteristics of metabolic acidosis are given in the Summary of Metabolic Acidosis. An example of blood gases in patients with metabolic acidosis is presented below.

Example: Patient with diabetic ketoacidosis:

pH = 7.05
HCO_3 = 5 mEq/L (primary disturbance, excess of ketones)
$PaCO_2$ = 12 mmHg (represents compensatory hyperventilation)
Base excess (BE) = −30 mEq/L

Acidemia depresses myocardial contractility, lowers the fibrillation threshold, and blunts the pressor

TABLE 9–3

Expected Directional Changes in Blood Gases in Metabolic Acidosis

IMBALANCE	pH	HCO_3	$PaCO_2$	BASE EXCESS
Uncompensated metabolic acidosis	↓	↓	N	↓
Partly compensated metabolic acidosis	↓	↓	↓	↓
Completely compensated metabolic acidosis	N	↓	↓	↓

N, normal.

Summary of Metabolic Acidosis (Base Bicarbonate Deficit)

ETIOLOGICAL FACTORS	DEFINING CHARACTERISTICS
Normal anion gap: • Diarrhea • Intestinal fistulas • Ureterosigmoidostomy • Acidifying drugs (such as ammonium chloride) • Renal tubular acidosis (RTA) High anion gap: • Diabetic ketoacidosis • Starvational ketoacidosis • Alcoholic ketoacidosis • Lactic acidosis • Renal failure • Ingestion of toxins (such as salicylates, ethylene glycol, and methanol)	Headache Confusion Drowsiness Increased respiratory rate and depth (may not become clinically evident until HCO_3 is quite low) Nausea and vomiting Peripheral vasodilatation (may be present, causing warm, flushed skin) Decreased cardiac output when pH falls below 7.1 Arterial blood gases: • Fall in pH (<7.35) • HCO_3 < 22 mEq/L (primary) • $PaCO_2$ < 35 mmHg (compensation by lungs)

response to catecholamines,[28] but it also enhances tissue oxygenation by shifting the oxyhemoglobin dissociation curve to the right.

TREATMENT

Because there are many conditions that lead to the development of metabolic acidosis, it is reasonable that treatment must vary, at least somewhat, according to the cause of the imbalance. For example, dialysis may be needed for the extremely acidotic renal failure patient. Insulin administration and fluid replacement are frequently sufficient to correct even very low pH values in patients with ketoacidosis. The need for alkali therapy is influenced by the severity of acidosis. Although the precise level to which the pH must drop before alkali therapy is necessary is somewhat controversial, it is generally considered prudent to keep the blood pH above 7.1 to 7.2 to avoid the adverse cardiovascular effects of severe acidemia.[29] Acidosis to this degree can result in myocardial depression, hypotension, and resistance to vasopressor therapy.[30] Generally, there are three types of alkali that can be used for the treatment of metabolic acidosis: bicarbonate, salts of organic acids (such as lactate, acetate, and citrate) that are metabolized to bicarbonate, and tromethamine (THAM).[31] Most frequently used is sodium bicarbonate because it is effective immediately and requires no metabolic activation, unlike lactate, acetate, and citrate.[32] Care must be taken during bicarbonate administration to avoid overalkalinization of the plasma, which could result in cardiac arrhythmias and tetany. Thus, frequent monitoring of the acid–base status is warranted during treatment. No further bicarbonate should be given once the pH reaches 7.2.[33] The response to the administration of alkali partially depends on the cause of the metabolic acidosis. The reader is referred to Chapter 18 for a discussion of the use of alkali in the treatment of ketoacidosis, and to Chapter 16 for a discussion of the use of alkali during cardiac resuscitation.

METABOLIC ALKALOSIS

Metabolic alkalosis (HCO_3 excess) is a clinical disturbance characterized by a high pH (decreased hydrogen concentration) and a high plasma bicarbonate concentration. It can be produced by a gain of bicarbonate or a loss of hydrogen ion. In compensation, the lungs hypoventilate to increase the $PaCO_2$ concentration (movement in the same direction as the primary bicarbonate disturbance).

ETIOLOGICAL FACTORS

Probably the most common cause of metabolic alkalosis is vomiting or gastric suction (results in loss of hydrogen and chloride anions). Metabolic alkalosis occurs frequently in pyloric stenosis as only gastric fluid is lost in this disorder. Recall that gastric fluid has an acid pH (usually 1–3); loss of acidic fluid, of course, increases alkalinity of body fluids. (Vomiting related to other conditions sometimes involves loss of both gastric and alkaline upper small-intestinal fluid. When this occurs, the severity of the pH change is tempered.)

Other factors predisposing to metabolic alkalosis include the loss of potassium, such as that caused by certain diuretics (e.g., thiazides, furosemide, and ethacrynic acid) and the presence of excessive adrenal corticoid hormones (as in hyperaldosteronism and Cushing's syndrome). Hypokalemia produces alkalosis in two ways: (1) In the presence of hypokalemia, the kidneys conserve potassium and thus increase hydrogen ion excretion (recall that these ions compete for renal excretion). (2) Cellular potassium moves out into the ECF in an attempt to maintain near normal serum levels (as potassium leaves the cell, hydrogen must enter to maintain electroneutrality).

Excessive alkali ingestion, as in the use of bicarbonate-containing antacids (e.g., Alka-Seltzer) can also cause metabolic alkalosis. Metabolic alkalosis due to high-dose sodium bicarbonate administration during cardiopulmonary resuscitation was a common finding a decade ago.[34]

Abrupt relief of chronically high CO_2 level in plasma (e.g., assisted ventilation) results in a "lag period" before the chronically high serum bicarbonate level can be corrected by the kidneys.

DEFINING CHARACTERISTICS

Alkalosis is manifested primarily by symptoms related to decreased calcium ionization, such as tingling of the fingers and toes, dizziness, and hypertonic muscles. Respirations are depressed as a compensatory action by the lungs.

Arterial blood gases show an increased pH (>7.45) and an elevated bicarbonate level (>26 mEq/L), the primary disorder. To help temper the severity of the imbalance, compensatory hypoventilation occurs (elevating the $PaCO_2$) and is more pronounced in semiconscious, unconscious, or debilitated patients than in alert patients. Debilitated patients may develop marked hypoxemia as a result of hypoventilation. The BE is always positive.

Example: Patient with vomiting:

pH = 7.62
HCO_3 = 45 mEq/L
$PaCO_2$ = 48 mmHg
BE = 16 mEq/L

Other laboratory values are also disrupted in metabolic alkalosis. The serum potassium concentration is often, although not always, below 3.5 mEq/L. This is especially likely if the cause of the alkalosis is also associated with potassium loss (as in use of potassium-losing diuretics or vomiting). The serum chloride is relatively lower than sodium, as an elevation in the serum bicarbonate level causes the chloride level to drop. (Recall that as one anion increases, another tends to decrease to maintain electroneutrality.)

The ionized fraction of serum calcium decreases in the presence of alkalosis as more calcium combines with serum proteins. Because it is the ionized fraction of calcium that influences neuromuscular activity, it is understandable why symptoms of hypocalcemia are often the predominant ones of alkalosis.

Urinary chloride concentration is sometimes measured to determine the cause of metabolic alkalosis. It is usually less than 15 mEq/L when metabolic alkalosis is due to vomiting or gastric suction or prolonged diuretic use. Conversely, it is usually greater than 20 mEq/L when metabolic alkalosis is due to hyperaldosteronism, Cushing's syndrome, or profound potassium depletion (serum potassium <2.0 mEq/L).

Metabolic alkalosis can be acute or chronic. Expected directional changes in blood gases for uncompensated, partly compensated, and completely compensated metabolic alkalosis are listed in Table 9-4. The Summary of Metabolic Alkalosis lists the etiological factors and defining characteristics of metabolic alkalosis.

TREATMENT

Treatment is aimed at reversal of the underlying disorder. Sufficient chloride must be supplied for the kidney to absorb sodium with chloride (allowing the excretion of excess bicarbonate). Treatment also includes restoration of normal fluid volume by administration of sodium chloride fluids (because continued volume depletion serves to maintain the alkalosis).

TABLE 9-4

Expected Directional Changes in Blood Gases in Metabolic Alkalosis

IMBALANCE	pH	HCO_3	$PaCO_2$	BASE EXCESS
Uncompensated (acute) metabolic alkalosis	↑	↑	N	↑
Partly compensated (subacute) metabolic alkalosis	↑	↑	↑	↑
Completely compensated (chronic) metabolic alkalosis	N	↑	↑	↑

N, normal.

Summary of Metabolic Alkalosis (Base Bicarbonate Excess)

ETIOLOGICAL FACTORS

Vomiting or gastric suction

Hypokalemia

Hyperaldosteronism

Cushing's syndrome

Potassium-losing diuretics (e.g., thiazides, furosemide, ethacrynic acid)

Alkali ingestion (bicarbonate-containing antacids)

Parenteral $NaHCO_3$ administration for cardiopulmonary resuscitation

Abrupt relief of chronic respiratory acidosis

DEFINING CHARACTERISTICS

Those related to decreased calcium ionization, such as
- Dizziness
- Tingling of fingers and toes
- Circumoral paresthesia
- Carpopedal spasm
- Hypertonic muscles

Depressed respiration (compensatory action by lungs)

Arterial blood gases:
- pH > 7.45
- Bicarbonate > 26 mEq/L (primary)
- $PaCO_2$ > 45 mmHg (compensatory)

Serum Cl relatively lower than Na

RESPIRATORY ACIDOSIS

Respiratory acidosis (H_2CO_3 excess) can be either acute or chronic; the acute imbalance is particularly dangerous. When respiratory acidosis is acute, the bicarbonate level remains in the normal range because renal compensation is very slow. Therefore, the high $PaCO_2$ can quickly produce a sharp decrease in plasma pH. When respiratory acidosis is chronic, as in COPD, the kidneys compensate for the elevated $PaCO_2$ by increasing the bicarbonate level. (Compensatory renal bicarbonate generation takes several hours to days to develop.)

ETIOLOGICAL FACTORS

Respiratory acidosis is always due to inadequate excretion of CO_2 (inadequate ventilation), resulting in increased plasma CO_2 levels and therefore increased carbonic acid levels. In addition to an elevated $PaCO_2$ levels, hypoventilation usually causes a decrease in PaO_2.

Acute respiratory acidosis is associated with certain emergency situations (such as acute pulmonary edema, aspiration of a foreign object, atelectasis, pneumothorax, overdosage of sedatives, and severe pneumonia). Chronic respiratory acidosis is associated with chronic situations such as emphysema, bronchiectasis, and bronchial asthma. Other etiological factors are listed in the Summary of Respiratory Acidosis.

DEFINING CHARACTERISTICS

Clinical signs vary between acute and chronic respiratory acidosis and are listed in the Summary of Respiratory Acidosis.

Acute Respiratory Acidosis

Sudden hypercapnia (elevated $PaCO_2$) can cause increased pulse and respiratory rate, increased blood pressure, mental cloudiness, and a feeling of fullness in the head ($PaCO_2$ causes cerebrovascular vasodilatation and increased cerebral blood flow, particularly when more than 60 mmHg).

Ventricular fibrillation may be the first sign of respiratory acidosis in the anesthetized patient. Respiratory acidosis may occur as soon as 15 min after the start of anesthesia and is most likely to occur in patients with chronic pulmonary disease. As stated, arterial blood gas changes occur immediately when ventilation is abruptly altered. The pH may reach a level of 7 or less in a few minutes. The $PaCO_2$ is greater than 45 mmHg, and may reach 120 mmHg or higher. The bicarbonate is normal or only slightly elevated because there has been little time for renal compensation (an exception would be the patient with COPD who has a chronically elevated bicarbonate; in that situation, it would not be high enough to compensate for the sudden increase in $PaCO_2$). The PaO_2 is below normal when the patient is breathing room air and is the result of hypoventilation.

Example: Patient with acute respiratory acidosis:

pH = 7.26
$PaCO_2$ = 56 mmHg
HCO_3 = 24 mEq/L

Chronic Respiratory Acidosis

The patient with chronic respiratory acidosis may complain of weakness, dull headache, and the symptoms of the underlying disease process. The arterial blood gases reveal a pH less than 7.35 or within the lower limit of normal (if complete compensation has occurred). The $PaCO_2$ is greater than 45 mmHg (frequently between 50 and 60 mmHg or greater). Patients with COPD who gradually accumulate CO_2 over a prolonged period (days to months) may not develop symptoms of hypercapnia (listed previously under Acute Respiratory Acidosis) because compensatory changes have had time to occur. For example, an emphysematous patient kept alive with oxygen therapy for more than 1 year was mentally alert although his $PaCO_2$ was 140 mmHg. In the healthy person, a rapid rise in the $PaCO_2$ to 140 mmHg would surely produce unconsciousness. The patient with chronic respiratory acidosis has had time for partial or complete renal compensation; therefore, the bicarbonate is above normal, as is the BE.

Example: Patient with chronic respiratory acidosis:

pH = 7.38
$PaCO_2$ = 76 mmHg
HCO_3 = 42 mEq/L
BE = +14 mEq/L

Remember that when the $PaCO_2$ is chronically elevated above normal, the respiratory center becomes relatively insensitive to CO_2 as a respiratory stimulant, leaving hypoxemia as the major drive for respiration. Excessive oxygen administration removes the stimulus of hypoxemia and the patient develops acute ventilatory failure unless the situation is quickly reversed.

Expected directional changes in blood gases in uncompensated, partly compensated, and completely compensated respiratory acidosis are listed in Table 9-5.

TREATMENT

Treatment is directed at improving ventilation; exact measures vary with the cause of inadequate ventilation. Pharmacological agents are used as indicated. For example, bronchodilators help reduce

Summary of Respiratory Acidosis (Carbonic Acid Excess)

ETIOLOGICAL FACTORS

Acute respiratory acidosis:
- Acute pulmonary edema
- Aspiration of a foreign body
- Atelectasis
- Pneumothorax, hemothorax
- Overdosoge of sedatives or anesthetic
- Position on OR table that interferes with respirations
- Cardiac arrest
- Severe pneumonia
- Laryngospasm
- Mechanical ventilation improperly regulated

Chronic respiratory acidosis:
- Emphysema
- Cystic fibrosis
- Advanced multiple sclerosis
- Bronchiectasis
- Bronchial asthma

Factors favoring hypoventilation:
- Obesity
- Tight abdominal binders or dressings
- Postoperative pain (as in high abdominal or chest incisions)
- Abdominal distention from cirrhosis or bowel obstruction

DEFINING CHARACTERISTICS

Acute respiratory acidosis:
- Feeling of fullness in the head ($PaCO_2$ causes cerebrovascular vosodilatation and increased cerebral blood flow, particularly when higher than 60 mmHg)
- Mental cloudiness
- Dizziness
- Palpitations
- Muscular twitching
- Convulsions
- Warm, flushed skin
- Unconsciousness
- Ventricular fibrillation may be first sign in anesthetized patient (related to hyperkalemia)
- ABGs:
  - — pH < 7.35
  - — $PaCO_2 > 45$ mmHg (primary)
  - — HCO_3 normal or only slightly elevated

Chronic respiratory acidosis:
- Weakness
- Dull headache
- Symptoms of underlying disease process
- ABGs:
  - — pH < 7.35 or within lower limits of normal
  - — $PaCO_2 > 45$ mmHg (primary)
  - — $HCO_3 > 26$ mEq/L (compensatory)

TABLE 9–5

Expected Directional Changes in Blood Gases in Respiratory Acidosis

IMBALANCE	pH	$PaCO_2$	HCO_3	BASE EXCESS
Uncompensated respiratory acidosis (acute)	↓	↑	N	N
Partly compensated respiratory acidosis	↓	↑	↑	↑
Completely compensated respiratory acidosis	N	↑	↑	↑

N, normal.

bronchial spasm; antibiotics are used for respiratory infections. Pulmonary hygiene measures are used, when necessary, to rid the respiratory tract of mucus and purulent drainage. Adequate hydration (2–3 L/day) is indicated to keep the mucous membranes moist and thereby facilitate removal of secretions. Supplemental oxygen is used as necessary.

A mechanical respirator, used cautiously, may improve pulmonary ventilation. Remember that overzealous use of a mechanical respirator may cause such rapid excretion of CO_2 that the kidneys will be unable to eliminate excess bicarbonate with sufficient rapidity to prevent alkalosis and convulsions. For this reason, the elevated $PaCO_2$ must be decreased slowly.

RESPIRATORY ALKALOSIS

ETIOLOGICAL FACTORS AND DEFINING CHARACTERISTICS

Respiratory alkalosis (H_2CO_3 deficit) is always due to hyperventilation, which causes excessive "blowing off" of CO_2 and, hence, a decrease in plasma H_2CO_3 content. Etiological factors associated with respiratory alkalosis and defining characteristics are listed in the Summary of Respiratory Alkalosis.

As with respiratory acidosis, acute and chronic conditions can occur in respiratory alkalosis. In the acute state, the pH is elevated above normal as a result of a low $PaCO_2$ and a normal bicarbonate level. (Recall that the kidneys cannot alter the bicarbonate level quickly.)

Example: Patient with acute respiratory alkalosis:

pH = 7.52
$PaCO_2$ = 30 mmHg
HCO_3 = 24 mEq/L
BE = +2.5 mEq/L

In the compensated state, the kidneys have had time to lower the bicarbonate level.

Example: Patient with chronic respiratory alkalosis:

pH = 7.40
$PaCO_2$ = 30 mmHg
HCO_3 = 18 mEq/L
BE = −5 mEq/L

Expected directional changes in blood gases in uncompensated, partly compensated, and completely compensated respiratory alkalosis are listed in Table 9-6.

TREATMENT

If the cause of respiratory alkalosis is anxiety, the patient should be made aware that the abnormal breathing practice is responsible for the symptoms accompanying this condition. Instructing the patient to breath more slowly (to cause accumulation of CO_2) or to breath into a closed system (such as a paper bag) is helpful. Usually a sedative is required to relieve hyperventilation in very anxious patients. (If alkalosis is severe enough to cause fainting, the increased ventilation will cease and respirations will revert to normal.) Treatment for other causes of respiratory alkalosis is directed at correcting the underlying problem.

TABLE 9–6

Expected Directional Changes in Arterial Blood Gases in Respiratory Alkalosis

IMBALANCE	pH	$PaCO_2$	HCO_3	BASE EXCESS
Uncompensated respiratory alkalosis	↑	↓	N	N
Partly compensated respiratory alkalosis	↑	↓	↓	↓
Completely compensated respiratory alkalosis	N	↓	↓	↓

N, normal.

Summary of Respiratory Alkalosis (Carbonic Acid Deficit)

ETIOLOGICAL FACTORS

Extreme anxiety (most common cause)

High fever

Hypoxemia

Early salicylate intoxication (stimulates respiratory center)

Gram-negative bacteremia

Central nervous system lesions involving respiratory center

Pulmonary emboli

Thyrotoxicosis

Excessive ventilation by mechanical ventilators

Pregnancy (high progesterone level sensitizes the respiratory center to CO_2; physiological)

DEFINING CHARACTERISTICS

Lightheadedness (a low $PaCO_2$ causes cerebral vasoconstriction and thus decreased cerebral blood flow)

Inability to concentrate

Those of decreased calcium ionization (numbness and tingling of extremities and circumoral paresthesia; more likely to occur if respiratory alkalosis develops rapidly)

Hyperventilation syndrome:

- Tinnitus
- Palpitations
- Sweating
- Dry mouth
- Tremulousness
- Precordial pain (tightness)
- Nausea and vomiting
- Epigastric pain
- Blurred vision
- Convulsions and loss of consciousness (may be partly due to cerebral ischemia, caused by cerebral vasoconstriction)

ABGs:

- pH > 7.45
- $PaCO_2 < 35$ mmHg (primary)
- $HCO_3 < 22$ mEq/L (compensatory)

MIXED ACID–BASE IMBALANCES

The preceding discussions have described single acid–base imbalances. These single imbalances do occur; however, one should be aware that in some clinical situations the patient may have two or more primary acid–base disturbances simultaneously. Some examples are given in Table 9-7 and at the end of the chapter. A number of steps and formulas are available to evaluate blood gas changes and determine whether they are purely compensatory in nature or represent a *second* primary imbalance. These are listed here in Clinical Tip: Systematic Assessment of Arterial Blood Gases and Table 9-8.

SAMPLE MIXED ACID–BASE PROBLEMS

Use rules in Table 9-8 and Clinical Tips: Systematic Assessment of Arterial Blood Gases to analyze the following situations:

Respiratory Alkalosis Plus Metabolic Acidosis

Example: A patient has taken an overdose of aspirin. Recall that early in salicylate poisoning, the medulla is stimulated to produce hyperventilation (respiratory alkalosis results). Later, due to disrupted glucose metabolism, metabolic acidosis may result.

pH = 7.4
$PaCO_2$ = 18 mmHg
HCO_3 = 16 mEq/L
BE = −10 mEq/L

Note in the above situation that the simultaneous appearance of respiratory alkalosis and metabolic acidosis has produced a normal pH. (This is not always the case; one imbalance may be stronger than the other and cause an abnormal pH in its favor.)

TABLE 9–7

Examples of Combinations of Mixed Acid–Base Disorders

Metabolic acidosis/respiratory acidosis	
Cardiopulmonary arrest	Hypoxemia produces lactic acidosis with decrease in HCO_3 Respiratory arrest causes CO_2 retention
Metabolic acidosis/respiratory alkalosis	
Salicylate intoxication	Salicylate alters peripheral metabolism and causes overproduction of organic acids with resultant decrease in HCO_3 Salicylate stimulates respiratory center and causes decrease in CO_2
Metabolic acidosis/metabolic alkalosis	
Renal failure with vomiting	Renal failure causes retention of acid metabolites with decrease in HCO_3 Vomiting causes loss of H^+ and Cl^- and thus increase in HCO_3
Metabolic alkalosis/respiratory alkalosis	
Vomiting during pregnancy	Vomiting causes loss of H^+ and Cl^- and thus increase in HCO_3 Progesterone increase during pregnancy stimulates respirations and causes decrease in CO_2
Metabolic alkalosis/respiratory acidosis	
Vomiting with COPD	Vomiting causes loss of H^+ and Cl^- and thus increase in HCO_3 Chronic obstructive pulmonary disease is associated with sustained elevation of CO_2

COPD, chronic obstructive pulmonary disease.

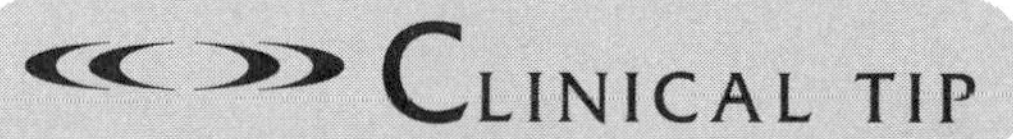

Systematic Assessment of Arterial Blood Gases

The following steps are recommended to evaluate arterial blood gas values. They are based on the assumption that the average values are

pH = 7.4
$PaCO_2$ = 40 mmHg
HCO_3 = 24 mEq/L

I. *First,* look at the pH. It can be high, low, or normal as follows:

pH > 7.4 (alkalosis)
pH < 7.4 (acidosis)
pH = 7.4 (normal)

A normal pH may indicate perfectly normal blood gases, or it may be an indication of a compensated imbalance. A compensated imbalance is one in which the body has been able to correct the pH by either respiratory or metabolic changes (depending on the primary problem). For example, a patient with primary metabolic acidosis starts out with a low bicarbonate level but a normal carbon dioxide level. Soon afterward, the lungs try to compensate for the imbalance by exhaling large amounts of carbon dioxide (hyperventilation).

Another example, a patient with primary respiratory acidosis starts out with a high carbon dioxide level; soon afterward, the kidneys attempt to compensate by retaining bicarbonate. If the compensatory maneuver is able to restore the bicarbonate: carbonic acid ratio back to 20:1, full compensation (and thus normal pH) will be achieved.

II. *The next step is to determine the primary cause of the disturbance. This is done by evaluating the $PaCO_2$ and HCO_3 in relation to the pH.*

pH > 7.4 (alkalosis)

1. If the $PaCO_2$ is <40 mmHg, the primary disturbance is respiratory alkalosis. (This situation occurs when a patient hyperventilates and "blows off" too much carbon dioxide. Recall that carbon dioxide dissolved in water becomes carbonic acid, the acid side of the "carbonic acid:base bicarbonate" buffer system.)

2. If the HCO_3 is >24 mEq/L, the primary disturbance is metabolic alkalosis. (This situation occurs when the body gains too much bicarbonate, an alkaline substance. Bicarbonate is the basic, or alkaline side of the "carbonic acid:base bicarbonate" buffer system.)

pH < 7.4 (acidosis)

1. If the $PaCO_2$ is >40 mmHg, the primary disturbance is respiratory acidosis. (This situation occurs when a patient hypoventilates and thus retains too much carbon dioxide, an acidic substance.)

2. If the HCO_3 is <24 mEq/L, the primary disturbance is metabolic acidosis. (This situation occurs when the body's bicarbonate level drops, either because of direct bicarbonate loss or because of gains of acids such as lactic acid or ketones.)

III. *The next step involves determining if compensation has begun.*

This is done by looking at the value other than the primary disorder. If it is moving in the same direction as the primary value, compensation is under way. Consider the following gases:
Example:

	pH	$PaCO_2$	HCO_3
(1)	7.20	60 mmHg	24 mEq/L
(2)	7.40	60 mmHg	37 mEq/L

The first set (1) indicates acute respiratory acidosis without compensation (the $PaCO_2$ is high, the HCO_3 is normal). The second set (2) indicates chronic respiratory acidosis. Note that compensation has taken place; that is, the HCO_3 has elevated to an appropriate level to balance the high $PaCO_2$ and produce a normal pH.

TABLE 9–8

Compensatory Changes Related to Primary Acid–Base Disturbances

IMBALANCE	PRIMARY CHANGE	COMPENSATORY CHANGE
Metabolic acidosis (base bicarbonate deficit)	HCO_3 decreased	$1.5(HCO_3) + 8 \pm 2$
Metabolic alkalosis (base bicarbonate excess)	HCO_3 increased	0.6 mmHg increase in $PaCO_2$ for every 1 mEq/L rise in HCO_3
Respiratory acidosis (carbonic acid excess)		
• Acute	$PaCO_2$ increased	1.0 mEq/L increase in HCO_3 for every 10 mmHg rise in $PaCO_2$
• Chronic	$PaCO_2$ increased	3.5 mEq/L increase in HCO_3 for every 10 mmHg rise in $PaCO_2$
Respiratory alkalosis (carbonic acid deficit)		
• Acute	$PaCO_2$ decreased	2.0 mEq/L decrease in HCO_3 for every 10 mmHg fall in $PaCO_2$
• Chronic	$PaCO_2$ decreased	5.0 mEq/L decrease in HCO_3 for every 10 mmHg fall in $PaCO_2$

If the only problem in this situation were respiratory alkalosis, the HCO_3 would be expected to be approximately 20 mEq/L. Note that it is lower than expected (indicating metabolic acidosis). If the only problem were metabolic acidosis, the $PaCO_2$ would be expected to be approximately 32 mEq/L. Note that it is lower than expected (indicating respiratory alkalosis).

Respiratory Acidosis Plus Metabolic Acidosis

Example: A patient has lactic acidosis secondary to cardiac failure and hypercapnia secondary to pneumonia.

$$\begin{aligned} pH &= 7.10 \\ PaCO_2 &= 50 \text{ mmHg} \\ HCO_3 &= 15 \text{ mEq/L} \\ BE &= -6 \text{ mEq/L} \end{aligned}$$

Because both primary disturbances produce acidosis, the pH is quite low. If the only problem were acute respiratory acidosis, the HCO_3 level would increase to slightly above normal (instead, it has decreased). If the only problem were metabolic acidosis, the $PaCO_2$ would decrease (instead, it has increased).

REFERENCES

1. Guyton A: Textbook of Medical Physiology, 8th ed, p 447. Philadelphia, WB Saunders, 1991
2. Ibid, p 449
3. Narins R: Clinical Disorders of Fluid and Electrolyte Metabolism, 5th ed, p 669. New York, McGraw-Hill, 1994
4. Rose B: Clinical Physiology of Acid–Base and Electrolyte Disorders, 4th ed, p 778. New York, McGraw-Hill, 1994
5. Ibid
6. Ibid
7. Chernow B (ed): The Pharmacologic Approach to the Critically Ill Patient, 3rd ed, p 963. Baltimore, Williams & Wilkins, 1994
8. Rose, p 512
9. Narins, p 669
10. Narins, p 790
11. Rose, p 512
12. Rose, p 828
13. Narins, p 669
14. Ibid
15. Ibid
16. Chernow, p 963

17. Pemberton L, Pemberton D: Treatment of Water, Electrolyte, and Acid–Base Disorders in the Surgical Patient. New York, McGraw-Hill, 1994
18. Narins, p 762
19. Shapiro B, Peruzzi W, Templin R: Clinical Application of Blood Gases, 5th ed, p 238. St. Louis, CV Mosby, 1994
20. Ibid, p 173
21. Ibid
22. Iberti T, et al: Low sensitivity of the anion gap as a screen to detect hyperlactatemia in critically ill patients. Crit Care Med 18:275–277,1990
23. Mechta K, Kruse J, Carlson R: The relationship between anion gap and elevated lactate (Abstract). Crit Care Med 14:405,1986
24. Shapiro, p 172
25. Ibid, p 238
26. Hoffman R, Goldfrank L: Ethanol-associated metabolic disorders. Endocrinol Metabol Emerg 7(4):943, 1989
27. Kokko J, Tannen R: Fluids and Electrolytes, 2nd ed, p 31. Philadelphia, WB Saunders, 1990
28. Kearns T, Wolfson A: Metabolic acidosis. Endocr Metabol Emerg 7(4):823,1989
29. Chernow, p 965
30. Woodley M, Whelan A: Manual of Medical Therapeutics, 27th ed, p 56. Boston, Little, Brown, 1992
31. Chernow, p 965
32. Pemberton L, Pemberton D: Treatment of Water, Electrolyte, and Acid–Base Disorders in the Surgical Patient, p 324. New York, McGraw-Hill, 1994
33. Woodley, Whelan, p 57
34. Shapiro, p 240

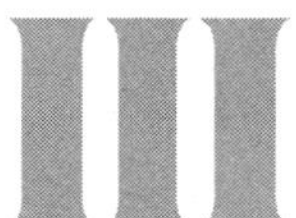

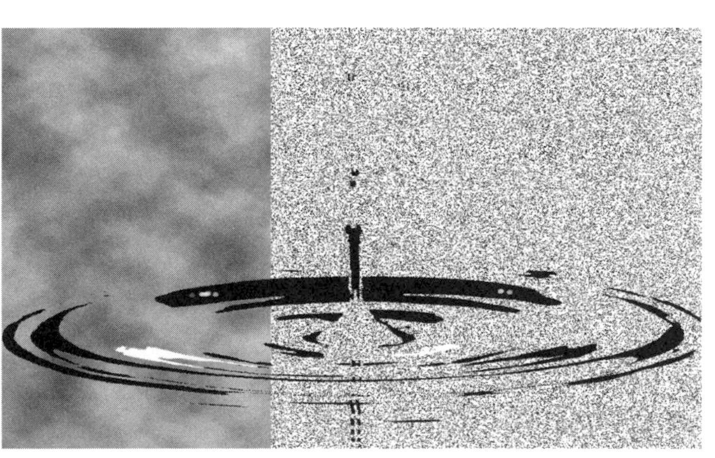

Parenteral and Enteral Nutrition

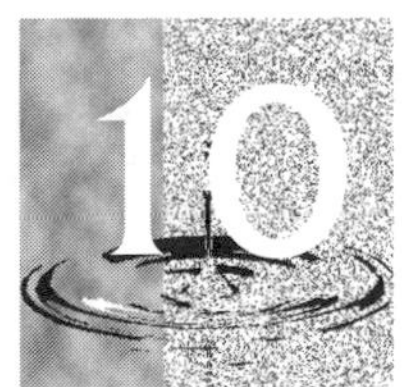

Parenteral Fluids

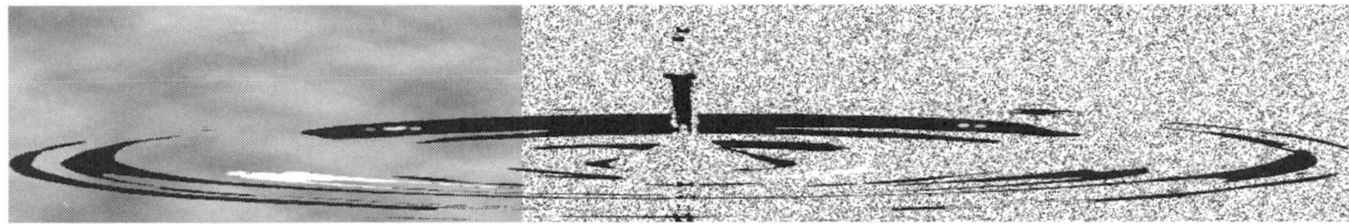

The nurse's role in parenteral fluid therapy is crucial because it is the nurse who usually initiates fluids and, almost invariably, is responsible for monitoring the patient's response. One must be knowledgeable about the contents of parenteral fluids, their purposes, and the contraindications and complications associated with their uses.

Before discussing the types of parenteral fluids available and the factors to be considered with their administration, it is helpful to review some basic facts.

There are essentially three major purposes for parenteral fluid therapy: (1) providing fluids to meet daily maintenance needs; (2) providing fluids to replace ongoing losses; and (3) providing electrolytes to correct any existing disturbances. Each of these purposes is briefly discussed.

PURPOSES OF FLUID THERAPY

PROVISION OF USUAL MAINTENANCE NEEDS

As noted in Table 2-1, the average healthy adult requires approximately 2600 mL/day of fluid to replace fluid lost in urine, stool, exhalation, and radiation from the skin. Many patients require parenteral fluids for only a few days while they are temporarily unable to ingest food and fluid during a limited illness or after surgery. In these patients, the typical fluid prescription for maintenance needs ranges between 2000 and 3000 mL/day.

Of course, the body needs more than water for maintenance. Electrolytes are also needed. The average adult needs approximately 50 to 150 mEq of sodium and approximately 40 to 60 mEq of potassium each day.[1] An example of a 24-hr fluid prescription to meet these needs is 2 L of 0.45% NaCl with 20 mEq of KCl added to each liter. Because each liter of 0.45% NaCl contains 77 mEq of sodium, 2 L would provide 154 mEq (easily meeting the daily sodium requirement of most adults). Addition of 20 mEq of KCl to each liter of fluid would provide the typically needed 40 mEq of potassium per day.

Because 0.45% NaCl is a hypotonic solution, it provides some free water to aid in the renal excretion of solutes. Free water can also be supplied in the form of 5% dextrose in water. Calories are needed in parenteral fluids to minimize protein catabolism and prevent ketosis of starvation. Thus, the above example would more likely be 2 L of 5% dextrose in 0.45% NaCl (rather than 0.45% NaCl alone). Because each liter of a 5% dextrose solution provides 50 g of carbohydrate with approximately 170 calories, 2 L would provide 100 g of carbohydrate with 340 calories. Although this is a small fraction of the daily caloric need, it is far better than none in terms of warding off ketosis of starvation. As discussed in Chapter 11, sophisticated solutions are available to meet the nutritional needs of patients requiring prolonged parenteral therapy or of those needing a large caloric intake due to hypermetabolism (as occurs with trauma or burns).

Maintenance needs for sodium and potassium were discussed briefly. Remember that calcium, magnesium, and phosphorus may be necessary after 1 week of parenteral therapy.[2]

Although 2000 to 3000 mL/day of water for the average healthy adult is a useful figure to keep in mind, it is important to realize that it may need to be adjusted downward for smaller adults. Furthermore, children need entirely different volumes based on their body size and age. To avoid the possibility of fluid volume error, some clinicians favor the use of fluid volume replacement based on body surface area.

The above discussion of needed fluid volume is predicated on the assumption that the patient has normal renal function. If this is not the case, fluid volume as well as sodium and potassium replacement must be adjusted according to severity of the renal impairment. For example, an oliguric renal failure patient might logically receive the same amount of fluid as the sum of urinary output and estimated insensible losses.

REPLACEMENT OF ABNORMAL FLUID LOSSES

If the patient is losing fluid by an abnormal route (such as gastric suction, vomiting, or diarrhea), more than maintenance fluids must be provided to prevent fluid volume deficit (FVD). In addition, the electrolyte content of the parenteral fluid will need to be modified to correct imbalances. The need for a carefully kept intake and output (I&O) record is evident to identify lost water and electrolytes. It is also important to record elevated body temperature because this increases fluid needs. Free water needs are increased in individuals with unusual insensible water losses, such as those who are hyperventilating or exposed to low environmental humidity. Water needs are also greater in patients with decreased renal concentrating ability because relatively more water is required to eliminate wastes. Finally, fluid requirements are greatly increased by shock, multiple trauma, and sepsis (either because of direct fluid loss or pooling of fluid in the capillaries or interstitial space). See Chapters 13 through 25 for discussion of fluid therapy in patients with specific clinical problems.

CORRECTION OF EXISTING ELECTROLYTE DISTURBANCES

Providing maintenance fluid and electrolytes is more complicated if the patient has electrolyte disturbances that need correction. The task becomes one of safely providing needed electrolytes in conjunction with maintenance needs. (For discussion of fluid therapy for specific electrolyte disturbances, see Chapters 3 through 9.)

ASSESSMENT OF PATIENTS RECEIVING PARENTERAL FLUID THERAPY

Before parenteral fluid therapy is initiated for a patient with a real or potential fluid balance problem, renal status must be evaluated. There is danger of causing other imbalances if the kidneys are not functioning adequately. For example, administration of potassium-containing fluids to a patient with inadequate renal function can induce serious hyperkalemia.

If the patient with a severe FVD is oliguric, it is necessary to determine if the depressed renal function is due to prerenal azotemia secondary to decreased renal perfusion or, more seriously, to actual renal parenchymal damage (acute tubular necrosis) after prolonged untreated FVD. To differentiate between these conditions, a fluid load is infused over a short period and the patient is observed closely. If urine output improves, the problem was simple FVD; if urine flow is not reestablished, the problem is likely to be renal insufficiency. A fluid challenge test to distinguish simple FVD from a deficit complicated by acute tubular necrosis (ATN) is described in Chapter 3. These two conditions must be differentiated because prompt treatment of prerenal azotemia can prevent ATN. Treatment of a patient with adequate renal function is simplified greatly. If sufficient water and electrolytes are provided, healthy kidneys can select needed substances and maintain normal fluid and electrolyte balances.

Although physicians are responsible for writing fluid orders, nurses share in the responsibility for safe fluid replacement therapy. A major nursing responsibility is the provision of precise I&O records and daily weight charts. The accuracy of this information is crucial to correct formulation of fluid replacement regimens. In addition, nurses must share the responsibility for detecting undesirable trends in these data.

Parameters to be considered in assessment include the following:

- Comparison of I&O measurements
- Daily or more frequent body weights
- Vital signs
- Skin turgor
- Hemodynamic measurements (such as central venous pressure [CVP], pulmonary arterial pressure [PAP], pulmonary capillary wedge pressure [PCWP], cardiac output [CO])
- Urinary specific gravity
- Laboratory values

The reader is referred to Chapter 2 for a review of these indices and to later Chapters 13 thru 25 dealing with specific clinical conditions. Chapters 3 through 9 also present specific information regarding assessment of patients receiving parenteral fluids.

To summarize, giving the right amount of fluid depends on calculating measurable fluid losses, estimating insensible and third-space losses, factoring in the functional ability of key homeostatic organs, and revising fluid prescriptions according to current indicators of the patient's fluid and electrolyte status. Thus, standing fluid orders are never acceptable. For typical patients, fluid orders are readjusted every 24 hr. However, this is not sufficient for many critically ill patients whose fluid status is subject to rapid change. For these patients, it may be necessary to readjust fluid directives every 8 hrs (or even more frequently).

WATER AND ELECTROLYTE SOLUTIONS

Table 10-1 lists some commercially available water and electrolyte solutions. Examples of these fluids are discussed.

DEXTROSE SOLUTIONS

Five percent dextrose in water (D_5W) is a roughly isotonic (278 mOsm/L) fluid given to provide free water. (Distilled water without additives cannot be infused intravenously [IV] because it would cause hemolysis of red blood cells as it entered the vein.) The dextrose in D_5W is metabolized to carbon dioxide and water, leaving a solution physiologically equivalent to distilled water but without the hemolysis. Water given IV as D_5W is distributed evenly into every body compartment. For each liter of free water given IV, no more than 100 mL remains in the intravascular space after 1 hr.[3] Thus, D_5W is used to replace deficits of total body water but is never used alone to expand the extracellular fluid (ECF) volume. Too much D_5W can seriously dilute serum sodium, especially in a patient who has excess antidiuretic hormone (ADH) activity.

Dextrose and water solutions are also available in 2.5%, 10%, 20%, and 50% concentrations. Theoretically, because each gram of carbohydrate supplies 4 calories, the 50 g in 1 L of D_5W should supply 200 calories. However, because dextrose in parenteral solution provides only 3.4 calories per gram, 1 L of D_5W provides 170 calories and 1 L of $D_{10}W$ provides 340 calories. Although 50 or 100 g of dextrose is a small portion of an adult's daily caloric requirements, either amount is often enough to stave off the ketosis of starvation, which is why dextrose is often added to electrolyte solutions until the patient can assume oral intake. (Electrolyte solutions without added nutrients have essentially no calories.) Examples of dextrose and electrolyte solutions are 5% dextrose in 0.9% NaCl, 5% dextrose in 0.45% NaCl, and 5% dextrose in lactated Ringer's solution (LR). As discussed in Chapter 11, a typical total parenteral nutrition (TPN) solution for central vein administration consists of 500 mL of 50% dextrose mixed with 500 mL of amino acid solution (for a net 25% dextrose solution). Because concentrated solutions of dextrose can cause hyperglycemia, they must be infused slowly.

SODIUM CHLORIDE SOLUTIONS

Isotonic Saline

Also called normal saline, 1 L of isotonic saline (0.9% NaCl) contains 154 mEq of sodium and 154 mEq of chloride. Total cations (Na^+) and anions (Cl^-) amount to 308 mEq/L, an isotonic concentration. Solutions are considered roughly isotonic if the total electrolyte content (i.e., anions plus cations) approximates 310 mEq/L; hypotonic if the total is less than 250 mEq/L; and hypertonic if electrolyte content exceeds 376 mEq/L. (These are arbitrary figures but are useful as a basis for comparing solutions.)

Although 0.9% sodium chloride is isotonic, it is not considered physiological. That is because ECF normally contains 140 mEq/L of sodium and 103 mEq/L of chloride, amounts that are smaller and in different proportions from those in isotonic saline. Although the excess chloride in isotonic saline could theoretically cause hyperchloremic acidosis, this does not seem to be a problem clinically because the excess chloride ions are excreted by the kidney.[4]

When infused IV, isotonic saline is distributed in the ECF compartment; none enters the intracellular fluid. One liter of isotonic saline adds 1 L to the ECF, theoretically expanding the plasma volume in the average adult by one fourth of a liter and the interstitial volume by three fourths of a liter 1 hr after administration.[5] In the critically ill or injured patient, only one-fifth or less of the volume may remain in the circulation 1 to 2 hrs after infusion.[6]

Isotonic saline is ideal for correcting ECF deficits, especially in patients who have hyponatremia, hypochloremia, and metabolic alkalosis (such as patients with excessive vomiting or gastric suction loss). Because of its high sodium content, however, the solution is used cautiously in patients

TABLE 10–1

Contents of Selected Water and Electrolyte Solutions with Comments About Their Use

SOLUTION	COMMENTS
5% dextrose in water (D_5W): No electrolytes 50 g of dextrose	Supplies approximately 170 cal/L and free water to aid in renal excretion of solutes Should not be used in excessive volumes in patients with increased ADH activity or to replace fluids in hypovolemic patients
0.9% NaCl (isotonic saline): Na^+ 154 mEq/L Cl^- 154 mEq/L	Isotonic fluid commonly used to expand the extracellular fluid in presence of hypovolemia Because of relatively high chloride content, it can be used to treat mild metabolic alkalosis
0.45% NaCl (½-strength saline): Na^+ 77 mEq/L Cl^- 77 mEq/L	A hypotonic solution that provides Na^+, Cl^-, and free water (Na^+ and Cl^- provided in fluid allow kidneys to select and retain needed amounts) Free water desirable as aid to kidneys in elimination of solutes
0.33% NaCl (1/3-strength saline): Na^+ 56 mEq/L Cl^- 56 mEq/L	A hypotonic solution that provides Na^+, Cl^-, and free water Often used to treat hypernatremia (because this solution contains a small amount of Na^+, it dilutes the plasma sodium while not allowing it to drop too rapidly.)
3% NaCl: Na^+ 513 mEq/L Cl^- 513 mEq/L	Grossly hypertonic solutions used only to treat severe hyponatremia See Clinical Tip (p 75) for summary of important nursing considerations in administration
5% NaCl: Na^+ 855 mEq/L Cl^- 855 mEq/L	Dangerous solutions
Lactated Ringer's solution: Na^+ 130 mEq/L K^+ 4 mEq/L Ca^{2+} 3 mEq/L Cl^- 109 mEq/L Lactate (metabolized to bicarbonate) 28 mEq/L	A roughly isotonic solution that contains multiple electrolytes in approximately the same concentrations as found in plasma (Note that this solution is lacking in Mg and PO_4.) Used in the treatment of hypovolemia, burns, and fluid lost as bile or diarrhea Useful in treating mild metabolic acidosis
Sodium lactate solution, 1/6 M: Na^+ 167 mEq/L Cl^- 167 mEq/L	A roughly isotonic solution used to correct severe metabolic acidosis (Lactate is metabolized to bicarbonate in 1–2 hr by the liver.) Not used in patients with liver disease (lactate cannot be converted to bicarbonate in such individuals), also not used in patients with oxygen lack (unable to adequately convert lactate to bicarbonate)
Sodium bicarbonate, 5% Na^+ 595 mEq/L Cl^- 595 mEq/L	A very hypertonic solution used to correct severe metabolic acidosis Should be cautiously administered at a slow rate, under careful volume control Should be administered only with extreme caution to salt-retaining patients (e.g., those with cardiac, renal, or liver damage)
Ammonium chloride, 2.14%	Acidifying solution used to correct severe metabolic alkalosis Due to high ammonium content, must be administered cautiously to patients with compromised hepatic function
Potassium chloride, 0.15% K^+ 20 mEq/L Cl^- 20 mEq/L	Premixed potassium chloride solution
Potassium chloride, 0.30% K^+ 40 mEq/L Cl^- 40 mEq/L	Premixed potassium chloride solution

whose renal or other regulatory mechanisms are compromised.

Half-Strength Saline (0.45% NaCl)

As its name implies, 1 L of half-strength saline provides half the electrolytes found in 1 L of isotonic saline, therefore, 77 mEq each of sodium and chloride. If this hypotonic solution is understood as a mixture of 500 mL of isotonic saline and 500 mL of free water, it is obvious why it is a good choice to provide some sodium to adjust serum levels plus free water to replace insensible losses. As pointed out earlier in the chapter, it is frequently used as a basic fluid for maintenance needs. It is also used to treat hypovolemic patients who have hypernatremia; that is, those who have a greater water deficit than solute deficit.

Other even more hypotonic sodium chloride solutions are available commercially. Examples of these are 0.11% NaCl (furnishing about 19 mEq/L each of sodium and chloride), 0.2% (34 mEq/L of each), 0.225% (39 mEq/L of each), and 0.33% (56 mEq/L of each). Excessive use of these hypotonic solutions can cause dilutional hyponatremia, especially in people who tend to retain water.

Hypertonic Saline

On relatively rare occasions, 3% or 5% sodium chloride (hypertonic saline solutions) is used to treat severe symptomatic hyponatremia. Small volumes are infused slowly and with great caution to avoid inducing a severe volume overload, along with pulmonary edema. Patients with cardiovascular compromise or severe volume overload may need a diuretic to help remove hypotonic fluid as soon as the concentrated saline solution is infused. Hypertonic saline should be used only in settings where the patient can be closely monitored because it requires frequent assessment for pulmonary edema, worsening neurological signs, and serum sodium levels. The 3% solution provides 513 mEq/L each of sodium and chloride and the 5% solution provides 855 mEq/L of each. The reader is referred to Clinical Tip in Chapter 4 (p 75) for a summary of important nursing considerations in the administration of hypertonic saline solutions to treat hyponatremia.

There are indications that a 7.5% sodium chloride solution is useful in the resuscitation of hemorrhagic shock and burns. This hypertonic fluid provides resuscitation with less volume than do isotonic crystalloids (such as isotonic saline or lactated Ringer's solution). After infusion, hypertonic saline pulls fluid away from the intracellular into the extracellular space. Apparently this action provides about 7 mL of free water for every 1 mL of hypertonic saline administered.[7] Thus, resuscitation with 200 mL of hypertonic saline (7.5% NaCl) expands the extracellular space by 1600 mL (the 200 mL infused plus 1400 mL pulled from the cellular space).[8] To keep the fluid within the intravascular space, the hypertonic saline has usually been added to a hyperoncotic agent (such as 6% dextran) in clinical trials. There are indications that hypertonic saline is more useful than isotonic fluids (0.9% NaCl or lactated Ringer's solution) in the volume resuscitation of head-injured patients because it improves systemic cerebral blood flow without a concomitant increase in the intracranial pressure.[9] Use of 7.5% sodium chloride and 6% dextran 70 for resuscitation is still pending approval by the U.S. Food and Drug Administration.[10] Possible side effects include hypernatremia, hyperchloremia, and hypokalemia.

BALANCED ELECTROLYTE SOLUTIONS

One of the most frequently prescribed balanced solutions, lactated Ringer's, carries the same name regardless of the commercial supplier. One liter of this commonly used fluid provides 130 mEq of sodium, 4 mEq of potassium, 3 mEq of calcium, 28 mEq of lactate, and 109 mEq of chloride. Lactated Ringer's solution contains 137 mEq/L each of cations and anions, for a total concentration of 274 mEq/L. It behaves similarly to isotonic saline in terms of expanding the extracellular fluid volume.

Considered a near-physiological solution, the electrolyte content of lactated Ringer's solution is quite similar to that of plasma. It is often used to correct isotonic fluid volume deficits (as in hypovolemia due to third-space fluid shift after major trauma or surgery). Because each liter of lactated Ringer's solution contains 28 mEq of lactate that normally is quickly metabolized into bicarbonate, the solution can be used to treat many forms of metabolic acidosis. The bicarbonate source in lactated

Ringer's solution may be useful in patients with metabolic acidosis due to renal failure; however, it should probably be avoided when hyperkalemia is present as it contains 4 mEq of potassium per liter. Lactated Ringer's solution should generally not be given to a patient who has lactic acidosis because the ability to convert lactate into bicarbonate is impaired in this disorder. However, the lactate load in lactated Ringer's solution does not potentiate the lactic acidosis associated with shock; also, the use of lactated Ringer's solution does not affect the reliability of laboratory blood lactate measurements.[11] Although lactated Ringer's solution may seem more physiological than isotonic saline, there is no evidence that it offers any advantage when compared with isotonic saline.[12] For fluid resuscitation, isotonic (normal) saline and lactated Ringer's solutions can be used interchangeably.[13] Isotonic saline is preferred for the treatment of hypercalcemia and hyponatremia.

Numerous other balanced electrolyte solutions are available commercially in a wide array of electrolyte combinations. (See Table 10-2 for a description of some of these fluids.) Some solutions are designed for maintenance needs, whereas others are formulated to replace specific body fluids. Each manufacturer usually affixes its own trade name to these solutions, making it necessary to refer to the label to review the specific content. As noted earlier, one

TABLE 10–2

Commercially Available "Balanced" Electrolyte Solutions (approximate concentrations, mEq/L)

SOLUTION	Na^+	K^+	Ca^{++}	Mg^{++}	Cl^-	$HPO_4^=$	BICARBONATE OR PRECURSOR
Plasma-Lyte 148 (Baxter)	140	5		3	98		27 acetate 23 gluconate
Normosol R (Abbott)	140	5		3	98		23 gluconate 27 acetate
Plasma-Lyte R (Baxter)	140	10	5	3	103		47 acetate 8 lactate
Isolyte E (McGaw)	140	10	5	3	103		49 acetate 8 citrate
Isolyte S (McGaw)	140	5		3	98		27 acetate 23 gluconate
Ionosol B (Abbott)	57	25		5	49	7	25 lactate
Isolyte H (McGaw)	42	13		3	39		17 acetate
Isolyte R (McGaw)	41	16	5	3	40		24 acetate
Ionosol T (Abbott)	40	35			40	15	20 lactate
Electrolyte #75	40	35			48	15	20 lactate
Plasma-Lyte M (Baxter)	40	16	5	3	40		12 acetate 12 lactate
Plasma-Lyte 56 (Baxter)	40	13		3	40		16 acetate
Normosol M (Abbott)	40	13		3	40		16 acetate
Isolyte M (McGaw)	38	35			44	15	20 acetate
Ionosol MB (Abbott)	25	20		3	22	3	23 lactate
Isolyte P (McGaw)	25	20		3	23	3	23 acetate
Electrolyte #48	25	20		3	24	3	23 lactate

of the most frequently prescribed balanced solutions, lactated Ringer's, carries the same name regardless of the supplier.

POTASSIUM SOLUTIONS

Premixed potassium-replacement solutions are available in a variety of strengths furnishing from 10 to 40 mEq of potassium per liter. Concentrated potassium solutions are available in ampules for addition to parenteral fluids (such as D_5W, 0.9% NaCl, or 0.45% NaCl). Of course, concentrated solutions from ampules are *not* meant for direct IV injection because they would cause fatal cardiac arrhythmias. See Clinical Tip (pp 101–103) for a list of critical points in administering potassium intravenously.

MAGNESIUM ADMINISTRATION

Magnesium is not present in most routine IV solutions. However, it is found in some of the commercially available balanced electrolyte solutions (see Table 10-1). Magnesium is also available in concentrated form in ampules for addition to parenteral fluids when deemed necessary. The reader is referred to Clinical Tip (p 138) for a review of nursing considerations in administering IV magnesium solutions.

CALCIUM ADMINISTRATION

Calcium is not present in most routine IV solutions; however, it is found in some balanced electrolyte solutions (see Table 10-1). Calcium is also available in concentrated form in ampules for addition to parenteral fluids as deemed necessary. The reader is referred to Clinical Tips in Chapter 6 for a review of nursing considerations in administering IV calcium solutions.

SOLUTIONS TO CORRECT ACID–BASE DISORDERS

Alkalinizing Solutions

Alkalinizing solutions (such as sodium lactate or sodium bicarbonate) are available to correct severe metabolic acidosis. Sodium bicarbonate is available as a 5% solution, furnishing 595 mEq/L each of sodium and bicarbonate.[14] Some clinicians elect to mix their own solutions by adding a concentrated $NaHCO_3$ solution (44.6 mEq per 50-mL ampule) to existing parenteral fluids. Sodium bicarbonate should not be added to lactated Ringer's solution or any other calcium-containing fluid, because calcium and bicarbonate combine to form the insoluble salt, calcium chloride.[15] As described in Chapter 9, controversy exists about when bicarbonate replacement is indicated in the treatment of acidosis. However, because severe acidosis can cause myocardial depression, it is generally considered prudent to keep the blood pH above 7.1 to 7.2.[16] Bicarbonate therapy must be instituted cautiously because overalkalinization can induce tetany, seizures, and cardiac arrhythmias. To avoid problems, bicarbonate therapy should cease when the pH reaches 7.2.[17] The use of sodium bicarbonate during cardiorespiratory arrest is discussed in Chapter 16.

Acidifying Solutions

When metabolic alkalosis is due to chloride deficiency, the use of isotonic saline (0.9% NaCl) may suffice as treatment. If hypokalemia is a contributing factor, the administration of potassium chloride is indicated.

If sodium chloride and potassium chloride solutions are unable to correct the metabolic alkalosis, consideration is given to using ammonium chloride (NH_4Cl) as an acidifying salt. However, NH_4Cl should be avoided in patients with impaired hepatic function as it might cause hepatic coma.[18] A solution of 0.1 normal (N) hydrochloric acid (HCl) is said to be the ideal acidifying agent for treating metabolic alkalosis. However, because it is not available commercially, it must be specially prepared in the pharmacy. This fluid is very corrosive and must be administered through a central catheter (after the catheter's position has been radiographically confirmed).[19] The 0.1 N HCL solution is filtered and poured into a glass IV bottle for administration; because the solution reacts with the plastic administration tubing, the tubing should be changed every 12 hrs.[20] Frequent monitoring of blood gases, pH, and serum electrolytes is indicated for patients receiving treatment for severe alkalosis.

COLLOIDS

In addition to the water and electrolyte solutions described previously, occasionally patients with fluid and electrolyte disturbances may require treatment with colloids. Colloids are fluids containing proteins or starch molecules that remain uniformly distributed in fluid and do not form a true solution. Examples of colloids are albumin, plasma protein fraction, dextran, and hetastarch. By increasing the osmotic pressure within the bloodstream, colloids draw fluid in from other compartments to increase the vascular volume.

ALBUMIN

Albumin provides about 80% of the plasma colloid osmotic pressure (COP) in healthy adults. Albumin for therapeutic uses is prepared from donor plasma and treated for approximately 10 hrs at 60 °C. There is no risk for hepatitis with albumin or any known risk for AIDS.[21] Normal human serum albumin (NHSA) is available as either 5% or 25% solutions. Five percent albumin solution is osmotically and oncotically equivalent to plasma; 25% albumin solution is hyperoncotic. The sodium content of albumin preparations is 145 ± 15 mEq/L.[22]

Albumin's major clinical use is as a plasma volume expander in the treatment of shock owing to blood or plasma loss. For example, the intravascular volume can be expanded by 500 mL by administering 500 mL of 5% albumin with a suitable crystalloid fluid, or by administering 100 mL of 25% albumin (causing 350 mL of water to be pulled into the vascular space from the interstitial fluid). The use of the 25% albumin is particularly helpful in patients in whom there is clinical evidence of both edema and hypovolemia.

Albumin may be useful in treating burns and third-space fluid shifts due to acute peritonitis, intestinal obstruction, or postoperative radical surgical procedures. It is also prescribed for acute volume depletion associated with paracentesis, dialysis, or overaggressive diuresis in patients with chronic diseases such as cirrhosis and nephrotic syndrome.

Albumin will *not* correct chronic hypoalbuminemia due to malnutrition, cirrhosis, or nephrotic syndrome and should not be used for this purpose. In these situations, the decreased albumin level reflects basic underlying problems that need to be corrected. Using albumin as a source of nutritional protein is not only inefficient, it is expensive; nutritional repletion is best accomplished with parenteral fluids designed for this purpose (see Chapter 11). Also, the only use for albumin in wound healing may be to reduce peripheral edema in a hypoproteinemic patient.

Albumin costs about 30 times more than crystalloid solutions, therefore, unless specifically needed, albumin is less likely to be used. The ability of albumin to remain in the vascular space is also a consideration. For example, colloid use during capillary leak (as occurs in burns, intestinal obstruction, sepsis, or adult respiratory distress syndrome [ARDS]) should be minimized until the capillary leak has been resolved.[23] In patients with burns and intestinal obstruction, the capillary integrity is restored in approximately 24 hrs; however, in sepsis or ARDS, the "leak" may persist for longer periods.

Reported side effects of albumin include urticaria, flushing, chills, fever, and headache.[24] Albumin should be used with caution in patients likely to develop fluid overload.

DEXTRAN AND HETASTARCH

Other colloid substitutes used for volume expansion include dextran and hetastarch (hydroxyethyl starch). These substances are not derived from donor plasma and therefore, are relatively nontoxic and inexpensive. They also are free of the risk of transfusion-related diseases.[25]

Dextrans are polysaccharides that behave as colloids; they are available as low molecular weight dextran (dextran 40) and high molecular weight dextran (dextran 70). Dextran is used clinically as a plasma volume expander and has favorable hemodynamic effects in restoring intravascular volume in shock patients when compared with other plasma volume expanders. It also has some specific beneficial effects on blood flow through the microvasculature, which is beneficial in shock patients; by coating endothelial surfaces, dextran reduces the interaction with the cellular elements in blood.[26] Dextran 70 is available as a 6% solution of dextran in isotonic saline, D_5W, or 10% invert sugar; dextran 40 is available as a 10% dextran solution in either isotonic saline or D_5W.

Anaphylactoid reaction may be a complication of dextran administration; the incidence is estimated to be between 1%[27] and 5.3%.[28] This adverse reaction usually occurs within the first one-half hour of the infusion and is characterized by urticaria, rash, nausea, bronchospasm, and shock.[29]

Dextran can interfere with the cross-matching of blood. Thus, if it is necessary to draw blood for typing and cross-matching, it should be done before dextran is started. If this is not possible, the laboratory should be notified that dextran is in use.

Dextran may interfere with blood coagulation, thus increasing the risk for bleeding. To minimize this risk, the total administered dosage should remain less than 1.5 g/kg/day of dextran 40 and 2 g/kg/day of dextran 70.[30]

An osmotic diuresis occurs early during the infusion of any dextran preparation, but is greater with dextran 40 than with dextran 70. Because of this obligate osmotic diuresis, urinary volume should *not* be used as a gauge for the adequacy of intravascular volume replacement. Failure to note inadequate intravascular volume replacement may greatly increase the risk for renal failure associated with dextran administration. The mechanism for this complication is concentration and precipitation of dextran in the renal tubules.[31]

Hetastarch (hydroxyethyl starch) is a synthetic colloid made from starch. Properties of hetastarch make it useful as a plasma volume expander in the treatment of shock due to hemorrhage, trauma, sepsis, or burns.[32] Its ability to expand the plasma volume is similar to that of a 5% albumin solution; however, it costs about two-thirds as much as an equivalent volume of 5% albumin. Like albumin and dextran, hetastarch is not a substitute for blood in patients requiring the oxygen-carrying properties of red blood cells. Like dextran, an osmotic diuresis can occur and the urinary volume increase should not be interpreted as a sign of adequate peripheral perfusion.[33] Bleeding complications associated with hetastarch are avoided by administering doses <1500 mL/24 hrs. Because serum amylase levels will be approximately twice normal after hetastarch infusion and elevation may persist for 5 days postinfusion, blood for serum amylase testing should be drawn before initiation of the infusion. The elevated serum amylase does not indicate pancreatitis.

CRYSTALLOID VERSUS COLLOID RESUSCITATION

For a variety of conditions, both crystalloids and colloids are widely used in clinical practice. The debate regarding which is superior in a given situation is likely to continue, as there is clinical evidence supporting the use of both types of fluids. Proponents of crystalloids (primarily isotonic saline and lactated Ringer's solutions) point to their quick availability and low cost, and the fact that they are reaction-free. These investigators also point out that clinical trials have shown these fluids to be effective plasma volume expanders in a wide range of conditions. As noted above, only about one-fifth of each liter of isotonic saline (sometimes referred to as "normal" saline) or lactated Ringer's solution administered to a critically ill patient remains in the intravascular space after 1 hr; the rest shifts into the tissue (interstitial) space. Because of this, as much as 5 L of normal saline or lactated Ringer's solution may be needed to expand the blood volume by 1 L, resulting in the accumulation of significant tissue edema. Despite this, proponents of crystalloids argue that although some tissues may be prone to edema, in most cases the lung has sufficient safety factors to prevent pulmonary edema from developing.[34]

Much greater volumes of crystalloids (as compared to colloids) are required to achieve the same hemodynamic end points; in fact, it may be necessary to administer two to six times more volume when crystalloids are used.[35] Proponents of colloids thus argue that a good clinical response can be accomplished with less fluid volume and greater precision with colloids, resulting in less accumulation of edema fluid. A study reported by Hankeln et al.[36] confirmed that substantially more fluid was required when crystalloids (versus colloids) were used in a critically ill patient, but that there did not appear to be any measurable difference in the development of pulmonary edema or other complications between the two groups.

Because there are advantages associated with both types of resuscitation, the question becomes one of which type is best in a given situation. Generally, the choice of fluids should be guided by considering the urgency and pathophysiology of the condition requiring fluid resuscitation.[37] It is helpful to review some common clinical conditions to compare the efficacy of both crystalloids and colloids.

HEMORRHAGIC SHOCK

In this situation, resuscitation with crystalloids (isotonic saline and lactated Ringer's solution) is prudent and of proved efficacy.[38] There is *no* place for salt-free crystalloid solutions (plain dextrose in water) in resuscitation of acutely hypovolemic patients.[39] Lactated Ringer's solution and normal saline are readily available and are commonly administered while blood is being cross-matched. These solutions can limit the total amount of blood eventually needed for patients with major blood loss. As a rule, several liters are administered quickly while the patient's clinical status is further assessed. How much more is needed depends on the patient's response to the fluids as well as the hematocrit level. Large volumes of crystalloids may ultimately be required to maintain peripheral perfusion (as evidenced by a mean arterial pressure between 70 and 80 mmHg, a heart rate <100 beats/min, warm extremities with good capillary refill, adequate central nervous system function, a urine output between 0.5 and 1 mL/kg/hr, and the absence of increasing lactic acidosis).[40] The visible edema that will develop as a major portion of the infused fluid shifts into the interstitial space should *not* be used as an indicator of adequate intravascular volume expansion. The reader is referred to Chapter 15 for a more thorough discussion of fluid resuscitation in hemorrhagic shock.

ADULT RESPIRATORY DISTRESS SYNDROME

The ARDS refers to an acute lung injury that can be caused by a variety of insults. Significant risk factors are sepsis, aspiration of gastric contents, major trauma, and drug overdose.[41] Shock is associated with loss of capillary wall integrity, resulting in "capillary leak." This is especially problematic in the lung because of the subsequent development of ARDS. In ARDS, the increased vascular permeability to large molecular weight proteins results in pulmonary edema. Invasive monitoring with a pulmonary artery catheter is helpful in guiding the clinician in maintaining the lowest intravascular volume that is compatible with adequate tissue perfusion. In this way, the microvascular hydrostatic pressure in the lung can be kept as low as practical. An attempt is made to maintain the PCWP at the lowest value required to maintain adequate cardiac output (generally 10 to 12 cm of water).[42]

Considerably differing thoughts exist regarding which fluid is superior in resuscitating patients with ARDS. Those who favor crystalloids believe that the use of colloids is counterproductive because the colloids "leak" through the damaged pulmonary capillaries into the pulmonary interstitium. Those who favor colloids believe that the sometimes massive volumes of crystalloids needed to achieve adequate tissue perfusion add to the pulmonary edema. Although it is known that crystalloids dilute the plasma oncotic pressure, it is debatable whether this decreases lung function. It appears that neither crystalloids nor currently available colloids have any preferential effects to minimize edema in patients with ARDS.[43] It seems that the development of ARDS is more related to the presence of sepsis than to the type of fluid used in shock resuscitation.[44]

OTHER CONDITIONS

It appears that neither colloids nor crystalloids are superior in the treatment of sepsis, as the use of both can be supported in the literature.[45] Colloids may have a greater role than crystalloids in managing patients with burns, anaphylaxis, and venom injuries.[46] Patients with burns, peritonitis, and pancreatitis may need colloid replacement early.[47]

FLUID AND ELECTROLYTE DISTURBANCES ASSOCIATED WITH BLOOD TRANSFUSIONS

Principal indications for blood transfusion are to correct the diminished oxygen-carrying capacity of the blood, to replace hemostatic components, or to replenish or expand the circulating intravascular volume. Although blood transfusion can be life-saving when indicated, it should not be undertaken lightly because there are a number of inherent risks with the transfusion process. Among these are immune-mediated reactions to the transfused substances, infections (such as malaria, hepatitis, and acquired immunodeficiency syndrome), and fluid/electrolyte/acid–base disturbances. Only the electrolyte/acid–base disturbances are discussed in this chapter.

Chemical and physical changes in blood are brought about by preservatives and prolonged storage. These changes in stored blood can cause electrolyte problems and other related complications.

HYPERKALEMIA

Continual destruction of red blood cells occurs when blood is stored, perhaps reaching a concentration as great as 25 mEq/L after 21 days.[48] Potassium is released from the destroyed red blood cells and is also transferred from intact red blood cells into the surrounding plasma. This leakage of potassium is related to loss of cell membrane integrity resulting from hypoxia. When the stored blood is infused into the recipient, the blood cells are reoxygenated and take up the leaked potassium; however, before this occurs, there can be a transient hyperkalemia if blood administration is extremely rapid.

Although hyperkalemia associated with even rapid transfusion is rarely a problem, it has the potential to be very serious. Hyperkalemia is accentuated in patients with metabolic acidosis, renal dysfunction, or both. Hypocalcemia, if also present, decreases cardiac tolerance to the hyperkalemia and increases the risk for arrhythmias.[49] Fatal hyperkalemia has been reported with as little as 2 units of blood administered over a 1-hr period.[50] In situations where hyperkalemia may be of concern, fresher units of blood (<10 days old) or washed cells should be used.[51] Twenty-four hours after massive transfusion, *hypo*kalemia can occur as the red blood cells are reoxygenated and take up potassium from the plasma.[52]

HYPOCALCEMIA

Citrate-phosphate-dextrose (CPD)-preserved bank blood contains excessive amounts of citrate ions. In some situations, the excess citrate may combine with ionized calcium in the recipient's blood, producing a deficiency of ionized calcium. (Recall that it is ionized calcium that controls neuromuscular irritability.) However, the excess citrate usually causes no difficulty because the liver rapidly converts it to bicarbonate. Another safeguard to protect the body from hypocalcemia is the rapid mobilization of calcium from bone when needed.

Citrate-induced decreases in calcium ionization are usually transient and cause no hemodynamic effect in most patients receiving blood transfusions.[53] For example, in a study of 100 patients who received blood during a variety of surgical procedures, only 1 patient developed cardiovascular problems related to hypocalcemia, although 10% of the patients had ionized calcium levels below 2 mg/dL.[54]

Current recommendations are to administer calcium only to patients in whom symptomatic hypocalcemia develops.[55] Calcium chloride or calcium gluconate may be administered intravenously as needed. Because infusions of calcium can be associated with ventricular dysrhythmias, it should not be used indiscriminately.[56]

Although the overall incidence of transfusion-related hypocalcemia is thought to be quite small, certain patients are at increased risk. For example, most liver transplant patients are anhepatic for part of the surgical procedure and thus cannot metabolize the citrate they receive in blood transfusions during this time.[57] In such patients, calcium supplementation may be needed to prevent decreased ventricular function and hypotension.[58]

Hemodynamic parameters remain stable in most patients with transfusion-related hypocalcemia; however, in patients with underlying cardiac problems, there is increased risk for complications such as hypotension or heart failure. This group of patients may required calcium replacement therapy.[59]

ACID–BASE CHANGES

The pH of 2-week-old bank blood decreases to approximately 6.5 (due to leakage of lactate and pyruvate into the plasma as a result of red cell hypoxia during storage).[60] Because banked blood is acidic, a metabolic acidosis is expected to occur in the massively transfused recipient.[61] Historically, this led to the prophylactic administration of bicarbonate to patients who received massive blood transfusions. However, this practice was shown to be detrimental, often leading to a more severe metabolic alkalosis.[62] Now, it is considered prudent to monitor the arterial blood pH and correct metabolic defects as they are discovered. Because it is more likely that the acidosis seen in massively transfused patients is due to hypoxemia and poor tissue perfusion than it is to the blood itself, the key is to provide adequate volume restoration and perfusion (which will correct any transient acidosis).[63,64]

Although an initial metabolic acidosis may occur during rapid transfusion, metabolic alkalosis may eventually result due to metabolism of citrate to bicarbonate. This is because blood is stored in a solution containing citrate (which eventually is converted to bicarbonate by the liver). Although patients with normal renal function can readily excrete the excess bicarbonate load, those who require large volumes of blood usually also have decreased renal perfusion due to decreased intravascular volume. Thus, patients requiring massive transfusions may have impaired ability to excrete bicarbonate through the kidneys.[65] Also, the presence of renal failure reduces the patient's ability to excrete the excess alkali load. In addition to metabolic alkalosis, patients requiring massive transfusions may develop respiratory alkalosis. This is because of a combination of catecholamine release, hypoxemia, and noncardiogenic pulmonary edema.[66]

HYPERAMMONEMIA

Ammonia concentration in stored blood begins to rise after 5 days to a week and reaches high levels after 2 to 3 weeks of storage.[67] Healthy patients can tolerate the extra ammonia with no difficulty; however, the ammonia content in stored blood may be of concern in patients with liver failure who require large amounts of blood. Washed cells can be considered as an alternative to stored blood, although there is no documented advantage to giving washed cells.[68]

FLUID VOLUME OVERLOAD

Fluid volume overload and congestive heart failure are frequent complications of blood transfusions. The onset of circulatory overload is usually gradual, with symptoms becoming more severe as the transfusion continues. Symptoms include cough, shortness of breath, neck vein distention, and pulmonary congestion. Many physicians request hemodynamic monitoring during rapid blood administration. (See procedures for hemodynamic monitoring in Chapter 2.)

Individuals with compromised cardiovascular status should be monitored especially closely for fluid volume overload. Packed red blood cells (PRBC) are frequently used for such patients to reduce the volume of the infusion (recall that packed cells are obtained by centrifuging whole blood and drawing off approximately 200–225 mL of plasma). Although PRBC have a reduced plasma volume, it is necessary to use a slow infusion rate for high-risk patients. At times it may be necessary to ask the blood bank to split a unit of PRBC into two containers and administer each half unit over 4 hrs. Prophylactic diuretic therapy (such as 10–20 mg IV furosemide) may also be helpful in the management of these patients.

REFERENCES

1. Woodley M, Whelan A: Manual of Medical Therapeutics, 27th ed, p 43. Boston, Little, Brown, 1992
2. Ibid
3. Narins R (ed): Clinical Disorders of Fluid and Electrolyte Metabolism, 5th ed, p 1466. New York, McGraw-Hill, 1994
4. Chernow B (ed): The Pharmacologic Approach to the Critically Ill Patient, 3rd ed, p 274. Baltimore, Williams & Wilkins, 1994
5. Smith E K: Fluids and Electrolytes: A Conceptual Approach, 2nd ed, p 151. New York, Churchill Livingstone, 1991
6. Chernow, p 274
7. Ibid, p 276
8. Ibid, p 277
9. Walsh J, et al: A comparison of hypertonic to isotonic fluid in the resuscitation of brain injury and hemorrhagic shock. J Surg Res 50(3):284–292,1991
10. Chernow, p 277
11. Ibid, p 274
12. Rose B: Clinical Physiology of Acid-Base and Electrolyte Disorders, 4th ed, p 406. New York, McGraw-Hill, 1994
13. Chernow, p 274
14. Rose, p 405
15. Ibid, p 406
16. Chernow, p 965
17. Woodley, Whelan, p 56
18. Condon R, Nyhus L: Manual of Surgical Therapeutics, 8th ed, p 174. Boston, Little, Brown, 1993
19. Woodley, Whelan, p 56
20. Pemberton L, Pemberton D: Treatment of Water, Electrolyte, and Acid-Base Disorders in the Surgical Patient. p 154. New York, McGraw-Hill, 1994
21. Chernow, p 280
22. Ibid
23. Ibid, p 281
24. Wilson B et al: Nurses Drug Guide. p 995. Stamford, CT, Appleton & Lange, 1996
25. Deglin J, Vallerand A: Davis's Drug Guide for Nurses, 4th ed. p 549. Philadelphia, F.A. Davis, 1995
26. Chernow, p 285
27. Ring J, Messmer K: Incidence and severity of ana-

phylactoid reactions to colloid volume substitutes. Lancet 1:466–469,1977
28. Thompson W: Rational use of albumin and plasma substitutes. Johns Hopkins Med J 136:220–225,1975
29. Chernow, p 284
30. Ibid, p 285
31. Ibid, p 284
32. Ibid, p 286
33. Ibid, p 287
34. Ibid, p 281
35. Narins, p 1468
36. Hankeln K, et al: Comparison of hydroxethyl starch and lactated Ringer's solution on hemodynamics and oxygen transport of critically ill patients in prospective crossover studies. Crit Care Med 17:133,1989
37. Narins, p 1469
38. Ibid
39. Condon, Nyhus, p 6
40. Chernow, p 275
41. Chernow, p 281
42. Narins, p 1469
43. Ibid
44. Chernow, p 274
45. Narins, p 1469
46. Ibid, p 1470
47. Condon, Nyhus, p 6
48. Ibid, p 241
49. Narins, p 708
50. Ibid
51. Condon, Nyhus, p 241
52. Woodley, Whelan, p 355
53. Chernow, p 778
54. Howland W, et al: Factors influencing the ionization of calcium during major surgical procedures. Surg Gynecol Obstet 58:274,1976
55. Condon, Nyhus, p 240
56. Ibid
57. Chernow, p 335
58. Ibid
59. Narins, p 1484
60. Condon, Nyhus, p 241
61. Chernow, p 335
62. Condon, Nyhus, p 241
63. Chernow, p 335
64. Condon, Nyhus, p 241
65. Narins, p 999
66. Ibid
67. Condon, Nyhus, p 241
68. Ibid

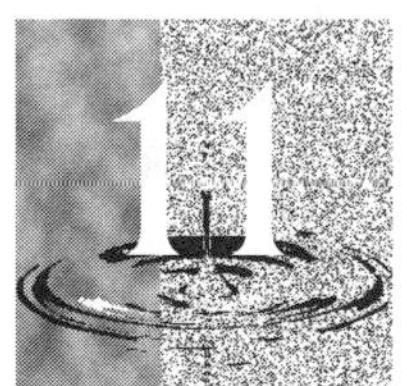

Parenteral Nutrition

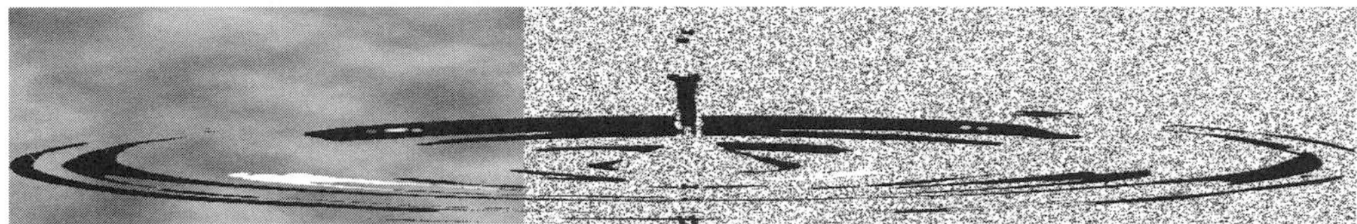

This chapter reviews the effects of parenteral nutrition on fluid and electrolyte balance and describes the nurse's role in caring for patients with imbalances and other metabolic abnormalities caused by this treatment.

INDICATIONS FOR PARENTERAL NUTRITION

Clinicians generally agree that "when the gut works, use it."[1] That is, if gastrointestinal function is present, enteral feedings should be favored over parenteral nutrition. Aside from being less expensive, benefits of enteral feedings compared with parenteral nutrition include better preservation of both immune function and intestinal function.[2] Despite the preference for enteral feedings, however, certain patients require parenteral nutrition because they are unable to meet their nutritional needs by the gastrointestinal tract. Candidates for parenteral nutrition include patients with inadequate small bowel surface area to absorb nutrients (as in massive small bowel resection or severe radiation enteritis), and those in need of temporary "bowel rest" during recovery from a primary gastrointestinal disease condition. Others who may benefit from parenteral nutrition includes those who are unable to consume (or use) sufficient enteral calories to meet their total nutritional needs.

PERIPHERAL PARENTERAL NUTRITION

Occasionally patients need parenteral nutrition support for only a relatively short period of time, making it impractical to access a central vein. Some clinicians have reported success in providing nutrients through peripheral parenteral nutrition (PPN) to a number of patients[3]; other researchers have found that relatively few patients benefit substantially from this form of support.[4]

The typical PPN solution consists of 5% to 10% glucose, 2% to 5% amino acids, and variables quantities of electrolytes (according to individual need). This glucose–amino acid solution is mixed with a 10% or 20% fat emulsion as a "three-in-one" mixture, or the fat emulsion is piggybacked simultaneously. The final osmolality of such a solution is usually 600 to 900 mOsm/kg and it is administered at a rate of 2 to 3 L/day.[5]

Candidates for PPN should have good peripheral veins. Even then, because of the high osmolality of the PPN solution, phlebitis at the infusion site will eventually occur. The onset of this complication may be slowed by decreasing the nutrient density of the formula or by decreasing its flow rate. Unfortunately, these maneuvers also serve to decrease the caloric intake. Peripheral parenteral nutrition usually involves daily re-siting of the cannula as a prophylactic measure to avoid phlebitis.[6] A study of the incidence and severity of infusion phlebitis with PPN in 142 surgical patients found that the administration of an "all-in-one"" solution (dextrose, amino acids, and fat emulsions) resulted in significantly less phlebitis than when the PPN was administered in separate containers (with the fat emulsion piggybacked into the infusion site of the glucose and amino acid solution).[7]

The large fluid volume needed for PPN as the sole source of calories limits its use to patients requiring only short-term support (such as 5 to 7 days). Usually, PPN is used to supplement the nutrient intake of patients who are consuming inadequate nutrients orally or by tube feeding.[8]

TOTAL PARENTERAL NUTRITION FOR CENTRAL ADMINISTRATION

When prolonged parenteral nutritional support is needed, a central vein is the necessary delivery site. Phlebitis is not a problem because central veins have high volume flow and can rapidly dilute very hypertonic solutions. Patients may receive total parenteral nutrition (TPN) as a continuous infusion or by cycling the solution on for 10 to 12 hrs and then off for the remainder of the 24-hr period. The cyclic method frees the patient from the infusion for a major part of the day and allows for normal activities. In a report of 36 patients receiving home cyclic TPN through Broviac or Hickman catheters, it was noted that 80% were able to return to work, school, or housekeeping activities, or at least to care for themselves unaided.[9] The cyclic method of infusion is generally limited to patients who are metabolically stable, such as those in home or outpatient settings.

In acute care facilities, a central venous catheter is usually inserted via the right subclavian vein into the superior vena cava. For patients receiving TPN at home, a Silastic central venous catheter threaded through a subcutaneous tunnel is preferred; examples of such catheters are Broviac and Hickman catheters (see Figure 11-1).

In today's cost-conscious environment, many TPN patients are cared for outside of acute care facilities. Patients receiving TPN at home tend to adjust fairly well, provided there is adequate social and technical support available.[10] To assist patients in home settings, a number of home nutrition support educational materials are available.[11]

An example of a typical TPN solution is presented in Table 11-1 (usually 2 or 3 L are infused daily in adults). Typically, 500 mL of a 50% dextrose solution is added to 500 mL of a 8.5% amino acid solution for a final concentration of 25% dextrose and 4.25% amino acids. However, individual needs may necessitate varying these concentrations. The most concentrated intravenous nutrients available commercially are 70% dextrose in water, 20% fat emulsion, and 15% amino acid solution.[13] The desired proportions of these nutrients are prepared by a pharmacist under a laminar-flow hood to maintain strict sterility. Obviously, patients requiring fluid restriction receive more concentrated formulas than contained in a typical TPN formula. Electrolytes, trace elements, vitamins, and other substances are added according to need.

TABLE 11–1

Example of a Typical 1-L Total Parenteral Nutrition Solution for Adults

Dextrose, 25%	(500 mL of 50% dextrose solution)
Amino acids, 4.25%	(500 mL of 8.5% amino acid solution)
Electrolytes (includes electrolyte content of amino acid solution)[12]	
Sodium	35 mEq
Potassium	30 mEq
Chloride	35 mEq
Magnesium	5 mEq
Calcium	5 mEq
Phosphate	15 mmol
Acetate	70 mEq
Vitamins	
MVI-12 (10 mL/day)	
Trace element solution	
1–5 mL/day	
Other additives as indicated	

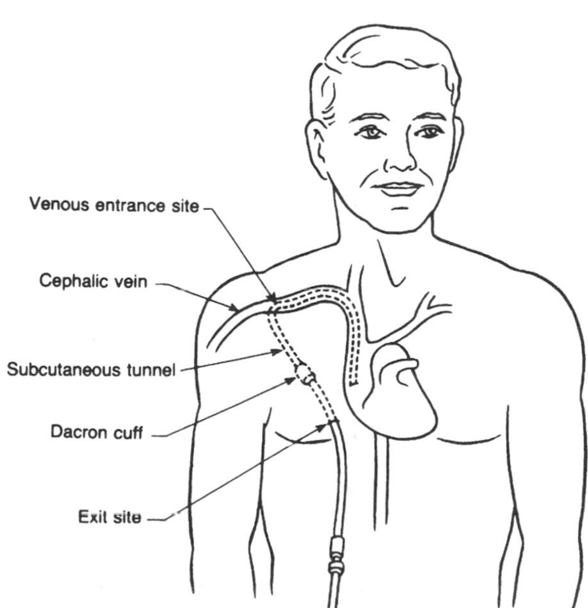

Figure 11–1. Indwelling central venous catheter for prolonged total parental nutrition or chemotherapy.

Glucose (dextrose) is the primary carbohydrate used in parenteral nutrition solutions. The dextrose used in parenteral nutrition solutions is hydrated with a caloric yield of 3.4 kcal/g (see Table 11-2). Glucose is the carbohydrate of choice for TPN because it is readily metabolized by all tissues, stimulates secretion of the anabolic hormone insulin, and usually, it is well-tolerated in large quantities.[14]

Crystalline amino acids are the usual source of proteins for intravenous administration. In addition to standard amino acid solutions, there are special amino acid formulations containing higher essential amino acids (for patients with renal failure), and more branched-chain amino acids (for patients with liver failure). However, the diagnosis of a specific disease does not necessitate the use of a specialty product in all instances.[15] For example, patients with

TABLE 11–2

Caloric Content and Osmolality of Selected Dextrose Solutions*

	DEXTROSE		
DEXTROSE CONCENTRATION	**g/L**	**Kcal/L**	**OSMOLALITY/L**
5%	50	170	252
10%	100	340	505
15%	150	510	758
20%	200	680	1010
25%	250	850	1263
30%	300	1020	1515

*Each gram of dextrose provides 3.4 kcal.

chronic stable renal failure without dialysis may benefit from a solution with a higher proportion of essential amino acids to prevent worsening of uremia while promoting positive nitrogen balance. However, when dialysis is initiated, standard amino acid solutions should be used.[16]

Fat emulsions made from soybean or a combination of soybean and safflower oil are available as 10% and 20% emulsions providing 1.1 and 2.0 kcal/mL, respectively. The only advantage of a 20% emulsion is its lower fluid volume for a given caloric yield. Fat emulsions can be delivered via piggyback or as part of a "three-in-one" mixture (depending on the TPN formulation). TPN formulas with 20% to 30% of the nonprotein calories as fat are associated with fewer complications than when formulas contain more glucose.[17] Patients with diabetes may require a higher percentage of fat calories to prevent hyperglycemia and patients with respiratory failure may require more fat (and less glucose) calories to minimize carbon dioxide (CO_2) production. The latter is particularly important when attempting to wean patients off ventilators. Both 10% and 20% fat emulsion contain between 4.3 and 8.0 mM bound phosphate per 500-ml bottle.[18]

Standard electrolyte formulations for TPN exist and are suitable for 50% to 80% of patients receiving TPN.[19] These standard solutions are not suitable for patients with preexisting conditions such as renal failure or congestive heart failure or those with specific electrolyte deficits associated with other clinical problems. Mineral allowances may need to be adjusted during parenteral nutrition as the patient's clinical status fluctuates. Specific electrolyte requirements are discussed in the next section.

Before TPN is initiated, the patient's caloric need is calculated and the appropriate percentage of macronutrients (dextrose, protein, and fat) as well as electrolytes and vitamin needs are determined. Caloric intake is based on actual weight unless the patient is more than 120% of ideal body weight; beyond 40 kcal/kg/day, the excess calories may be a stress to the patient and lead to CO_2 retention and fatty infiltration of the liver.[20] Daily weights are measured; weight gain as lean body mass occurs at a maximum rate of ¼ to ½ lb/day; any increase beyond this value is either as fat or water.[21]

METABOLIC DERANGEMENTS ASSOCIATED WITH TPN

Virtually any fluid and electrolyte or metabolic disturbance may occur during parenteral nutrition. Specific imbalances are largely reflective of the patient's underlying disease state that can interfere with the ability to metabolize or excrete the infused nutrients (see Table 11-3). Essentially, expected abnormalities fall into two categories. First, the electrolytes or nutrients in the parenteral solution may lead to toxicity when they exceed the body's normal metabolic and excretory capacity. Second, the addition of too little of an essential element or nutrient can result in a deficiency state.

Electrolyte abnormalities in TPN patients are primarily detected by evaluating daily laboratory

(text continues on page 200)

TABLE 11–3

Summary of Selected Metabolic Disturbances Associated With Total Parenteral Nutrition

PROBLEM	CAUSES	SIGNS/SYMPTOMS	MANAGEMENT
Hyperglycemia	Too rapid flow rate Increased production of stress hormones, as in sepsis or surgical trauma Patients with diabetes mellitus at high risk	Elevated blood sugar Glucosuria Polyuria: Acute weight loss and other signs of fluid volume deficit are associated with severe polyuria	Attempt made to maintain serum glucose < 200 mg/dL (preferably <140 mg/dL) unless blood sugar is so labile that careful control carries high risk for hypoglycemia If insulin is needed, it is usually added directly to the TPN solution. Less often, it is given SQ according to a sliding scale; if the patient is markedly fluid volume depleted, insulin should not be given SQ because of erratic absorption. Stable patients who suddenly develop a blood sugar >200 mg/dL, or who require increasing amounts of insulin, should be evaluated for sepsis or other stressors. Administration rate of TPN solution should be temporarily reduced if serum glucose is markedly elevated (such as >350 mg/dL) and not advanced until <200 mg/dL. If hyperglycemia has caused significant osmotic diuresis, fluid volume deficit must be corrected with appropriate electrolyte solutions. Management of nonketotic hyperglycemic hyperosmolar syndrome is described in Chapter 18. TPN flow rate is generally slowed or TPN solution is temporarily replaced with a 10% dextrose solution when patient is scheduled for surgery (see text).

(continued)

TABLE 11–3 (cont.)

PROBLEM	CAUSES	SIGNS/SYMPTOMS	MANAGEMENT
Hyperglycemia (cont.)			Prevention: • Initiate infusion slowly and increase gradually (Example: rate of a 35% dextrose solution might be initiated at 30 mL/hr/day and increased by the rate of 20 mL/hr/day until the desired flow rate is achieved. • Infuse via a volumetric infusion pump. • Monitor flow rate at least hourly. • If infusion rate falls behind, do not attempt to "catch up" by increasing the flow rate.
Hypoglycemia	Sudden discontinuance of TPN solution	Diaphoresis Confusion Agitation	Bolus injection of 50% dextrose; further management determined by serum glucose and clinical response. Prevention: • Discontinue TPN gradually (over hours) when possible. If not possible, infuse a 5% or 10% dextrose solution at same rate as TPN for several hours. • Ensure adequate caloric intake by GI route before stopping TPN, if feasible.
Hypophosphatemia	Anabolism increases demand for intracellular phosphorus (if inadequate amount is provided in TPN solution, phosphorus is pulled from the extracellular fluid) Factors increasing risk are severe malnourishment and alcoholism	Paresthesias Muscle weakness Muscle pain and tenderness Mental changes	Provide adequate phosphorus in TPN solution; required amount is determined by serum phosphorus levels and clinical indicators. (See text for usual requirements.) Significant hypophosphatemia (<1 mg/dL) requires supplemental phosphorus in a separate IV line. For emergency treatment of hypophosphatemia, 0.16 mmol/kg body weight may be given IV over 6 hr (followed by re-evaluation of serum phosphorus level).[57] Phosphate is supplied as either a sodium or a potassium salt; the most appropriate form is selected based on the patient's serum potassium concentration and state of renal function.

TABLE 11–3 (cont.)

PROBLEM	CAUSES	SIGNS/SYMPTOMS	MANAGEMENT
Hypokalemia	Anabolism increases demand for intracellular potassium	Fatigue Muscular weakness Decreased bowel motility	Provide adequate potassium in TPN solution; required amount is determined by serum potassium levels and clinical indicators. (See text for usual requirements.)
	Factors increasing risk are severe malnutrition, drugs such as amphotericin and furosemide, as well as loss of GI fluids	Cardiac arrhythmias ECG changes	When hypokalemia is present, consider peripheral IV or oral route for immediate potassium replacement and then adjust potassium in TPN solution.[58] Potassium replacement is described in Chapter 5.
Hypomagnesemia	Anabolism increases demand for intracellular magnesium	Increased reflexes Disorientation Cardiac arrhythmias	Provide adequate magnesium in TPN solution; required amount is determined by serum magnesium levels and clinical indicators. (See text for usual requirements.)
	Factors increasing risk: alcoholism, drugs such as aminoglycosides and cisplatin, and loss of GI fluids		Severe hypomagnesemia requires magnesium replacement via a separate IV line. Magnesium replacement is described in Chapter 7.
Hypercapnia (excessive $PaCO_2$)	Infusion of calories in excess of patient's need Infusion of TPN solution with a high dextrose concentration (end-product of CHO metabolism is CO_2 and water). Patients at increased risk are those with compromised respiratory function.	Respiratory decompensation (increasing $PaCO_2$) Difficulty weaning from ventilator	If patient is being overfed, reduce caloric intake to tolerable level. Provide more calories as fat and reduce glucose concentration in TPN formula (up to 60% of calories may need to be provided as fat).[59]

Abbreviations: TPN, total parenteral nutrition; SQ, subcutaneous; GI, gastrointestinal; ECG, electrocardiogram.

results. When caught early, the imbalance(s) can usually be rectified by altering the electrolyte composition of the formula. For this reason, it is customary to monitor serum electrolytes at least daily during early TPN and at less frequent, but regular, intervals thereafter. Of course, baseline electrolyte values should be obtained before the initiation of central TPN and serious abnormalities corrected before TPN is initiated.

Of great importance during parenteral nutrition therapy are the major intracellular ions (potassium, phosphate, and magnesium). During nutritional repletion, these ions, derived from the serum, are incorporated in newly synthesized cells. Failure to supplement these ions adequately can lead to hypophosphatemia, hypokalemia, and hypomagnesemia.

PHOSPHATE IMBALANCES

Hypophosphatemia is probably the most common imbalance in patients receiving parenteral nutrition. In one study, 30 of 100 patients receiving TPN had serum phosphorus concentrations less than 2 mg/dL; in six of these patients, the phosphorus concentration was less than 1 mg/dL.[22] Hypophosphatemia occurs as a result of new tissue synthesis and a shift from the extracellular to the intracellular compartment caused by glucose. It is most likely to develop when large volumes of hypertonic dextrose are administered, particularly with insulin, in severely malnourished patients or those with intestinal malabsorption, alcoholism, or thermal burns. The intracellular consumption of phosphate during protein synthesis may produce a striking deficit in the serum phosphate level if adequate phosphate supplements are not given. Although phosphorus requirements vary, the TPN solution usually provides 15 to 45 mmol of phosphorus per day.[23] Larger amounts are needed for high-risk patients (such as those who are severely malnourished or chronic alcoholics). To avoid precipitation of calcium phosphate, the amount of calcium and phosphorus that can be added to a TPN mixture must be controlled. Significant hypophosphatemia (<1 mg/dL) should be corrected with supplemental phosphorus in a separate intravenous line. Intravenous preparations containing either sodium phosphate or potassium phosphate are available and selection of the most appropriate salt is based on the patient's serum potassium concentration and the state of renal function.[24] The reader is referred to Chapter 8 for a review of the severe metabolic abnormalities associated with hypophosphatemia.

Although rare, hyperphosphatemia is possible if excessive phosphate is added to the TPN solution (particularly in patients who have impaired renal ability to excrete phosphate).

POTASSIUM IMBALANCES

Potassium abnormalities are common in patients receiving parenteral nutrition. A study of 100 patients receiving TPN found that 18 of them had a serum K level of less than 3 mEq/L.[25] Hypokalemia in patients receiving parenteral nutrition is related to a shift of potassium from the extracellular to the intracellular compartment under the influence of glucose during tissue synthesis. If insufficient potassium is contained in the solution, a significant fall in the serum concentration may occur as early as 6 to 12 hrs after beginning TPN.[26] For this reason, serum potassium levels must be monitored closely during the initiation of TPN. Patients who receive insulin for hyperglycemia need to be monitored especially closely for hypokalemia because insulin facilitates transport of potassium into cells and further depresses the serum potassium concentration. (The reader is referred to Chapter 5 for a review of the clinical signs of hypokalemia as well as its treatment.)

It has been recommended that TPN patients whose serum potassium concentration and renal function are normal should receive 60 to 90 mEq of potassium per day[27]; occasionally up to 150 to 200 mEq is needed per day.[28] Even patients with advanced renal failure who receive TPN usually require potassium, although in a reduced amount.[29] The actual amount needed is determined by serial monitoring of serum potassium levels.

Of course, addition of too much potassium to the TPN solution, or large intake from other sources without cutting back the amount added to the solution can lead to hyperkalemia (particularly in patients with impaired renal ability to excrete potassium). Hyperkalemia is more likely in TPN patients who are not sufficiently anabolic to use the relatively high potassium load administered in the TPN solution. Tissue necrosis and systemic sepsis also predispose to hyperkalemia.

MAGNESIUM IMBALANCES

Hypomagnesemia is less common than hypophosphatemia or hypokalemia in patients receiving parenteral nutrition. When it occurs, it is usually in patients who are chronic alcoholics, severely malnourished, receiving drugs associated with renal magnesium wasting (such as diuretics, amphotericin, or cisplatin), or experiencing large losses of intestinal fluid. Other causes of hypomagnesemia as well as clinical signs are described in Chapter 7. Severe hypomagnesemia requires treatment with up to 100 mEq of magnesium sulfate administered over 24 hrs through a separate intravenous line.[30] *Hyper*magnesemia can occur if excessive magnesium is supplied in the parenteral formula of patients with renal failure.

The daily requirement for magnesium in TPN patients has not been established and recommendations vary from 4 to 42 mEq/day.[31] In the absence of renal insufficiency, patients on TPN seem to tolerate 16 to 30 mEq of magnesium per day.[32]

SODIUM IMBALANCES

Hyponatremia ($<$125 mEq/L) was reported in 6% of TPN patients in a study by Weinsier et al.[33]; this was compared with only a 1% incidence of hypernatremia ($>$160 mEq/L) in the same population. It is important to recognize all factors that predispose patients receiving TPN to hyponatremia and hypernatremia and to remember that although the focus is often on the sodium content of the TPN solution, sodium and fluid administered by other means, including medication admixtures and maintenance intravenous fluids, influence sodium balance.

The typical TPN solution contains 30–50 mEq of sodium per liter[34]; this amount may be decreased when fluid retention is a problem or increased when sodium is being lost in excessive amounts (as from diarrhea or fistula drainage). However, hyponatremia in TPN patients is most commonly associated with excessive antidiuretic hormone (ADH) levels and excessive free water intake.[35] A case was recently reported in which a young adult trauma patient receiving TPN became hyponatremic because of the daily administration of almost 3 L of D_5W in a peripheral vein as a diluent for antimicrobial agents administered for sepsis.[36] Dilutional hyponatremia is usually managed by decreasing the fluid intake.

Hypernatremia, as indicated above, is less common than hyponatremia in TPN patients. It will occur when excessive water loss is present; in this situation, the free water intake should be increased (either in the TPN solution or through another route).

CALCIUM IMBALANCES

Because most patients receiving parenteral nutrition are malnourished and thus have low serum albumin levels, it is likely that their total serum calcium levels will also be below normal. (There is approximately a 0.8 mg/dL decrease in calcium per 1 g/dL drop in serum albumin below normal.) However, because ionization of calcium usually remains normal in hypoalbuminemic patients, this "hypocalcemia" is not physiologically significant and will not result in paresthesias or other signs of tetany. Other causes of hypocalcemia, such as hypomagnesemia, are discussed in Chapter 6. The usual TPN solution contains 5 to 10 mEq/L of calcium. A daily calcium supplement in TPN is needed to prevent bone demineralization.

Hypercalcemia can occur in patients receiving parenteral nutrition for extended periods. Possible causes are metabolic bone disease associated with long-term parenteral nutrition, or the excessive infusion of calcium or vitamin A and D supplements. When hypercalcemia occurs, it is necessary to consider other causes, such as neoplasms or primary or secondary hyperparathyroidism.

ACID–BASE IMBALANCES

Metabolic Disturbances

Either metabolic alkalosis or acidosis can occur in patients receiving TPN. These imbalances are largely a consequence of the basic underlying disease, although they may be influenced by the composition of the TPN solution. For example, metabolic alkalosis can result from excessive acetate in the

TPN solution (because acetate is converted to bicarbonate). Or, complete metabolism of the sulfur-containing acids (methionine, cysteine, and cystine) results in production of hydrogen ions (predisposing to metabolic acidosis).[37]

Respiratory Acidosis

Respiratory acidosis can result from excessive carbohydrate infusion (causing increased CO_2 production as a result of excessive glucose metabolism). In this case, patients with respiratory dysfunction may have difficulty eliminating the high CO_2 load. Covelli et al.[38] observed a rise in $PaCO_2$ within 12 hrs after TPN was initiated in a patient maintained on a fixed mechanical ventilator setting; the $PaCO_2$ rose from 43 to 93 mmHg and the serum pH fell from 7.4 to 7.25 within 24 hrs after the carbohydrate intake was increased from 1500 to 2500 kcal/day. To minimize excessive CO_2 production, an effort is made to avoid administering excessive calories (particularly in the form of glucose) to patients at risk for hypercapnia (excessive $PaCO_2$).[39]

TRACE ELEMENT IMBALANCES

Trace elements have a major effect on body function; deficiencies are clearly reported more frequently than are toxicities.[40] To prevent trace element deficiencies, selected trace elements are routinely added to TPN solutions. Trace elements typically added to TPN include zinc, copper, manganese, and chromium; some hospitals also add selenium and perhaps molybdenum.[41]

There have been numerous reports of zinc deficiency in patients receiving parenteral nutrition without zinc supplementation. One reason is that massive losses of zinc can occur in the urine of patients with catabolic illnesses. Also, tissue demand for zinc during anabolism quickly depletes plasma stores. Thus, it is conceivable that patients with normal serum zinc levels can develop a deficiency during rapid accretion of tissue, even when supplements are given. Patients with diarrhea or other large fluid losses from the intestine may require significantly more zinc than typical patients. Clinically significant zinc deficiency may occur within the first few weeks of parenteral nutrition. Signs of hypozincemia may include diarrhea, delayed wound healing, alopecia, mental changes, abnormalities in taste and smell, and a characteristic dermatitis. As with other additives to parenteral nutrition solutions, it is possible to cause toxicity if too much zinc is added (particularly in patients with renal failure).

Copper deficiency states (such as hypochromic anemia and neutropenia) have been observed in patients receiving parenteral nutrition. Most often, deficiency states are not observed until many months of treatment have elapsed; however, subnormal serum copper values may occur within weeks in some patients if copper intake is inadequate. On the other hand, copper excess can result if too much copper is added to the parenteral solution.

Chromium deficiency can occur in patients receiving long-term parenteral nutrition and cause glucose intolerance (as chromium is necessary for proper use of glucose). This glucose intolerance is reversible with chromium replacement. Other signs of chromium deficiency include mental confusion and a peripheral sensory neuropathy.

Selenium deficiency can occur during long-term parenteral nutrition therapy with solutions lacking this element, but clinical manifestations (primarily cardiomyopathy) are uncommon.

Although rare, molybdenum deficiency states may also occur during long-term parenteral nutrition; one patient reportedly developed tachycardia, tachypnea, and several neurological abnormalities. Clinical signs associated with these deficits usually resolve with supplementation of the needed substances.

HYPERGLYCEMIA

Hyperglycemia is one of the most common metabolic derangements caused by TPN. For example, one prospective study of 100 patients receiving parenteral nutrition found that 47 patients had serum glucose concentrations greater than 300 mg/dL.[42] Hyperglycemia is more likely to occur in patients receiving more than the required number of calories. Of course, patients with diabetes mellitus are at higher risk. Common causes of hyperglycemia include too rapid or uneven administration of the high dextrose solution and increased levels of glucose-elevating stress hormones (associated with a number of illnesses and injury states). The development or worsening of a glucose intolerance may be a harbinger of sepsis or another complicating condition (such as myocardial infarction). Indeed, hyperglycemia may precede other signs of infection by 18 to 24 hrs.[43] When hyperglycemia occurs despite careful management, the cause should be investigated carefully.

Uncontrolled hyperglycemia can lead to hyperosmotic hyperglycemic nonketotic syndrome (HHNS). Fortunately, due to frequent monitoring for glucosuria and hyperglycemia, this complication is less frequent than in the past. In a study of 200 patients receiving TPN, 6 patients were found to have developed HHNS; all had familial histories of diabetes mellitus and had negative water balance with hyperglycemia for several days preceding the development of the syndrome.[44] See Chapter 18 for a detailed discussion of HHNS and its management.

Prevention

To prevent hyperglycemia, infusion of the TPN solution must begin slowly and gradually be increased as tolerated. For example, for a patient receiving a 25% dextrose solution, on day 1 the rate might be 40 mL/hr for a total of 960 mL (40 mL × 24 hrs). On day 2, the rate might be increased to 80 mL/hr (for a total of 1920 mL). On day 3 the rate might be increased to 120 mL/hr. An infusion pump should be used to ensure even flow of the solution at the correct rate. If the patient falls behind in TPN administration, the rate of infusion should *not* be abruptly increased to compensate for the deficiency. A common cause of transient hyperglycemia in TPN patients is inadvertent rapid administration of the TPN solution due to equipment malfunction or operator error.

For patients receiving cyclic TPN, it is customary to begin with a reduced flow rate for 2 hrs before initiating the full infusion rate and then to taper the rate of flow for 2 hrs before discontinuance. As described earlier, this method is usually reserved for patients who are metabolically stable.

When patients receiving TPN are scheduled to go to surgery for a major operation, orders should be clear about what to do with the infusion rate. The rate may be maintained as is or reduced by one-half, or the solution may be replaced with a 10% dextrose solution immediately before, during, and shortly after the surgery.[45] Although recommendations vary, the rate of glucose infusion is usually decreased because patients often become less glucose tolerant when subjected to the major stress of surgery. The preoperative infusion rate can usually be resumed within 48 hrs postoperatively.[46]

Detection

During TPN administration, the patient should be closely monitored for glucose intolerance, especially during the early days. In acute care settings, glucose tolerance is usually measured by checking capillary blood sugars every 6 to 8 hrs. An attempt is made to maintain blood glucose levels at less than 200 mg/dL (preferably <140 mg/dL) unless the blood sugar level is so labile that careful control carries a high risk for hypoglycemia.[47] If the patient's renal threshold is known, it may be possible to monitor for hyperglycemia by checking urinary glucose content every 6 hrs. Urinary glucose levels are not reliable for some patients. For example, patients with renal disease may have glucosuria despite normal blood glucose levels, or they may have high blood sugars and little or no glucosuria.[48]

Insulin Therapy

In the presence of hyperglycemia, it is usually necessary to administer insulin. Regimens vary somewhat but most centers favor adding regular insulin to the TPN solution to achieve more even blood sugar control. For example, mild or moderate hyperglycemia may be managed by adding 1 to 2.5 units of regular insulin per 25 g of glucose in the TPN solution; greater quantities may be needed for patients with more severe glucose intolerance.[49] Although variable levels of insulin adsorption to the parenteral fluid container and tubing have been demonstrated in laboratory settings, this does not appear to be a clinically significant problem. That is, clinical experience has indicated that blood glucose concentrations can be controlled effectively by adding insulin to the TPN solution.

The administration rate of the TPN solution should be temporarily reduced if the serum glucose concentration is more than 350 mg/dL; the TPN administration rate should not be increased until the serum glucose level is less than 200 mg/dL.[50] If hyperosmolar hyperglycemic nonketotic syndrome occurs, the TPN solution is stopped until the fluid volume deficit is corrected (usually with isotonic saline) and hyperglycemia is treated intravenously with low-dose insulin. The reader is referred to Chapter 18 for a discussion of the treatment of HHNS.

HYPOGLYCEMIA

Hypoglycemia is always a possibility when exogenous insulin is supplied directly in the TPN solution or subcutaneously by sliding scale. Also, hypoglycemia is a possible complication of abrupt discontinuance of TPN (especially after the infusion rate has recently been increased, resulting in increased endogenous insulin production). Presumably, the high glucose infusion stimulates hyperinsulinism; abrupt discontinuance of the high glucose fluid may temporarily allow the serum glucose level to fall precipitously.

One study indicated that when TPN was stopped abruptly, serum insulin and glucose concentrations returned quickly to normal levels and no reactive hypoglycemia was observed.[51] The researchers reported that hypoglycemia only occurred when the rate of the TPN solution was transiently increased and then was abruptly stopped. Several other small studies have suggested that TPN can be discontinued abruptly without the risk of hypoglycemia.[52,53] However, many authorities still believe that TPN solutions should be tapered in all patients who receive 200 to 300 g or more of intravenous glucose per day.[54] Clinically, there is rarely a reason to discontinue TPN abruptly. In most instances, an effort is made to ensure that adequate nutrients (i.e., 75% of maintenance calories) are consumed by the enteral route before TPN is stopped. Even when quick discontinuance is needed, there is usually time to taper the solution's flow rate over several hours. If this is not possible, there is no risk and little cost involved in providing coverage with a 5% or 10% dextrose solution in a peripheral vein. For example, 10% dextrose in water may be ordered for 4 hrs at the same rate the TPN solution was infusing when stopped.[55]

OTHER PROBLEMS

Fat intolerance is a problem in patients unable to clear intravenously administered fat emulsions. When giving fat emulsion in conjunction with TPN therapy, it is customary to obtain a baseline plasma triglyceride level and then to monitor the levels two or three times per week when TPN is initiated (and once or twice a week thereafter).[56] Other possible complications of TPN are fatty liver and cholecystitis. For this reason, liver function tests are performed on a regular basis.

REFERENCES

1. Kudsk K, Minard G: Enteral nutrition. In Zaloga G: Nutrition in Critical Care, p 331. St. Louis, Mosby, 1994
2. Heizer W, Holcombe B: Approach to the patient requiring nutritional supplementation. In Yamada T, et al (eds): Textbook of Gastroenterology, Volume One, p 975. Philadelphia, JB Lippincott, 1991
3. Payne-James J, Khawaji H: First choice for total parenteral nutrition: The peripheral route. J Parenter Enter Nutr 17:468–478,1993
4. Heizer, Holcomb, p 969
5. Ibid
6. Taylor M: Total parenteral nutrition. Part 1. Nursing Standard 8(23):25–28,1994
7. Nordenstrom J, et al: Peripheral parenteral nutrition: Effect of a standardized compounded mixture on infusion phlebitis. Br J Surg 78(11):1391–1394,1991
8. Nussbaum M, Fischer J: Parenteral Nutrition. In Zaloga G: Nutrition in Critical Care. St. Louis, CV Mosby, 1994
9. Freund H, et al: A decade of experience with home total parenteral nutrition. Harefuah 12(9):294–297, 1991
10. Freeman F: Home infusion for the 1990s: A patient's perspective. N Engl J Med 89(1):60–62,1992
11. Evans M, Czopek S: Home nutrition support materials. Nutrit Clin Pract 10(1):37–39,1995
12. Thomas Jefferson University Hospital: Formulary and Regulations Governing Drugs, 28th ed. Philadelphia, Thomas Jefferson University Hospital, 1987
13. Heizer, Holcombe, p 971
14. Inadomi D, Kopple J: Fluid and electrolyte disorders in total parenteral nutrition. In Narins R (ed): Clinical Disorders of Fluid and Electrolyte Metabolism, 5th ed, p 1438. New York, McGraw-Hill, 1994
15. Andris D, Krzywda E: Nutrition support in specific diseases: Back to basics. Nutrit Clin Pract 9(1):28–32, 1994
16. Clouse R: Parenteral nutrition. In Wyngaarden J,

Smith L, Bennett J (eds): Cecil Textbook of Medicine, 19th ed, p 1189–1193. Philadelphia, WB Saunders, 1992
17. Heizer, Holcombe, p 971
18. Kovacevich D, Braunschweig C, August D (eds): The University of Michigan Medical Center: Parenteral and Enteral Nutrition Manual, 7th ed, p 24. 1994. Prepared by the Parenteral and Enteral Nutrition Team at the University of Michigan Medical Center 94-3434-5-May, 1994
19. Heizer, Holcombe, p 971
20. Mirtallo J: TPN composition. Postgraduate Course I. Fundamentals I. Total Parenteral Nutrition, p 52. American Society for Parenteral and Enteral Nutrition. 19th Clinical Congress, 1995
21. Ibid
22. Weinsier R, Bacon J, Butterworth C: Central venous alimentation: a prospective study of the frequency of metabolic abnormalities among medical and surgical patients. J Parenter Enter Nutr 6:421,1982
23. Heizer, Holcombe, p 974
24. Sacks G, et al: Observation of hypophosphatemia and its management in nutrition support. Nutrit Clin Pract 9(3):105–108,1994
25. England B, Mitch W: Acid-base, fluid, and electrolyte aspects of parenteral nutrition. In Kokko J, Tannen R (eds): Fluids & Electrolytes, 2nd ed, p 1024. Philadelphia, WB Saunders, 1990
26. Heizer, Holcombe, p 971
27. Inadomi, Kopple, p 1449
28. Heizer, Holcombe, p 974
29. Inadomi, Kopple, p 1449
30. Heizer, Holcombe, p 974
31. Inadomi, Kopple, p 1475
32. Ibid
33. Weinsier et al, p 422
34. Seshardri V, Meyer-Tettambel O: Electrolyte and drug management in nutritional support. Crit Care Nurs Clin North Am 5(1):31–36,1993
35. Inadomi, Kopple, p 1448
36. Sunyecz L, Mirtallo J: Sodium imbalances in a patient receiving total parenteral nutrition. Clin Pharm 12(2):138–149,1993
37. England, Mitch, p 1029
38. Covelli H, et al: Respiratory failure precipitated by high carbohydrate loads. Ann Intern Med 95:579,1981
39. DeMeo M, et al: The hazards of hypercaloric nutritional support in respiratory disease. Nutrit Rev 49(4):112–115,1991
40. Baumgartner T: Trace elements in clinical nutrition. Nutrit Clin Pract 8(6):251–263,1993
41. Hak L: Nutrition/Fluid & Electrolytes. Fundamentals I. Total Parenteral Nutrition, p 41. American Society for Parenteral and Enteral Nutrition, 19th Clinical Congress. January 15–18,1995
42. Weinsier et al, p 425
43. Inadomi, Kopple, p 1440
44. Kaminski M: A review of hyperosmolar hyperglycemic nonketotic dehydration: Etiology, pathophysiology and prevention during intravenous hyperalimentation. J Parenter Enter Nutr 2:690,1978
45. Kovacevich et al, p 39
46. Ibid, p 43
47. Inadomi, Kopple, p 1440
48. Ibid
49. Ibid
50. Heizer, Holcombe, p 974
51. Sanderson I, Deitel M: Insulin response in patients receiving concentrated infusions of glucose and casein hydrolysates for complete parenteral nutrition. Ann Surg 179:387,1974
52. Krzywda E, et al: Glucose response to abrupt initiation and discontinuance of total parenteral nutrition. J Parenter Enter Nutr 17:64–67,1993
53. Wagman et al: The effect of acute discontinuation of TPN. Ann Surg 204:524,1986
54. Inadomi, Kopple, p 1438
55. Heizer, Holcombe, p 975
56. Ibid
57. Hak, p. 35
58. Ibid, p 34
59. Kovacevich et al, p 45

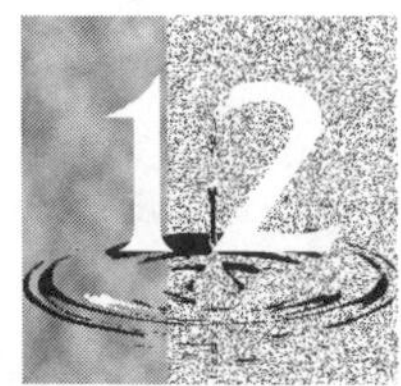

Tube Feedings

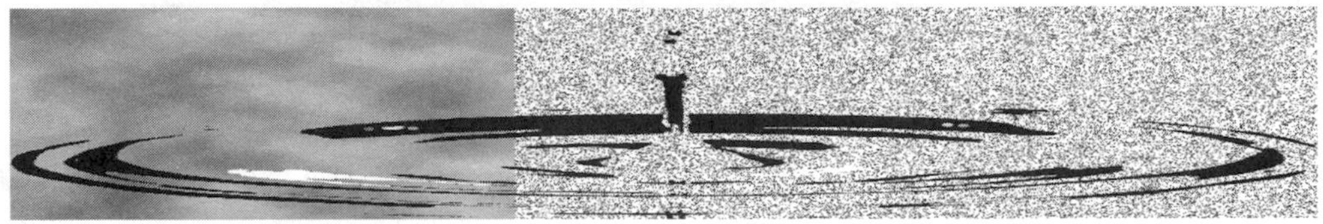

Enteral feedings are commonly used to provide nutritional support for patients who, for some reason, cannot consume adequate nutrients although they have functional gastrointestinal (GI) tracts. Indeed, enteral feedings are believed to be more beneficial physiologically and more cost-effective than total parenteral nutrition (TPN). More specifically, enteral nutrition is associated with improved gut and liver function, enhanced immune function, reduced infection rates, and better survival rates in critically ill patients.[1] However, there are problems associated with enteral feedings just as there are with most therapies. Those related to fluid and electrolyte balance are discussed in this chapter.

CHARACTERISTICS OF FORMULAS

Before discussing specific problems, it is helpful to review briefly some characteristics of tube feeding solutions. Formulas have evolved from the blenderized whole foods used several decades ago to a multitude of commercially available preparations that can provide total nutrient needs. Whereas commercially available standardized formulas have many advantages, they must be selected carefully to meet the patient's individual needs. Formulas differ in osmolality, protein and carbohydrate sources, fat content, caloric density, and electrolyte content.

OSMOLALITY

An important characteristic of a tube feeding formula is its osmolality (concentration). Osmolality is primarily a function of the number and size of molecular and ionic particles in a given volume. Most enteral products range in osmolality from 270 mOsm/kg to approximately 700 mOsm/kg.[2] Commercially prepared feedings usually have this value printed on the product label. If this information is not on the product label, as well as the information on the renal solute load, it is usually available in product brochures. Major determinants of a formula's osmolality include protein, carbohydrate, and electrolyte concentrations as well as the protein form (intact versus partially hydrolyzed). The more a formula is predigested, the higher is its osmolality.[3] Table 12-1 shows the wide variance in osmolalities of some commercially available tube feeding formulas. Whereas some formulas approximate the osmolality of plasma (and therefore are deemed isotonic), others have considerably higher osmolalities (hypertonic). (Recall that plasma osmolality is approximately 300 mOsm/kg.)

A formula's osmolality affects tolerance to the feeding in several ways. First, it often affects the renal solute load and water requirements. (The primary determinants of renal solute load are protein, sodium, potassium, and chloride.[4]) A high renal solute load (formed during nutrient use) requires a large water volume for excretion. Another way in which osmolality affects tolerance to feedings is in its effect on gastric function. If given too quickly, hypertonic solutions slow gastric emptying and can lead to gastric retention, nausea, and vomiting. This effect is believed to be regulated by osmoreceptors in the duodenum.[5] Hypertonic solutions may also cause diarrhea if given too rapidly, especially into the small intestine (due to large shifts of fluid into the small bowel to dilute the hypertonic bowel contents).

ELECTROLYTES

Standard enteral formulas have fixed electrolyte contents, based on usual requirements. This can be a source of fluid and electrolyte problems in tube-fed patients as some patients require additional electrolytes whereas other patients cannot tolerate the preestablished amounts.

As with TPN, either deficiencies or excesses of electrolytes can occur, varying with the patient's underlying disease condition, general clinical status, and the electrolyte content of the formula being used. For example, starving patients beginning vigorous refeeding may suffer extracellular deficits of potassium, phosphorus, and magnesium as these electrolytes are pulled into the cells during anabolism. Such patients need more of these electrolytes than those who are not undergoing this process. Conversely, patients with renal failure often need limitations on potassium, phosphorus, and magnesium intake. (The electrolyte content of selected enteral formulas is listed in Table 12-1.)

SPECIALIZED FORMULAS

Commercial sources supply specialized products targeted to patients with specific problems, such as renal, hepatic, and respiratory failure. Because numerous products are available, it is important to study the literature supplied by the manufacturer. In summary, to avoid complicating existing metabolic derangements, nutritional prescriptions must be tailored in the direction of restoring homeostasis.

Renal Failure

Patients with renal failure tend to be malnourished because of poor dietary intake, particularly when coupled with nutrient losses from dialysis treatments. Although GI problems (such as nausea, vomiting, diarrhea, and GI bleeding) may preclude enteral feedings in some patients, others may benefit from enteral nutrition. When enteral feedings are tolerated, the content of the formula is partly dependent on whether dialysis is used. For patients with acute renal failure, specialized enteral formulas containing only essential amino acids may be necessary; however, once dialysis is instituted, standard enteral formulas may be used to provide a full complement of amino acids.[6] Characteristically, renal enteral formulas have low to absent mineral content and are calorically dense. (An example of a renal formula is Travasorb Renal; see Table 12-1.)

Although patients with acute renal failure require less sodium than patients with normal renal function, they still require sodium replacement as a result of obligatory losses from the GI tract and skin. Sodium intake should be matched to output. Potassium, phosphorus, and magnesium are restricted in patients with acute renal failure as these minerals are normally excreted in the urine.[7] When patients are highly catabolic, intracellular electrolytes escape from the cells and cause significant elevations in serum levels. However, when these individuals become anabolic, the opposite occurs (perhaps rendering the patient

TABLE 12–1

Selected Characteristics of Some Commercially Available Enteral Formulas

FORMULA	mOsm/ Kg	Cal/ mL	% WATER	TOTAL DIETARY FIBER (g/L)	Na (Mg/L)	K (Mg/L)	Cl (Mg/L)	Ca (Mg/L)	P (Mg/L)	Mg (Mg/L)
Ensure (R)	470	1.06	85.0	0	846	1564	1312	530	530	212
Ensure Plus (R)	690	1.50	77.0	0	1055	1943	1904	704	704	282
Entrition.5 (C)	120	0.50	92.6	0	350	600	500	250	250	100
Glucerna (R)	375	1.00	87.3	14.4	928	1561	1435	704	704	282
Hepatic Aid II (M)	560	1.10	87.3	0	288	196	—	—	—	—
Isocal (M)	270	1.06	84.0	0	530	1320	1061	630	530	210
Isocal HN (M)	270	1.06	84.0	0	930	1610	1440	850	850	340
Jevity (R)	310	1.06	83.3	14.4	933	1567	1314	912	759	303
Nepro (R)	635	2.00	70.0	0	829	1057	1011	1373	686	211
Magnacal (SM)	590	2.00	83.0	0	1000	1250	950	1000	1000	400
Osmolite (R)	300	1.06	84.0	0	636	1018	848	530	530	212
Pulmocare (R)	520	1.50	78.6	0	1311	1733	1688	1056	1056	423
Sustacal (MJ)	650	1.06	85.0	0	930	2100	1480	1010	930	380
Travasorb Hepatic (C)	600	1.10	82.0	0	235	892	697	491	491	197
Travasorb Renal (C)	590	1.35	77.0	0	—	—	—	—	—	—
Two Cal HN (R)	690	2.00	71.2	0	1306	2422	1642	1052	1052	422
Vivonex TEN (S)	630	1.00	85.0	0	460	782	819	500	500	200

C, Clintec Nutrition Company; M, McGaw; MJ, Mead Johnson; S, Sandoz Pharmaceutical; SM, Sherwood Medical; R, Ross Laboratories. Information from Zaloga G (ed): Nutrition in Critical Care, pp 450–468. St. Louis, CV Mosby, 1994, with permission.

hypokalemic, hypophosphatemic, and hypomagnesemic).[8] In patients with acute renal failure, it is obvious that nutritional requirements must be evaluated on a daily basis and modifications made as needed.

Hepatic Failure

Some patients with hepatic insufficiency may be able to tolerate the protein contained in standard enteral formulas without developing hepatic encephalopathy. For those who cannot, specialized products are available. Branched-chain amino acid supplements may help prevent encephalopathy in protein-intolerant patients. Because hepatic formulas have low electrolyte content, it may be necessary to supplement electrolytes when needed (as determined by laboratory analyses). (Examples of hepatic formulas are Hepatic Aid II and Travasorb Hepatic; see Table 12-1.)

Respiratory Failure

Patients with compromised respiratory function are frequently malnourished. Although these patients often need nutritional support, they may be unable to tolerate high caloric intake if ventilator weaning is in progress. This is because high caloric intake (especially from carbohydrates) causes increased carbon dioxide production (a problem in patients who are already hypercapneic). To meet the needs of patients with compromised respiratory function, special formulas are available that are lower in carbohydrate content and higher in fat than standard enteral products. These diets reduce the respiratory quotient of pulmonary patients by lowering the production of carbon dioxide and thereby the partial pressure of carbon dioxide in arterial blood ($PaCO_2$). (An example of such a formula is Pulmocare; see Table 12-1.)

FLUID AND ELECTROLYTE DISTURBANCES ASSOCIATED WITH TUBE FEEDINGS

Tube-fed patients tend to have the fluid and electrolyte disturbances associated with their underlying disease and treatment conditions. Therefore, theoretically it is possible to observe all types of electrolyte disturbances in tube-fed patients. Understandably, fluid and electrolyte disturbances are more common in patients with severe illness than in relatively healthy persons requiring tube feedings for only short periods. The discussion of imbalances in this chapter is limited to the more commonly encountered disturbances.

SODIUM IMBALANCES

Hypernatremia

Hypernatremia has been described as a possible electrolyte abnormality in tube-fed patients.[9] However, it is less common today than in the past when high-protein, high-osmolality formulas (approximately 1000 mOsm/kg) were often used.[10] Ingestion of large solute loads without a sufficient amount of water to excrete the metabolic products from these solutes can result in dehydration (hypernatremia) and azotemia.[11] Although formulas in use today tend to have lower osmolalities, hypernatremia can still develop in patients given inadequate water supplements. This problem is most prevalent in patients unable to make their thirst known (such as those who are unconscious, very young, aphasic, elderly, or debilitated). Elderly patients are more prone to develop hypernatremia with hyperosmolar feedings because of their decreased renal ability to conserve needed water.[12] The very young may also have difficulty in concentrating urine because of immature renal function. With decreased ability to concentrate urine, patients need more fluid to eliminate body wastes. If not provided through the feeding tube or the IV route, it is taken from internal fluid reserves.

Clinical studies have reported variable rates of hypernatremia in tube-fed patients. In one study it occurred in 10% of the tube-fed population (primarily in neurosurgical patients who were unable to conserve free water because of transient diabetes insipidus).[13] In another study, a higher incidence (18%) was reported in an acutely ill tube-fed population, being greatest in patients older than 60 years of age who were receiving feedings with osmolalities greater than 400 mOsm/kg.[14]

Hyponatremia

In two recent studies of tube-fed patients, the incidence of hyponatremia was higher than that of hypernatremia (24%–31% versus 10%–18%).[15,16] In both studies, the condition was often associated with the concomitant use of IV dextrose and water solutions for parenteral drug administration.

Factors contributing to hyponatremia in tube-fed patients include water-retaining states, such as occurs with syndrome of inappropriate antidiuretic hormone (SIADH) and abnormal routes of sodium loss, such as diarrhea or diuretic use. Note in Table 4-2 that a number of conditions predispose to this condition. In the presence of excessive ADH activity, large water supplements (by any route) can cause dilution of the serum sodium level, particularly when hypotonic or isotonic feedings are used. Although water added to the formula is usually charted, it is often difficult to determine the amount of fluid used as flushes to maintain tube patency and to administer medications by the tube.[17] The administration of medications by tube can be a significant source of fluid intake, which is particularly important in patients with a water-retaining state (such as SIADH).

FLUID VOLUME IMBALANCES

Fluid Volume Overload

It is possible to cause fluid volume overload when attempting to provide sufficient calories to a patient with renal, cardiac, or hepatic disease. For such patients, a formula supplying 2 kcal/mL is often selected (as opposed to one supplying only 1 kcal/mL). In addition, special low-sodium formulas are available for such patients. As noted in Table 12-1, some formulas have considerably more sodium than others. However, in most situations, the volume of formula needed to provide 2000 kcal will deliver 40 to 80 mEq of sodium.[18]

Edema can also occur when a high-carbohydrate formula is fed to a previously fasting patient. Weight gains of 20 lbs in a single week have been reported, accompanied by massive pedal edema.[19] Refeeding with carbohydrate causes an abrupt decrease in urinary sodium excretion in patients who have fasted for as little as 3 days.[20] Fluid retention is most pronounced during the first few days of refeeding.[21] Contributing to edema in tube-fed patients may be the presence of hypoalbuminemia, which favors shifting of fluid from the vascular to the interstitial space. One study of tube-fed patients found the incidence of edema to be 20% to 25%.[22]

Fluid Volume Deficit Associated With Hyperglycemia

Tube-fed patients are at risk for hyperglycemia because of the high carbohydrate content of some formulas and because of the relative insulin resistance commonly present in acute illness.[23] Patients with mild to moderate hyperglycemia need extra fluid to replace increased urinary fluid losses until the disorder can be controlled by hypoglycemic agents. (When insulin is administered, it is important to remember its contributory effect on the shifting of potassium, phosphorus, and magnesium from the extracellular fluid into the cells.) Occasionally, tube feedings will cause severe hyperglycemia that may progress to a hyperosmolar reaction.[24] In this situation, vigorous hydration is warranted (see Chapter 18).

REFEEDING SYNDROME

When starving (catabolic) patients are started on vigorous enteral feedings, there is a shift of potassium, phosphorus, and magnesium from the extracellular space into the cells. This shift occurs as protein synthesis (anabolism) is initiated. Insulin administration further favors intracellular shifting of these electrolytes. Failure to detect early hypokalemia, hypophosphatemia, and hypomagnesemia, and to furnish replacements as needed, can result in serious consequences as these electrolytes have vital functions.

Although parenteral nutrition has received more attention as a precipitator of the refeeding syndrome, enteral feedings are not without risk.[25] For example, the sudden death of four malnourished children within 6 to 9 days of starting high caloric enteral feedings has been reported.[26] Interventions for dealing with the refeeding syndrome are discussed later in this chapter. Other causes for hypokalemia, hypophosphatemia, and hypomagnesemia exist and are discussed below.

POTASSIUM IMBALANCES

Hypokalemia

Hypokalemia is a common metabolic complication of enteral feeding that reportedly occurs in up to 50% of tube-fed patients.[27] Therefore, close attention should be paid to the potassium content of the formula as well as to other conditions predisposing to hypokalemia (such as diarrhea or use of potassium-losing diuretics). Note in Table 12-1 that there is variability in the potassium content in tube feeding formulas. Clinical indicators of hypokalemia are described in Chapter 5.

Hyperkalemia

Hyperkalemia also may occur in the tube-fed patient. If excessive supplements are given in addition to the formula, hyperkalemia could result, particularly in high-risk patients. As explained in Chapter 5, a number of factors predispose to hyperkalemia (such as metabolic acidosis and advanced renal failure). In one study, hyperkalemia was observed in 40% of tube-fed patients; most of these had renal insufficiency and metabolic acidosis.[28] Holcombe and Adams[29] observed hyperkalemia in 16% of their tube-fed population. It usually developed secondary to potassium supplementation after tube feedings were initiated. In a study of 13 patients receiving tube feedings, Primrose et al.[30] reported a rise in serum potassium from a mean of 4.2 ± 0.5 mmol/L before feeding to 5.1 ± 0.5 mmol/L after 1 week. Two patients had increases that were considered hazardous, necessitating discontinuance of the feedings. The researchers concluded that careful attention should be paid to monitoring serum potassium levels in patients receiving tube feedings.

PHOSPHORUS IMBALANCES

Hypophosphatemia

Hypophosphatemia is less common in enterally fed patients than in those fed intravenously. This is because enteral nutrition solutions usually contain adequate phosphate for patients with normal phosphate stores. However, as described previously, there is danger of hypophosphatemia during aggressive enteral feeding of starving patients as refeeding causes phosphates to shift into the cells where they are used for glucose phosphorylation and protein synthesis.[31] When this happens, the plasma phosphate level may drop precipitously. A recent report described two patients with protein-energy malnutrition who developed severe hypophosphatemia during enteral feeding with phosphorus-containing formulas.[32] Additional risk factors in these two patients were present (one had chronic alcoholism and the other had malabsorption because of Crohn's disease). The researchers pointed out that patients with depleted phosphate stores and high metabolic demand have a higher daily requirement for phosphorus than is available in routine isotonic enteral formulas.[33] These case reports emphasize the importance of monitoring daily serum phosphate concentration for at least 1 week after commencement of feeding.[34]

In another study of tube-fed patients, a 30% incidence of hypophosphatemia was observed, even when phosphate-containing solutions were used.[35] This occurred primarily in patients who received insulin for treatment of hyperglycemia; thus, the hypophosphatemia was probably secondary to a shift of phosphorus into the cells. Other investigators reported hypophosphatemia in malnourished patients receiving glucose infusions (again, related to a cellular shift).[36] Clinical indicators of hypophosphatemia are described in Chapter 8.

Hyperphosphatemia

Hyperphosphatemia has also been observed in tube-fed patients. A 14% incidence of hyperphosphatemia was reported by Vanlandingham et al.[37]; the elevated phosphate levels correlated with renal failure (a common cause of this imbalance). This is reflective of the close parallel between electrolyte abnormalities and underlying disease states in tube-fed patients.

MAGNESIUM IMBALANCES

Hypomagnesemia

During anabolism, magnesium requirements increase as the intracellular mass expands. As with the other primary cellular electrolytes (potassium and phosphorus), extracellular deficiency may result if inadequate amounts are present in the formula or added as supplements (either enterally or parenterally). In a study by Holcombe and Adams,[38] 46% of the patients had lower than normal serum magnesium levels (11 had the problem before the initiation of tube feedings and 9 patients became hypomagnesemic during the course of tube feedings). Clinical indicators of hypomagnesemia are described in Chapter 7.

Hypermagnesemia

Patients with renal failure are at risk for hypermagnesemia if the amount of magnesium contained in the formula exceeds the kidneys' ability to excrete magnesium. Use of magnesium-containing medications adds to the risk.

ZINC DEFICIENCY

Although several trace element deficiencies may occur in patients receiving long-term enteral feedings as their only nutritional source, zinc deficiency has probably received the most attention. Zinc deficiency has been described in two patients who received tube feedings for 4 and 7 months.[39] Both patients developed skin rashes around the groin and under the breasts and axilla; after supplementation with zinc sulfate, the rashes disappeared and the serum zinc levels returned to normal. Below-normal serum zinc levels occurred in 11% of the tube-fed patients in the study by Vanlandingham et al.[40]

ASSESSMENT FOR FLUID AND ELECTROLYTE DISTURBANCES IN TUBE-FED PATIENTS

ROUTINE LABORATORY AND CLINICAL MONITORING

Although clinical assessment is important, electrolyte disturbances are usually detected by laboratory analyses. Although recommendations vary regarding the frequency of metabolic monitoring in tube-fed patients, it seems reasonable to measure serum sodium, potassium, glucose, blood urea nitrogen (BUN), and creatinine daily for the first week and once a week thereafter; and serum phosphorus, magnesium, and calcium at least twice weekly during the first week and once a week subsequently. As stabilization evidence is gathered, the testing frequency can be gradually decreased. In many situations, the severity of illness dictates how frequently laboratory values are obtained. For example, it may be necessary to check all electrolytes daily in critically ill patients.

Fluid intake and output (I&O) should be monitored and recorded every 8 hrs (or hourly in acute situations such as an hyperosmolar reaction). Body weight should be measured and recorded daily. Vital signs should be monitored at least once per shift. Urine glucose and acetone should be checked every 6 hrs for the first 48 hrs and then once daily if normal. If the renal threshold is in question (as it frequently is in elderly and very ill patients), capillary blood glucose should be measured.

RISK FACTORS FROM UNDERLYING DISEASE AND TREATMENT CONDITIONS

As indicated earlier, virtually any electrolyte imbalance can occur in tube-fed patients, usually reflecting abnormalities associated with their primary disease condition(s). Factors related to enteral nutrition (such as the formula itself) can add to the patient's chance of developing fluid and electrolyte problems. Some risk factors for specific imbalances are summarized in Table 12-2.

HYDRATION STATUS

Because tube-fed patients may develop either fluid volume deficit (FVD) or fluid volume excess (FVE), with or without sodium imbalances, it is necessary to monitor the hydration status closely (see Table 12-3).

NURSING INTERVENTIONS

PREVENTING THE REFEEDING SYNDROME

Some recommendations suggested by Solomon and Kirby[44] to avoid the refeeding syndrome include:

1. Recognize "at-risk" patients (such as those with chronic cachexia due to prolonged starvation or any patient who has been chronically deprived of adequate nutrition).
2. Test for and correct electrolyte abnormalities before initiating nutritional support in at-risk patients, either orally, enterally, or intravenously.
3. Begin nutritional repletion slowly and keep increases in calories modest during the first week.
4. Monitor serum sodium, potassium, magnesium, and phosphorus levels and administer supplements as indicated (especially during the first

(text continues on page 215)

TABLE 12–2

Summary of Fluid and Electrolyte Imbalances in Tube-Fed Patients: Risk Factors and Interventions

FLUID/ELECTROLYTE IMBALANCE	EXAMPLES OF RISK FACTORS	POSSIBLE INTERVENTIONS
Hyponatremia	Excessive water retention associated with increased ADH activity: • Disease conditions such as oat-cell lung tumor and head injury • Medications such as Cytoxan, Oncovin, Diabenese, and Mellaril	Adjust water intake according to serum sodium levels Avoid hypotonic formulas or large water intake in patients at risk for hyponatremia
	Excessive water administration in form of hypotonic enteral formula, water flushes of the feeding tube, or D_5W to administer IV medications	Use calorie-dense formula to limit water intake, as indicated Administer IV medications in isotonic saline (instead of D_5W) if compatible
	Abnormal routes of sodium loss, as in diarrhea or diuretic use	Administer sodium supplements via enteral route, if indicated (If NaCl supplements are prescribed, it is safer to obtain predetermined quantities of NaCl in capsule form from a pharmacist than it is to measure table salt in a teaspoon at the bedside.) Sodium may also be supplemented by IV route, if indicated.
Hypernatremia	Excessive water loss, as in: • Diabetes insipidus • Fever • Hyperventilation	Adjust water intake according to serum sodium levels Change to isotonic formula (if problem is a hyperosmolar formula)
	Use of hyperosmolar enteral formulas with insufficient water supplements	Administer water supplements as boluses via feeding tube, as indicated
	Decreased renal concentrating ability (as in very old and very young patients)	Administer IV medications in D_5W (instead of normal saline), if compatible
	Decreased level of consciousness, inability to recognize or respond to thirst	Rehydrate gradually over a period of several days if severe hypernatremia is present; too rapid correction can cause brain edema.[41]

(continued)

TABLE 12–2 (cont.)

FLUID/ELECTROLYTE IMBALANCE	EXAMPLES OF RISK FACTORS	POSSIBLE INTERVENTIONS
Hypokalemia	Aggressive refeeding of starving patients	Initiate feedings cautiously in starving patient
	Use of potassium-losing medications: • Furosemide, thiazide diuretics • Aminoglycosides • Amphotericin	Monitor serum potassium levels and administer potassium supplements as indicated (intravenous route may be necessary)
	Insulin administration	
	Severe diarrhea	
Hypomagnesemia	Aggressive refeeding of starving patients	Initiate feedings cautiously in starving patients
	Use of magnesium-losing medications such as aminoglycosides, cisplatin, and mannitol	Monitor serum magnesium levels and provide magnesium supplements as indicated (intravenous route may be necessary)
	Insulin administration	
	Chronic alcoholism	
	Diarrhea	
Hypophosphatemia	Aggressive refeeding of starving patients	Initiate feedings cautiously in starving patients
	Insulin administration Chronic alcoholism Malabsorption Respiratory alkalosis Diarrhea	Monitor serum phosphorus levels and provide supplements as indicated: Fleet Phospho-Soda is sometimes added to the enteral formula to treat mild to moderate hypophosphatemia; parenteral phosphorus should be used to treat patients with serum phosphorus concentrations <1.5 mg/dL.[42]
Hyperkalemia	Use of potassium-conserving diuretics Renal failure	Monitor serum potassium levels; if elevated, consider potassium content of enteral formula, IV fluids, and medications
		Reduce potassium intake
Hypermagnesemia	Use of magnesium-containing antacids Renal failure	Monitor serum magnesium levels; if elevated, consider magnesium content of enteral formula, IV fluids, and medications
		Reduce magnesium intake

TABLE 12–2 (cont.)

FLUID/ELECTROLYTE IMBALANCE	EXAMPLES OF RISK FACTORS	POSSIBLE INTERVENTIONS
Hyperphosphatemia	Use of phosphate-containing antacids Renal failure	Monitor serum phosphorus levels; if elevated, consider phosphorus content of enteral formula, IV fluids, and medications Reduce phosphorus intake
Fluid volume deficit	Osmotic diuresis from hyperglycemia	Monitor serum glucose level every 6 hr after feedings are initiated (until stable) Control hyperglycemia by adjusting formula or administering hypoglycemic agent
Fluid volume excess	Use of standard formula with relatively high sodium content in patients with renal, cardiac, or hepatic failure Early period (especially first few days) of refeeding of patients with chronic malnutrition	Assess for fluid excess by daily body weights, I&O measurement, looking for edema, listening to breath sounds Consider use of low-sodium or calorie-dense formula. Initiate refeeding cautiously in chronically malnourished patients; assess fluid volume carefully, monitor for signs of cardiac stress

week of refeeding when most of the serious electrolyte problems are likely to occur).

It may be helpful to monitor the pulse rate as a noninvasive method to assess fluid replacement. Most severely malnourished patients have bradycardia; if during nutritional repletion the intravascular volume is increased too rapidly, the heart rate may increase markedly. For example, a heart rate of 80 to 100 beats/min in a previously malnourished, bradycardic patient may be a sign of cardiac stress and warrants close observation.[45]

MANAGING ELECTROLYTE IMBALANCES

A brief summary of interventions for specific electrolyte imbalances associated with tube feedings in present in Table 12-2. See Chapters 3 through 9 for more detailed information regarding assessment for these imbalances and treatment recommendations.

WATER SUPPLEMENTATION

A perplexing problem for the nurse is determining how much free water is needed for each tube-fed patient. The previous discussion identified several variables affecting this decision. To reiterate, clinical assessment helps to determine whether a patient has normal volume status, or is fluid volume deficient or overloaded. Review of the underlying disease condition(s) is imperative. For example, is there a need for fluid restriction due to SIADH or renal or cardiac disease? Is extra fluid required due to delivery of high-osmolality, high-protein feedings, or increased loss from other routes, such as diarrhea, fistula or wound drainage, hyperventilation, or fever? Is the patient receiving sizable amounts of fluid through the IV

TABLE 12–3

Summary of Assessment of Hydration Status of Tube-Fed Patients

ASSESSMENT	DESCRIPTION
Fluid I&O	Record volume and type of all fluids given by mouth, tube, and intravenously. (include water used to flush tube to maintain patency and to administer medications) Record all fluid losses, including: • Urine • Liquid feces • Vomitus • Drainage from fistulas, wounds, etc. Consider fluid losses associated with fever, perspiration, hyperventilation, and dry environmental conditions.
Urine concentration	In addition to volume of urine, record its color (ranging from dark amber to pale or colorless). If necessary, measure urinary specific gravity with urinometer. (If glucosuria is present, specific gravity will be abnormally high; urinary osmolality is a more accurate measure in this instance.)
Urinary glucose	Monitor for glucosuria at least 3 times daily throughout initial feeding period, particularly in middle-aged and elderly patients. If present, check capillary blood sugar. If renal threshold is in question, omit urinary tests and check capillary blood sugars.
Body weight	Measure body weight daily (using same scales and same clothing). A slight increase in weight is anticipated in the anabolic patient. This gain should not exceed 0.7 kg/day, roughly 1.5 lbs/day.[43] A gain greater than this amount probably indicates fluid volume overload.
Edema	Look for dependent edema in feet and ankles of ambulatory patients and in the backs of bedfast patients. Assess breath sounds for pulmonary edema.
Sensorium	Assess for changes in sensorium (from baseline) after feedings are initiated. Severe sodium derangements (either high or low) can affect the patient's level of alertness and responsiveness.
Blood chemistries	Examine BUN:creatinine ratio; if elevated, possibility of fluid volume deficit exists. Examine serum sodium level (if high, indicates need for free water; if low, indicates need for restriction of free water). Look for elevated blood sugar level; if present, patient is at increased risk for osmotic diuresis and fluid volume deficit.

route? How does the I&O record look? All of these factors must be considered individually.

Given these qualifiers, a few rough guidelines may be considered. Some suggest that adults need 1.0 mL of fluid per calorie delivered, whereas children require 1.5 mL per calorie.[46] Another method suggests that adults require from 25 to 35 mL of water per kilogram of body weight per day.[47] See Table 12-4 for a sample problem to calculate water needs of a hypothetical tube-fed patient. (Water requirements for children of various ages are presented in Chapter 24.)

TABLE 12-4

Sample Calculation for Estimating Daily Fluid Requirements

A 56-year-old patient weighing 70 kg is being fed Osmolite HN, 75 mL/hr/day (75 x 24 = 1800 mL/day)

Step 1. Estimated daily fluid requirement = Estimated water need (mL) times body weight (kg). For a person of this age, 30 mL per kg of water is generally accepted as adequate. For this patient, therefore, estimated daily fluid requirement equals 30 mL times 70 kg = 2100 mL.

Step 2. Fluid provided by enteral formula = mL water/L times volume of formula/day (L). Fluid provided by enteral formula = 841 mL/L times 1.8 L. (See Table 12-1 for water content of formula.) Fluid provided by enteral formula = 1514 mL.

Step 3. Additional fluid required = Result 1 – Result 2
Additional fluid required = 2100 mL – 1514 mL
Additional fluid required = 586 mL/day.

Adapted from Enteral Nutrition Handbook, p 14. Ross Products Division, Abbott Laboratories, March 1989. With permission of Ross Laboratories, Columbus, OH 43216.

MANAGING DIARRHEA

Severe diarrhea leads to fluid, electrolyte, and nutrient depletion.[48] Although the true prevalence of diarrhea in tube-fed patients is difficult to pinpoint (largely because clinicians use varying definitions of diarrhea), it is generally agreed that diarrhea is a potential problem in tube-fed patients that must be reckoned with to avoid serious fluid and electrolyte problems. Researchers have attempted to identify causes of diarrhea and have often found multiple factors. Among these are osmolality of the formula, rate of delivery, site of delivery (gastric versus intestinal), formula contamination, malnutrition, severity of illness, antibiotics, hyperosmolar medications, fecal impaction, *Clostridium difficile* infection, and mechanical ventilation.

Reported incidences range from as low as 2% in some populations to as high as 68% in others.[49–51] When GI function is normal, the incidence of diarrhea in tube-fed patients is reported to be 12% to 25%.[52,53] In contrast, about half of the patients in intensive care units develop diarrhea.[54] Several factors may account for this higher incidence, such as increased rates of malnutrition (causing decreased ability of the intestinal mucosa to absorb nutrients), multiple-system organ disease, multiple medications, and infectious processes. Apparently, critically ill patients who are mechanically ventilated are at even greater risk for diarrhea. A study of 73 critically ill, mechanically ventilated patients reported a 63% incidence of diarrhea.[55] Another study of tube-fed patients found that 26% had documented diarrhea (defined as stools greater than 500 mL/day for at least 2 consecutive days).[56] A single cause was specified in 29 of the 32 episodes of diarrhea. Medications were directly responsible in 61%, whereas tube feeding formulas were responsible in only 21%, and *Clostridium difficile* in 17%. In yet another study, antibiotic usage was most strongly associated with the incidence of diarrhea.[57]

Because multiple factors can cause diarrhea, it is reasonable to try a variety of measures to prevent or at least minimize this problem. Some of these are described below.

Formula Selection

High-Fiber Formulas

Because the colon is the final site of water and electrolyte absorption and ultimately determines fecal composition, diarrhea associated with enteral feedings may result from altered colonic function.[58] In patients who can tolerate high-residue formulas, use of a high-fiber formula is thought to increase the sodium and water absorptive ability of the colon and thus, minimize fecal fluid loss. Commercially available fiber-supplemented formulas are often prescribed to either prevent or treat diarrhea.

Peptide-Based Formulas

Hypoalbuminemia is commonly cited as a cause of diarrhea. Theoretically, hypoalbuminemia results in a decrease in oncotic pressure that produces intestinal edema and therefore, a malabsorptive state. Some clinicians favor correcting hypoalbuminemia by parenteral nutrition before starting enteral feedings. Several studies have indicated that peptide-based formulas are helpful in avoiding diarrhea in hypoalbuminemic, critically ill patients.[59,60] However, a larger prospective study did not demonstrate any advantage in a peptide-based formula over a standard, polymeric formula.[61]

Lactose-Free Formulas

Formulas with little or no lactose are indicated for very ill patients with small-bowel conditions that predispose to lactose intolerance (such as intestinal resection, radiation enteritis, and malnutrition). The presence of mucosal damage reduces the total intestinal surface area available for absorption and produces secondary lactose deficiency. Most commercially available feedings are lactose-free. Of course, any feeding prepared with milk contains lactose.

Formula Dilution and Rate of Delivery

Formulas that are isotonic (approach the osmolality of plasma, 280–300 mOsm/kg) are usually administered at full strength. Even those that are moderately hyperosmotic can often be administered at full strength. An example of an administration schedule for formulas having osmolalities between 300 and 600 mOsm/kg is presented in Table 12-5. When hyperosmolar feedings are thought to be the cause of diarrhea, it may be necessary to dilute the formula or decrease the volume infused.[62] If dilution is necessary, it should be performed as aseptically as possible. Generally, attempts are made to avoid diluting formulas; instead, the nutrient density delivery to the site may be decreased by lowering the rate of flow. Hyperosmolar solutions are less well tolerated in the small intestine than in the stomach.

Although some institutions still routinely dilute formulas to one-half strength when enteral feedings are first started ("starter regimens"), there is growing evidence that this is not necessary. Studies have demonstrated that full-strength isotonic to hypertonic formulas can be used safely and effectively in a variety of patient populations.[63] In fact, starter regimens requiring formula dilution may result in greater GI complications and poorer nutritional outcomes.[64] In addition, diluting feedings has the potential for introducing microbial contamination.[65]

If the cause of diarrhea is too rapid administration of the formula, it is customary to decrease the rate of flow to the point where no diarrhea occurs.[66] Then, the rate is gradually increased until the desired rate is achieved. Feedings may be administered either intermittently or continuously in the stomach, but only continuously in the intestine.

Medications

It is helpful to assess whether medications (such as sorbitol or elixirs) received by the tube-fed patient might be responsible for the development of diarrhea. For example, aminophylline given in a sorbitol-containing elixir is a major cause of diarrhea.[67] Although liquid preparations of medications are frequently useful in enterally fed patients to avoid clogging of feeding tubes, it may be necessary to consult with the pharmacist and physician to find a more suitable method for administering agents suspected of causing diarrhea.

TABLE 12–5

Example of an Administration Schedule for Formulas Having Osmolalities of 300–600 mOsm/kg Water

CONTINUOUS SCHEDULE				
DAY	TIME	STRENGTH	RATE (ML/HR)	VOLUME (ML)
1	1st 8 hrs	Full	25–50	200–400
	2nd 8 hrs	Full	50	400
	3rd 8 hrs	Full	75	600
2	24 hrs	Full	Adjust volume fed and rate administered to meet specific nutritional goals	

From Pendley F, Geckle R, Campbell S: Enteral Nutrition Support in Critical Care, p 22, May 1994. With permission of Ross Products Division, Abbott Laboratories. Columbus, OH 43216.

In measurements of 58 commercial preparations available as liquid formulations, investigators reported that the range of average osmolalities was between 450 and 10,950 mOsm/kg.[68] Indeed, a number of medications are hyperosmolar and can cause osmotic diarrhea if given undiluted, especially into the small intestine. Examples of osmolalities of such medications include 10% potassium chloride solution (Adria), 3000 mOsm/kg; acetaminophen elixir, 65 mg/mL (Roxanne), 5400 mOsm/kg; and sodium phosphate liquid, 0.5 g/mL (Fleet), 7250 mOsm/kg.[69]

Hyperosmolar medications should be diluted before administration and water flushes given through the tube before and after delivery.[70] This not only dilutes the medication but enhances its absorption. (This should be done with the patient's fluid requirements in mind.) Hyperosmolar preparations should only be administered in the stomach to minimize GI intolerance.[71] At times, the parenteral route may be necessary for electrolyte supplements when they are not tolerated well by the GI tract. Use of magnesium-containing antacids may also cause diarrhea. When antacids are necessary, it may be helpful to alternate magnesium-containing antacids with magnesium-free antacids[72] or to change to calcium or aluminum antacids.[73] Other medications frequently implicated in diarrhea are penicillin-like antibiotics.

Another possible cause of diarrhea is the administration of metoclopramide, an agent often prescribed to stimulate gastric emptying. It is possible that stopping treatment with this drug will cause the diarrhea to resolve.[74]

Temperature of Solution

Recently refrigerated formulas should be started at a slow rate to permit them time to warm to room temperature. Research findings by Kagawa-Busby et al.[75] suggest that cold feedings can predispose to cramping and diarrhea in some patients.

Preventing Contamination of Formula/Feeding System

Recent studies indicate that enteral nutritional solutions may be an important source of nosocomial infection.[76] This can be particularly dangerous in severely ill, immunocompromised patients.[77] Thus, enteral formulas should be handled with sanitary technique to prevent microbial contamination. The complete delivery set (except the feeding tube itself) should be changed every 24 hrs for patients in a hospital setting to reduce the incidence of contamination.[78,79] When powdered formulas are used, all of the preparation equipment needs to be cleaned meticulously. Some researchers recommend the use of sterile water (versus tap water) when it is necessary to reconstitute or dilute enteral nutrition solutions.[80] It has been recommended that dilution of liquid formulas be avoided whenever possible because of the risk for contamination.[81] Although formulas prefilled by manufacturers into large-volume containers can hang for 24 hrs, formulas decanted into other containers for administration should hang no more than 8 to 12 hrs.[82]

REFERENCES

1. Zaloga G: Nutrition in Critical Care, p 675. St. Louis, CV Mosby, 1994
2. Ibid, p 446
3. MacBurney M, Russell C, Young L: Formulas, p 167. In Rombeau J, Caldwell M (eds): Clinical Nutrition: Enteral and Tube Feeding, 2nd ed. Philadelphia, WB Saunders, 1990
4. Ibid
5. Ibid
6. Matarese L: Rationale and efficacy of specialized enteral nutrition. Nutr Clin Pract 9(2):58–68,1992
7. Zaloga, p 673
8. Ibid
9. Gault et al: Hypernatremia, azotemia, and dehydration due to high-protein feeding. Ann Intern Med 68:778,1968
10. Silk D, Payne-James J: Complications of enteral nutrition. In Rombeau J, Caldwell M (eds): Clinical Nutrition: Enteral and Tube Feeding, 2nd ed, p 525. Philadelphia, WB Saunders, 1990
11. Pemberton L, Pemberton D: Treatment of Water, Electrolyte and Acid-Base Disorders in the Surgical Patient, p 99. New York, McGraw-Hill, 1994
12. Walike J: Tube feeding syndrome in head and neck surgery. Arch Otolaryngol 89:117,1969
13. Vanlandingham et al: Metabolic abnormalities in patients supported with enteral tube feeding. J Parenter Enter Nutr 5:322,1981
14. Bowman M: Sodium Imbalances in Tube-Fed Patients. Master's Thesis. St. Louis University, 1986
15. Vanlandingham et al, p 323
16. Bowman et al: Sodium imbalances in tube-fed patients. Crit Care Nurs 9(1):22,1989

17. Bowman
18. Alpers D, Clouse R, Stenson W: Manual of Nutritional Therapeutics, 2nd ed, p 226. Boston, Little, Brown, 1988
19. Havala T, Shronts E: Managing the complications associated with refeeding. Nutrit Clin Pract 5(1):27,1990
20. Zaloga, p 770
21. Ibid, p 771
22. Heymsfield et al: Enteral hyperalimentation: An alternative to central venous hyperalimentation. Ann Intern Med 90:63,1979
23. Silk, Payne-James, p 525
24. Condon R, Nyhus L: Manual of Surgical Therapeutics, 8th ed. Boston: Little, Brown, 1992
25. Zaloga, p 776
26. Patrick J: Death during recovery from severe malnutrition and its possible relationship to sodium pump activity in the leukocyte. Br Med J 1:1051,1977
27. Silk, Payne-James, p 525
28. Vanlandingham et al, p 324
29. Holcombe B, Adams M: Metabolic complications associated with enteral nutritional support. Nutritional Support Services 5(3):26,1985
30. Primrose et al: Hyperkalemia in patients on enteral feedings. J Parenter Enter Nutr 5:130,1981
31. Silk, Payne-James, p 525
32. Maier-Dobersberger T, Lochs H: Enteral supplementation of phosphate does not prevent hypophosphatemia during refeeding of cachectic patients. J Parenter Enter Nutr 18(2):182–184,1994
33. Ibid
34. Ibid
35. Vanlandingham et al, p 324
36. Hayek M, Eisenberg P: Severe hypophosphatemia following the institution of enteral feedings. Arch Surg 124(11):1325–1328,1989
37. Vanlandingham et al, p 324
38. Holcombe, Adams
39. Jhangiana et al: Clinical zinc deficiency during long-term total enteral nutrition. J Am Geriatr Soc 34: 385,1986
40. Vanlandingham et al, p 324
41. Rombeau, p 168
42. Zaloga, p 490
43. Heymsfield et al, p 69
44. Solomon S, Kirby D: The refeeding syndrome: A review. J Parenter Enter Nutr 14:90–97,1990
45. Ibid
46. Anonymous: Enteral Nutrition Handbook, p 13. Columbus, OH, Ross Laboratories, 1989
47. Ibid
48. Guenter P, Settle G, Perlmutter S, et al: Tube feeding-related diarrhea in acute ill patients. J Parenter Enter Nutr 15(3):277–280,1991
49. Kelly T, et al: Study of diarrhea in critically ill patients. Crit Care Med 11:7–9,1983
50. Bliss D, et al: Defining and reporting diarrhea in tube-fed patients—What a mess! Am J Clin Nutr 55:753–759,1992
51. Heimburger D: Diarrhea with enteral feeding: Will the real cause please stand up? Am J Med 88: 89–90,1990
52. Cataldi-Betcher et al: Complications occurring during enteral nutrition support: A prospective study. J Parenter Enter Nutr 7:546,1983
53. Jones et al: Comparison of an elemental and polymeric enteral diet in patients with normal gastrointestinal function. Gut 24:78,1983
54. Brinson R, Anderson W, Singh M: Hypoalbuminemia-associated diarrhea in critically ill patients. J Crit Illness 2(9):72,1987
55. Smith et al: Diarrhea associated with tube-feeding in mechanically ventilated critically ill patients. Nurs Res 39(3):148,1990
56. Edes T, Walk B, Austin J: Diarrhea in tube-fed patients: Feeding formula not necessarily the cause. Am J Med 88:91,1990
57. Guenter et al: Administration and delivery of enteral nutrition. In Rombeau J, Caldwell M (eds): Clinical Nutrition: Enteral and Tube Feeding, 2nd ed, p 199. Philadelphia, WB Saunders, 1990
58. Palacio J, Rombeau J: Dietary fiber: A brief review and potential application to enteral nutrition. Nutr Clin Pract 5(3):99–106,1990
59. Brinson R, et al: Diarrhea in the intensive care unit: The role of hypoalbuminemia and the response to a chemically defined diet. J Am Coll Nutr 6:517–523,1987
60. Brinson R, Kolts B: Diarrhea associated with severe hypoalbuminemia: A comparison of a peptide-based chemically defined diet and standard enteral alimentation. Crit Care Med 16:130–136,1988
61. Mowatt-Larssen C, et al: Comparison of tolerance and nutritional outcome between a peptide and a standard enteral formula in critically ill, hypoalbuminemic patients. JPEN 16:20–24,1992
62. Zaloga, p 825
63. Ibid, p 822
64. Keohane P, et al: Relation between osmolality of diet and gastrointestinal side effects in enteral nutrition. Br Med J 288:678–680,1984
65. Pendley F, Geckle R, Campbell S: Enteral Nutrition Support in Critical Care, p 5. Ross Products Division, Abbott Laboratories, 1994
66. Eisenberg P: Causes of diarrhea in tube-fed patients: A comprehensive approach to diagnosis and management. Nutr Clin Pract 8(3):119–123,1993
67. Zaloga, p 341
68. Dickerson R, Melnik G: Osmolality of oral drug solutions and suspensions. Am J Hosp Pharm 45:832–834,1988
69. Melnik G: Pharmacologic aspects of enteral nutrition. In Rombeau J, Caldwell M (eds): Clinical Nutrition: Enteral and Tube Feeding, 2nd ed, p 493. Philadelphia, WB Saunders, 1990

70. Edes et al, p 91
71. Seshadri V, Meyer-Tettambel O: Electrolyte and drug management in nutritional support. Crit Care Nurs Clin North Am 5(1):31–36,1993
72. Zaloga, p 572
73. Eisenberg, p 121
74. Zaloga, p 342
75. Kagawa-Busby K, Heitkemper M, Hansen B: Effects of diet temperature on tolerance of enteral feedings. Nurs Res 29:276,1980
76. Thurn et al: Enteral hyperalimentation as a source of nosocomial infection. J Hosp Infect 15:203,1990
77. Moe G: Enteral feeding and infection in the immunocompromised patient. Nutr Clin Pract 6:55–64,1991
78. Perez S, Brandt K: Enteral feeding contamination: Comparison of diluents and feeding bag usage. J Parenter Enter Nutr 13(3):306,1989
79. Kohn C: The relationship between enteral formula contamination and length of enteral delivery set usage. J Parenter Enter Nutr 15:567–571,1991
80. Fagerman K: Microbiological monitoring of enteral nutrition solutions needed (Letter). J Parenter Enter Nutr 13(6):670,1989
81. Pendley et al, p 23
82. Ibid

IV

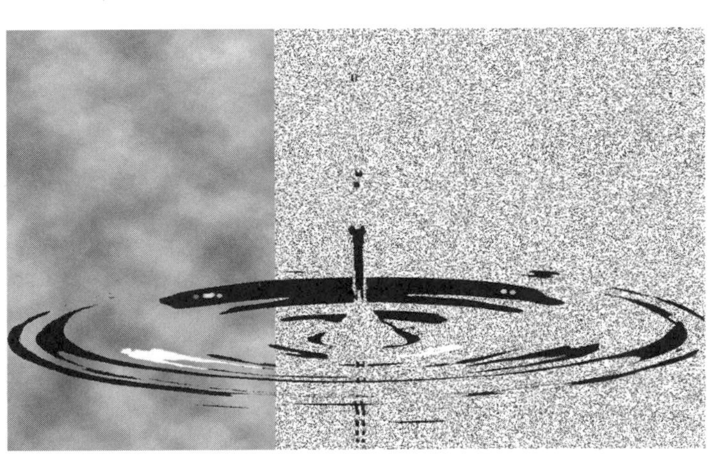

Clinical Situations Associated With Fluid and Electrolyte Problems

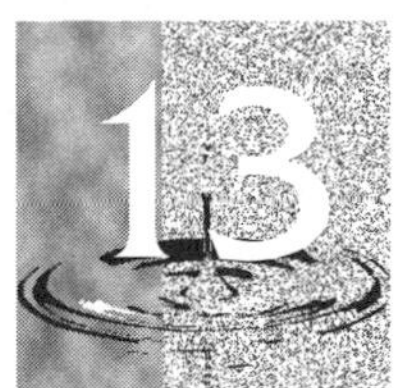

Gastrointestinal Problems

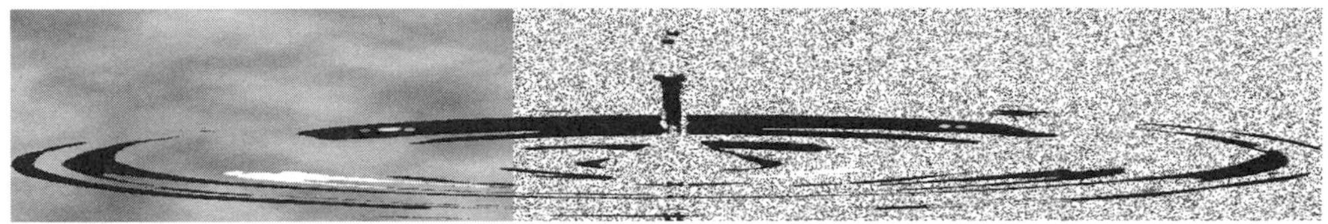

Gastrointestinal (GI) fluid loss is the most common cause of water and electrolyte disturbances. This is evident because of the large fluid volumes in the GI tract and the many ways in which these fluids can be lost, such as vomiting, diarrhea, suction drainage, fistulas, and sequestration into an obstructed bowel. Along with the possibility of fluid volume deficit (FVD), there is the potential for various electrolyte imbalances. Nursing considerations related to these GI fluid and electrolyte losses are discussed in this chapter.

CHARACTER OF GASTROINTESTINAL FLUIDS

In healthy individuals, approximately 3 to 6 L of gastric, pancreatic, biliary, and intestinal secretions are secreted into the GI lumen each day.[1] Counting normal fluid intake and endogenous GI secretions, approximately 9 L/day enter the upper intestinal tract. Most of these fluids are then reabsorbed in the ileum and proximal colon, resulting in daily loss of only 100 to 200 mL of water in feces.

With the exception of saliva, the GI secretions are isotonic with the extracellular fluid (ECF). In addition, material entering the GI tract tends to become isotonic during the course of its absorption. Because many liters of ECF pass into the GI tract and back again, as part of the normal digestive process, this movement is sometimes referred to as the "gastrointestinal circulation." The electrolyte content of GI secretions is summarized in Table 13-1. The usual pH of GI secretions is listed in Table 13-2.

VOMITING AND GASTRIC SUCTION

FLUID AND ELECTROLYTE DISTURBANCES

Major electrolytes in gastric juice are hydrogen (H^+), chloride (Cl^-), potassium (K^+), and, to a lesser extent, sodium (Na^+). Gastric juice is the most acidic of the GI secretions with a pH of 1.0 to 3.5 in the fasting state in most individuals not receiving H_2-receptor antagonists. Imbalances most often associated with the loss of gastric juice include the following:

- Fluid volume deficit
- Metabolic alkalosis
- Hypokalemia
- Sodium imbalances
- Hypomagnesemia

Fluid Volume Deficit

If vomiting is prolonged and fluid replacement therapy is inadequate, severe FVD may result, manifested by decreased urinary output, postural hypotension, tachycardia, elevated hematocrit, and elevated blood urea nitrogen (BUN)/creatinine ratio. It is not uncommon to see a 10-point drop in the hematocrit level during the first 12 to 24 hrs after fluid replacement.[2] Also, because many liters can be removed daily by gastric suction (depending on the underlying disease process), FVD can easily occur in this situation if fluids are not replaced parenterally.

Metabolic Alkalosis

Excessive loss of gastric juice by vomiting or suction causes metabolic alkalosis (base bicarbonate excess) for several reasons. First, secretions from the stomach contains high concentrations of H^+ and Cl^- ions. With loss of Cl^-, there is a compensatory increase in bicarbonate ions. (Each mEq of hydrochloric acid [HCl] lost from the stomach represents 1 mEq of bicarbonate added to the ECF.)[3] The kidneys add to the metabolic alkalosis by failing to excrete all the excess circulating bicarbonate (HCO_3^-).[4] Symptoms are generally those of decreased calcium ionization related to the alkaline plasma. (Recall that calcium ionization is decreased in alkalosis.) Because it is the ionized fraction of calcium that controls neuromuscular excitability, symptoms of tetany can occur. Metabolic alkalosis is less common in patients with gastric suction than it was 20 years ago, largely because of the widespread use of H_2-receptor antagonists.[5] By suppressing HCl production, these drugs minimize the amount of HCl that needs to be removed by the suction apparatus.

Hypokalemia

As noted in Table 13-1, gastric fluid contains approximately 10 mEq/L of potassium. With the loss of several liters of gastric fluid, it is clear that

TABLE 13–1

Approximate Electrolyte Composition of Gastrointestinal Secretions

SECRETION	USUAL MAXIMUM VOLUME/DAY	SODIUM (mEq/L IN ADULTS)	CHLORIDE (mEq/L IN ADULTS)	POTASSIUM (mEq/L IN ADULTS)
Normal				
Saliva	1000	100	75	5
Gastric juice (pH <4.0)	2500*	60	100	10
Gastric juice (pH >4.0)	2000*	100	100	10
Bile	1500	140	100	10
Pancreatic juice	1000	140	75	10
Succus entericus (mixed small-bowel fluid)	3500	100	100	20
Abnormal				
New ileostomy	500–2000	130	110	20
Adapted ileostomy	400	50	60	10
New cecostomy	400	80	50	20
Colostomy (transverse loop)	300	50	40	10
Diarrhea	1000–4000	60	45	30

*Nasogastric suction volume is usually much less than this unless pyloric obstruction exists.

From Condon R, Nyhus L. Manual of Surgical Therapeutics, 8th ed, p 183. Boston, Little, Brown, 1993, with permission.

hypokalemia could easily develop. In addition to the direct loss of potassium with vomiting and gastric suction, there is a transient renal wasting of potassium early in the period of gastric fluid loss. The metabolic alkalosis described previously accompanies hypokalemia.

Recall that an adult, not eating, requires the daily addition of approximately 40 to 60 mEq of potassium to intravenous (IV) fluids. A patient with large gastric fluid losses may require substantially more.

TABLE 13–2

Gastrointestinal Secretions and Their Usual pH

SECRETION	pH
Saliva	6.0–7.0
Gastric juice	1.0–3.5*
Pancreatic juice	8.0–8.3
Bile	7.8
Small intestine	7.5–8.0
Large intestine	7.5–8.0

*Gastric pH will probably be higher than 3.5 in patients receiving H_2-receptor antagonists.

Sodium Imbalances

The plasma sodium level varies in patients losing gastric fluid by vomiting and gastric suction. Recall that gastric fluid is usually isotonic or mildly hypotonic; therefore, the plasma sodium level will remain essentially normal unless other factors are present. For example, in the hospital setting, if excessive amounts of free water (such as 5% dextrose in water) are given, the plasma sodium concentration may drop below normal. This is particularly likely to occur because vomiting is a potent stimulus for the release of antidiuretic hormone (ADH), thus causing water retention. Hyponatremia is less likely to occur in the home-bound patient because vomiting usually precludes oral fluid intake until the problem is resolved. Of course, in the presence of other factors that increase free water loss (eg, fever and hyperventilation), it is possible that the plasma sodium level could be elevated.

Hypomagnesemia

Prolonged vomiting or gastric suction can result in magnesium deficit, an imbalance not as likely as those listed previously because the magnesium concentration in gastric juice is relatively low (1.4 mEq/L). However, it is likely to occur if losses are prolonged (lasting several weeks) and no magnesium is supplied in the IV fluids. Unfortunately, most routine electrolyte replacement solutions do not contain magnesium (e.g., lactated Ringer's solution and isotonic saline have none).

MANAGEMENT OF GASTRIC FLUID LOSS

Treatment of gastric fluid loss requires correction of both the hypokalemia and the hypochloremic alkalosis with adequate amounts of fluid, potassium, and sodium chloride.[6] One author recommends replacing gastric fluid losses with 5% dextrose in 0.45% NaCl/0.45% NaCl with 20 mEq KCl, given milliliter for milliliter of gastric fluid lost in the previous 24 hrs.[7] For gastric fluid losses more than 1500 mL in 24 hrs, it has been recommended that the electrolyte content of the lost fluid be analyzed and treatment planned accordingly.[8]

Examples of nursing diagnoses related to loss of gastric fluid loss in vomiting or nasogastric suction include:

- Fluid volume deficit related to loss of isotonic gastric fluid
- Alteration in acid–base balance (metabolic alkalosis) related to loss of hydrogen and chloride ions

Examples of nursing interventions for patients with vomiting are listed in Table 13-3, and those for nasogastric suction in Clinical Tip: Nursing Interventions for Patients With Gastric Suction.

DIARRHEA

FLUID AND ELECTROLYTE DISTURBANCES

Diarrhea is characterized by increased frequency of stools with excessive water content. It can have many causes, such as infectious agents (viral, bacterial, and parasitic), toxins, and certain drugs. Viral enteritis and bacterial infections (such as enterotoxigenic *Escherichia coli*, *Shigella*, and *Salmonella)* are the most common causes of diarrhea in the United States.[9] Common causes in hospitalized patients who develop diarrhea are antibiotics and fecal impactions. Diarrhea is classified into several categories, including osmotic, secretory, structural, and primary motility disorders. Examples of causes of osmotic diarrhea are ingestion of poorly absorbable solutes (eg, lactulose, sorbitol, mannitol, magnesium sulfate, magnesium hydroxide, and sodium phosphate), generalized malabsorption or maldigestion, and certain infections. Secretory diarrhea is caused by abnormal secretion of water and electrolytes into the bowel lumen. Examples of causes of secretory diarrhea include enterotoxigenic bacteria (e.g., *Escherichia coli* and *Vibrio cholerae*) and partial or recently relieved intestinal obstruction.[10] Diarrhea secondary to structural changes occur in inflammatory bowel disease, collagen vascular disease, and sprue. Imbalances likely to be associated with diarrhea include the following:

- Fluid volume deficit
- Metabolic acidosis
- Hypokalemia
- Hypomagnesemia
- Sodium imbalances

Fluid Volume Deficit

Volume depletion is secondary to sodium and water loss in the diarrheal fluid. Severe diarrhea can lead to a daily loss of 2 to 10 L of fluid, together with large quantities of electrolytes.[11] Obviously, prolonged diarrhea is a serious threat to water and electrolyte balance.

Metabolic Acidosis

The incidence of acid–base disorders in patients with severe diarrhea is about 70%, and the entire spectrum of disturbances may be seen.[12] However, metabolic acidosis is by far the most common disorder and is especially likely to occur in pediatric patients and in those with secretory or infectious diarrhea. Recall that intestinal fluids are relatively alkaline because of their bicarbonate content, as a result loss

TABLE 13–3

Nursing Interventions for Patients With Vomiting

1. Discourage the intake of plain water if vomiting is prolonged. Instead, encourage the frequent intake of small volumes of fluids containing electrolytes. (See Table 3-1 for a summary of the electrolyte content of commonly available oral fluids.)
2. Report vomiting early so that appropriate treatment can be started before fluid and electrolyte disturbances become severe. The physician will likely prescribe a medication to relieve nausea. If vomiting is prolonged and oral fluids are not retained, parenteral fluids are indicated .
3. Alter physical environment as much as possible to lessen stimuli for nausea (e.g., remove sources of unpleasant odors).
4. Promote bedrest when vomiting is severe; avoid quick movements because they often make nausea more severe.
5. Measure, or estimate as accurately as possible, the amount of vomitus so that lost water and electrolytes can be replaced by the parenteral route. In fact, all fluids lost and gained from the body should be measured.
6. Measure body weight daily to detect significant changes in fluid balance. Daily weights are helpful in detecting FVD, particularly if vomitus has not been measured. A patient on a starvation diet should lose about ½ lb/day; a loss in excess of this amount probably implies FVD. A weight gain in this situation implies FVE. Routine IV fluids are low in calories; for example, a liter of 5% dextrose solutions contains only 170 calories.
7. Monitor for imbalances associated with loss of gastric fluid (see preceding discussion).
8. Be familiar with parenteral fluids commonly used to replace gastric fluid. Solutions that may be prescribed include routine solutions (such as isotonic or half-strength saline) with added potassium and magnesium, or special gastric replacement solutions (see Chapter 10).

FVD, fluid volume deficit; FVE, fluid volume excess.

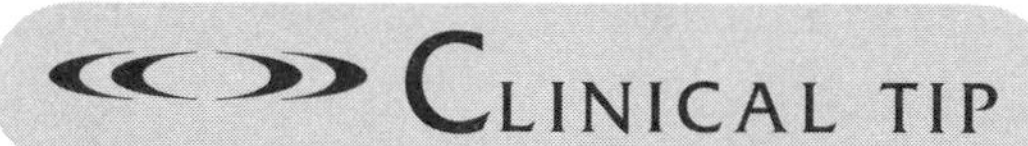

Nursing Interventions for Patients With Gastric Suction

1. Irrigate suction tube with isotonic saline (0.9% NaCl) if available. If tap water is used, limit volume to least amount possible to keep tube patent. When large amounts of plain water are instilled into the tube, gastric secretions are increased in an attempt to make the water "isotonic" for absorption. However, before the fluid can be absorbed, the gastric suction apparatus triggers on and pulls both the water and electrolytes out through the tube. This phenomenon is sometimes referred to as "electrolyte washout."
2. Prohibit the intake of large quantities of water or ice chips by mouth because water washes electrolytes from the stomach. Profound states of metabolic alkalosis and sodium deficit have been caused by the unwise practice of giving large quanitites of plain water to a patient undergoing gastric suction. (Metabolic alkalosis is less likely in patients receiving H_2-receptor antagonists.)
   Be aware that some physicians prefer that patients with gastric suction receive nothing by mouth; others allow small quantities of ice chips (such as 1 oz/hr). Be particularly careful when orders are written to give ice chips "sparingly"; this term is open to interpretation by the staff, and more ice may be given than was intended, especially if the patient asks frequently. Occasionally physicians will prescribe ice chips made from electrolyte solutions for patients experiencing great discomfort (dry mouth or thirst). Remember that true thirst should not be present if the patient is adequately hydrated via the parenteral route. The patient's desire for ice chips may be lessened by supplying a wet washcloth to apply to the lips and mouth.
3. Measure and record the amount of fluid lost by suction, as well as by all other fluid losses and gains.
4. Measure daily weight variations to help detect early fluid volume deficit (or excess related to excessive fluid replacement).
5. Monitor for imbalances associated with loss of gastric fluid (see previous discussion in this chapter).

of intestinal fluid is likely to lead to metabolic (hyperchloremic) acidosis. (The plasma chloride level increases as the bicarbonate level decreases.)

Hypokalemia

Diarrhea, due to a multitude of causes, can be associated with excessive stool losses of potassium and result in hypokalemia. The typical electrolyte disorder in patients with diarrhea is hypokalemia with hyperchloremic metabolic acidosis.[13] A clinically significant depletion of total body potassium is likely only when severe chronic diarrhea is present.[14] A profound potassium depletion can occur in patients with colonic villous adenomas that secrete a profuse amount of potassium-rich, watery mucus.

Hypomagnesemia

Magnesium deficit can occur with prolonged diarrhea, particularly if magnesium is not adequately replaced. Most routine electrolyte solutions do not contain magnesium (e.g., lactated Ringer's solution and isotonic saline have none).

Sodium Imbalances

The plasma sodium concentration varies in patients with diarrhea, depending on the cause of the problem and related clinical events. As discussed below, the diarrheal fluid may have a sodium content that is similar to, higher than, or lower than that of plasma. Extraneous factors also affect the plasma sodium concentration; among these are the amount of water intake (orally or IV) and the presence of fever or hyperventilation. Fever increases water loss in perspiration, and the compensatory hyperventilation associated with metabolic acidosis increases water loss from the lungs.

When the sodium content of the diarrheal fluid is similar to that of plasma, its loss causes an isotonic FVD (with no change in the plasma sodium level). This is often the case with diarrheal conditions classified as secretory diarrhea.[15] In contrast, diarrhea caused by osmotic conditions tends to be associated with relatively greater losses of water than sodium, resulting in a tendency toward an elevated plasma sodium concentration.[16] Hypernatremic dehydration due to watery diarrhea is most often seen in children less than 2 years of age.[17] In some types of diarrhea, sodium is lost in excess of water, causing a tendency toward hyponatremia. See Chapter 24 for a discussion of diarrhea in children.

MANAGEMENT OF DIARRHEAL FLUID LOSS

Most acute diarrheal episodes of viral or bacterial origin are self-limited and do not require specific therapy. If diarrhea is due to accumulation of poorly absorbed solutes in the intestine (osmotic diarrhea), it usually subsides with fasting. However, the diarrhea will usually persist despite fasting if it is a form of secretory diarrhea.[18]

Oral rehydration with glucose and electrolytes in infantile diarrhea is described in Chapter 24. It has been found that glucose in the solution promotes small intestinal sodium reabsorption as well as calories.

If oral fluids are not tolerated, parenteral fluids are indicated. For moderate increases in stool fluid (500–1000 mL/24 hrs), a replacement fluid of 0.45% NaCl plus 20 mEq of potassium acetate (which the liver converts to bicarbonate) might be used.[19] If the stool volume increases to more than 1 L/day, the replacement fluid might be changed to lactated Ringer's solution plus 20 mEq of KCl.[20]

Examples of nursing diagnoses for patients with diarrhea include:

- Fluid volume deficit due to loss of isotonic diarrheal fluid
- Alteration in potassium balance (hypokalemia) related to loss of potassium-rich diarrheal fluid

See Clinical Tip: Nursing Interventions for Patients With Diarrhea.

IMBALANCES ASSOCIATED WITH LAXATIVES AND ENEMAS

Laxatives and enemas are frequently used to treat constipation and to cleanse the colon before diagnostic radiological studies and abdominal surgical procedures. Whenever possible, constipation should be treated by nonpharmacological means (Table 13-4). When

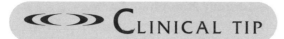

Nursing Interventions for Patients With Diarrhea

1. Measure, or estimate as accurately as possible, the amount of liquid feces so that lost water and electrolytes can be replaced (either by oral electrolyte solutions or via the parenteral route). All fluids gained and lost from the body should be measured and recorded on the I&O record. (See discussion of I&O measurement in Chapter 2.)
2. Measure body weight daily to detect significant changes in fluid balance. Daily weights are helpful in detecting fluid volume deficit, particularly if liquid stools have not been measured.
3. Monitor for clinical and laboratory indicators of imbalances commonly associated with the loss of intestinal fluid (see text). Specific imbalances are described in Chapters 3–9.
4. Offer oral electrolyte-containing liquids if allowed by the type of diarrhea present. (Some types of diarrhea respond better to temporary fasting and parenteral fluid replacement.)(See Table 24-1.)
5. Monitor response to parenteral fluids (if they are indicated) to replace fluid losses. Commonly used fluids for this purpose are lactated Ringer's solution and half strength saline (0.45% NaCl) with added potassium. Other electrolytes (such as magnesium) are replaced as indicated. Nursing responsibilities in fluid replacement therapy are described in Chapter 10.

I&O, intake and output.

these measures are not feasible or are ineffective, occasional use of laxatives or enemas may be indicated. However, the fluid and electrolyte problems that may accompany the injudicious use of laxatives and enemas must be considered. These fluid and electrolyte problems vary according to the nature of the laxative or enema solution used.

LAXATIVES

Patients with impaired renal function are at risk for hypermagnesemia and hyperphosphatemia when magnesium salts (such as magnesium citrate, magnesium sulfate, and milk of magnesia) or sodium phosphate solutions are administered because their kidneys are unable to excrete these substances adequately.[24] This can be a problem as magnesium-containing laxatives are frequently administered in quantities sufficient to cause toxic serum levels of magnesium when renal function is impaired.[25] Of interest, several instances have been described in which hypermagnesemia developed in patients with *normal* renal function (after administration of large doses of magnesium sulfate to facilitate poison removal from the GI tract).[26] Magnesium and phosphate cathartics are further contraindicated in patients with poor bowel motility (as occurs in adynamic ileus) because slowed motility increases the likelihood of absorption. A fatal case of hyperphosphatemia secondary to the administration of Fleet Phospho-Soda as a cathartic to a 64-year-old man with colonic ileus was recently reported.[27]

ENEMAS

Tap Water Enemas

Repeated tap water enemas can result in excessive water absorption by the colon and thus dilutional hyponatremia. Excessive water absorption from the colon has been observed in states of chronic constipation and megacolon. Especially at risk are young children. Also thought to be at increased risk are adults with congestive heart failure, AIDS, and malignancy.[28] A case of severe hyponatremia and irreversible brain damage associated with tap water

TABLE 13–4

Nursing Interventions Related to Laxative and Enema Abuse

1. Encourage patients to avoid the repeated use of cathartics and enemas and rely on other methods to achieve bowel evacuation regularity.
2. Encourage maximum level of tolerated physical activity. Regular exercise stimulates gut motility and is an important part of a bowel management program. Walking 20 to 30 minutes a day is a good form of exercise. For immobilized patients, even small increases in activity may be helpful. For example, modest activities such as sitting up in bed or turning and twisting in a chair cause changes in colonic motility.[21]
3. Encourage ingestion of a glass of warm fluid first thing in the morning to stimulate the evacuation reflex.
4. Encourage regular fluid intake to act as a stool softener. For example, a glass or two of water on rising, between meals, and before bedtime should be consumed if tolerated.[22]
5. Encourage adequate bulk in the diet. Wheat bran is an excellent source that is available in many cereals and breads; approximately 3 Tbs supplies roughly 10 g of dietary fiber.[23] Most fruits and vegetables are good sources of fiber. Dietary fiber holds water, causing stools to be softer, bulkier, and heavier. The increased bowel bulk causes quicker movement of stool through the colon.
6. Encourage patients to attempt to develop a regular bowel routine. The best time to attempt a bowel elimination is probably after breakfast because this is the time when the strongest propulsive contractions occur.

enemas in a patient with spinal cord injury was reported by Chertow and Brady.[29] Before receiving five tap water enemas of 1.5 to 3 L each over a 10-day period, the patient (a 65-year-old man with C-6 quadriplegia) had mild symptomless hyponatremia and a baseline glomerular filtration rate (GFR) of 82 mL/min. During the fifth enema, the patient became confused and developed seizures. Despite treatment with hypertonic saline, the patient remained comatose. The authors emphasized that the colonic mucosa can absorb life-threatening amounts of water in patients with ineffective renal water clearance ability.

Sodium Phosphate Enemas

Sodium phosphate enemas are available over the counter in pediatric (2.25 oz) and adult (4.5 oz) sizes (Fleet, C.B. Fleet Co., Lynchburg, VA). Because these enemas are composed of a hypertonic sodium phosphate solution, they act as an osmotic laxative by causing an increase in fluid volume of the colon, thus distending the colon and causing peristalsis to become more vigorous; ultimately, defecation occurs. However, if defecation does not occur before the hypertonic enema solution is absorbed by the colon, these enemas may produce a series of fluid and electrolyte problems (primarily hyperphosphatemia, hypernatremia, and hypocalcemia). The hyperphosphatemia and hypernatremia are a result of direct absorption of these electrolytes from the enema solution; hypocalcemia is a reciprocal response to hyperphosphatemia.

Imbalances occur primarily in patients unable to eliminate the enema solution adequately before significant absorption occurs. There have been reports of hyperphosphatemia, hypernatremia, and hypocalcemia after the use of sodium phosphate enemas in patients with GI disorders that interfere with prompt elimination of the enema solution (such as megacolon or fecal impaction).[30,31] Because of this finding, the manufacturer warns that sodium phosphate (Fleet) enemas should not be used in patients with conditions predisposing to retention of the enema solution (e.g., congenital megacolon, imperforate anus, or colostomy). The manufacturer of sodium phosphate enemas warns that if after the enema solution is administered there is no return of the liquid, a physician should be contacted immediately as dehydration could occur.[32] The manufacturer also advises caution in the use of sodium phosphate enemas in patients with impaired renal function, heart disease, or preexisting electrolyte disturbances or in patients on calcium channel blockers, diuretics, or other medications that can affect electrolyte levels because hyperphosphatemia, hypocalcemia, and hypernatremia and acidosis may occur.[33]

Risks in Children

Most published reports of adverse effects from sodium phosphate enemas involve small children; usually the children had GI or renal problems, but sometimes they did not. It is helpful to review some of these cases to fully grasp the potential seriousness of the use of sodium phosphate enemas in young children.

Use of adult-sized sodium phosphate enemas for constipation or bowel cleansing before surgery or diagnostic procedures in children can produce disastrous results. A case of hypocalcemia and severe hyperphosphatemia was reported in a 4-year-old boy who received adult-sized sodium phosphate enemas for the treatment of constipation.[34] Due to tetany from the hypocalcemia, the child's extremities were stiff and could not be actively or passively moved. After treatment with IV calcium gluconate and oral calcium supplements, and hydration to promote diuresis, the child's condition improved. A similar case was described in which a previously healthy 5-month-old child suffered severe hyperphosphatemia, hypocalcemia, acidosis, and shock after administration of an adult-sized sodium phosphate enema for the treatment of constipation.[35] Still another tragic occurrence involved the administration of four adult-sized sodium phosphate (Fleet) enemas to an 11-month-old male infant admitted for surgical correction of an imperforate anus.[36] The child had a sigmoid colostomy constructed shortly after birth. Two enemas were given in each barrel of the colostomy. Before the enemas, the child also received 800 mL of GI lavage solution (GoLytely). Approximately 2.5 hrs after the enemas were administered, cardiac arrest occurred. Despite extensive resuscitative efforts with IV calcium, phosphate-binding resins per ostomy, and peritoneal dialysis, the child died. The marked hypernatremia, acidemia, hyperphosphatemia, and hypocalcemia observed before the child's death were replicated in an animal model in which the same enemas were administered before anal obstruction with balloon catheters. In the pig model, the retained enema solution was lethal at a dose of 20 to 30 mL/kg. The manufacturer of sodium phosphate (Fleet) enemas warns that adult-sized enemas should not be used in children under 12 years of age and that the children's size should not be administered to children less than 2 years of age.[37]

Not all cases of serious electrolyte disturbances in children after sodium phosphate enemas involve the use of adult-sized enemas. A situation was reported in which two sodium phosphate *pediatric* enemas were administered to a girl aged 2 years, 6 months in preparation for a radiographic procedure.[38] Subsequently she developed coma, tetany, dehydration, hypotension, tachycardia, and hyperpyrexia. Laboratory results indicated severe hyperphosphatemia, hypocalcemia, hypernatremia, and acidosis. Apparently about one-third of the administered enema solution was absorbed systemically.

Although more likely in high-risk patients, electrolyte disturbances from sodium phosphate enemas have also been reported in patients with no obvious underlying disease process.[39–41] Because most of the adverse effects with these enemas involve small children, some investigators reiterate that sodium phosphate enemas should be avoided in children under 2 years of age and that they should be used only with caution in those 2 to 5 years of age, especially if underlying bowel or renal dysfunction exists.[42] Still other researchers recommend against the use of sodium phosphate enemas entirely in small children and infants, indicating that it is incorrect to assume that sodium phosphate solutions are not absorbed by the colon.[43] Because sodium phosphate enemas are available over the counter, it has been recommended that parents be made aware that these enemas can be dangerous to infants, and that prominent labeling be provided on the enema containers to indicate the potential dangers associated with their administration to infants.[44] Nurses should take an active part in educating parents about the dangers of nonjudious use of enemas. Many clinicians favor the use of isotonic saline (0.9% NaCl) as an enema solution for patients of all ages to minimize fluid and electrolyte changes associated with absorption of the enema solution.

Risks in the Elderly

The elderly are also at increased risk for electrolyte disturbances associated with sodium phosphate enemas, particularly if they have atonic colons and/or renal failure. A recent case report of a 77-year-old woman who developed severe hyperphosphatemia and hypocalcemia after the administration of multiple sodium phosphate (Fleet) enemas to relieve fecal impaction indicates the potential problem in elderly patients.[45] (See Case Study 8-2.) The investigators cautioned against the over-aggressive use of sodium phosphate enemas in elderly patients with fecal impactions because of the potential for prolonged retention of the enema solution; they further recommended that isotonic enemas be used instead whenever possible.[46]

A study of 14 elderly subjects (mean age, 78.5 years) indicated that sodium phosphate (Fleet) enemas carry a potential risk for acutely ill elderly patients.[47] To avoid untoward effects due to hyperphosphatemia and hypocalcemia, these researchers recommended that the phosphate load be adjusted to the patient's level of renal function. In that way, the amount of phosphate that could conceivably be retained by the colon could ultimately be safely excreted by the kidneys.

STANDARD BOWEL PREPARATIONS VERSUS POLYETHYLENE GLYCOL LAVAGE FOR DIAGNOSTIC STUDIES AND SURGERY

Two commonly used regimens to cleanse the colon before colonoscopy or colon surgery consist of (1) a clear liquid or low-residue diet for 1 to 3 days, plus laxatives and enemas, and (2) the rapid ingestion (either orally or by nasogastric tube) of a balanced electrolyte-polyethylene glycol (PEG) solution. Polyethylene glycol is a nonabsorbed osmotic agent. Among the commercially available PEG lavage solutions are GoLytely (Braintree Laboratories, Inc., Braintree, MA) and Colyte (Reed and Carnrick, Jersey City, NJ). When reconstituted with water, Colyte contains 125 mEq/L sodium, 10 mEq/L potassium, 20 mEq/L bicarbonate, 80 mEq/L sulfate, 35 mEq/L chloride, and 18 mEq/L PEG 3350.[48] Approximately 1.5 L/hr of a PEG lavage solution are ingested in adults until the rectal effluent is clear or up to 4 L are consumed. According to the manufacturers, large volumes may be administered without significant changes in fluid and electrolyte balance because the osmotic activity of the PEG lavage results in virtually no net absorption or excretion of ions or water.

A survey of 206 physicians regarding preferences for a primary mechanical bowel cleansing method indicated that 51% preferred cathartics and enemas, 43% the PEG lavage method, and the rest preferred less commonly used methods.[49] The same group of physicians estimated the incidence of fluid and electrolyte complications at 10% for patients receiving cathartics and enemas and 5% for patients receiving the PEG lavage method. The investigators noted that complications are usually underreported in survey research.

Several studies indicated that neither of the two commonly used methods (traditional bowel preparation and PEG lavage) results in clinically significant changes in body weight, blood chemistries, and hematological values. In the studies, changes associated with PEG lavage were less pronounced than those associated with the traditional mechanical method.[50–52] For example, Beck et al.[51,52] described an average weight loss of 2.2 lb with a standard bowel preparation as opposed to 0.1 lb loss with PEG lavage (GoLytely). Ambrose et al.[53] found that the serum sodium increased an average of 0.35 mEq/L with the PEG lavage method and decreased an average of 1.2 mEq/L with a cathartic and rectal washout method.

Compared with the traditional method, the major advantage of PEG lavage is the considerably shorter time needed for preparation. Because the food restriction period is shortened by as much as 2 or 3 days, hunger and associated weakness are less problematic. A disadvantage is nausea, abdominal fullness, and bloating (occurring in up to 50% of patients) associated with rapid ingestion of the PEG lavage.[54] Some patients complain that the PEG lavage solution has a disagreeable mildly salty taste and refuse to drink it. Chilling the solution makes it more palatable. The manufacturers recommend that patients fast for approximately 3 or 4 hrs before ingesting the solution. They emphasize that solid food should not be allowed for at least 2 hrs before the solution is given. Only clear liquids are allowed during the interval between PEG lavage solution ingestion and examination.

A major disadvantage of the traditional method is the 1- to 3-day period of reduced food intake, resulting in hunger and weakness. Adding to the discomfort is the use of laxatives and enemas. Rigorous use of cathartics and numerous cleansing enemas after several days of dietary restrictions can present problems for elderly patients, particularly those with cardiovascular disease. Thus, the elderly patient undergoing rigorous bowel preparation should be observed closely for adverse reactions. Care should be taken to perform the procedure correctly the first time to avoid the need for repeated roentgenograms (requiring more cathartics, more enemas, and more fluid restriction). The elderly patient cannot afford to undergo one test after another without a rest period in between; it is frequently the nurse's responsibility to intervene in this area on the patient's behalf. The already-reduced GFR in the elderly potentiates the hazards of any further decrease in ECF volume (as occurs in vigorous catharsis). The aged patient having GI roentgenograms should probably receive IV fluids during the preparation period of reduced oral intake and increased fluid loss (caused by catharsis and enema). Note also that use of radiocontrast agents in diagnostic radiology (particularly in large doses) has been incriminated as predisposing to acute renal failure, especially when the patient has a severe FVD. See Chapter 25 for further discussion of the effect of standard bowel preparations on elderly patients.

In a clinical study, serum magnesium levels were found to be increased in patients receiving the standard preparation when compared with those in patients receiving a PEG lavage solution.[55] Presumably the higher magnesium levels resulted from use of magnesium citrate as a laxative. Although the serum magnesium concentrations remained within a normal range, the potential for hypermagnesemia could be an important consideration in patients with renal insufficiency because they lack the ability to excrete magnesium normally.

LOSS OF FLUID THROUGH FISTULAS

Fistulas are abnormal communications between the intestine and the skin (external fistula) or another hollow viscus (internal fistula). They can result from trauma or occur spontaneously as a complication of pancreatitis, inflammatory bowel disease, neoplasia, or other GI disorders. The majority of external GI fistulas that develop postoperatively are the result of technical complications.[56] Fistulas can develop at any level in the GI tract.

The three factors that are most associated with increased mortality in patients with GI fistulas are fluid and electrolyte disturbances, sepsis, and malnutrition.[57] Loss of fluid from fistulas can produce serious fluid and electrolyte disturbances. External gastric, duodenal, and jejunal fistulas can drain up to 5 L/day.[58] Failure to adequately replace large fistulous losses can lead to fluid volume deficit, hypoperfusion, and eventually multiple organ failure.[59]

The electrolytes lost in fistulous drainage depend on the exact site of the fistula. An educated guess regarding imbalances likely to accompany a specific fluid's loss can be made by reviewing the usual electrolyte content of fluid in the region of the fistula (see Table 13-1). When doubt about the fistula's origin exists, sending a sample of the drainage fluid to the laboratory for analysis of pH and electrolyte composition can aid in determining replacement therapy.

Intestinal fluids, including pancreatic and biliary secretions, are relatively alkaline because of their bicarbonate content. Thus, loss of these fluids would likely lead to metabolic acidosis. In contrast, loss of chloride-rich gastric fluid predisposes to metabolic alkalosis.

Although fluid and electrolyte problems are possible with any fistula, they are most likely to be substantial in patients with pancreatic, duodenal stump, and gastrojejunal anastomotic fistulas.[60] Biliary and pancreatic fistulous drainage contains sizable amounts of sodium and bicarbonate, predisposing to FVD and metabolic acidosis. Hyponatremia can easily occur if fluid replacement contains more free water than needed. High-output pancreatic fistulas produce more than 200 mL/day.[61]

Drainage from external fistulas can often be collected with a well-fixed stoma appliance. The volume of drainage collected in this device should be measured and recorded on the intake–output record. If the drainage cannot be obtained and directly measured, an estimate should be made of the volume absorbed by dressings and bed linens. Of course, skin care is essential to guard against the effects of autodigestion by GI enzymes. A variety of skin barrier films and other preparations are available for this purpose.

It seems prudent to provide aggressive nutritional support for patients with fistulas.[62] Nutritional support can be in the form of total parenteral nutrition (TPN) or enteral feedings. When tolerated, enteral feedings are preferred because they are more effective in maintaining intestinal integrity and therefore in decreasing bacterial translocation and infection. When enteral feedings are used, the feeding tube is inserted about 30 to 40 cm past the fistula.[63]

Several studies have reported increased spontaneous closure rates of fistulas as well as decreased mortality rates when IV hyperalimentation was used.[64,65] Data exist to suggest that somatostatin used in conjunction with nutritional support allows spontaneous closure of fistulas to occur earlier.[66,67]

IMBALANCES ASSOCIATED WITH ANOREXIA NERVOSA

Anorexia nervosa can be subdivided into the "restricting" form in which the patient loses weight by self-induced starvation and perhaps compulsive exercising, and the "bulimic" form, in which there is a combination of marked dietary restriction and episodes of binging, vomiting, and diuretic/laxative abuse.[68] Serious, even life-threatening, fluid and electrolyte problems are understandably possible in patients with eating disorders. The prognosis for severe bulimia nervosa is less favorable than for uncomplicated anorexia nervosa.[69] One study of 168 patients with bulimia or related eating disorders found about 50% had some sort of electrolyte abnormality.[70]

The type of electrolyte abnormalities in anorexic patients depends on whether or not self-induced vomiting is the predominant behavior, or whether laxative or diuretic abuse is dominant.[71] A careful history is needed to determine which methods are used by the patient to lose weight. Among the more frequent fluid and electrolyte problems observed in patients with eating disorders are FVD, hypokalemia, hypomagnesemia, hypophosphatemia, hyponatremia, hypocalcemia, and either metabolic alkalosis or metabolic acidosis.

FLUID VOLUME DEFICIT

This condition is most likely in patients who take large doses of diuretics and laxatives. Clinically, hypotension (<90/60 mmHg) and postural dizziness or syncope may be present. Also, the BUN is elevated out of proportion to the serum creatinine level. Skin turgor may appear normal despite FVD in adolescents or young adults who characteristically have good skin elasticity.

HYPOKALEMIA

Hypokalemia is possible due to excessive losses from vomiting and laxative abuse, coupled with poor dietary intake. If the patient has access to potassium-losing diuretics, such as the thiazides, the likelihood of hypokalemia is even greater. (Chlorothiazide and hydrochlorothiazides are commonly abused diuretic agents.)[72] Hypokalemia is a particularly dangerous imbalance because of the possibility of cardiac arrhythmias. One researcher recommends that patients with serum potassium concentrations less than 2.5 mEq/L be hospitalized for bedrest and treatment.[73] Hypokalemic nephropathy can follow prolonged potassium depletion in anorectics and be associated with the development of polyuria, polydipsia, and elevated serum creatinine levels.[74]

HYPOMAGNESEMIA

Like hypokalemia, hypomagnesemia is possible because of excessive losses from vomiting and diuretic or laxative abuse, coupled with poor dietary intake. Hypomagnesemia has been reported in up to 25% of patients and is often associated with refractory hypokalemia and hypocalcemia that may not resolve unless the hypomagnesemia is corrected simultaneously.[75]

HYPOPHOSPHATEMIA

Hypophosphatemia is an ominous sign in eating disorder patients.[76] The etiology of hypophosphatemia is not clear, but is most likely the result of inadequate oral intake and absorption of phosphorus. It is most problematic during aggressive refeeding when rapid glucose-rich hyperalimentation causes extracellular phosphorus to shift into the cells, thus further lowering the serum phosphorus levels. This may result in myocardial dysfunction and neurological complications, such as convulsions.[77] Thus, plasma phosphorus levels should be monitored for several days in any malnourished patient during refeeding and supplements administered as indicated.

HYPONATREMIA

Hyponatremia may result from excessive sodium losses from diuretic and laxative abuse, as well as from self-induced vomiting. However, it may also result from excessive water intake. Several cases have recently been reported in which patients affected by anorexia nervosa presented with seizures secondary to self-induced water intoxication. One of these was a 17-year-old girl who ingested an average water intake of 7 to 8 L/day.[78] Her history did not include abuse of laxatives or diuretics. Upon admission to the hospital with a generalized tonic–clonic seizure, her serum sodium level was found to be 116 mEq/L.

HYPOCALCEMIA

Hypocalcemia can result from poor dietary intake and diminished bone stores of calcium after prolonged malnutrition. Ionized levels of calcium are decreased in patients with metabolic alkalosis, a common imbalance in those with vomiting and potassium-losing diuretic abuse.

ACID–BASE IMBALANCES

In a study of 168 bulimic patients, metabolic alkalosis was found to be the most frequent acid–base imbalance.[79] It is commonly associated with loss of gastric fluid from vomiting and with the abuse of potassium-losing diuretics.

Metabolic acidosis (due to the loss of alkaline intestinal fluid) may be the predominant acid–base disturbance if the patient is a heavy abuser of laxatives. Some patients have been reported to take as many as 100 laxative doses per day.[80] Most commonly taken are stimulant-type laxatives that are available over-the-counter (such as Correctol, Ex-Lax, and Senokot).[81] The most common diuretic agent used by adolescents and young adults is ammonium chloride (available without a prescription); abuse of this drug compounds the metabolic acidosis caused by laxative abuse.[82]

In summary, patients with eating disorders must be observed closely for life-threatening electrolyte abnormalities. As pointed out by Hofland and Dardia,[83] bulimia is a psychiatric disorder, but morbidity and mortality can occur because of the physical problems. For example, sudden death with unexplained cardiovascular collapse may occur secondary to electrolyte-induced arrhythmias. These arrhythmias may result from imbalances such as hypokalemia, hypomagnesemia, and altered pH disturbances, all of which are commonly present in eating disorder patients. Although these risks are present in the purely "restrictive" forms of the disease, they are even greater in those who abuse laxatives and diuretics. Refeeding the starving patient also carries increased risks for cardiac dysfunction, especially if performed too aggressively. In general, a cautious and gradual approach with regular blood electrolyte analyses is indicated in the initial period of refeeding.[84]

IMBALANCES ASSOCIATED WITH INTESTINAL OBSTRUCTION

Intestinal obstruction causes interference with the normal progression of intestinal contents. A common indication for emergency intervention, small bowel obstruction accounts for 20% of all acute surgical admissions.[85] Intestinal obstruction may be termed either complete or incomplete. A mechanical obstruction is defined as an actual physical barrier (e.g., adhesions, hernia, tumor, or diverticula) blocking normal passage of intestinal contents. A mechanical obstruction is termed *simple* when there is no compromise in vascular supply; it is termed *strangulated* when the vascular supply is inhibited. A functional obstruction is sometimes referred to as *paralytic ileus*, or an *adynamic* or *neurogenic ileus*. As the name implies, the obstruction is caused by ineffective or nonpropulsive peristalsis. Although motor activity is slowed, it is not completely absent. Causes of paralytic ileus can include intraabdominal conditions such as peritonitis, appendicitis, cholecystitis, and pancreatitis. Other causes involve trauma and systemic conditions such as hypokalemia, uremia, and septicemia.

Simple mechanical obstruction results in a striking accumulation of intestinal fluid and gas above the obstruction. Most of the gas is due to swallowed air, although some results from bacterial fermentation within the gut. Because of distention, large quantities of water and electrolytes are secreted into the bowel lumen, even in the absence of oral intake. Fluid also accumulates within the bowel wall. The edematous bowel wall is not able to absorb the large volume of intestinal secretions; therefore, distention becomes progressively greater, leading to isotonic contraction of the ECF compartment as fluid is sequestered in the bowel (third-space effect). Ten liters or more of fluid can collect in this third space and lead to hypovolemic shock. Vomiting or nasogastric suctioning add to the fluid losses. (Nursing assessment for third-space fluid shift is described in Chapter 3.)

In adynamic ileus, decreased propulsive motility can affect the small intestine and colon, separately or together. As in mechanical obstruction, gas accumulates in the involved intestine, producing marked distention. Fluid also accumulates in the intestine because of decreased absorption. Although third-space fluid loss may be significant, it is not likely to be as great as in mechanical obstruction.

Plasma concentrations of electrolytes are initially preserved because the fluid lost is primarily isotonic; however, the patient usually becomes thirsty and drinks water, thereby developing hyponatremia.[86] Contributing to hyponatremia is the endogenous release of water produced by oxidation. Sodium and other electrolytes (such as potassium and magnesium) are also lost by vomiting or as a result of GI suction after treatment is initiated. If the lost electrolytes are not replaced, deficits will eventually result.

The type of acid–base imbalance likely to be encountered is largely determined by the site of the obstruction. Metabolic alkalosis is common with pyloric or high small intestinal obstruction in which copious vomiting produces loss of acidic gastric juice. Sometimes in upper small-intestinal obstruction, the patient will vomit approximately equal volumes of gastric and intestinal juice, thus preventing serious disturbances in pH levels. If the obstruction is in a distal segment of the small intestine, the patient may vomit larger quantities of alkaline fluids than of acid fluids. (Recall that secretions below the pylorus are mainly alkaline.) Thus, metabolic acidosis can result from a low intestinal obstruction. If the obstruction is below the proximal colon, most of the GI fluids will be absorbed before reaching the point of obstruction, and thus acid–base balance may remain intact. In this situation, solid fecal matter accumulates until symptoms of discomfort develop. Respiratory acidosis can develop in patients with abdominal distention because respirations are compromised by upward pressure on the diaphragm, resulting in carbon dioxide retention. Impairment of renal function due to severe hypovolemia can lead to metabolic acidosis, as can starvation with subsequent ketoacidosis.[87]

CASE STUDIES

13-1. A 16-year-old high school student was brought to the Emergency Room after experiencing a seizure within a few minutes of complaints of dizziness and faintness. According to her parents, she had a history of restrictive dietary intake (interspersed with brief periods of binge eating) and self-induced vomiting, as well as heavy abuse of laxatives. At the time of admission, her body weight was 79 lbs (height, 63 inches). Lying flat, her blood pressure (BP) was 88/54 mmHg and her pulse rate was 98/min; upon standing, her BP dropped to 64/46 mmHg and her pulse rate increased to 130/min. Blood chemistries revealed the following:

Sodium	=	128 mEq/L
Chloride	=	90 mEq/L
Potassium	=	2.5 mEq/L
CO_2 content	=	29 mEq/L
Magnesium	=	1.8 mEq/L
BUN	=	30 mg/dL
Calcium	=	8.5 mg/dL
Creatinine	=	1.2 mg/dL
Phosphorus	=	2.6 mg/dL

The patient was treated with 0.9% NaCl with added KCl intravenously. After stabilization, she was cautiously started on TPN. Several days after treatment was initiated, the patient experienced fluid retention (as evidenced by mild puffiness and bloating).

COMMENTARY: Probably the seizure was caused by FVD, which was associated with cerebral hypoperfusion and hyponatremia (which predisposed to a reduced seizure threshold because of mild brain swelling). Note that several typical indicators of FVD were present in this patient (namely, postural hypotension, tachycardia, and a BUN elevated out of proportion to the serum creatinine level).

Isotonic saline was not only effective in expanding her ECF volume, it helped correct the lower than normal serum sodium and chloride levels. Both the FVD and hyponatremia were probably due to self-induced vomiting, laxative abuse, and poor dietary intake.

The low serum potassium level (2.5 mEq/L) was quite serious and required admission to an intensive care unit for cardiac monitoring until corrected.

It is not uncommon for anorexics who are chronically fluid volume depleted to develop a compensatory increased production of aldosterone (which causes the kidneys to conserve sodium and water). This compensatory renal mechanism begins slowly but once initiated persists after FVD is corrected, resulting in temporary fluid retention during purgation-free periods.[88] Eating disorder patients usually find this phenomenon highly distressing and often renew their pattern of vomiting and laxative/diuretic abuse to relieve bloating.

13-2. An 80-year-old woman was admitted to the hospital with a history of diarrhea (average of six watery stools per day) over a period of several weeks. The following laboratory data were obtained:

Sodium	=	135 mEq/L
Arterial pH	=	7.25
Potassium	=	3.0 mEq/L
$PaCO_2$,	=	28 mmHg
Chloride	=	111 mEq/L
HCO_3,	=	12 mEq/L

COMMENTARY: Note the presence of metabolic acidosis, as indicated by the low pH and bicarbonate concentration. This is a normal anion gap acidosis: $Na - (HCO_3 + Cl) = 12$ mEq/L [135 − (12 + 111) = 12]. The $PaCO_2$ is appropriately reduced as a compensatory change.

13-3. A 40-year-old woman was admitted with a 5-day history of nausea and episodic vomiting. She complained of feeling lightheaded upon standing. Lying flat, her BP was 102/68 mmHg and her pulse rate was 92/min; standing up, her BP fell to 92/60 mmHg and her pulse rate rose to 110/min. The following laboratory data were observed:

Sodium	=	143 mEq/L
Arterial pH	=	7.53
Potassium	=	2.9 mEq/L
$PaCO_2$,	=	47 mmHg
Chloride	=	85 mEq/L
HCO_3,	=	36 mEq/L

COMMENTARY: This patient had a fluid volume deficit, as evidenced by the postural changes in BP and pulse rate. She also had metabolic alkalosis (secondary to loss of Cl^- and H^+ from vomiting), as evidenced by the greater than normal arterial pH and elevated HCO_3 level. The $PaCO_2$ was elevated as a compensatory mechanism. The low serum potassium was related to loss of potassium in vomitus and in the urine (see text for further explanation).

REFERENCES

1. Rose B: Clinical Physiology of Acid-Base and Electrolyte Disorders, 4th ed, p 389. New York, McGraw-Hill, 1994
2. Kokko J, Tannen R: Fluids and Electrolytes, 2nd ed, p 924. Philadelphia, WB Saunders, 1990
3. Narins R: Clinical Disorders of Fluid and Electrolyte Metabolism, 5th ed, p 947. New York, McGraw-Hill, 1994
4. Kokko, Tannen, p 924
5. Szerlip H, Goldfarb S: Fluid and Electrolyte Disorders, p 138. New York, Churchill Livingstone, 1993
6. Narins, p 680
7. Pemberton L, Pemberton D: Treatment of Water, Electrolyte and Acid-Base Disorders in the Surgical Patient, p 54. New York, McGraw-Hill, 1994
8. Ibid
9. Woodley M, Whelan A (eds): Manual of Medical Therapeutics, 27th ed, p 290. Boston, Little, Brown, 1992
10. Narins, p 1143
11. Ibid
12. Ibid, p 1145
13. Szerlip, Goldfarb, p 92
14. Narins, p 1143
15. Rose, p 644
16. Ibid
17. Narins, p 1143
18. Woodley, Whelan, p 291
19. Pemberton, Pemberton, p 55
20. Ibid
21. Ellickson E: Bowel management plan for the homebound elderly. J Gerontol Nurs 14(1):16,1988
22. Yakabowich M: Prescribe with care: The role of laxatives in the treatment of constipation. J Gerontol Nurs 16(7):4,1990
23. Preece G, Judd C: Constipation in the elderly: Are drugs the only alternative to irregularity? Canadian Pharmaceutical J 115(4):136,1982
24. Yakabowich, p 4
25. Shires G: Fluids, Electrolytes, and Acid-Base, p 16. New York, Churchill Livingstone, 1988
26. Jones et al: Cathartic-induced magnesium toxicity during overdose management. Ann Emerg Med 15: 1214,1986

27. Fass R, et al: Fatal hyperphosphatemia following Fleet Phospho-Soda in a patient with colonic ileus. Am J Gastroenterol 88(6):929–932,1993
28. Chertow G, Brady H: Hyponatremia from tap-water enema. Lancet 344(8924):748,1994
29. Ibid
30. Moseley P, Segar W: Fluid and serum electrolyte disturbances as a complication of enemas in Hirchsprung's disease. Am J Dis Child 115:714,1968
31. Korzets A, et al: Life-threatening hyperphosphatemia and hypocalcemic tetany following the use of fleet enemas. J Am Geriatr Soc 40(6):6210–6211,1992
32. Physician's Desk Reference, 48th ed, p 945. Oradell, NJ, Medical Economics Company, 1994
33. Ibid
34. Edmondson S, Almquist T: Iatrogenic hypocalcemic tetany. Ann Emerg Med 19:938,1990
35. Wason S, et al: Severe hyperphosphatemia, hypocalcemia, acidosis, and shock in a 5-month old child following the administration of an adult Fleet enema. Ann Emerg Med 18:696,1989
36. Martin et al: Fatal poisoning from sodium phosphate enema: Case report and experimental study. JAMA 257(16):2190,1987
37. PDR, p 945
38. Sotos et al: Hypocalcemic coma following two pediatric phosphate enemas. Pediatrics 60(3):305,1977
39. Swerdlow D, et al: Tetany and enemas: Report of a case. Dis Colon Rectum 17:786,1974
40. Davis et al: Hypocalcemia, hyperphosphatemia, and dehydration following a single hypertonic phosphate enema. J Pediatr 90:484,1977
41. Levitt M, et al: Inorganic phosphate (laxative) poisoning resulting in tetany in an infant. J Pediatr 82:479,1973
42. Craig J, et al: Phosphate enema poisoning in children. Med J Austr 160(6):347–351,1994
43. Martin, p 2192
44. Wason et al, p 696
45. Korzets et al, p 620
46. Ibid
47. Grosskopf et al: Hyperphosphatemia and hypocalcemia induced by hypertonic phosphate enema—An experimental study and review of the literature. Hum Exper Toxicol 10(5):351–355,1991
48. PDR, p 1836
49. Beck D, Fazio V: Current preoperative bowel cleansing methods. Dis Colon Rectum 33:12,1990
50. Fleites et al: The efficacy of polyethylene glycol- electrolyte lavage solution versus traditional mechanical bowel preparation for elective colonic surgery: A randomized prospective, blinded clinical trial. Surgery 98(4):708,1985
51. Beck D, et al: Comparison of oral lavage methods for preoperative colonic cleansing. Dis Colon Rectum 29:699,1986
52. Beck et al: Comparison of cleansing methods in preparation for colonic surgery. Dis Colon Rectum 28:491,1985
53. Ambrose et al: A physiological appraisal of polyethylene glycol and a balanced electrolyte solution as bowel preparation. Br J Surg 70:428,1983
54. PDR, p 635
55. DiPalma et al: Comparison of colon cleansing methods in preparation for colonoscopy. Gastroenterology 86:856,1984
56. Schwartz S, Shires G, Spencer F: Principles of surgery, 6th ed, p 476. New York, McGraw-Hill, 1994
57. Fischer J (ed): Total Parenteral Nutrition, 2nd ed, p 153. Boston, Little, Brown, 1991
58. Edmunds L, et al: External fistulas arising from the gastrointestinal tract. Ann Surg 152:445,1960
59. Zaloga G (ed): Nutrition in Critical Care, p 625. St. Louis, CV Mosby, 1994
60. Kokko, Tannen, p 937
61. Schwartz, p 478
62. Zaloga, p 625
63. Ibid, p 316
64. Chapman R, et al: Management of intestinal fistulas. Am J Surg 108:157–164,1964
65. MacPhayden B, et al: Management of gastrointestinal fistulas with parenteral hyperalimentation. Surgery 74:100–105,1973
66. diCostanzo J, et al: Treatment of external gastrointestinal fistulas by a combination of total parenteral nutrition and somatostatin. J Par Ent Nutr 11:465–467,1987
67. Torres A, et al: Somatostatin in the management of gastrointestinal fistulas: A multicenter trial. Arch Surg 127:97–100,1992
68. Sharp C, Freeman C: The medical complications of anorexia nervosa. Br J Psych 162:452--462,1993
69. Comerco G: Medical complications of anorexia nervosa and bulimia nervosa. Med Clin North Am 74(5):1293–1310,1990
70. Mitchell et al: Electrolyte and other physiological abnormalities in patients with bulimia. Psychol Med 13a:273,1983
71. Comerci, p 1298
72. Ibid, p 1306
73. Sharp, Freeman, p 459
74. Hall R, Beresford T: Medical complications of anorexia and bulimia. Psychiatr Med 7:165–192,1989
75. Sharp, Freeman, p 454
76. Comerci, p 1301
77. Sharp, Freeman, p 454
78. Cuesto M, et al: Secondary seizures from water intoxication in anorexia nervosa. Gen Hosp Psychiatr 14:212–213,1992
79. Mitchell J: Medical complications of anorexia nervosa and bulimia. Psychiatr Med 1:229–255,1984
80. Edelstein C, et al: Early clues to anorexia and bulimia. Patient Care 23:155–175,1989
81. Mitchell J, Boutacoff L: Laxative abuse complicating bulimia: Medical and treatment implications. Int J Eating Disorders 5:325–334,1986
82. Comerci, p 1306
83. Hofland S, Dardia P: Bulimia nervosa: Associated

physical problems. J Psychosoc Nurs 30(2):23–27, 1992
84. Sharp, Freeman, p 458
85. Schwartz, p 1028
86. Narins, p 1147
87. Ibid
88. Comerci, p 1304

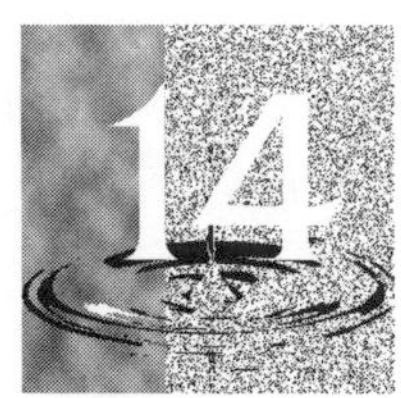

Fluid Balance in the Surgical Patient

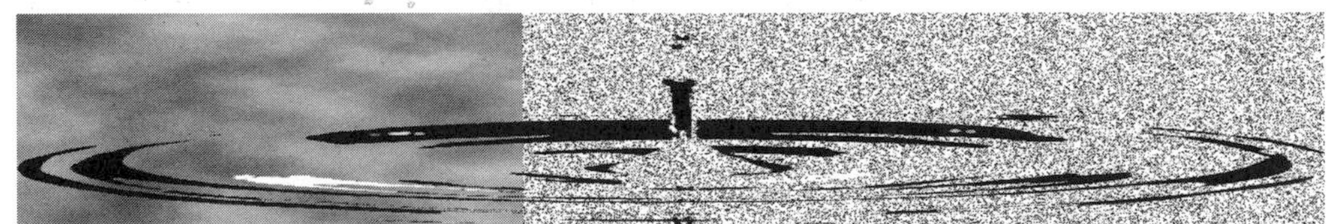

Although surgical patients are at great risk for fluid and electrolyte imbalances, these disturbances can often be prevented or minimized by appropriate intervention. Assessment and management of the patient's fluid and electrolyte status begins in the preoperative period and continues into the postoperative recovery period.

PREOPERATIVE PERIOD

Before surgery, potential perioperative problems should be identified by reviewing the patient's history and assessment for specific indicators of potential problems. Preoperative assessment in the ambulatory surgical setting presents a special challenge to the nurse. Various methods (such as telephone interviews and mailed questionnaires) have been used to gain needed information. Some ambulatory surgery centers require previsits for all patients (or at least those who will have general anesthesia); others rely on voluntary previsits.[1] At times, the needed assessment is performed in the surgeon's office or clinic. In any event, the nurse must work with the surgeon and anesthesia department to manage potential problems before or on the day of surgery.

FLUID AND ELECTROLYTE DISTURBANCES

Laboratory data should be reviewed carefully to detect fluid and electrolyte problems. (See Tables 2-3 and 2-4 for blood and urine tests useful in determining fluid balance status. Any abnormalities should be called to the attention of the medical staff for early correction. (Specific fluid and electrolyte imbalances are discussed in Chapters 3 through 9.)

Hypokalemia

Hypokalemia is the most frequent cause for cancellation of elective surgery because this imbalance predisposes to cardiac arrhythmias during the intraoperative period, especially in those with cardiac disease.[2] Patients with hypokalemia due to diuretics should also be screened and treated for hypomagnesemia because of its arrhythmogenic capacity and its ability to worsen renal potassium wasting.[3] Correction of potassium deficit should be started only after adequate urine output is established.

Fluid Volume Deficit

Surgical patients are at risk for fluid volume deficit (FVD) for a number of reasons. Prolonged periods of "nothing per os" (NPO) are not uncommon in patients who have undergone numerous diagnostic tests before surgical intervention. This is particularly problematic as diagnostic tests may require the use of cathartics and enemas (promoting fluid loss through the intestine) or use of contrast agents (producing osmotic diuresis). In addition, the patient may have suffered fluid losses related to the primary illness requiring surgical intervention.

Fluid volume deficit should be detected and corrected before induction of anesthesia as it is more difficult to correct intraoperatively. Before surgery, sufficient fluid must be given to stabilize blood pressure and pulse and increase hourly urine volume to an acceptable range (preferably 50 mL/hr in an adult). The rate of fluid administration varies considerably, depending on severity and type of fluid disturbances, presence of continuing losses, and cardiac status.

Preoperative Fluid Restriction

Various methods have been used to reduce the risk of nausea and vomiting in surgical patients; among these are NPO regimens, preanesthesia and postanesthesia suctioning of gastric contents, and ingestion of antacids.[4] It is still common practice to restrict hospitalized patients to NPO status at midnight before the day of surgery; however, this practice is coming into question in ambulatory care settings. This is partly because currently used anesthetic agents cause less nausea and vomiting than those used in the past.[5,6] It has been suggested that prolonged liquid fasts are unnecessary in healthy patients before ambulatory surgery; ingestion of coffee and pulp-free orange juice (250 mL) 2 to 3 hrs before surgery apparently does not increase gastric volume.[7] Goresky and Maltby[8] have offered the following recommendations for elective surgical patients: (1) permission for unrestricted intake of clear liquids until 3 hrs before the scheduled time of surgery; (2) allowing oral medications to be taken with 30 mL of water up to 1 hr before surgery; and (3) use of an H_2 blocker preoperatively for patients at increased risk for regurgitation and aspiration of gastric contents.

Other Imbalances

Patients with hypotension, sepsis, or tissue ischemia often demonstrate metabolic (lactic) acidosis from hypoxia and may require alkali administration.[9] Calcium and magnesium replacements may be needed for patients with massive subcutaneous infections, acute pancreatitis, or chronic starvation. Correction of anemia is also important; a hematocrit increase of approximately 3% should follow the infusion of a unit of packed red blood cells in an average-sized adult.[10] In a patient with a contracted intravascular volume, a significantly greater increase may occur, indicating the need for concurrent fluid volume replacement.

CHRONIC CONDITIONS

Certain chronic illnesses predispose to fluid, electrolyte, and acid–base disturbances during the stressful perioperative period. For example, patients with renal failure are at risk for hyperkalemia, metabolic acidosis, hypermagnesemia, and hyponatremia and may require emergent hemodialysis before emergency surgery.[11] Those with chronic obstructive pulmonary disease are predisposed to respiratory acidosis and hypoxemia. Patients who have experienced a myocardial infarction in the last 6 months or those with uncompensated congestive heart failure are at high risk for perioperative myocardial infarction and death and therefore are not acceptable candidates for elective surgery.[12] Patients with chronic cardiac conditions should be in the best metabolic control possible before surgery and often require preoperative insertion of a pulmonary artery catheter for monitoring during and after surgery.

MEDICATIONS

As discussed in Chapters 3 through 9, a number of medications can cause fluid and electrolyte disturbances. Some of the more problematic are potassium-losing diuretics. Examples of others include antibiotics predisposing to renal potassium wasting (such as carbenicillin and amphotericin B) and renal magnesium wasting (such as gentamicin).

Altered Adrenal Response

Factors that can interfere with the expected adrenal response to the stress of surgery must be identified preoperatively. One such factor is altered adrenal function related to use of therapeutic doses of corticosteroids. To review, the usual daily secretion of cortisol ranges from 15 to 30 mg/day.[13] However, increased secretion is needed to withstand the stress of surgery. (Estimates of endogenous cortisol production in patients undergoing major surgery vary from 75–150 mg/day.)[14] The adrenal glands of patients who have used corticosteroids for prolonged periods may not be able to respond during periods of high stress. Thus, patients maintained on chronic corticosteroid therapy or who have received them in the past 2 years will require steroid replacement in the perioperative period to prevent acute adrenocortical insufficiency (adrenal crisis).[15] Symptoms of this relatively rare but dangerous complication may include lethargy, disorientation, confusion, hypotension, hyponatremia, and hyperkalemia. These signs, with or without cardiovascular collapse, in any intraoperative or postoperative patient should raise the suspicion of adrenocortical insufficiency.[16]

Controversy exists as to the steroid dosage needed in at-risk patients to prevent acute adrenocortical insufficiency in the postoperative period without producing other complications (such as impaired wound healing, increased catabolism, electrolyte disturbances, and more frequently, infectious complications). In general, however, remember that short-term excess of glucocorticoids is relatively harmless, but short-term deficiency during stress may be fatal.[17]

NUTRITIONAL STATUS

The reasonably well nourished and otherwise healthy individual undergoing an uncomplicated major surgical procedure has sufficient body fuel reserves to withstand the catabolic insult and partial starvation for at least 1 week. However, the nutritionally depleted patient undergoes surgery with a serious handicap. It has been shown that operative morbidity and mortality are increased enormously in malnourished patients.[18] Atrophy of the mucous membrane linings of the respiratory and gastrointestinal (GI) tracts predispose to infection, as does diminished ability to form antibodies. Hypoproteinemia follows prolonged negative nitrogen balance and increases susceptibility to shock. Diminished supplies of protein and vitamin C retard wound healing.

Because malnutrition greatly increases perioperative risk, the malnourished patient should be identified early so that appropriate intervention can be undertaken. The patient's nutritional history must be reviewed. For example, consider whether the weight is 20% above or below normal, 10% of usual body weight has been recently lost or gained, physical problems are present that interfere with eating, and the patient has been maintained for more than a week on "routine" intravenous (IV) fluids. (One liter of fluid with 5% dextrose contains only 170 calories, all from carbohydrates; electrolyte solutions without dextrose have essentially no calories.)

Early institution of nutritional support provides essential nutrients for maintenance of gut integrity, prevention of bacterial translocation, and preservation of organ function, wound healing, and immune function.[19] However, research findings do not justify routine use of preoperative total parenteral nutrition (TPN) to decrease surgical complications or to improve outcome.[20] It is probably more prudent to provide perioperative nutrients for high-risk patients through the enteral route whenever possible.

INTRAOPERATIVE PERIOD

INTRAOPERATIVE FLUID MANAGEMENT

Hypotension may develop promptly with the induction of anesthesia if preoperative correction of extracellular FVD has been inadequate. Other factors predisposing to hypotension in the operative period are fluid loss due to bleeding, shifting of intravascular fluid into the surgical site (third-space edema), evaporation of fluid from the exposed peritoneum during abdominal surgery, and inhalation of dry gases. Most patients tolerate a 500-mL blood loss without difficulty, as albumin synthesis and erythropoiesis will usually compensate for such minor losses. However, when this volume is exceeded, blood replacement must be considered. In patients at high risk for congestive heart failure, intraoperative deviation of 40 mmHg in mean arterial pressure (increases or decreases) in relation to the baseline pressure may increase the risk of congestive heart failure postoperatively, whereas IV administration of greater net volumes may decrease the risk.[21] The risk of adult respiratory distress syndrome in the critically ill patient may also be increased in the setting of low net fluid balance and hypovolemia.[22]

Third-space fluid shift (which cannot be measured directly) can be substantial after extensive dissection of tissue; fluid can also sequester into the lumen and wall of the small bowel and accumulate in the peritoneal cavity. Judicious intraoperative correction of third-space fluid losses with an electrolyte solution (such as lactated Ringer's solution) markedly reduces postoperative oliguria. Although no accurate formula for intraoperative fluid administration is known, balanced salt solution needed during surgery is approximately 0.5 to 1 L/h (but only to a maximum of 2–3 L during a 4-hr major abdominal procedure unless there are other measurable losses).[23] Intraoperative assessment of wedge and central venous pressures may be needed to optimally guide fluid replacement in high-risk patients. (Debate on the best type of fluid replacement [crystalloids versus colloids] has continued for many years; isotonic crystalloids, colloids, and hypertonic saline solutions have advantages and disadvantages, depending on the setting.) The reader is referred to Chapter 10 for a review of various fluids and to Chapter 15 for further discussion of parenteral fluids used in resuscitation for hypovolemia.

EFFECT OF CARDIOPULMONARY BYPASS ON FLUID AND ELECTROLYTE BALANCE

Cardiopulmonary bypass, used for patients undergoing cardiac surgery, has unique effects on body fluids and electrolytes. The hypooncotic solution used to prime the pump dilutes plasma proteins and increases movement of water from the vascular space to the interstitial space. Intravascular fluid loss is further enhanced by increased capillary permeability associated with kinin and prostaglandin release from the damaged blood cells and platelets.[24] This fluid loss may persist for up to 8 hrs postoperatively, requiring close monitoring of the hemodynamic status with fluid replacement.[25] Because massive extracellular fluid (ECF) volume expansion is required for patients undergoing cardiopulmonary bypass, a 5- to 15-lb weight gain is expected.[26] It has been shown that patients undergoing cardiopulmonary bypass without weight gain during the procedure develop significant postoperative problems (such as hypovolemia and poor cardiac function).[27] The expanded ECF can persist for up to 10 days postoperatively.[28] Management of this problem in the postoperative period includes use of diuretics and colloids (such as albumin or hetastarch) to help mobilize the accumulated fluid. (See Chapter 10 for a discussion of colloids.)

There is a tendency to hyponatremia because plasma antidiuretic hormone (ADH) levels during cardiopulmonary bypass are higher than in other types of surgery (causing excessive water retention with sodium dilution).[29] During the postoperative period, free-water intake is minimized to avoid hyponatremia. In patients with preoperative congestive heart failure, both fluid and sodium restriction may be indicated. The serum sodium level is influenced to some extent by the type of cardiac surgery. For example, hyponatremia has been reported after mitral commissurotomy, whereas hypernatremia has been reported in a subset of patients undergoing tricuspid valve replacement.[30]

Hypokalemia commonly occurs during bypass and requires treatment.[31] This is especially important in patients who were taking digoxin before surgery (because hypokalemia intensifies the action of digoxin on the myocardium). Conditions aggravating the decrease in serum potassium concentration during cardiopulmonary bypass include the preoperative use of potassium-losing diuretics, urinary potassium losses, and shifting of potassium into the intracellular space. The obvious danger of hypokalemia is increased risk of arrhythmia. Potassium replacement may be delivered by slow infusion into the extracorporeal circulation or intermittently through a central venous catheter.[32] Intraoperative *hyper*kalemia has been associated with the preoperative use of nonselective beta-blockers (because of prevention of $beta_2$-mediated uptake of potassium by muscles).[33]

Hypomagnesemia is also common during and after cardiopulmonary bypass (due to dilution of plasma magnesium by ECF volume expansion, and binding of magnesium by chelating agents in administered stored blood products).[34] Indicators of hypomagnesemia in the postoperative period can include hyperreflexia, enhanced digitalis toxicity, and cardiac arrhythmias. Hypomagnesemia is associated with increased risk of dysrhythmias and prolonged need for mechanical ventilatory support.[35]

Lactic acidosis can result from cardiopulmonary bypass. Mild increases to levels of approximately 3 to 4 mEq/L may occur in uncomplicated cases, returning to normal by 18 hrs.[36]

EFFECT OF IRRIGATING SOLUTIONS ON FLUID AND ELECTROLYTE BALANCE

Irrigation solutions used during transurethral resection of the prostate (TURP), ultrasonic lithotripsy, and uterine endoscopic laser surgery may be absorbed intravascularly and result in fluid and electrolyte disturbances.[37] Because saline is an electrically conductive solution, fluids that contain no electrolytes must be used. Among the solutions used for irrigating purposes in these surgical procedures are glycine, sorbitol, and mannitol.

The TURP Syndrome

The TURP syndrome consists of a variety of symptoms related to absorption of hypoosmotic irrigating fluid during transurethral prostatectomy. It has been reported to occur in 5% to 10% of TURP cases.[38] Risk factors for the TURP syndrome include preoperative hyponatremia, chronic obstructive pulmonary disease, congestive heart failure, anemia, and malnutrition.[39]

During transurethral prostatectomy, the prostatic veins are opened and the irrigant solutions, which are used to distend the urethra and clear fragments and blood from the operative field, can be absorbed. In the United States, 1.5% glycine is the most commonly used irrigating solution during TURP.[40] On average during a TURP procedure, 10 to 30 mL/min[41] are absorbed, with a range of 300 mL to 4 L reported.[42] The fundamental pathology in the TURP syndrome is volume overload and dilutional hyponatremia. The severity and rapidity of the hyponatremia is proportional to the volume of the absorbed irrigant.[43]

Symptoms are often first noticed in the operating room or the recovery area when the patient complains of headache or visual changes. Other signs may include agitation or lethargy, vomiting, muscle twitching, bradycardia, diminished pupillary reflexes, hypertension, and respiratory distress.[44] The appropriate treatment consists of supportive care, fluid restriction, and diuretics; when extreme hyponatremia (<110 mEq/L) is present, hypertonic saline may be needed.[45] Measures that can be taken to prevent the TURP syndrome include using low-pressure irrigation and limiting the procedure to less than 1 hr to decrease the degree of volume overload.[46] Also, use of epidural or spinal anesthesia allows earlier symptom recognition.

Endometrial Ablation

Endometrial ablation is a surgical technique used for management of a variety of problems, including menorrhagia, leiomyoma uteri, or dysfunctional uterine bleeding.[47] During this procedure, an irrigating solution is infused into the uterine cavity to wash away operative debris. Because uterine veins are opened during this procedure, there is the possibility of intravenous absorption of substantial quantities of fluid. Hyponatremia may result and is especially problematic in women of childbearing age because this group is most susceptible to hyponatremic encephalopathy.[48] Indeed, women undergoing elective endometrial ablation can develop severe symptomatic hyponatremia.

The presence of symptoms suggesting hyponatremia should lead to immediate testing of the plasma sodium level; if below normal, early and appropriate therapy for the hyponatremia should be instituted before respiratory insufficiency occurs. In patients with general anesthesia during endometrial ablation, the possiblity of hyponatremia should be suspected if the patient has a drop in body temperature, decreased oxygen saturation, or displays tremulousness or dilated pupils.[49]

Arieff and Ayus[50] described four patients with hyponatremia due to endometrial ablation. Hyponatremia in three of the women was detected early and treated (mean sodium levels were corrected from 102 to 123 mEq/L within the first 24 hrs); all three recovered completely. Unfortunately, the fourth patient suffered respiratory arrest before therapy could be initiated; she never regained consciousness and died several days later. Autopsy revealed cerebral edema with tonsillar herniation.

POSTOPERATIVE PERIOD

NEUROENDOCRINE RESPONSE

The neuroendocrine response stimulated by many anesthetic agents is further heightened by surgical stress. Secretion of adrenocorticotrophic hormone (ACTH) and cortisol is increased according to the magnitude of surgery or trauma. Cortisol and ACTH levels generally remain elevated for 2 to 4 days after surgery; however, with extensive trauma or the complications of sepsis or shock the levels may remain elevated for weeks.[51]

Circulatory instability related to fluid losses during surgery and trauma produces decreased renal perfusion, which in turn stimulates production of substances (renin, angiotensin, and aldosterone) that support the blood pressure through vasoconstriction and sodium and water conservation.[52] In humans, isotonic fluid volume reduction (as occurs in simple blood loss) is one of the most potent stimuli to aldosterone and ADH secretion. Surgery and trauma also cause increased release of ADH through vasoconstriction of the renal artery and stimulation of the hypothalamus; these effects may persist for 12 to 24 hrs into the postoperative period. Reduced volumes of concentrated urine can be expected in the early postoperative period due to these hormonal changes. Unfortunately, increased aldosterone secretion results in greater urinary loss of potassium, predisposing to hypokalemia if potassium replacement is inadequate. In elderly surgical patients, the neuroendocrine response to the stress of surgery may result in increased morbidity.[53] Cerebrovascular surgical patients may have either prolonged inappropriate secretion of ADH (resulting in dilutional hyponatremia) or possibly suppression of ADH secretion (resulting in diabetes insipidus with hypernatremia). Therefore, careful monitoring of plasma osmolality and sodium levels is required (see Chapter 19).

METABOLIC CHANGES

During the first hours after surgical trauma, increased blood glucose levels may result from secretion of growth hormone and glucagon and suppression of insulin release. The extent of negative nitrogen balance that occurs postoperatively is largely related to the magnitude of the injury.[54] Normally, the patient should lose ¼ to ½ lb/day during the acute injury phase. Finally, the altered metabolism is associated with a slow but progressive reaccumulation of protein followed by a reaccumulation of body fat.

HEMODYNAMIC ALTERATIONS

With the increase in circulating catecholamines, an increase in heart rate and cardiac output occurs, as does vasoconstriction. A variety of undesirable changes can result from this physiological challenge in patients with heart disease who cannot increase cardiac output (or in older individuals with chronic coronary insufficiency) and in critically ill postoperative patients. These changes include acute congestive heart failure, acute cardiac arrhythmias, peripheral tissue anoxia and lactic acidoses, and visceral failure (brain or kidneys). As the circulating volume changes, the right and left atria and great veins of the mediastinum alter the production of aldosterone and ADH secretion. If alkalosis occurs, a left shift in the oxyhemoglobin curve results; reduced oxygen delivery may reduce cerebral function, causing disorientation, hallucinations, extreme restlessness, or coma.

FLUID AND ELECTROLYTE IMBALANCES

Fluid Volume Deficit

The most common fluid disorder in the postoperative patient is extracellular FVD.[55] Contributing factors to postoperative FVD include loss of GI fluids, continued third-space fluid shifts, fever, overzealous blood sampling for repeated chemical determinations, hyperventilation of greater than 35 respirations per minute, injudicious administration of diuretics, and an unhumidified tracheostomy with hyperventilation.

Among the indicators of FVD are decreased urine output, postural hypotension and tachycardia, diminished skin turgor, decreased capillary refill time, and blood urea nitrogen (BUN) elevated out of proportion to the serum creatinine (see Chapter 3). If fluids are directly lost from the body (as from vomiting or diuresis), body weight will decrease acutely. However, if FVD is due to third-spacing, decreased body weight does not occur because the fluid "lost" from the vascular space pools in another part of the body (such as the surgical site or bowel due to adynamic ileus). Actually, as parenteral fluids are administered to correct the vascular volume deficit, the patient will *gain* weight. Intake and output (I&O) measurements are mandatory when FVD is suspected; in general, in the adult an acceptable hourly urine volume is 30 to 50 mL. If the urine volume is decreased and is accompanied by tachycardia and depressed blood pressure, one should suspect a deficit of at least 2 to 3 L.

Of course, fluid replacement must be guided by the intravascular volume status (estimated by vital signs, urine output, and filling pressures when available). Remember that third-spacing from surgical trauma is not limited to the operative period; indeed, it may continue slowly for a few hours or more during the 1st day of injury.[56] Unrecognized deficits of ECF volume during the early postoperative period may be manifested as circulatory instability. Later, as the third-spacing resolves and fluid shifts back into the intravascular space, diuresis and weight loss will occur. In patients with cardiac or renal dysfunction, the shift of fluid back into the vascular bed may result in congestive heart failure or pulmonary edema.

Treatment of FVD depends on the composition of lost fluids. Generally, it can be accomplished with either lactated Ringer's solution or isotonic saline (0.9% NaCl). Use of a large volume of isotonic saline can theoretically produce hyperchloremic acidosis because it contains considerably more chloride than is normally present in plasma. In some situations, normal volume can be accomplished with albumin or other blood products. (See Chapter 10 for a discussion of IV replacement fluids and their recommended use.) Because fluid losses are only roughly estimated, careful monitoring of physiological indices must be done to warn of overhydration when large volumes of fluid are given rapidly. For example, a sudden increase in pulmonary artery occlusion pressure to greater than 20 mmHg may be an indicator of too much fluid given too rapidly.[57]

Urine Output

Preferably, urinary output should be at least 30 to 50 mL/hr in adults; an hourly urinary output of less than 25 mL should be investigated. The decreased urinary output of stress reaction (healthy physiological response to surgery) must be differentiated from pathological developments. Factors associated with decreased urinary volume in the postoperative patient may include the following:

- Inadequate preoperative fluid replacement
- Hypovolemia resulting from fluid loss incurred during surgery (either direct loss or subtle third-space accumulation at the surgical site or intestinal ileus)
- Disturbance in myocardial function causing decreased blood flow to the kidneys and thus decreased urine formation
- Renal failure (a serious cause of postoperative oliguria)

Postoperative renal failure is highest in the elderly patient undergoing cardiac surgery, aortic aneurysm repair, or biliary tract surgery for obstructive jaundice.[58] Although oliguric renal failure may occur postoperatively in the patient who has suffered poor renal perfusion during surgery, high-output renal failure is actually more frequent. High-output renal failure is characterized by uremia occurring with a daily urine volume greater than 1000 to 1500 mL. It probably represents the renal response to a less severe episode of renal injury than is required to cause the classic oliguric renal failure. Although it is generally easier to manage than oliguric renal failure, high-output failure is more difficult to recognize. Typically, the urine volume is normal or greater than normal (often reaching 3–5 L/day) and the BUN is increased. A real danger for hyperkalemia exists when potassium is administered to a patient with unrecognized high-output failure.

Fluid Volume Excess

In trauma and postoperative patients, there may be seepage of large volumes of fluid from the vascular space into a third space (such as the surgical site or a generalized interstitial space due to decreased plasma oncotic pressure after albumin loss). As fluids are administered to correct these vascular losses, the body takes on an added fluid load. Technically, this positive salt and water retention is not considered fluid volume overload. Instead, fluid volume overload is defined as overexpansion of the *intravascular* volume.[59]

In the surgical patient without renal failure, the most common causes of intravascular volume overload are iatrogenic (overcorrection of a previous volume deficit, a poorly guarded IV line, or a positive gain of water in patients receiving constant humidified ventilatory support). Morphine stimulates the release of vasopressin (antidiuretic hormone), causing decreased urine output and thus increased fluid retention.[60] Among the earliest signs is weight gain during the catabolic period when the patient is expected to lose ¼ to ½ lb/day. In addition to peripheral edema, overadministration of isotonic electrolyte solutions may cause pulmonary edema and increased local edema at the surgical site. The increased edema may be sufficient to cause partial obstruction in intestinal surgery.

Although volume overload can occur at any time in the postoperative period, it is more common soon after surgery. Daily weight measurement is necessary to detect excessive weight gain due to retained fluid. If pulmonary edema is present, diuretics may be indicated. Observation for pulmonary edema is important because eventually any retained third-space fluid will shift back into the vascular space.

Hyponatremia

A frequent imbalance in the postoperative period is hyponatremia related to excessive ADH secretion. In one study, hyponatremia was found to be present in 4.4% of postoperative patients within 1 week of surgery.[61] Predisposing factors included a temporary increase in ADH release after anesthesia and the stress of surgery. (Antidiuretic hormone is also referred to as arginine vasopressin [AVP].) Pain enhances the release of ADH by direct stimulation of the hypothalamus. Nausea, which is frequently present in postoperative patients, can increase ADH release as much as 1000-fold; the nausea does not have to be associated with vomiting.[62] Because of the tendency for hyponatremia in new postoperative patients, the excessive administration of electrolyte-free solutions during the first 2 to 4 postoperative days should be avoided. In fact, because elevated plasma levels of ADH are essentially a universal postoperative occurrence in the first few postoperative days, some investigators state that it may be important to avoid the use of any hypotonic IV solutions in the immediate postoperative period.[63] A serum sodium level between 130 to 135 mEq/L should be heeded; the simple act of restricting free water may be sufficient to avoid the full-blown syndrome of water intoxication (severe dilutional hyponatremia).[64] Cases of permanent brain damage related to profound hyponatremia have been reported in postoperative patients receiving excessive free water. The reader is referred to Case Study 4-5 and the section on postoperative hyponatremia in Chapter 4 for a discussion of the danger of postoperative hyponatremia in menstruant women, and to the section on endometrial ablation earlier in this chapter.

Potassium Imbalances

Hypokalemia is the most common potassium imbalance in surgical patients. However, it is unnecessary and probably unwise to administer potassium during the first 24 hrs postoperatively unless a definite potassium deficit exists.[65] This is because trauma causes release of potassium from cells at the surgical site into the extracellular space in the early postoperative period. For patients at risk for renal failure due to hypotensive episodes during the surgical procedure, even small potassium supplements can be detrimental. After the first 24 hrs, potassium is administered daily as necessary to replace urinary and GI potassium losses.[66] Generally, a daily supplementation of 60 to 100 mEq is required postoperatively.[67] The needed potassium should be distributed evenly in the total daily maintenance fluids. For example, if 2 L of fluid are prescribed over 24 hrs, and 80 mEq of potassium chloride is the required daily potassium supplement, 40 mEq/L should be added to each liter. This makes far more sense than routinely administering "K-runs" to meet maintenance potassium needs. (See the discussion of IV potassium replacement in Chapter 5.) Special considerations for patients undergoing cardiopulmonary bypass are discussed earlier in this chapter.

Hyperkalemia is rare in the postoperative patient, except when acute renal failure, rhabdomyolysis, massive hemolysis, or tissue necrosis is present. If hyperkalemia occurs at any time in the postoperative period, the possibility of impaired renal function (manifested by rising serum creatinine in the presence of low, normal, or high urine output) should be explored. Release of cellular potassium by crush injuries and electrical injuries, plus acute renal failure, can lead to lethal hyperkalemia within hours.

Hypocalcemia

Postsurgical hypocalcemia may accompany parathyroidectomy, thyroidectomy, or radical neck dissection. Hypocalcemia reportedly occurs in up to 70% of patients undergoing parathyroidectomy, particularly when a severe hyperparathyroid state was present before surgery.[68] Transient hypocalcemia reportedly occurs in 5% to 10% of patients undergoing thyroidectomy.[69] The hypocalcemia may occur immediately or 1 to 2 days postoperatively, and usually lasts less than 5 days.[70]

The most likely mechanism for hypocalcemia after thyroidectomy and radical neck dissection is reduced blood flow to the parathyroid glands after dissection and hemostatic maneuvers. Intraoperative release of calcitonin has also been suggested as a possible mechanism for hypocalcemia that complicates thyroid surgery.[71] It is possible that trauma to the parathyroid glands does not allow parathyroid hormone (PTH) to increase as needed to elevate the lower serum calcium level, thus contributing to the hypocalcemia. If permanent parathyroid damage has not occurred, parathyroid insufficiency resolves as edema at the surgical site lessens and revascularization occurs, allowing reestablishment of parathyroid gland integrity.

Although it has been postulated that the hypocalcemia after thyroidectomy is due to a temporary disruption in the blood supply to the parathyroid tissue, a group of researchers reported observing transient hypocalcemia despite preservation of parathyroid blood supply in a group of patients who underwent thyroid surgery.[72] These researchers studied serum levels of calcium, PTH, and proteins at regular intervals in 95 consecutive patients (30 with total thyroidectomy, 14 with subtotal thyroidectomy, and 51 with hemithyroidectomy). At nearly every time of blood withdrawal, when compared with preoperative levels, calcium concentrations were significantly lower after total thyroidectomy than after hemithyroidectomy. Severe hypocalcemia was found in 8 patients after total thyroidectomy, compared with 2 after hemithyroidectomy and was present in 3 of the 5 patients with thyroid carcinoma compared with 7 of the 90 with nonmalignant thyroid disease. No patients had persistent symptoms of hypocalcemia from 2 to 3 months after surgery.

Permanent hypocalcemia associated with thyroid surgery (which may be defined as a hypocalcemia lasting 2 months or longer) is due to accidental removal of the parathyroid glands or to vascular necrosis.[73] Fortunately, permanent post-surgical hypoparathyroidism occurs in only a small percentage of patients; the frequency of this complication is partially dependent on the technical skill of the surgeon.[74] Indeed, surgeons performing thyroidectomies and parathyroidectomies strive to preserve the blood supply to the parathyroid glands.[75] Extensive neck surgeries (as in radical neck dissection for cancer) are more likely to be associated with permanent hypoparathyroidism than are less involved surgical maneuvers.

Most patients who develop hypocalcemia after neck surgery are asymptomatic; however, some may develop paresthesias, laryngeal spasm, or tetany.[76] It has been recommended that the serum ionized calcium level be checked every 12 hrs after neck surgery (and more frequently if symptoms of hypocalcemia are present) until the serum ionized concentration begins to elevate, indicating recovery of the parathyroid glands.[77] Of course, symptomatic patients should receive supplemental calcium to increase the serum calcium level to the low normal range.

It is possible that postoperative hypoparathyroidism may manifest itself months to years after neck surgery; therefore, serum ionized calcium levels should be serially monitored on patients at risk. It is also possible that stress can induce hypocalcemia in these individuals; therefore, critically ill patients with a history of neck surgery should have a serum calcium test performed.[78]

Acid–Base Disorders

Surgical patients may have normal pH or develop virtually any acid–base abnormality (depending on individual circumstances). Respiratory acidosis may result from shallow respirations related to anesthesia, narcotics, abdominal distention, pain, or large cumbersome dressings. On assessment, decreased respirations and decreased breath sounds in the bases may be noted. Measures to increase gas exchange, such as frequent coughing and deep breathing, frequent suctioning of tracheobronchial secretions, avoidance of oversedation, and turning and ambulating the patient, will decrease the likelihood of respiratory acidosis.

Subclinical respiratory alkalosis is common in surgical patients.[79] Common causes include hyperventilation due to pain, hypoxia, central nervous system injury, and assisted ventilation. In fact, most patients who require ventilatory support in the post-operative period will develop varying degrees of respiratory alkalosis. Therefore, frequent measurement of arterial blood gases is performed to allow proper corrections of the ventilatory pattern when indicated. To prevent serious complications, the partial pressure of carbon dioxide in blood ($PaCO_2$) should not be allowed to drop below 30 mmHg.[80] This is particularly important in the presence of a complicating metabolic alkalosis (for which hypoventilation with subsequent carbon dioxide retention is needed for compensatory purposes).

The most common causes of metabolic acidosis in surgical patients include loss of alkali from biliary and pancreatic drainage, ketoacidosis, renal failure, and lactic acidosis associated with shock. Metabolic alkalosis generally results from loss of acid due to nasogastric drainage or vomiting, and therapy with potassium-losing diuretics.

PARENTERAL FLUID RESUSCITATION

Chapter 10 describes commonly prescribed water and electrolyte fluids and colloids (hetastarch, albumin, and other blood products) and Chapter 15 discusses fluid resuscitation for patients with hypovolemic shock after surgery or trauma.

AMBULATORY SURGERY CONSIDERATIONS

Ambulatory surgery patients will usually recover initially in a Post Anesthesia Care Unit and then in some type of Phase II Recovery or Discharge Unit. Procedures performed in ambulatory surgery seldom result in significant alterations in fluid and electrolyte status; however, because they do elicit the same stress response (to a much lesser extent), these patients require assessment and nursing interventions related to fluid and electrolyte balance.[81] Blood administration, autologous or donor, may be required.[82] Oral intake is encouraged after the

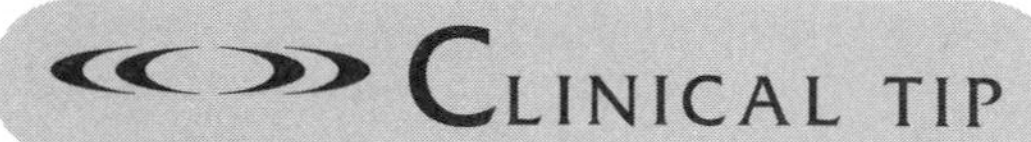

Examples of Nursing Diagnoses for a New Postoperative Patient After Abdominal Surgery

NURSING DIAGNOSIS	ETIOLOGICAL FACTORS	DEFINING CHARACTERISTICS
FVD related to actual fluid loss and third-space fluid shift during surgical procedure	Vomiting after reaction to anesthesia GI suction Third-space fluid shift at surgical site	Postural tachycardia Postural hypotension initially; later, low BP in all positions Decreased skin turgor Slowed capillary refill time Oliguria (<30 mL/hr in adult) Weight change depends on cause (decreased if actual fluid loss, as in GI suction; usually increased if fluid loss is due to third-space shift, provided parenteral fluids are given in an attempt to correct hypovolemia)
Altered tissue perfusion (renal) related to hypotension during surgical procedure	Hypotensive effects of anesthesia Hypovolemia due to direct or indirect loss of fluid Hypovolemia due to inadequate parenteral fluid replacement	Oliguria or polyuria in presence of elevated serum creatinine (see discussion of low-output and high-output renal failure in text)
Alteration in sodium balance (hyponatremia) related to excessive ADH activity	Major surgery with its premedication, anesthesia, decreased blood volume, and postoperative pain results in increased ADH release (causing water retention with sodium dilution)	Serum sodium <135 mEq/L May be asymptomatic if Na >125 mEq/L Lethargy, confusion, nausea, vomiting, anorexia, abdominal cramps, muscular twitching (see Chapter 5).
Alteration in acid–base balance (metabolic alkalosis) related to vomiting or gastric suction	Vomiting after reaction to anesthesia Gastric suction, particularly if patient is allowed to ingest ice chips freely	Tingling of fingers, toes, and circumoral region, due to decreased calcium ionization pH > 7.45, bicarbonate above normal, chloride below normal
Altered nutrition (less than body requirements) related to negative nitrogen balance after surgical stress, and inadequate caloric intake	Catabolic response to stress of surgery Inability to tolerate oral feedings during first few postoperative days due to decreased GI motility, anorexia, nausea, and general discomfort Failure of health-care providers to administer sufficient calories via the parenteral route	Weight loss of approximately ¼ to ½ lb/day in adult (provided fluids are not abnormally retained) Perhaps a decrease in serum albumin, transferrin, and retinol binding protein levels.

BP, blood pressure; FVD, fluid volume deficit; GI, gastrointestinal.

patient is sufficiently alert, able to protect the airway, and not nauseated. Nausea and vomiting can have multiple causes and require individual assessment and management. When IV fluids are used, they will be continued until the patient is able to tolerate oral fluids.[83] Assessment for ability to void as well as for bladder distention is also important.

Postoperative instructions for home are ideally given during the preadmission contact and reinforced in the discharge unit. Instructions related to fluid balance usually include:

- Increase oral fluids, especially after urologic procedures and spinal anesthesia.
- Do not drink any alcoholic beverages during the first 24 hrs.
- Methods for management of nausea and vomiting.
- Notify physician if uncomfortable due to inability to urinate.[84]

A follow-up phone call the day after surgery allows the nurse to assess the patient's status and address any questions or concerns.

NURSING DIAGNOSES

Clinical Tip: Examples of Nursing Diagnoses for a New Postoperative Patient After Abdominal Surgery lists some possible nursing diagnoses related to fluid and electrolyte balance for a patient who has undergone abdominal surgery.

CASE STUDIES

➤ **14-1.** A 60-year-old man underwent surgical repair of an abdominal aortic aneurysm and was brought to the surgical intensive care unit for follow-up care. He was mechanically ventilated with an inspired gas mixture containing 40% oxygen; tidal volume was set at 950 mL and breathing rate at 12 breaths/min. A nasogastric tube was connected to suction. He received 2 L of 5% dextrose in 0.11% sodium chloride solution every 24 hrs for the first 2 postoperative days. In addition, he received 20 mg of furosemide IV twice daily. On the morning of the third postoperative day the following laboratory results were obtained:

Serum sodium = 128 mEq/L
Serum potassium = 3.3 mEq/L
Arterial pH = 7.62
$PaCO_2$ = 26 mmHg
HCO_3 = 28 mEq/L
PaO_2 = 74 mmHg

COMMENTARY: Furosemide, a powerful diuretic, causes sodium loss in the urine. In addition, some sodium was lost in nasogastric suction. However, very little sodium was replaced via the intravenous route (5% dextrose in 0.11% sodium chloride solution contains only about 19 mEq of sodium per liter). In addition, pain and surgical stress stimulate production of antidiuretic hormone, which causes water retention (thus diluting the serum sodium level, especially when hypotonic fluids are supplied IV).

The arterial pH of 7.62 indicates alkalosis. A higher than normal bicarbonate level indicates metabolic alkalosis. A lower than normal $PaCO_2$ indicates respiratory alkalosis. Therefore, the patient has two primary acid–base problems (metabolic alkalosis and respiratory alkalosis). Possible causes of metabolic alkalosis include loss of acidic gastric fluid via suction and use of a potassium-losing diuretic. Because the patient was mechanically ventilated at a fixed volume and rate, he was unable to make the usual compensatory respiratory change (hypoventilation) seen when metabolic alkalosis exists. In fact, the high minute volume set by mechanical ventilation caused *hyper*ventilation and thus respiratory alkalosis.

➤ **14-2.** A 32-year-old woman presented with hypercalcemia and was diagnosed with primary hyperparathyroidism. Upon neck exploration, the surgeon found four enlarged parathyroid glands and removed three. On the first postoperative day, the total serum calcium was 8.6 mg/dL; it decreased to 6.8 mg/dL by the third postoperative day. At that time, she complained of feeling lightheaded and having paresthesias of the mouth, fingers, and toes. Upon examination, she was found to have a positive Chvostek's sign. Later, she developed twitching of the facial muscles. She was treated with 10 mL of 10% calcium gluconate IV over 10 min.

COMMENTARY: The hypocalcemia was caused by surgical hypoparathyroidism (after removal of three of the four parathyroid glands). A potential serious consequence that could have occurred with this degree of hypocalcemia is laryngeal spasm, which compromises the airway. This patient is likely to recover normal calcium balance after the operative injury heals.

REFERENCES

1. Burden N: Ambulatory Surgical Nursing, p 155. Philadelphia, WB Saunders, 1993
2. Narins RG (ed): Clinical Disorders of Fluid and Electrolyte Metabolism, 5th ed, p 1414–1413. New York, McGraw-Hill, 1994
3. Ibid
4. Epstein B: Preventing postoperative nausea and vomiting, Chapter 7, p 93–109. In Sleisenger M: The Handbook of Nausea & Vomiting. New York, Caduceus Medical Publishers by the Parthenon Publishing Group, 1993
5. Summers S, Ebbert DW: Ambulatory Surgical Nursing: A Nursing Diagnosis Approach, p 264. Philadelphia, JB Lippincott, 1992
6. Goodwin A, et al: The effect of shortening the preoperative fluid fast on postoperative morbidity. Anaesthesia 46:1066–1068,1991
7. Epstein, p 94
8. Goresky G, Maltby J: Fasting guidelines for elective surgical patients (Editorial). Can J Anaesthesia 37(5):493–495,1990
9. Narins, p 1417
10. Schwartz S (ed): Principles of Surgery, 5th ed, p 76. New York, McGraw-Hill, 1994
11. Narins, p 1409
12. Ibid
13. Condon R, Nyhus L: Manual of Surgical Therapeutics, 8th ed, p 246. Boston, Little, Brown, 1993
14. Schwartz, p 1577
15. Ibid
16. Ibid, p 1575
17. Condon, Nyhus, p 246
18. Pestana C: Fluids and Electrolytes in the Surgical Patient, 4th ed, p 174. Baltimore, Williams & Wilkins, 1989
19. Zaloga G: Nutrition in Critical Care, p 298. St. Louis, CV Mosby, 1994
20. The Veterans Affairs Total Parenteral Nutrition Cooperative Study Group: Perioperative total parenteral nutrition in surgical patients. N Engl J Med 325:525–532,1991
21. Charlson ME, MacKenzie R, Gold JP, Ales KL, Topkina M, Shires TG: Risk For postoperative congestive heart failure. Surg Gynecol Obstet 172: 95–104,1991
22. Bishop M, et al: The relationship between ARDS, pulmonary infiltration, fluid balance, and hemodynamics in critically ill surgical patients. Am Surgeon 57:785–792,1991
23. Schwartz et al, p 77
24. Vaska PL: Fluid and electrolyte imbalances after cardiac surgery. AACN Clin Issues 3:664–667,1992
25. Ibid
26. Kokko J, Tannen R: Fluids and Electrolytes, 2nd ed, p 1016. Philadelphia, WB Saunders, 1990
27. Ibid
28. Ibid
29. Ibid, p 1017
30. Narins, p 1419
31. Kokko, Tannen, p 1017
32. Narins, p 1422
33. Ibid
34. Kokko, Tannen, p 1017
35. Narins, p 1422
36. Ibid
37. Ibid, p 1419
38. Rhymer J: Hyponatremia following transurethral resection of the prostate. Br J Urol 57:450–202,1985
39. Ellis R, Carmichael J: Hyponatremia and volume overload as a complication of transurethral resection of the prostate. J Fam Pract 33(1):89–91,1991
40. Ibid
41. Gold MS: Perioperative Fluid Management. Crit Care Clin 8:409–421,1992
42. Narins, p 1414
43. Ibid, p 1419
44. Ellis, Carmichael, p 90
45. Ibid
46. Ibid
47. Arieff A, Ayus C: Endometrial ablation complicated by fatal hyponatremic encephalopathy. JAMA 279(10):1230–1232,1993
48. Ayus J, Wheeler J, Arieff A: Postoperative hyponatremic encephalopathy in menstruant women. Ann Intern Med 117:891–897,1992
49. Arieff, Ayus, p 1230
50. Ibid
51. Kokko, Tannen, p 993
52. Ibid
53. Beck LH: Perioperative renal, fluid, and electrolyte management. Clin Geriatr Med 6:557–567,1990
54. Schwartz, p 81
55. Ibid, p 65
56. Ibid, p 77
57. Shoemaker et al: Textbook of Critical Care, 3rd ed, p 261. Philadelphia, WB Saunders, 1995
58. Beck, p 56
59. Kokko, Tannen, p 1007
60. Clark J, Queener, S, Karb V: Pharmacologic Basis of Nursing Practice, 4th ed, p 665. St. Lous, Mosby, 1993
61. Chung et al: Postoperative hyponatremia. Arch Intern Med 146:333,1986
62. Narins, p 599

63. Ayus et al, p 891
64. Kokko, Tannen, p 1008
65. Schwartz, p 78
66. Ibid
67. Kokko, Tannen, p 1010
68. Condon, Nyhus, p 251
69. Ibid
70. Chernow B (ed): The Pharmacologic Approach to the Critically Ill Patient, 3rd ed, p 777. Baltimore, Williams & Wilkins, 1994
71. Narins, p 1025
72. Bourrel C, et al: Transient hypocalcemia after thyroidectomy. Ann Otol Laryngol 102:496,1993
73. Ibid
74. Narins, p 1025
75. Pemberton L, Pemberton D: Treatment of Water, Electrolyte, and Acid-Base Disorders in the Surgical Patient, p 216. New York, McGraw-Hill, 1994
76. Chernow, p 780
77. Ibid
78. Ibid
79. Shires G: Fluids, Electrolytes and Acid-Bases, p 8. New York, Churchill Livingstone, 1988
80. Ibid, p 9
81. Burden, p 287
82. Ibid
83. Ibid
84. Ibid, p 358–362

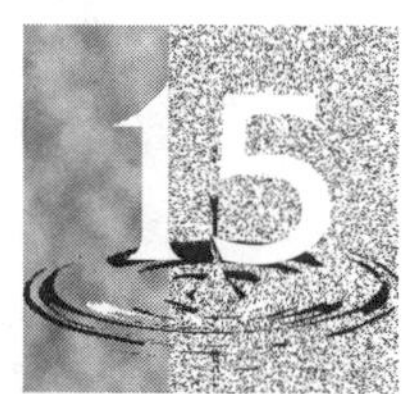

Hypovolemic Shock in Trauma and Postoperative Patients

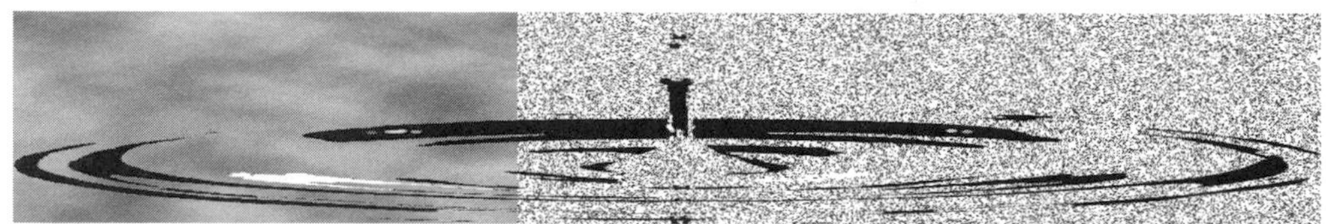

Trauma is one of the leading causes of death in the first four decades of life in the United States. Swift in onset and slow in recovery, trauma presents many pitfalls to the nurse caring for the injured patient. Trauma death has a trimodal pattern.[1] The first peak of death occurs within seconds to minutes of injury and is usually due to blood loss from lacerations of the heart, aorta or other large vessels, or trauma to the brain, brain stem, or high spinal cord. The second peak occurs within minutes to a few hours after injury and is usually due to epidural and subdural hematomas, hemopneumothorax, ruptured spleen, liver lacerations, pelvic fractures, or any injuries associated with significant blood loss. The third peak of death occurs several days or weeks after the initial injury and is primarily due to complications of shock including sepsis, adult respiratory distress syndrome (ARDS), and multiple system organ failure (MSOF). Every attempt should be made to prevent prolonged shock, as it can lead to MSOF and late death. Care of a patient in shock requires accurate assessment and timely interventions and continuous evaluation by the nurse. Management of the patient experiencing hypovolemic shock as a result of traumatic injury or after surgical procedures is the focus of this chapter.

DEFINITION OF SHOCK

Generally, shock has been defined as a state that develops when there is inadequate tissue perfusion.[2] More specifically, shock starts when oxygen delivery to the cells is inadequate to meet metabolic demands.[3] Most common in the injured patient is *hypovolemic shock* after acute blood loss, either externally or internally. External blood loss can result from lacerations, amputations, open fractures, or stab or gunshot wounds. Blood is also frequently lost at the injury site, especially after major closed fractures. For example, a fractured tibia or humerus may be associated with a blood loss of 755 mL, whereas a fractured femur may result in a 1.5-L blood loss.[4] Pelvic fractures may result in even greater blood losses. Depending on the injury site, a significant volume of blood may be sequestered into body cavities such as the thorax, intraperitoneal space, and retroperitoneal space. Two to three liters of blood may collect in the thoracic cavity after hemothorax, and the abdominal cavity may sequester as much as 6 L of blood. Fluid losses other than blood also occur as a result of tissue injury. Two liters of edema may be sequestered into soft tissues after a severe femur fracture.[5]

In *cardiogenic shock*, failure of the heart as a pump causes a decrease in tissue perfusion. In the trauma patient, cardiogenic shock may occur if compensatory mechanisms have failed or if cardiac tamponade, tension pneumothorax, or cardiac contusion is present.

Neurogenic shock results from the loss of vasomotor tone and vasodilation in much of the peripheral vascular system. Direct injury to the medullary vasomotor center or interruption of sympathetic innervation secondary to cervical or high thoracic spinal cord injury causes such a loss of vasomotor control.[6] Clinically, the patient with neurogenic shock will be hypotensive without tachycardia or cutaneous vasoconstriction. Patients with known or suspected neurogenic shock should be treated initially for hypovolemia; vasoactive drugs should not be administered until volume is restored. This directly inhibits compensatory vasoconstriction in response to intravascular fluid loss and thereby exacerbates the hypovolemic shock state. Intracranial injuries alone do not produce circulatory inadequacy until the brain stem and its reticular activating system are profoundly involved.[7] The presence of shock in a patient with a head injury indicates a search for another cause, such as internal bleeding from an abdominal injury.

For trauma patients surviving the first 3 postinjury days, sepsis is the principal cause of death.[8] *Septic shock* is uncommon immediately after a traumatic insult.[9] How the patient presents with septic shock depends partly on the volume status. For example, septic patients who are also hypovolemic are difficult to distinguish clinically from those in hypovolemic shock. In contrast, in the normovolemic septic patient, an elevated cardiac output, tachycardia, low systemic vascular resistance, and warm, flushed extremities may be evidence of septic shock.[10]

CLASSES OF SHOCK

The initial assessment and resuscitation of trauma patients is categorized into four classes of hypovolemic shock based on the amount of blood lost (Table 15-1).[11] The classes are related to physio-

TABLE 15–1

Estimated Fluid and Blood Losses* Based on Patient's Initial Presentation

	CLASS I	CLASS II	CLASS III	CLASS IV
Blood loss (mL)	Up to 750	750–1500	1500–2000	>2000
Blood loss (% BV)	Up to 15%	15–30%	30–40%	>40%
Pulse rate	<100	>100	>120	>140
Blood pressure	Normal	Normal	Decreased	Decreased
Pulse pressure (mmHg)	Normal or increased	Decreased	Decreased	Decreased
Respiratory rate	14–20	20–30	30–40	>35
Urine output (mL/hr)	>30	20–30	5–15	Negligible
CNS/mental status	Slightly anxious	Mildly anxious	Anxious and confused	Confused and lethargic
Fluid replacement (3:1 rule)	Crystalloid	Crystalloid	Crystalloid and blood	Crystalloid and blood

*For a 70-kg man.
From Advanced Trauma Life Support Course for Physicians. American College of Surgeons, 1993.

logical responses and can be helpful in understanding the clinical manifestations.

COMPENSATORY MECHANISMS

Circulatory reflexes and fluid shifts occur to compensate for the diminished blood volume. Circulatory reflexes trigger a response from the sympathetic nervous system when there is a blood loss greater than 10% of the total blood volume. This causes increased heart rate as well as constriction of arterioles and veins in the peripheral circulation. Fortunately, sympathetic stimulation does not cause significant constriction of either the cerebral or cardiac vessels, although blood flow in many areas of the body is markedly diminished. Thus, blood flow through the heart and brain is maintained at essentially normal levels until the arterial pressure falls below 70 mmHg.[12] Another compensatory mechanism that occurs over a number of hours involves a fluid shift from the interstitial space to the vascular space, thus increasing blood volume. Still another mechanism triggered by hypovolemia is increased release of the hormones aldosterone and antidiuretic hormone (ADH). Aldosterone increases renal sodium reabsorption and conserves intravascular water.[13] ADH functions to increase water reabsorption in the kidney.

MANAGEMENT

Treatment should be initiated early as prolonged shock leads to cellular swelling and damage, compounding the overall impact of blood loss and hypoperfusion. The overall goal of therapy is to reestablish adequate tissue perfusion and thus oxygen delivery to metabolically active cells. Nursing care is focused on restoring cellular perfusion rather than simply restoring the patient's blood pressure and pulse rate. Of course, active bleeding must be controlled by whatever means necessary.

INITIAL MEASURES

Securing Airway

To restore tissue oxygen delivery, first the airway must be secured. For some patients, a simple jaw thrust may suffice; for others (such as class III or class IV shock patients), endotracheal intubation is required. Once the airway is secured, assessment of respiratory rate and rhythm is performed. Spontaneous hyperventilation is initially noted in major shock, followed by a deterioration in ventilatory efforts. Supplemental high-flow oxygen should be administered to improve oxygen availability for transport to hypoxic tissues. This may be all that is necessary in the spontaneously breathing patient who maintains adequate arterial blood gases. Injury to the thorax or need for surgical intervention in the patient with significant traumatic shock usually necessitates mechanical ventilatory support.

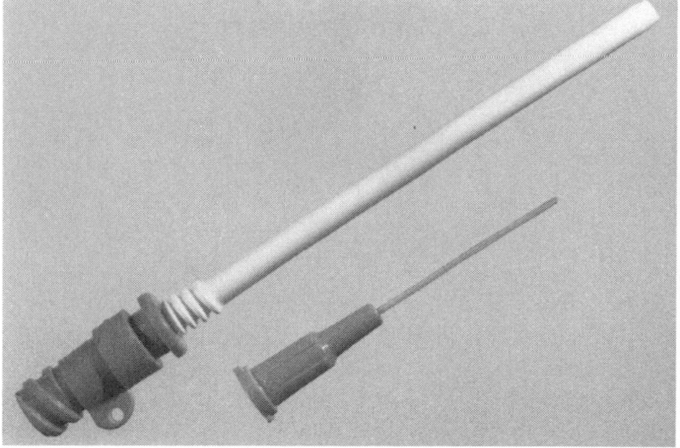

Figure 15–1. Arrow RIC 8.5 Fr (Rapid Infusion Catheter) compared with an ordinary 22-gauge device. Both are designed for the peripheral infusion of intravenous fluids; however, markedly higher infusion rates are possible with the wide-diameter device.

Initiating Intravenous Lines

Peripheral Sites

In the presence of severe hypovolemia, the aim of fluid resuscitation is to quickly infuse large volumes of fluid into the patient. Flow of intravenous fluids is directly dependent on the internal diameter of the administration device and inversely dependent on its length; other factors also greatly influence flow rates (see Table 15-2 below). It is possible to achieve high flow rates with a peripheral line. Large peripheral catheters have been developed that can deliver maximal fluid flow to hypovolemic patients. A peripheral access is preferred over a central site; if there is a 20-gauge or larger peripheral intravenous (IV) device already in place, a 7-Fr or 8.5-Fr catheter can be inserted over the existing catheter. (See Fig. 15-1 for a photograph of a 8.5-Fr Arrow RIC [Rapid Infusion Catheter] suitable for rapid peripheral fluid administration.) Percutaneous access in the upper extremities is preferred, primarily in the antecubital fossae or secondarily at the wrist.[14] If these veins cannot be accessed immediately, it is vital that another route be obtained. For example, cannulation of the saphenous vein in the leg or of the common femoral vein may be considered. Sites are needed both above and below the diaphragm if there are thoracic or abdominal injuries. Extremities that show evidence of proximal injury should not be used because of the potential for venous extravasation and fluid loss.[15] When a peripheral site is not available, cannulation of the subclavian vein with a central line introducer (usually 8-Fr) may also be considered.

Central Sites

Recommended central sites for rapid fluid resuscitation include the subclavian,[16] femoral, or internal jugular veins.[17] These sites, cannulated with large diameter devices, can accept rapid flow rates. A standard 8.5-Fr short introducer sheath is commonly used. Later, this same device can be used as an introducer for a hemodynamic monitoring catheter (see Fig. 2-8). It should be noted that typical central venous catheters are *not* suited for rapid fluid replacement because of their relatively small diameter and long length (causing resistance to rapid flow rate).[18] A wide variety of central venous catheters are in use, varying in length from 6 to 12 inches. Some have single lumens, but most have two or more lumens (see Fig. 15-2). Of course, the gauge of the lumen and length of the catheter influence the maximal flow rate through that particular IV line. For example, some catheters have triple lumens (two 18-gauge and one 16-gauge lumen; in that event, the 16-gauge lumen would facilitate flow rate more quickly than either of the 18-gauge ports). See Figure 15-3 for an explanation of the diameters of intravenous devices according to gauge and French sizes.

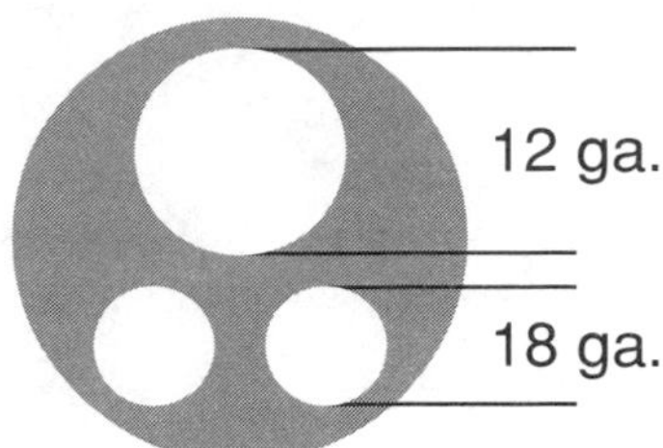

Figure 15–2. Cross-section diagram of triple-lumen central venous catheter having one 12-gauge and two 18-gauge ports.

FLUID ADMINISTRATION

Selection of Fluids

Crystalloids Versus Colloids

To some extent, volume replacement is essential in hypovolemic shock to restore intravascular volume and adequate tissue perfusion. Crystalloids are the primary treatment for a hemorrhaging patient who has adequate red cell mass. Crystalloids are defined as isotonic sodium-containing fluids (usually lactated Ringer's solution [LR] or 0.9% sodium chloride, also referred to as "normal saline" [NS]). The American College of Surgeons' Committee on Trauma recommends isotonic electrolyte solutions for initial replacement of fluid losses.[19] For trauma victims, fluid resuscitation is usually initiated in the field by medics. An initial fluid bolus of 1 to 2 L is given as rapidly as possible for an adult; a dose of 20 mL/kg is used for a pediatric patient.[20] For children, the dose of 20 mL/kg can be repeated once; if there is no response to these two fluid boluses, blood transfusion as well as ongoing crystalloid infusion is required. The patient's response to initial fluid administration must be observed and further action determined accordingly. If the shock state fails to show signs of resolution after aggressive fluid replacement, one should suspect continued blood loss, inadequate fluid delivery, or onset of complications.

After administration of the first few liters of a crystalloid, the question of when and if colloids should be added to the regimen frequently arises. The main factors considered when deciding between crystalloids and colloids are the hemodynamic and pulmonary effects of the fluids. As stated earlier, the volume of isotonic crystalloids required to attain adequate volume repletion varies from three to seven times the volume of colloids required to reach the same hemodynamic end point.[21] Studies regarding pulmonary status in the "colloid–crystalloid debate" have produced conflicting results. That is, some studies report that pulmonary injury is less likely with crystalloid resuscitation, whereas others state the reverse. Theoretically, based on Starling's law of fluid movement across a semipermeable membrane, excessive volumes of crystalloids might accumulate in the pulmonary interstitium because of a reduction in the colloid oncotic pressure–pulmonary capillary wedge pressure gradient. However, authorities disagree as to the clinical significance of this phenomenon. Some researchers point out that colloids may also extravasate into the interstitial space if there are damaged capillaries (endothelial leakiness). Protein-rich interstitial fluid can accumulate in the lungs and other tissues, causing ARDS and organ failure. However, it appears that the overall volume used and the presence or absence of sepsis affect pulmonary function to a far greater extent than does the type of resuscitation fluid used.[22] Despite continuing theoretical discussions, the available clinical data do not indicate that colloids have any advantage over crystalloids in initial fluid resuscitation; however, colloids are significantly more expensive and more complex to administer.[23] In a meta-analysis of eight published clinical studies in which patients were randomly assigned to receive either a colloid or a crystalloid regimen, Velanovich[24] found that mortality rates in trauma patients were about 12% less when crystalloid resuscitation was used. In contrast, mortality rates in nontrauma patients

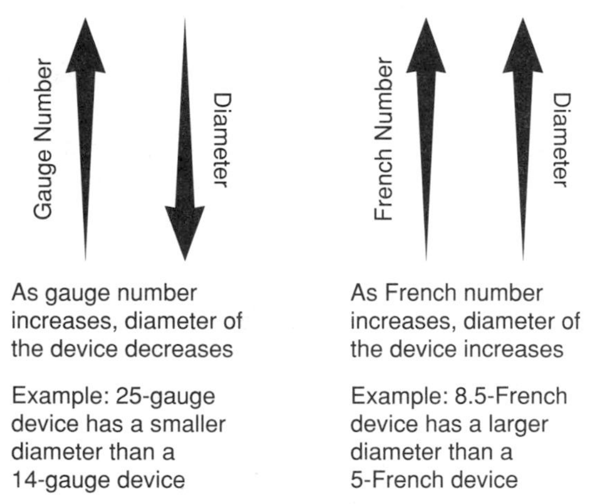

Gauge Number
Diameter
French Number
Diameter
As gauge number increases, diameter of the device decreases
Example: 25-gauge device has a smaller diameter than a 14-gauge device
As French number increases, diameter of the device increases
Example: 8.5-French device has a larger diameter than a 5-French device

Figure 15–3. Diameters of intravenous devices according to gauge and French sizes.

were found to be approximately 8% less when resuscitated with colloid regimens. The meta-analysis further indicated that colloid resuscitation was deleterious in septic trauma patients with capillary leak syndrome (leading to ARDS).

Hypertonic Saline

Hypertonic sodium chloride solutions contain large concentrations of sodium, ranging from 250 to 1200 mEq/L. Because of their high sodium content, these solutions are apparently capable of expanding the plasma volume by pulling fluid from the intracellular space into the extravascular space. The primary indication for the use of very hypertonic solutions is resuscitation of patients in the prehospital setting. It is difficult for paramedics in the field to administer the large volumes of isotonic salt solutions characteristically needed to treat shock. Recall that large volumes of isotonic salt solutions are needed because only about 25% of the administered fluid remain in the vascular space after 1 hr; thus, large quantities are required to achieve sustained vascular volume expansion. (The remaining 75% of each liter of balanced salt solution enters the interstitial space, causing edema.) Several studies have indicated good clinical response after hypertonic saline administration to trauma patients.[25–27] However, researchers have also warned that resuscitation with hypertonic saline can lead to hypernatremia and hyperosmolarity.[28]

In head-injured patients, there are indications that hypertonic saline is effective for volume resuscitation while decreasing brain water content in uninjured tissues, indicating that hypertonic saline might be useful in cases of combined hemorrhagic shock and head injury.[29] However, cerebral dehydration could develop rapidly with subsequent bleeding, as could central pontine myelinolysis due to rapid variations in serum sodium levels.[30]

In summary, small-volume resuscitation with hypertonic saline is an attractive alternative to large-volume replacement but is still at an early stage of experimental and clinical investigation. Hypertonic saline is not yet approved by the U.S. Food and Drug Administration (FDA) for shock resuscitation.

Blood Products

Blood replacement therapy is needed in patients with blood loss greater than 20% to 25% of their total blood volume (see Table 15-1). It is difficult to predict the actual percentage of blood loss in early treatment; this is generally accomplished by observing the patient's response to fluid resuscitation.

Early in the treatment of hemorrhagic shock, use of hematocrit to guide blood replacement therapy is unreliable (even massive blood loss produces a minimal acute decrease in hematocrit). Later on, after fluid shifts from the extravascular space have occurred, a hematocrit of less than 30% is usually viewed as need for blood replacement. Theoretically, it is at this point that red blood cell mass should be supplemented to provide adequate oxygen-carrying capacity to the tissues.[31] Although traditionally a hematocrit of 30% has been used as a marker of blood need, more recent clinical data have suggested that hematocrit be maintained at 33% to 35% in critically ill patients.[32] If the hematocrit is greater than 30% (or the designated level) and hemodynamic stability remains, further aggressive fluid resuscitation may be unnecessary. If the hematocrit falls below the designated level, packed red blood cells should be transfused. It is important to remember, however, that hemoglobin and hematocrit values alone are unreliable in initially gauging the degree of blood loss because up to 4 hrs may elapse before any significant changes are evident.[33] By 2 hrs, 14% to 26% of the ultimate drop in hematocrit occurs; a 36% to 50% change occurs in 8 hrs, and a 63% to 77% change occurs in 24 hrs.[34] Although a very low hematocrit suggests significant blood loss or preexisting anemia, an early near normal hematocrit does not rule out significant blood loss (see Case Study 15-1).

Packed red blood cells (PRBCs) are obtained by centrifuging whole blood and drawing off approximately 200 to 225 mL of plasma. Although whole blood is preferred, it is not available because of blood bank policies. Packed cells have a hematocrit level of approximately 70% and can be infused with little difficulty. In a 70-kg person, a unit of red blood cells will increase the hematocrit 3% to 4% (1 g/dL), or 1 mL/kg will result in a 1% increase in hematocrit.[35] There are two options for patients in urgent need of blood transfusion (i.e., those individuals who cannot wait the 30 to 45 min needed for full compatibility testing). One option includes the use of type-specific blood; this requires a blood sample from the patient to determine the ABO and Rh blood group and takes only a few minutes to perform. The second option is to use group O PRBCs (preferably

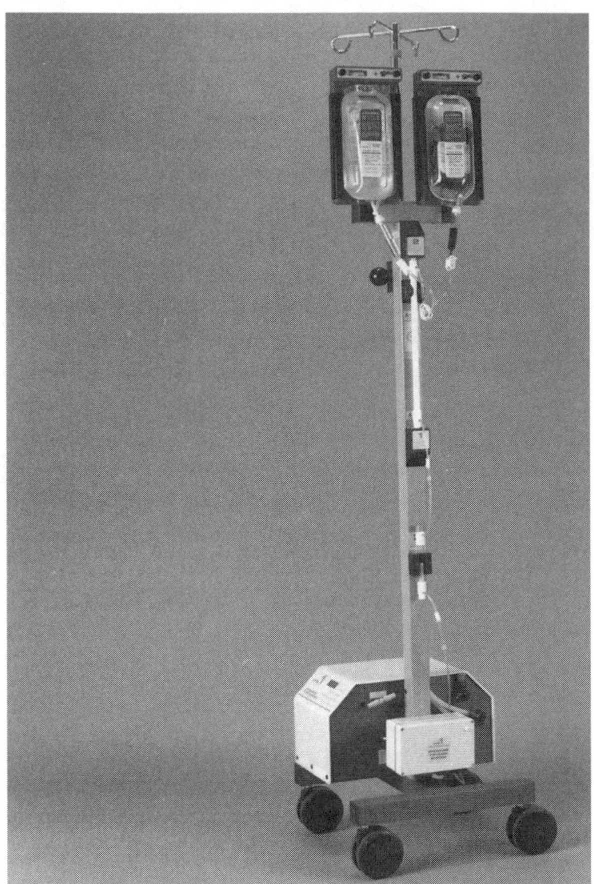

Figure 15–4. Fluid infusion warming system—Level 1 H500. Courtesy of Level One Technologies, Rockland, MA.

Rh negative).[36] Unstable patients with more than 40% blood loss (class IV) may require uncross-matched blood.

Warming Fluids/Infusion Techniques

Rapid infusion of cold fluids can predispose to hypothermia and cardiac dysrhythmias. Fluids should be heated before infusion if the patient requires a massive volume of crystalloids.[37] Werwath et al.[38] described a safe, efficient way of warming NS and LR solution by microwave if time permits. A 650-W microwave oven can be used to warm single liters of non-dextrose-containing crystalloids from room temperature to 101 °F in 120 sec. After 60 sec, the bag must be taken out and agitated, then warmed 1 min longer. The bag is agitated again, and the temperature is checked before administration. Blood, plasma, and glucose-containing solutions should *not* be warmed in a microwave oven.[39]

If a massive amount of fluid is needed rapidly, a fluid warming device that is also capable of pressure infusion may be necessary, such as the Level 1 H500 (Level One Technologies, Rockland, MA; see Fig. 15-4. This device has been shown to heat blood to $\geq$33 °C at flow rates of $\geq$500 mL/min.[40] It is also capable of administering crystalloids at a rate of 1000 mL/min. Studies suggest that many infusion pumps used today are not capable of warming fluids sufficiently when they are to be administered at a rate greater than 150 mL/min.[41] See Table 15-2 for a summary of strategies to facilitate rapid flow rates of intravenous fluids.

EVALUATING RESPONSE TO RESUSCITATION

Some patients (usually those who have lost $<$20% of their blood volume) respond rapidly to the initial fluid bolus and remain stable when the infusion is slowed. No further fluid bolus or immediate blood administration is indicated for this group of patients, although cross-matched blood should be made available. Other patients respond to the initial fluid bolus

(text continues on page 265)

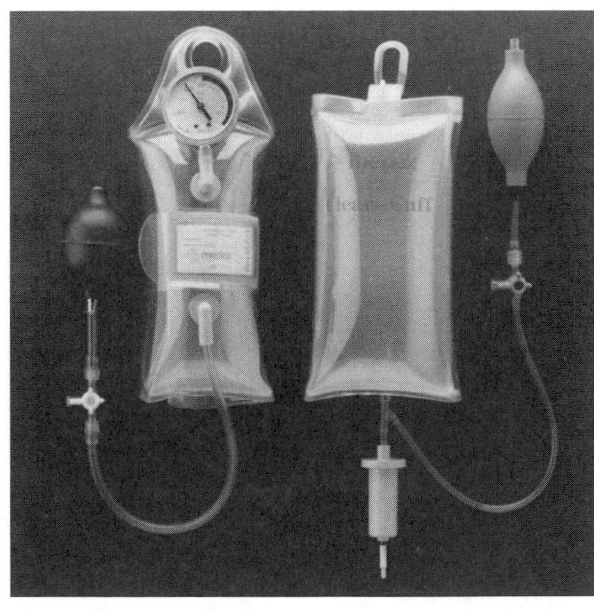

Figure 15–5. Pressure infusion cuff. Courtesy of Medex, Inc., Dublin, OH.

TABLE 15–2

Factors Affecting Flow Rate and Strategies to Increase Flow Rate

FACTORS AFFECTING FLOW RATE	STRATEGIES TO INCREASE FLOW RATE
Catheter diameter	Use largest diameter device available: Dutky 1989[42]: Demonstrated that in vitro* rate of flow increased as diameter of device increased (using crystalloid fluids administered by gravity drip): 18-ga: 87 mL/min 16-ga: 125 mL/min 14-ga: 147 mL/min 8.5-Fr: 160 mL/min See Figure 15-3 to compare the diameters of a rapid-flow infusion catheter and a typical small-diameter catheter
Catheter length	Use shortest large IV device available: Landow 1990[43]: Demonstrated that in vitro* flow rate increased as length of IV device decreased (using normal saline at a pressure of 50 mmHg): 14-ga 2 inch: 291 mL/min 14-ga 1.25 inch: 310 mL/min Note how approximate flow rates (mL/hr) are faster in shorter Arrow Multi-Lumen Central Venous Catheters (7 Fr x 20 cm vs 7 Fr x 30 cm) when normal saline is infused at room temperature through standard tubing under gravity (40 in. head height); under the same conditions, flow rates of up to 11,400 mL/hr can be achieved through the proximal (12 gauge) lumen of a two-lumen 12 Fr x 16 cm Arrow catheter:[44]

DISTAL LUMEN (16 GA) Brown Port		MIDDLE LUMEN (18 GA) Blue Port		PROXIMAL LUMEN (18 GA) White Port	
7 Fr x 20 cm	7 Fr x 30 cm	7 Fr x 20 cm	7 Fr x 30 cm	7 Fr x 20 cm	7 Fr x 30 cm
3107	2321	1506	993	1593	1086

FACTORS AFFECTING FLOW RATE	STRATEGIES TO INCREASE FLOW RATE
IV administration tubing diameter	Use largest possible IV tubing set available: Dutky et al 1989[45]: Demonstrated in vitro* flow rate increased with large-diameter tubing (as compared to regular tubing), using crystalloid fluid with gravity drip: Regular tubing with a 14-ga catheter: 268 mL/min Large tubing with a 14-ga catheter: 417 mL/min Regular tubing with a 8.5-Fr catheter: 316 mL/min Large tubing with a 8.5-Fr catheter: 805 mL/min
Pressure under which fluid is administered:	Consider variations in flow rate according to type of administration (gravity versus pressure device)
Gravity:	When gravity is used to deliver the solution, hang the container as high as possible to facilitate force of gravity
Gravity vs Pressure:	Use pressure method to administer fluid when possible

(continued)

TABLE 15–2 (cont.)

FACTORS AFFECTING FLOW RATE	STRATEGIES TO INCREASE FLOW RATE
Methods of Pressure	
• Pressure infusion cuff	Most facilities have pressure infusion cuffs available. (See Fig. 15-5.)
• Infusion pumps	Pumps for rapid fluid infusion are discussed in this chapter (see text) Landow 1990[46]: Demonstrated that pressure increases flow rate substantially in an in vitro* study using crystalloids and regular tubing with a 14-ga catheter: Gravity drip: 233 mL/min 300 mmHg pressure: 594 mL/min
Temperature of fluid to be administered	Warm fluids, as indicated. (See text.) Rapidly infused fluids are usually warmed to prevent hypothermia; this also increases rate of flow. For example, blood infusion flow rate increases by one half to one third after warming.[47]
Viscosity of fluid	Recognize that highly viscous fluids infuse more slowly than crystalloid fluids. If a filter is used in the administration set (as for blood), change it as frequently as indicated to avoid clogging and thus slowed fluid rate. A suggestion to speed the flow rate of viscous packed red blood cells is to mix them with warmed isotonic saline Comparison of flow rates (nonviscous versus viscous fluids): Flow rates (mL/min) of LR and whole blood with pressure infusion[48]

	LACTATED RINGER'S STANDARD TUBING (6 FT)	WHOLE BLOOD STANDARD TUBING (6 FT)
16-ga subclavian	158	60
16-ga Quik Cath	289	149
10-ga Angio Cath	496	261
8-Fr catheter introducer	492	265

FACTORS AFFECTING FLOW RATE	STRATEGIES TO INCREASE FLOW RATE
Kinking of IV device	Take precautions to prevent kinking of IV device; Dutky[49] recommends: • use a short catheter (such as a 3.5-inch, 8.5-Fr introducer) • use a lateral approach if the subclavian site is used • use jugular site if needed
Kinking of IV tubing	Use of a large-diameter IV infusion set minimizes the risk for kinking

*Note that these findings were obtained from studies conducted in a laboratory setting (*not* in actual patients); thus, the findings were not influenced by factors encountered during actual practice (such as the patient's intravenous pressure or catheter obstruction from venous valves, venous tortuosity, or occlusion of the catheter's orifice by the patient's venous wall).

but show signs of deterioration when the fluids are slowed; most of these patients have lost 20% to 40% of their blood volume, or are still bleeding and require continued crystalloid administration as well as blood transfusion and surgical intervention. Little or no response to fluid resuscitation is seen in a small but significant percentage of injured patients. For most of these, failure to respond to adequate crystalloid and blood administration indicates the need for unlimited blood and fluid resuscitation and immediate surgical intervention to control hemorrhage.

Noninvasive Clinical Signs

Traditionally, patient response to resuscitation therapy has been determined by noninvasive clinical indicators such as:

- Systolic blood pressure
- Heart rate
- Level of consciousness
- Pulse pressure
- Pulse rate
- Urine output

Although urine output is one of the primary indicators of response to fluid resuscitation, it should be recognized that it can be affected by variables other than adequate fluid replacement. For example, diuretics or vasopressors can increase urinary flow rate despite underlying tissue perfusion problems.

Adequate volume replacement should produce a urinary output of about 50 mL/hr in an adult and 1 mL/kg/hr in the pediatric patient; for children younger than 1 year of age, 2 mL/kg/hr should be maintained.[50]

It is recognized that hypoperfusion and thus poor cellular oxygen delivery can persist although the conventional signs are returned to a normal range. Because of this, current practice reflects an evolving view of how to monitor patients for an appropriate response to fluid resuscitation.[51] Recall that the hypoperfusion of shock creates a cellular oxygen debt and that the overall goal of volume resuscitation is to increase oxygen delivery to the cells. To determine whether this has occurred, it may be necessary to insert a pulmonary artery (PA) catheter (see discussion below in Oxygenation Measurements From a Pulmonary Artery Catheter). Other parameters to assess include hematocrit, blood pH, and lactate levels, which are discussed in the following sections.

During massive fluid resuscitation, it is possible to give too little or too much fluid. Inadequate fluid administration must be guarded against since prolonged hypovolemia predisposes to decreased perfusion of major organs.[52] Conversely, it is possible to administer too much fluid and thereby overwhelm the circulation, and perhaps cause pulmonary edema. Volume overload to some extent is common in shock patients during aggressive fluid resuscitation. As described earlier, because of compensatory increased secretion of hormones (aldosterone and ADH), injured patients have an impaired ability to excrete excessive fluid loads. Even when the intravascular volume is not excessive, it is common for skin, muscles, and subcutaneous tissue to become edematous after massive volume resuscitation. This is because approximately 75% of every liter of balanced salt solution shifts into the interstitial space within 1 hr after administration. Problems associated with the resulting soft tissue edema include a decreased rate of wound healing and an increased propensity to develop pressure sores.

Hemodynamic Parameters

Central Venous Pressure

Central venous pressures (CVP) can be used as a guide to assess the heart's ability to tolerate a fluid load; however, it is important to avoid overdependence on CVP monitoring.[53]

Some points to remember about CVP measurements include:

1. CVP is an indirect measure of volume.
2. Normal CVP is 0 to 7 mmHg when a transducer system is used; it is approximately 1 to 10 cm of water when a water manometer is used.
3. CVP is often low in hypovolemic shock because of inadequate filling of the right heart.
4. The initial CVP and actual blood volume are not necessarily related.
5. A high CVP may be observed even with a volume deficit; for example, patients with generalized vasoconstriction and fluid replacement may show a high pressure related to the appli-

cation of pneumatic antishock garment or inappropriate use of vasopressors.

6. A minimal rise in the initial, low CVP with fluid therapy suggests the need for further volume expansion.
7. A decrease in CVP suggests an ongoing fluid loss.
8. An abrupt or persistent elevation in CVP suggests volume replacement has been adequate or is too rapid, or that cardiac function has been compromised.
9. A malpositioned catheter or increased intrathoracic pressure from a pneumothorax may cause pronounced elevations of CVP.
10. CVP is best monitored in trends, especially in response to fluid therapy.

Pulmonary Capillary Wedge Pressure

The pulmonary catheter wedge pressure (PCWP) is a measure of preload, which reflects left ventricular end-diastolic volume; this measure is easily obtained at the bedside from the PA catheter. Although CVP and PCWP do not reflect blood volume accurately in all patients, they are useful in preventing acute volume overload during rapid fluid restoration and fluid challenges. In critically ill patients, a PCWP of 15 to 18 mmHg is the goal to increase cardiac output.[54]

New technology has allowed for the measurement of right ventricular end-diastolic volume (RVEDV) by way of a modified PA catheter. Research is underway to evaluate the efficacy of RVEDV as an improved measure of cardiac preload as compared to PCWP and CVP. The goal of RVEDV is a range of 160 to 180 mL.[55]

Cardiac Index

Cardiac index is more precise than cardiac output in reflecting left ventricular output because it takes into account the individual's body size. (Cardiac output expressed in liters per minute is the amount of blood pumped by the heart; cardiac index is the cardiac output per meter squared of body surface area.) A more specific measurement is available by calculating the cardiac output and then figuring the cardiac index according to the patient's height and weight. Factors that decrease or increase cardiac output will directly affect cardiac index. However, when blood loss exceeds 20% to 25% (class II shock) of the intravascular volume, these compensatory mechanisms are no longer effective, resulting in a decreased cardiac output and oxygen transport to the tissues.

There are indications that a cardiac index 50% greater than normal (>4.5 L/min/m^2) is associated with better outcomes in high-risk postoperative critically ill patients.[56] After intravascular volume repletion, inotropes may be added if further increases in cardiac output are needed. The first choice is low-dose dopamine because of its selective renal and mesenteric vasodilatory properties, and if further inotropic support is needed, dobutamine is added and titrated as needed.[57]

Oxygenation Measurements From a Pulmonary Artery Catheter

Oxygen Consumption and Oxygen Delivery

Oxygen consumption (VO_2) and oxygen delivery (DO_2) can be calculated from a PA catheter. VO_2 is defined as the amount of oxygen per m^2 consumed by the tissues. Normal values for VO_2 (indexed) are between 110 and 140 mL/min/m^2. Indexed DO_2 is defined as the amount of oxygen per m^2 delivered to the tissues from the arterial side of the circulation. Under normal circumstances, indexed DO_2 is much greater than oxygen demand. Normal indexed DO_2 is 520 ± 57 mL/min/m^2.

Oxygen demand is the amount of oxygen required by the tissues to maintain aerobic metabolism. Normally, oxygen delivery meets oxygen demand; however, during shock states, inadequate DO_2 causes tissues to convert to anaerobic metabolism, thereby causing the serum lactate concentration to rise. This results in irreversible damage to the cell after time. As more and more cells within an organ system are irreversibly damaged, the organ begins to fail, ultimately leading to multiorgan failure and death.

Studies have suggested that patients who are resuscitated to above normal values for DO_2 and VO_2 have a lower mortality and a lower incidence of multisystem organ failure. It is recommended that indexed DO_2 be increased to greater than normal (>600 mL/min/m^2) and indexed VO_2 to about 30% greater than normal (>170 mL/min/m^2).[58]

Oxygen delivery can be increased by (1) increasing cardiac output; (2) increasing hemoglobin concentration; and (3) increasing arterial oxygen saturation. To increase cardiac output, initial therapy is volume loading. If cardiac output remains low after volume loading, inotropic agents may be added. To increase hemoglobin, blood may be given to increase volume and to increase oxygen carrying capacity. To increase arterial oxygen saturation, mechanical ventilation with the use of increased inspired oxygen fractions and positive end-expiratory pressure are required.

Mixed Venous Oxygen Saturation

Mixed venous oxygen saturation (SVO_2) is measured in the PA. SVO_2 is a reflection of global tissue utilization of oxygen. It is the net result of overall cardiorespiratory function and tissue perfusion. It is determined by the arterial oxygen saturation (SaO_2), cardiac output, hemoglobin, and oxygen consumption.[59]

Other Oxygenation Indicators

Lactate Level

Lactate determinations have been used to assess the adequacy of tissue oxygenation in the critically ill. The most common cause of an elevated blood lactate concentration is hypoperfusion or circulatory shock.[60] When intracellular oxygen is not available, energy is produced by anaerobic metabolic pathways, resulting in increased lactate production. It has been shown that patients with blood lactate values below 2 mg/dL have a 90% survival, whereas those with values above 10 mg/dL have a 90% mortality.[61] Arterial or mixed venous blood specimens are favored for lactate analysis as peripherally obtained venous samples can yield falsely elevated values, depending on the techniques used.[62] If before obtaining the specimen the patient remains at complete rest, venous and arterial levels are virtually alike; however, if even minor movements such as hand clenching are performed, the lactate level in the sample can raise significantly.[63] (Venous stasis from applying a tourniquet has little effect.)[64] Measurement of lactate levels from arterial lines (when present) allows for monitoring of subtle but important serial changes that reflect the patient's response to therapy and provides the clinician with valuable feedback. If an arterial line is not present, a properly drawn specimen from a peripheral venous site is acceptable.

Interstitial pH of Gastrointestinal Tract

Measurements of oxygen consumption in specific organs could be helpful in determining the adequacy of resuscitation in patients in shock, especially organs at high risk (such as the gut and liver). A relatively new area of investigation to assess tissue oxygenation involves measuring the interstitial pH of the gastrointestinal (GI) tract using balloon tonometry. A tonometer consists of a saline-filled balloon attached to the distal end of a standard nasogastric tube. After the tube is inserted nasogastrically, anaerobic samples of the tonometer saline and of arterial blood are obtained simultaneously and analyzed by standard pH and blood-gas analyzers; intramucosal pH (pH_I) is then calculated by a modification of the Henderson-Hasselbach equation.[65] Normal pH_I is 7.35 or higher. Preliminary studies of critically ill patients suggest this measurement may merit further study.[66]

Acid–Base and Electrolyte Changes

The majority of acid–base abnormalities that develop in shock improve spontaneously once adequate ventilation and perfusion are achieved. Patients with severe traumatic injury and hemorrhagic shock are acidotic on admission as a result of loss of oxygen carrying capacity and decreased cardiac output.[67] As lactate and hydrogen ions accumulate in shock, a high anion gap metabolic acidosis develops. Respiratory acidosis will also develop as the number of functional pulmonary capillaries decrease, causing carbon dioxide (CO_2) retention. In the final stages of shock, there will be a combined metabolic and respiratory acidosis with an increase in the arterial carbon dioxide tension ($PaCO_2$), a low bicarbonate level, and a very low pH.[68] Metabolic acidosis or metabolic alkalosis may occur after massive blood transfusion (see Chapter 10).

Tissue injury or hemorrhage may cause catecholamine release, which in turn may cause an intracellular shift of potassium and cause hypokalemia.[69] Electrolyte disorders associated with massive transfusions are discussed in Chapter 10. In addition to treatment-related causes of electrolyte imbalances, underlying clinical problems can contribute to the development of specific imbalances.

CASE STUDIES

15-1. After undergoing a sigmoid colectomy and splenectomy, a 47-year-old man was returned to the postoperative recovery room at noon in good condition. At that time, he was receiving lactated Ringer's solution through an 18-gauge port of a triple lumen central venous catheter. His vital signs were normal, as was perfusion of the kidneys and brain (as evidenced by an adequate level of consciousness and urinary output). Approximately 4 hrs later, he developed seizure-type activity and became unresponsive; the following vital signs were obtained: blood pressure, 44/20 mm Hg; heart rate, 136 beats/min; CVP, 0 cm water; and rapid gasping respirations. Blood work was drawn and showed a hemoglobin of 11 g/dL and a hematocrit of 36%. No bleeding was noted from the abdominal incision. The physician was notified and the intravenous line was immediately turned to a "wide open" rate (under the influence of gravity). Over the next 5 hrs, the patient received LR "wide open" through the 18-gauge port of the central venous catheter (CVC), and two units of PRBCs were given through the 16-gauge port of the CVC (with the assistance of a pressure cuff). Despite this, the patient's vital signs remained extremely poor, urine output was almost nil, and full consciousness was never regained. The hemoglobin dropped to 6 g/dL and the hematocrit to 19%. The patient was returned to surgery where a short 14-gauge catheter was inserted in the external jugular vein; warmed blood and crystalloids were pumped in through this device. An exploratory laparotomy revealed that a ligature had slipped from the splenic artery and the patient's abdomen was filled with blood. Despite aggressive fluid resuscitation in the operating room and control of bleeding, the patient did not survive.

COMMENTARY: Because a major compensatory shift of fluid from the extravascular extracellular space into the vascular space (to help replace the diminished blood supply) had not had time to occur, the patient's hemoglobin and hematocrit values were close to normal at the time of the hemorrhagic event (see. Later, hemodilution from this process became more obvious (hemoglobin 6 g/dL and hematocrit 19%).

The patient's clinical status did not improve despite IV fluid given "wide open" because the fluids were administered via gravity with the flow control clamp wide open; because a small port (18-gauge) of a long, narrow CVC was used, the fluid met resistance as it attempted to flow through the catheter. (One could equate this to using a long, narrow ordinary garden hose to apply water to a major fire; instead, of course, one would want to use a wide short hose for this purpose, preferably with the water delivered under pressure). See Table 15-1 for strategies to administer fluids rapidly when severe hypovolemia is present. Failure of the patient to respond to the inadequate fluid regime described above was an indication that more aggressive fluid resuscitation (along with more rapid surgical intervention) was urgently needed.

A lack of visible incisional bleeding is insufficient to "rule out" hemorrhagic shock after abdominal surgery. In this instance, the patient was bleeding internally. All other clinical signs pointed to hemorrhagic shock; unfortunately, however, they were not recognized.

Although a PA catheter is often helpful in the early diagnosis of hypovolemic shock and to allow titration of fluids during resuscitation to achieve a satisfactory outcome, this patient could have been managed without a PA catheter. The blood pressure, 44/20 mmHg; heart rate, 136 beats/min; and CVP, 0 cm H_2O should have guided treatment to more aggressive fluid resuscitation along with more rapid surgical intervention. Hemodynamic parameters obtainable with the PA catheter are often indicated when the patient is stabilized and there is uncertainty of the volume status. However, a PA catheter was not actually needed in this case to detect hypovolemic shock because other clinical indicators were obvious, as was the inadequate clinical response to too little fluid resuscitation.

15-2. A 56-year-old man was trapped between two railroad cars in a mining accident. He was hypotensive at the scene of the accident and resuscitated with 3000 mL of lactated Ringer's solution before being transported to a trauma center. On arrival, he was anxious and confused and his vital signs were as follow: blood pressure, 98/60 mmHg; pulse rate, 120 /min; and respiratory rate, 40/min; estimated blood loss at this time, 2000 mL. He was given an additional 3000 mL of LR before being rushed to surgery. During surgery, he was found to have the following injuries: right diaphragmatic hernia, herniation of kidney and liver into the thoracic cavity, liver laceration, avulsion of the right ureter from the renal pelvis, injury to the lumbar vessels, crush injury to head of pancreas, and serosal tears of the duodenum. The surgical procedure consisted of an exploratory laparotomy with ligation of bleeding lumbar vessels, a repair of the right renal vein, a right nephrectomy, repair of the diaphragm, drainage of the pancreatic injury, and repair of the duodenal serosal tears. During surgery he received the following fluids:

5% albumin = 500 mL
Fresh frozen plasma = 785 mL
Hetastarch = 500 mL
Platelets = 200 mL
PRBCs = 12 units
0.9% sodium chloride = 1000 mL

Urinary output from the time of admission through the end of the surgical procedure was 2000 mL. The total estimated blood loss from the time of injury was 5000 mL. Because of the need for rapid fluid resuscitation, fluids were warmed and administered under pressure with the Level One Blood Warmer (see Fig. 15-4).

Vital signs and other data available from the time of admission through the first 24 hrs were as shown in Table 15-3. Arterial blood gas, lactate levels, and hematocrit levels were as shown in Table 15-4.

TABLE 15-3

	Hour 1 (ER)	Hour 3 (OR)	Hour 5 (OR)	Hour 10 (ICU)	Hour 16 (ICU)	Hour 22 (ICU)	Hour 24 (ICU)
Heart rate	120	130	118	98	110	118	113
Blood pressure	98/60	<60	110/70	166/90	138/78	136/76	140/80
CVP (mmHg)				6	2	5	13
PCWP (mmHg)				3	2	6	12

TABLE 15-4

	Hour 1 (ER)	Hour 2 (OR)	Hour 4 (OR)	Hour 5 (OR)	Hour 6 (OR)	Hour 10 (OR)	Hour 12 (ICU)	Hour 18 (ICU)	Hour 24 (ICU)
pH	7.26	7.23	7.15	7.18	7.3	7.26	7.25	7.35	7.36
$PaCO_2$ (mmHg)	46	44	40	45	47	43	43	37	43
HCO_3 (mEq/L)	20.2	18	20	18	13	16	23	20	24
Lactate (mg/dL)							5.8	3.6	1.8
Hematocrit	26%								33%

Total intake from the time of injury through the first 24 hrs was 20,035 mL; urine output during this time was 6900 mL. During this same period, he sustained an estimated blood loss of 5000 mL.

COMMENTARY: The patient experienced class III shock at the time of admission to the trauma center (based on estimated blood loss, vital signs, and mental status—see Table 15-1), which worsened during the surgical procedure. (Note the increased heart rate and lowered blood pressure at the third surgical hour.)

On admission, the patient had a combination of metabolic acidosis and respiratory acidosis. For example, the bicarbonate level was below normal (18 mEq/L). The expected $PaCO_2$ in this situation would be as follows (using Winter's formula, see Chapter 9): $1.5(18) + 8 \pm 2 = 33–37$ mmHg (instead, it was 44 mmHg, indicating an excess of $PaCO_2$).

Adding the urinary output to the estimated blood loss, the patient lost a total of approximately 12 L of fluid; during the same period, he gained approximately 20 L by the intravenous route. The discrepancy of approximately 8 L can partially be explained by third-spacing caused by the initial trauma as well as trauma sustained during the surgical procedures. The third spacing resulted in hypovolemia as fluid shifted from the vascular space into the injured tissues. Fluid was administered in sufficient quantities to keep the vital signs and other parameters within normal limits.

Serum lactate level may be used to assess adequacy of fluid resuscitation. Note how these readings improved from hour 14 to hour 24. Other parameters that improved with resuscitation were vital signs (blood pressure and pulse), hemodynamic readings (CVP and PCWP), hematocrit values, and arterial blood gas values.

REFERENCES

1. American College of Surgeons, Committee on Trauma, Advanced Trauma Life Support Course for Physicians. p 12. Chicago, American College of Surgeons, 1993
2. Kinney MR, Packa DR, Dunbar SB (eds): AACN's Clinical Reference for Critical-Care Nursing, 3rd ed, p 138. St. Louis, Mosby, 1993
3. Chernow B (ed): The Pharmacologic Approach to the Critically Ill Patient, 3rd ed. p 1110. Baltimore, Williams & Wilkins, 1994
4. ATLS, p 82
5. Ibid
6. Rice V: Shock, a clinical syndrome: An update. Part I. An overview of shock. Crit Care Nurse 11(4):20–27, 1991
7. Moore EE (ed): Early Care of the Injured Patient, 4th ed, p 77. Philadelphia, B.C. Decker, 1990
8. Cardona V, Hurn P, Mason P, Scanlon A, Veise-Berry S: Trauma Nursing, 2nd ed, p 152. Philadelphia, WB Saunders, 1994
9. Ibid
10. Ibid
11. ATLS, p 81–82
12. Guyton A: Textbook of Medical Physiology, 8th ed, p 264. Philadelphia, WB Saunders, 1991
13. Sabiston DC, Lyerly HK (eds): Sabiston Essentials of Surgery, 2nd ed, p 11. Philadelphia, WB Saunders, 1994
14. Moore, 1990, p 65
15. Ibid
16. Ibid
17. Dutky et al: Factors affecting rapid fluid resuscitation with large-bore introducer catheters. J Trauma 29:856–860, 1989
18. Moore, 1990, p 64
19. ATLS, p 84
20. Ibid
21. Chernow, p 275
22. Ibid, p 280
23. Moore, 1990, p 76
24. Velanovich V: Crystalloid versus colloid fluid resuscitation: A meta-analysis of mortality. Surgery 105:65–71, 1989
25. Holcroft et al: 3% NaCl and 7.5% NaCl/Dextran 70 in the resuscitation of severely injured patients. Anal Surg 206:278–288, 1987
26. Mattox et al: Prehospital hypertonic saline/dextran infusion for post-traumatic hypotension. Ann Surg 213:482–491, 1991
27. Vassar et al: Analysis of potential risks associated with 7.5% sodium chloride resuscitation of traumatic shock. Arch Surg 125:1309–1315, 1990
28. Soliman et al: Survival after hypertonic saline resuscitation from hemorrhage. Am Surgeon 56:749–751, 1990
29. Wisner K et al: Hypertonic saline resuscitation of head-injury: Effects on cerebral water content. J Trauma 30:75, 1990
30. Griffel M, Kaufman B: Pharmacology of colloids and crystalloids. Crit Care Clin 8:235–253, 1992
31. Clochesy J (ed): Critical Care Nursing, p 1237. Philadelphia, WB Saunders, 1993
32. Moore FA et al: Incommensurate oxygen consumption in response to maximal oxygen availability pre-

dicts postinjury multiple organ failure. J Trauma 33:58–67, 1992
33. Clochesy, p 1237
34. Chernow, p 274
35. Rossi E, Simon T, Moss G (eds): Principles of Transfusion Medicine, p 97. Baltimore, Williams & Wilkins, 1991
36. Ibid, p 82
37. ATLS, p 89
38. Werwath et al: Microwave ovens. A safe new method of warming crystalloids. Am Surgeon 50:656–659, 1984
39. ATLS, p 89
40. Uhl L, Pacini D, Kruskall M: A comparative study of blood warmer performance. Anesthesiology 77:1022–1028, 1992
41. Ibid, p 1026
42. Dutky et al, p 856–860
43. Landow L, Shahnarian A: Efficacy of large bore intravenous fluid administration sets designed for rapid volume resuscitation. Crit Care Med 18:540–543, 1990
44. Arrow Multi-Lumen Central Venous Catheter: Nursing Care Guidelines, p 13. Arrow International Inc; Reading, PA, December, 1994
45. Dutky et al, p 856–860
46. Landow, Shahnarian, p 540–543
47. Dula D et al: Flow rate variance of commonly used intravenous infusion techniques. J Trauma 21:480–482, 1981
48. Millikan J, Cain T, Hansbrough J: Rapid volume replacement for hypovolemic shock: A comparison of techniques and equipment. J Trauma 24(5):428–431, 1984
49. Dutky et al, p 856–860
50. ATLS, p 85
51. Annas C: Changing technology and research shape critical care trauma nursing. Intern J Trauma Nurs Fall:20–22,1994
52. Ibid, p 20–22
53. ATLS, p 85
54. Packman M, Rachow C: Optimum left heart filling pressure during fluid resuscitation of patients with hypovolemic and septic shock. Crit Care Med 11:165–169,1983
55. Durham R et al: Right ventricular end diastolic volume as a measure of preload. Crit Care Med Abstract S200, 1993
56. Shoemaker W: Pathophysiology, monitoring, and therapy of acute circulatory problems. Crit Care Nurs Clin N Am 6(2):295–307, 1994
57. Moore, 1992, p 58–67
58. Moore F, Moore E: Evolving concepts in the pathogenesis of postinjury multiple organ failure. Surgical Clinics of North America 75(2):267, 1995
59. Kinney, p 81
60. Kruse JA, Carlson RW: Lactate metabolism. Crit Care Med 5:725, 1987
61. Narins RG (ed): Maxwell and Kleeman's Clinical Disorders of Fluid and Electrolyte Metabolism, 5th ed, p 147. New York, McGraw-Hill, 1994
62. Ibid, p 1473
63. Henry J: Clinical Diagnosis and Management by Laboratory Methods, 18th ed, p 186. Philadelphia, WB Saunders, 1991
64. Ibid
65. Gutierrez G et al: Gastric intramucosal pH as a therapeutic index of tissue oxygenation in critically ill patients. Lancet 339:195–199, 1992
66. Dantzker D: Adequacy of tissue oxygenation. Crit Care Med 21(2):S40–43, 1993
67. Ferrera A, McArthur JD, et al: Hypothermia and acidosis worsen coagulopathies in the patient requiring massive transfusion. Am J Surg 160:515–518, 1990
68. Ibid, p 152
69. Dunham CM, Cowley RA: Shock Trauma/Critical Care Manual. Rockville, MD, Aspen Publishers, 1991

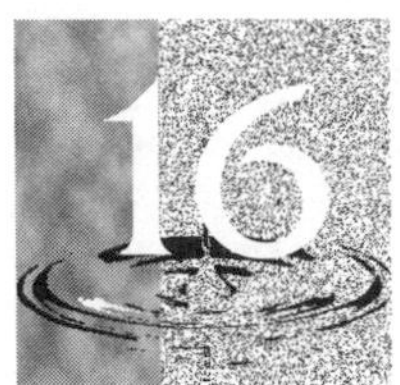

Heart Failure

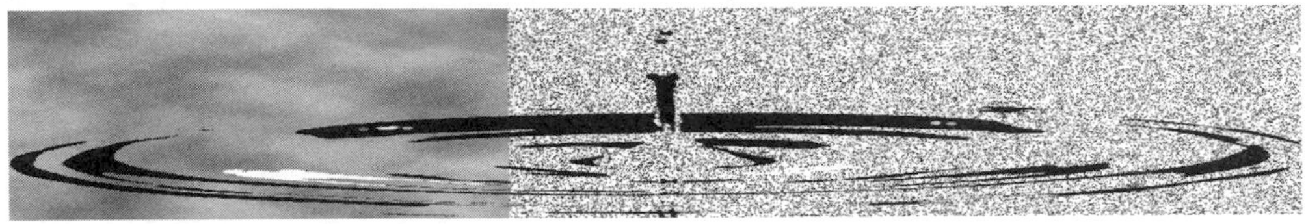

DEFINITION

Heart failure refers to an inability of the heart to pump enough blood to meet the metabolic needs of tissues throughout the body. Common causes of heart failure (often referred to as congestive heart failure [CHF]) include hypertension, myocardial infarction, cardiomyopathies, and valvular disease.

Left-ventricular failure, as seen in hypertensive heart disease or mitral stenosis, typically presents with pulmonary but not peripheral edema. In contrast, pure right-ventricular failure initially seen in patients with cor pulmonale, typically presents with edema in the lower extremities and perhaps ascites. Failure of one ventricle often leads to failure of the other, therefore both types of failure are present. Patients with cardiomyopathies tend to have simultaneous failure of both ventricles, presenting with both pulmonary and peripheral edema. Heart failure can be chronic or become acutely manifested in the form of pulmonary edema or cardiogenic shock.

MAJOR FLUID AND ELECTROLYTE IMBALANCES

The reader is referred to Table 16-1 for a summary of fluid and electrolyte disturbances associated with CHF. The primary imbalances include fluid volume overload with hyponatremia, hypokalemia, and hypomagnesemia.

FLUID VOLUME EXCESS

The patient with heart failure presents with the classic picture of an expanded extracellular fluid (ECF) volume, that is, swollen legs, engorged neck veins, congested liver, and pulmonary crackles. Although the ECF is increased, the kidneys respond as if a reduced blood volume is present. The decrease in cardiac output and increase in ventricular end-diastolic pressure set the stage for sodium retention. Decreased cardiac output and increased systemic resistance produce decreased organ flow, especially to the kidney.

Shunting of blood away from the kidneys stimulates secretion of renin, which acts on angiotensinogen to produce angiotensin I, which is subsequently converted to angiotensin II. Angiotensin II is a strong arterial vasoconstrictor that helps to support arterial blood pressure when cardiac output decreases. This arterial vasoconstriction increases the work of the left ventricle as it pumps against the increased pressure (increased afterload). Angiotensin II also stimulates the secretion of aldosterone, which strongly promotes the reabsorption of sodium in the distal tubules and collecting ducts of the kidney. Another effect is venous vasoconstriction, which tends to increase venous return to the heart (increased preload).

Treatment

The reader is referred to the section on methods to decrease preload, presented later in this chapter.

HYPONATREMIA

In addition to activation of the renin-angiotensin-aldosterone mechanism, responses to circulatory failure include stimulation of hormones such as arginine vasopressin (antidiuretic hormone [ADH]), and stimulation of the sympathetic nervous system. Antidiuretic hormone acts on the distal tubules to cause water retention, which can lead to an increased preload as well as *hyponatremia*. Although there is a total excess of sodium and water (due to aldosterone effect), the added water retention produced by ADH can cause dilutional hyponatremia. Thus, the patient has a fluid volume excess with a relatively greater retention of water than sodium (see Figure 4-2A). Patients with hyponatremia tend to be more ill and have a relatively unstable clinical course.[1] With the exception of those with hyponatremia due to overdiuresis (combined with hypotonic fluid replacement), hyponatremia in CHF usually indicates a severe clinical stage.[2] Most patients with CHF who have hyponatremia are clinically compromised, have disease of New York Heart Association functional class IV, and are volume-overloaded.[3] Consequences of severe hyponatremia are primarily neurological in nature (see Chapter 4). Contributing to hyponatremia in some patients is the tendency of sodium to shift from the ECF into the cells to replace the potassium loss associated with hyperaldosteronism and use of potassium-losing diuretics.

TABLE 16–1

Fluid and Electrolyte Disturbances Associated With Congestive Heart Failure

FLUID AND ELECTROLYTE DISTURBANCE	ETIOLOGY
Fluid volume excess	Secondary hyperaldosteronism (result of decreased renal blood flow associated with decreased cardiac output) Excessive aldosterone causes sodium and water retention
Hyponatremia	Although total body sodium content is above normal, excessive secretion of ADH causes relatively greater retention of water, diluting the serum level (see Figure 4-2A) Contributing to the hyponatremia is loss of sodium in, for example, vomiting, diarrhea, and paracentesis; most hazardous if patient is on severely restricted sodium diet and large doses of diuretics Contributing to hyponatremia can be the movement of extracellular sodium into the cells to replace the potassium so frequently lost in treatment of heart failure
Hypokalemia	Excessive aldosterone levels predispose to potassium excretion Excessive use of potassium-losing diuretics and prolonged loss of potassium by vomiting or diarrhea represent typical causes of potassium deficit
Hypomagnesemia	Similar mechanisms to those described for hypokalemia Most likely to be problematic in patients with moderately severe to severe CHF receiving chronic or aggressive thiazide or loop-diuretic therapy Frequently contributes to the development of hypokalemia that is resistant to correction by potassium replacement alone
Hyperkalemia	Excessive use of potassium supplements, potassium-sparing diuretics, or angiotensin-converting enzyme inhibitors, in patients with renal dysfunction
Metabolic alkalosis if potassium-losing diuretics are used	Potassium-losing diuretics cause loss of chloride ions and compensatory increase in bicarbonate ions (hence metabolic alkalosis)
Metabolic (lactic) acidosis	Increased liberation of lactic acid from anoxic tissues and failure of body to metabolize it rapidly Slowing of circulation interferes with the excretion of metabolic acids
Respiratory acidosis	Pulmonary congestion interferes with elimination of CO_2 from lungs

ADH, antidiuretic hormone.

Treatment

Fluid restriction may be necessary to deal with hyponatremia and fluid volume overload. Water intake is usually not restricted in the long-term management of heart failure unless there is dilution of the serum sodium to less than 130 mEq/L by excessive water retention. Most patients who present with significant hyponatremia are clinically compromised and usually require hospitalization. For inpatients, the total hypotonic fluid intake may be restricted to less than 1000 mL in 24 hrs.[4] In some patients with marked edema, oral diuretics may be ineffective because of poor absorption by the edematous gastrointestinal (GI) tract; thus, a "loop" diuretic may need to be given intravenously. If necessary, cardiovascular drug support (eg, dobutamine) may be used to improve the clinical state and increase the renal response to the loop diuretic.[5] The mainstay of chronic management of hyponatremia is use of a converting enzyme inhibitor; for mild hyponatremia (serum sodium concentration, 131–136 mEq/L), simply adding or increasing the dose of the converting enzyme inhibitor is often sufficient.[6]

HYPOKALEMIA

In the patient with CHF numerous conditions predispose to hypokalemia. Among these are increased aldosterone levels, which causes increased loss of potassium in the urine, and frequent use of potassium-losing diuretics. The metabolic alkalosis associated with diuretic use decreases the serum potassium level by driving potassium into the cells and by increasing renal potassium excretion. In volume-overloaded patients, the hypokalemia is in part "dilutional."

Treatment

Regardless of the serum potassium level, patients with CHF (who have good renal function) tend to have reduced total body potassium levels. Therefore, almost all patients with CHF should receive potassium supplementation, a potassium-sparing diuretic (such as spironolactone, amiloride, or triamterene), or an angiotensin-converting enzyme inhibitor; this is especially true if the patient is receiving a potassium-losing diuretic.[7] Hypokalemia is a serious threat because it increases the risk for arrhythmias and sudden death, especially in patients with CHF (because of diseased myocardium and use of arrhythmogenic drugs).[8] A serum potassium concentration of 4.5 to 5.0 mEq/L is favored by most investigators.[9] In the presence of serious dysrhythmias, intravenous (IV) administration of potassium chloride is best. When hypokalemia does not respond to potassium replacement, it may be necessary to administer magnesium concomitantly.

As is always the case, it is possible to over-correct an imbalance. Patients with renal dysfunction should be monitored closely for hyperkalemia, especially when receiving potassium supplementation or potassium-sparing agents. Also, the effects of potassium supplementation or potassium-sparing diuretics on patients chronically receiving angiotensin-converting enzyme inhibitors should be followed closely; when the serum potassium levels reach the upper end of the optimal maintenance range, potassium supplements and potassium-sparing diuretics should be discontinued.[10] See Table 16-2 for a description of common adverse effects of diuretics.

HYPOMAGNESEMIA

Magnesium depletion is most likely to occur in patients with severe CHF who are receiving chronic or aggressive therapy with thiazide or loop diuretics. Most of the causes of magnesium deficiency parallel those described above for the development of hypokalemia. It should be noted that serum magnesium levels do not correlate strongly with tissue magnesium concentrations; that is, serum magnesium levels may be normal despite the presence of a tissue magnesium deficit. Therefore, supplemental magnesium or other magnesium-retaining agents (e.g., potassium-sparing diuretics or angiotensin-converting enzyme inhibitors) should be considered for patients with moderately severe to severe CHF.[11] Hypomagnesemia and whole-body magnesium depletion in CHF patients are thought to be arrhythmogenic and probably increase the risk of morbidity and mortality, especially in the presence of digitalis toxicity, acute myocardial infarction, and after surgery.

Treatment

Routine magnesium supplementation is probably unnecessary for patients with mild to moderate CHF

TABLE 16–2

Common Adverse Eeffects of Diuretics

ELECTROLYTE ABNORMALITIES	METABOLIC ABNORMALITIES
Hypokalemia	Glucose intolerance (diabetes)*
Hyponatremia	Lipid changes (raised LDL and VLDL, unchanged HDL)
Hypomagnesemia	Hyperuricemia (gout)*
Variable calcium excretion	Thrombocytopenic purpura
Hyperkalemia with K-retaining diuretics	Increased platelet aggregation
	Activation of the renin-angiotensin system*
Metabolic alkalosis	Increased blood viscosity
GENERAL EFFECTS PARTICULARLY COMMON IN THE ELDERLY	
Hypovolemia with fatigue and even dizziness*	
Azotemia*	
Urinary incontinence*	
CARDIAC EFFECTS	
Arrhythmias*	
?? Effect on contractility	

*Important side effects

Reprinted from Poole-Wilson P: Diuretics for the treatment of heart failure. in: Barnett D, Poueur H, Francis G (eds): Congestive Cardiac Failure: Pathophysiology and Treatment; p 107, New York, Marcel Dekker, 1993. By courtesy of Marcel Dekker, Inc.

who are normokalemic and who are receiving an angiotensin-converting enzyme (ACE) inhibitor or a potassium-sparing diuretic. However, patients with advanced CHF who require aggressive thiazide or loop diuretic therapy and those with uncomplicated hypomagnesemia should be considered as candidates for long-term orally administered magnesium.[12] According to Leier et al.,[13] magnesium is a safe and potentially effective agent in the treatment of CHF, provided there is no significant renal dysfunction and reasonable clinical follow-up is performed. When magnesium is needed as an acute intervention, 10 to 20 mL of 10% magnesium sulfate may be prescribed IV over 5 to 10 min, usually followed by a 250- to 500-mL infusion of 2% solution during the subsequent 4 to 8 hrs.[14]

As mentioned above, magnesium administration is important in the management of hypokalemia that does not respond to simple potassium replacement. Presumably magnesium provides the necessary cofactor required for normal potassium utilization.[15]

METABOLIC ACIDOSIS

Stimulation of the sympathetic nervous system increases heart rate and contractility, which, in turn, increases cardiac output (Fig. 16-1). Blood is preferentially shunted to the brain and heart (away from the skin, skeletal muscles, abdominal organs, and kidneys). This shunting increases arteriovenous oxygen extraction, which can become so severe that the cells shift to anaerobic metabolism, leading to metabolic (lactic) acidosis.

ASSESSMENT

Knowledge of the pathophysiological mechanisms associated with the usual signs and symptoms of heart failure, especially those affecting fluid and electrolyte balance, contributes to effective management of this complex situation (Tables 16-1 and 16-3). The following discussion of assessment of patients with heart failure includes both noninvasive and invasive measures.

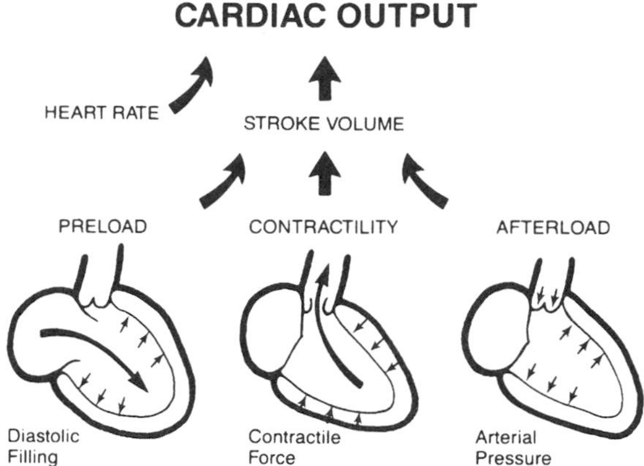

Figure 16–1. Factors determining cardiac output.

NONINVASIVE MONITORING

Left ventricular failure is associated with decreased cardiac output. It remains a challenge for clinicians to assess for a decrease in cardiac output without the benefit of invasive hemodynamic monitoring. It is, however, not impossible. Cardiac output is defined as the amount of blood pumped by the heart in 1 min. Normal cardiac output is 4 to 8 L/min. The two components of cardiac output are heart rate and stroke volume. Therefore, an indirect or noninvasive assessment of cardiac output would consist of analyzing these two components. For example, a heart rate that is too fast may indicate a decrease in cardiac output. The heart rate may be increased to make up for a loss of stroke volume in a failing heart. Assessment of a decrease in stroke volume is also challenging. Stroke volume is the amount of blood ejected with each beat. Therefore, stroke volume is one of the three components of systolic blood pressure; the other components are aortic distensibility and left ventricular ejection rate. If there is a drop in systolic blood pressure and you can assume that there has been no change in aortic distensibility or ejection rate, then the drop is most likely due to a decrease in stroke volume. This is particularly true at lower systolic pressures. Therefore, a noninvasive assessment of cardiac output would consist of a close observation for changes in heart rate and systolic blood pressure.

A decrease in cardiac output leads to symptoms of weakness and fatigue because tissue oxygenation is impaired. Dyspnea is also always present, at first experienced only with exercise. As heart failure worsens, dyspnea show up with progressively less exercise and finally even at rest.

Other pulmonary symptoms associated with left ventricular failure include orthopnea, paroxysmal nocturnal dyspnea, dry cough, and fine moist crackles in the lungs. Typically, crackles in the lungs that are induced by cardiac failure are described as gravity-dependent. For example, if the patient is sitting up, the crackles will be heard in the bases of the lungs, but if the patient is lying on the left side, they are heard throughout the left lung. Cardiac failure-induced crackles are due to fluid accumulation in the lungs. Clinicians must be able to distinguish these from pulmonary crackles. Crackles that are pulmonary in origin are due to weak airway walls. Typically, they are heard in all the lung fields. Pulmonary crackles are not gravity-dependent. Patients with left ventricular failure may also demonstrate expiratory wheezing and Cheyne-Stokes respirations. Severe left ventricular failure results in acute pulmonary edema, a potentially life-threatening condition characterized by severe dyspnea and profound anxiety.

Physical signs associated with left ventricular failure may include third and fourth heart sounds, systolic murmur, sinus tachycardia, or any dysrhythmia. The point of maximal impulse is shifted to the left when cardiomegaly occurs. Patients may also demonstrate pulsus alternans.

Right-sided heart failure is associated with jugular vein distention and hepatojugular reflux, which reflect increased venous pressure. The degree of jugular vein distention provides important data regarding fluid volume status and cardiac function; of importance, it can be performed noninvasively (see Fig. 2-1).

Dependent pitting edema (see Fig. 2-3) reflects excessive fluid in the interstitial space and is a major indication in right-sided heart failure. As such, the degree of peripheral edema should be assessed at regular intervals. This can be accomplished by measuring the extremities with a millimeter tape. The patient should be taught to monitor for fluid retention by noting, for example, tight shoes or tight clothing as the day progresses.

Weight gain usually occurs with heart failure because of abnormal retention of sodium and water. Early in the therapeutic period, a baseline body

TABLE 16–3

Signs and Symptoms of Congestive Heart Failure and Their Causes

SYMPTOM OR SIGN	CAUSE
Fatigue with little exertion or at rest, confusion, headache	Tissue anoxia due to decreased cardiac output
Dyspnea on exertion, later at rest	Cardiac output inadequate to provide for increased oxygen required by exertion (results in increased breathing effort)
PND in left-sided heart failure	When recumbent, edema fluid from the dependent parts returns to the bloodstream, increasing preload and causing decompensation
Cough; sputum may at times be brownish or blood-tinged Adventitious lung sounds (especially crackles)	Pulmonary capillary pressure greater than 30 mmHg causes transudation of serum with hemosiderin-filled macrophages into the alveoli, which causes pulmonary congestion and diminished oxygen–carbon dioxide exchange
Tachycardia, various dysrhythmias	Effort to compensate for decreased cardiac output; arrhythmias may be stimulated by hypoxia, digitalis toxicity, hypokalemia, or hypomagnesemia
Presence of third/fourth heart sounds	Associated with rapid ventricular/atrial filling in noncompliant ventricles/atria
Cardiomegaly	Hypertrophy of myocardium helps to maintain stroke volume
Decreased urinary output	Decreased cardiac output and renal blood flow
	Sodium and water retention caused by excess aldosterone level
	Increased water retention caused by excess antidiuretic hormone (ADH) secretion
Nocturia	While resting at night, deficit in cardiac output in relation to oxygen demands is reduced, leading to decreased renal vasoconstriction and increased glomerular filtration rate (GFR)
Elevated pulmonary capillary wedge pressure or left ventricular end-diastolic pressure	Left ventricle cannot maintain stroke volume in face of increased venous return
Edema (initially in dependent parts, later generalized)	Hydrostatic pressure is greatest in dependent parts of body
	Progressive cardiac failure causes substantial increase in hydrostatic pressure in all parts of body
Distention of peripheral veins, most noticeable on face, neck, and hands Elevated CVP (greater than 11 cm H_2O in vena cava)	Elevated venous pressure secondary to cardiac failure
Palpable liver, positive hepatojugular reflex	Decreased cardiac output causes damming of venous blood
	Increase in total blood volume and interstitial fluid volume
Nausea and vomiting	Edema of liver and intestines
	Impulses arising from the dilated myocardium in acute heart failure
	Digitalis toxicity
Anorexia	Potassium deficit
	Digitalis toxicity

TABLE 16–3 (cont.)

SYMPTOM OR SIGN	CAUSE
Constipation	Poor nourishment and inadequate bulk in diet Lack of activity Depression of motor activity by hypoxia
Orthopnea	Increased interstitial edema decreasing lung compliance and increasing work of breathing; upright position fosters air exchange in upper lungs
Pulmonary edema with severe dyspnea, profound anxiety, coughing of pink frothy fluid, cyanosis, shock, and death	Increased pulmonary venous pressure, which cause serum and blood cells to transudate into the alveoli

PND, paroxysmal nocturnal dyspnea; CVP, central venous pressure.

weight should be obtained to compare with subsequent weight measurements to monitor response to treatment. For accuracy, it is best to use the same scale and perform the procedure at the same time each day. Any change in daily weight of more than 0.25 kg (0.5 lb) can be assumed to have resulted from alterations in total body fluid and these measures can be used to monitor therapy with diuretics and other medications. The patient can be taught to monitor daily weight changes at home.

An important measurement during hospitalization is daily fluid intake and output (I&O). With diuretic administration, urinary output is expected to increase significantly. This increase should parallel the decrease in body weight. Discrepancies in these findings are an indication to check for errors in measurement.

INVASIVE HEMODYNAMIC MONITORING

Hemodynamic monitoring by means of multilumen flow-directed catheters has made it possible to assess pressures directly within the heart chambers and great vessels and to monitor cardiac output. Arterial pressure, central venous pressure (CVP), pulmonary artery pressure (PAP), pulmonary capillary wedge pressure (PCWP), and cardiac output (CO) can be measured. The obtained pressure measurements provide information concerning the fluid volume status of both sides of the heart. Several other hemodynamic indices can be derived from these measurements (eg, stroke volume, stroke volume index, and systemic and pulmonary vascular resistance). All these findings are used to monitor the patient's initial status and response to therapy.

In the patient experiencing heart failure, CVP is used to monitor the intravascular volume status. This measurement will decrease during periods of hypovolemia (which may occur with overdiuresis) and will increase with hypervolemia, increased venous return, and when right-sided failure worsens.

As indicators of the left ventricle's status in the absence of mitral valve disease, chronic obstructive pulmonary disease, or pulmonary hypertension, PAP and PCWP are more sensitive than is the CVP. The pulmonary artery end-diastolic pressure (PAEDP) and the PCWP reflect the left ventricular end-diastolic pressure (LVEDP). Left ventricular end-diastolic pressure represents the left ventricular filling pressure (preload), which is one of the determinants of stroke volume. An increase in PAEDP or PCWP is the result of the diminished ability of the left ventricle to empty its contents. Symptoms of pulmonary congestion occur when the PAEDP or PCWP exceeds 18 mmHg. This is the usual situation in pulmonary edema. Cardiac output is another hemodynamic measurement that can be obtained with flow-directed catheters. Decrease in CO can indicate the degree of failure and help determine needed therapy to increase the heart's contractility.

NURSING DIAGNOSES

Clinical Tip: Examples of Nursing Process in Care of Patients With Heart Failure presents three nursing diagnoses that occur at a high frequency in patients experiencing acute or chronic heart failure. Also included is information needed for assessment, intervention, and evaluation.

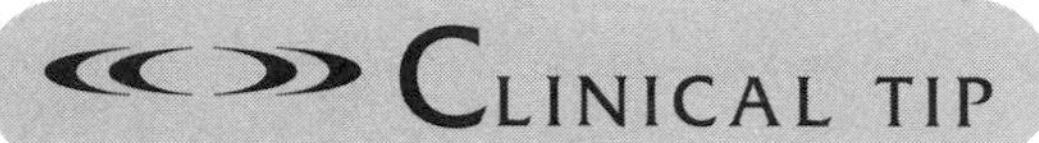

Examples of Nursing Process in Care of Patients With Heart Failure

NURSING DIAGNOSIS	ASSESSMENT	INTERVENTIONS	EXPECTED OUTCOMES
Fluid volume excess related to compromised regulatory mechanisms (cardiac failure) *Pathophysiology:* Decreased GFR; kidneys respond by retaining sodium and water (under the influence of aldosterone and ADH)	Weight gain Peripheral edema Intake greater than output Decreased urinary volume, increased urinary specific gravity Peripheral venous distention Paroxysmal nocturnal dyspnea Increased CVP, PCWP, LVEDP Abnormal breath sounds (crackles) Orthopnea and dyspnea Tachypnea Frothy sputum Hepatomegaly	Assess for fluid volume excess: • Measure I&O; look for I > O • Weigh daily (same scale, same amount of clothing, and same time each day) • Assess lung fields for crackles (compare to baseline) • Monitor changes in vital signs (compare to baseline) Instruct in dietary restrictions (sodium restriction favors diuresis) Restrict fluids as prescribed (may be necessary in patients with severe heart disease to decrease ECF volume) Monitor response to diuretics: • Weight should decline no faster than 1 kg/day (2.2 lb) with diuretic administration • Look for inadequate response to diuretics • Look for excessive response to diuretics (such as weight loss exceeding 2.2 lb/day and BUN elevated out of proportion to serum creatinine) Instruct patient to weigh self daily and report significant weight variations to health care provider Encourage rest periods in which patient lies down (rest, particularly in supine position, favors diuresis) Promote calm environment to decrease sympathetic nervous system stimulation (again, rest favors diuresis) Place in Fowler's position (reduced upward pressure on diaphragm, facilitating ease of breathing) Measures for management of acute pulmonary edema are described in text	Urine output will increase Weight will decrease to baseline as diuresis occurs Peripheral edema will lessen Peripheral venous distention will lessen Crackles will be absent or diminished Sputum production will diminish Dyspnea and tachypnea will diminish Liver size will diminish Patient and significant other will verbalize understanding of sodium-restricted diet Patient will demonstrate ability to weigh self and will verbalize significant variations requiring reporting to health care provider

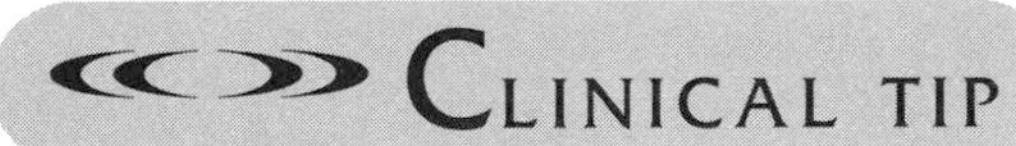

Examples of Nursing Process in Care of Patients With Heart Failure (con't.)

NURSING DIAGNOSIS	ASSESSMENT	INTERVENTIONS	EXPECTED OUTCOMES
Activity intolerance related to decreased cardiac reserve *Pathophysiology:* Decreased contractility and increased preload lead to decreased cardiac output and tissue hypoxia	Heart rate increased more than 10% over baseline with activity Heart rate remains increased 2 minutes after exercise Increased LVEDP	Provide bedrest during acute phase of failure (reduces metabolic requirements and thus myocardial workload) Encourage patient to sit in chair when tolerated (pooling of blood in legs decreases venous return and thus preload) Encourage rest 1 hour after meals (since digestion increases metabolic requirements, tolerance to activity is diminished at this time) Monitor response to increases in activity; encourage rest when heart rate increases significantly over baseline and when heart rate remains elevated for longer than 2 minutes after exercise Promote emotional rest (decreases workload of heart by decreasing sympathetic nervous system stimulation) Instruct patient and significant other in prescribed activity regimen Institute measures to maintain normal body temperature, such as avoiding extremes in environmental temperature and prevention of fever (decrease tissue metabolic needs and thus the myocardial workload)	Heart rate will not increase more than 10% above baseline with allowed activity Heart rate will return to baseline within 2 minutes after allowed activity Patient or significant other will verbalize understanding of balance between rest and activity
Impaired gas exchange related to pulmonary congestion *Pathophysiology:* Decreased cardiac output, increased preload, transudation of fluid into alveoli	Dyspnea, orthopnea, PND Crackles (dependent) Cough PaO_2 <80 mmHg $PaCO_2$ >45 mmHg pH <7.35 ↑LVEDP ↑PCWP Alveolar congestion (radiograph)	Elevate head of bed (facilitates ventilation by allowing full chest expansion, draining uppermost alveoli) Tracheal suctioning (removes secretions and thus increases alveolar surface area for gas exchange) Lower feet (decreases venous return and thus preload) Implement medical regimen as appropriate: • Bronchodilators (increases airway diameter) • Oxygen (maintains PaO_2 greater than 80 mmHg to reduce hypoxia and work of breathing)	Absence or diminishing of dyspnea, crackles PaO_2 >80 mmHg $PaCO_2$ <45 mmHg pH $\geq$7.35 (important to correct acidemia since it predisposes to decreased myocardial contractility) Hemodynamic parameters within normal limits

ADH, antidiuretic hormone; CVP, central venous pressure; BUN, blood urea nitrogen; ECF, extracellular fluid; GFR, glomerular filtration rate; LVEDP, left ventricular end-diastolic pressure; I&O, intake and output; PCWP, pulmonary capillary wedge pressure; PND, paroxysmal nocturnal dyspnea.

INTERVENTIONS/TREATMENTS

Because the nurse works closely with physicians in the management of fluid balance problems in heart failure patients, the principles of treatment are presented with collaborative actions as a focus.

When possible, therapy is directed at eliminating the disease condition producing heart failure (e.g., surgical correction of a valvular disorder). When this is not possible, therapy must focus on making the most efficient use of the remaining cardiac function. Unfortunately, most persons with CHF have irreversible cardiac damage. There is some evidence, however, that relief of pressure or volume overload (preload and afterload) may lessen or even reverse the decline in contractility; thus, this is an important therapeutic objective.[16] It is now well recognized that a variety of neurohormonal responses, which are initially activated to support the gradually failing heart, may eventually contribute to the progressive nature of the disease and further reduce cardiac function.[17]

DECREASING MYOCARDIAL WORKLOAD

Rest causes a reduction in oxygen need and therefore decreases cardiac workload. It also produces a physiological diuresis. Sometimes rest alone is sufficient to alleviate the symptoms of CHF because it diminishes the discrepancy between the heart's ability to pump blood and the tissues' oxygenation needs. The amount of rest required varies with the person and may range from complete bedrest to only slight restriction of activity.

The patient should be helped to identify an appropriate level of activity that is as nondisruptive to the usual lifestyle as possible. Even somewhat strenuous activities may be tolerated if they are done slowly and are accompanied with frequent rest periods.

Another important nursing responsibility involves monitoring the patient's response to exercise, including changes in pulse and respiratory rate. An increase in heart rate more than 10% over the baseline indicates that an activity may exceed the capacity of the failing heart to respond. Careful reporting of these observations helps to determine the desired amount of activity and aids in the evaluation of the therapeutic regime.

Other interventions to ensure decreased myocardial workload include relief of pain and reduction of fever, if present. Also, patients with heart failure often receive oxygen therapy to maintain a partial pressure of oxygen in arterial blood (PaO_2) of at least 80 mmHg. This reduces hypoxia and the work of breathing. Positioning the patient in a semi-Fowler's position facilitates ventilation by allowing full chest expansion and diaphragmatic excursion. The upright position may also decrease venous return by sequestering blood in the dependent areas.

DECREASING PRELOAD

Venous return is one of the most important determinants of ventricular preload. As preload is increased, so are peripheral edema and pulmonary congestion.

Dietary Sodium/Fluid Restriction

Restriction of dietary sodium is a valuable aid in the management of heart failure (see Chapter 3). In general, the fewer sodium ions are in the body, the less water is retained. The degree of sodium restriction necessary to control edema varies with the severity of heart failure. Often the dietary sodium intake can be cut in half by not adding salt at the table and in cooking and avoiding foods with a high salt content (see Chapter 3). Limiting sodium intake to 2 g daily, in conjunction with diuretic therapy, is sufficient to control congestive symptoms while maintaining a reasonably palatable diet.[18] A stricter diet limited to only 0.5 to 1 g of sodium may be required; if so, the patient will need help to achieve the knowledge and motivation necessary to adhere to the recommended diet.

The degree of sodium restriction necessary to control edema also varies with the degree of rest, dosage, and type of diuretic. For example, an ambulatory patient requires more sodium restriction than a patient at bedrest because rest in itself encourages diuresis. A patient receiving potent diuretics has less need for severe sodium restriction than one not receiving diuretics. Indeed, a drastic reduction of sodium intake can be dangerous to the patient receiving a potent diuretic, particularly during bouts of abnormal sodium loss, such as occurs with vomiting or diarrhea.

At times it may be necessary to reduce fluid intake in patients with CHF. Primarily this is done to deal with fluid volume overloaded patients who also have hyponatremia. (See discussion of treatment of hyponatremia earlier in this chapter.)

Diuretics

Diuretics are a valuable aid in the symptomatic treatment of heart failure. Their primary purpose is to promote the excretion of sodium and water from the body, thus lowering intravascular volume. If hemodynamic monitoring is being used, it may be noted that diuretics produce a decrease in LVEDP (preload) and move the heart's function to a more favorable portion of the Starling curve (Fig. 16-2). This effect decreases pulmonary and systemic congestion and also decreases the degree of backward failure. These effects, in turn, will tend to decrease myocardial need for oxygen. Another advantage of certain diuretics (e.g., furosemide) is an increase in venous capacitance with decreased venous return. At times, it is necessary to administer diuretics by the IV route to achieve a positive therapeutic result. This is because orally administered medications may be poorly absorbed when right-sided heart failure causes congested abdominal organs.

Because thiazides (e.g., hydrochlorothiazide) and loop diuretics (furosemide, bumetanide, and

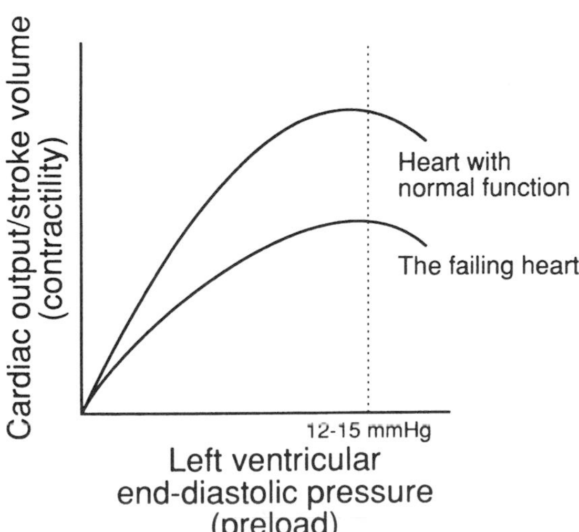

Figure 16–2. The Starling mechanism in normal heart function and heart failure.

ethacrynic acid) predispose to hypokalemia, potassium supplementation is often needed. A potassium-sparing diuretic (e.g., spironolactone) may also be indicated, particularly as secondary hyperaldosteronism often plays a significant role in advanced heart failure. (Recall that spironolactone is an aldosterone-blocking agent.) It should be remembered that ACE inhibitors (such as captopril) cause potassium retention and should not be given simultaneously with potassium-retaining diuretics or with potassium supplements.

As discussed above, possible side effects of diuretics are disturbances in potassium balance. For example, thiazides and loop diuretics promote renal potassium loss, whereas spironolactone, amiloride, and dyrenium promote potassium retention. Acid–base disturbances usually accompany disruptions in potassium balance (metabolic alkalosis with hypokalemia, and metabolic acidosis with hyperkalemia). Excessive reduction in the intravascular volume caused by too vigorous diuresis may actually worsen heart failure by diminishing the preload stimulus to cardiac contractility. As CO decreases, so do renal blood flow and glomerular filtration rate (GFR), resulting in prerenal azotemia and increased blood urea nitrogen (BUN).

In intractable heart failure, the kidney is unable to respond to the usual diuretics. At that point treatment may consist of a combination of things involving more severe sodium restriction, more potent diuretics in higher dosage, and fluid restriction to 1000 mL/day.

Priority nursing responsibilities in the care of patients with heart failure include keeping an accurate account of fluid I&O and daily weight measurements. Data obtained from the measurements, in addition to revealing changes in edema accumulation, are invaluable in regulating diuretic dosage and dietary sodium restriction.

Although fluid restriction may be indicated at times, the patient should not be allowed to become volume depleted. As described above, volume depletion further impairs cardiac output by decreasing the preload's stimulus on cardiac contractility. It is desirable to use hemodynamic monitoring to guide fluid replacement therapy in seriously ill heart failure patients. Frequent checks of venous pressure and PCWP during fluid administration can give an early warning of circulatory overload or underload and guide the safe administration of needed water and electrolytes. Administration of fluids to patients with CHF requires individualized and cautious attention. Generally, fluid may be given until the LVEDP rises no higher than 15 mmHg. This level assures maximum CO while preventing pulmonary edema caused by increased preload. This level is meant to be a guideline for administration of fluids. Individuals with long-standing CHF may have baseline pressures that are much higher than normal due to overstretching of the left ventricle. In these cases the LVEDP may already exceed 15 mmHg. Therefore, treatment goals should be individualized. The patient at home must understand the precise fluid regimen best suited for his or her condition, and situations that can complicate this regimen (such as increased fluid loss in vomiting and diarrhea).

Monitoring volume, speed, and composition of IV fluids given to CHF patients is important. Oral fluids should also be monitored carefully in those requiring fluid restriction; the patient's cooperation in this endeavor should be sought. As is the case with most patients, an ongoing assessment of response to fluid intake must occur, and alterations made as indicated in the treatment plan.

Vasodilators

Vasodilator drugs are used to inhibit vascular tone in the veins and/or arteries. Venous vasodilators act on vascular smooth muscle to increase venous pooling. This effect reduces venous return and preload. This would be noted by a decrease in CVP and PCWP and a subsequent improvement in stroke volume. As a result, there is decreased pulmonary congestion and dyspnea. Nitrates are the most common venous vasodilators used to treat heart failure. Drugs in this classification include IV nitroglycerin, sustained-release nitroglycerin preparations, topical nitroglycerin ointment and patches, and isosorbide dinitrate. Vasodilators are now considered one of the first-line medications to treat CHF because clinical studies have shown that isosorbide in combination with hydralazine (an arterial vasodilator) can decrease mortality.[19]

Other vasodilators used in the treatment of CHF include ACE inhibitors and hydralazine. These drugs also have an effect on afterload reduction and are discussed later in this chapter. Several vasodilators that are not generally recommended for the treatment of CHF include minoxidil, prazosin, and calcium channel blocking agents.[20]

DECREASING AFTERLOAD

Afterload refers to the pressure against which the ventricle must work to achieve blood flow during systole. In heart failure, even in the presence of normal arterial blood pressure, there is a relative worsening of the relationship between contractility and afterload that causes an even greater workload and oxygen need. To reduce the resistance against which the heart must work and to increase cardiac output, arterial vasodilators are one of the first-line medications used in the treatment of heart failure.

Hydralazine is one of the most effective arterial vasodilators. It works by reducing systemic vascular resistance (SVR). By decreasing the SVR it leads to an increase in CO. When used in combination with nitrates it results in a decrease in mortality.

Angiotensin-converting enzyme inhibitors are indirect vasodilators that are also used in treatment of CHF. ACE inhibitors interfere with the conversion of angiotensin I to angiotensin II and thereby decrease the vasoconstricting action of angiotensin II. Another effect of ACE inhibitors includes a reduction in aldosterone. The overall effect is a decrease in filling pressures and systemic vascular resistance. Drugs in this class include captopril, enalapril, and lisinopril. ACE inhibitors have been shown to improve cardiac function and to decrease mortality.[21] Because aldosterone is inhibited, there is retention of potassium and magnesium; therefore, supplement of these electrolytes should not be given. Blood pressure must be monitored when therapy is initiated because the patient may experience hypotension due to the effect of the drug. This hypotensive effect is heightened by the concurrent presence of a low intravascular volume (as occurs with too vigorous use of diuretics). An additional consideration before initiating ACE inhibitor therapy is to check serum sodium levels. Patients with serum sodium levels less than 130 mmol/L may be predisposed to an acute drop in blood pressure.[22]

The calcium channel blockers (nifedipine, verapamil, and diltiazem) are not indicated for the routine treatment of systolic heart failure because they demonstrate a negative inotropic effect. These agents may be helpful in the less frequent diastolic failure (e.g., dilated cardiomyopathy). These agents inhibit the influx of extracellular calcium during muscular contraction, producing arterial vasodilation and decreased afterload. They may also improve myocardial relaxation during diastole, thus allowing more complete filling when diastolic compliance is impaired.[23]

INCREASING MYOCARDIAL CONTRACTILITY

Administration of positive inotropic agents (medications that increase the strength of cardiac contractility) affects one factor contributing to stroke volume and, therefore, to CO.

Digitalis

The most commonly used inotropic agent is digitalis. This medication increases the force and velocity of myocardial contraction. As the heart contracts more forcefully, tissue perfusion increases and the compensatory responses caused by hypoxia decrease, allowing a corresponding improvement in renal function with diuresis. Digitalis increases the intracellular calcium concentration by inhibiting the sodium-potassium-adenosine triphosphatase (Na-K-ATPase) pump, resulting in increased intracellular sodium, which then exchanges with calcium. The role of digitalis in heart failure has been evaluated.[24] It was found that digitalis is effective in treating patients with heart failure complicated by atrial fibrillation with a rapid ventricular response. It is now recommended that CHF patients be treated selectively based on the severity of ventricular dysfunction, symptoms, degree of neuroendocrine activation, and risk of toxicity.[25]

When digitalis preparations are used, be alert for toxic symptoms, such as aversion to food, nausea and vomiting, blurred or distorted vision, confusion, and dysrhythmias. Increased myocardial automaticity may reflect alterations in transmembrane concentrations of sodium, potassium, and calcium. Conduction disturbances can occur secondary to changes in the refractory period.

Remember that symptoms of digitalis toxicity may be induced by hypokalemia, hypomagnesemia, hyponatremia, or hypercalcemia because these imbalances sensitize the heart to digitalis. Hypokalemia occurs frequently in patients with heart failure because of the simultaneous administration of potassium-losing diuretics. Often, a potassium supplement (see Chapter 5) or potassium-sparing diuretics will be used to prevent hypokalemia in a digitalized patient. Potassium replacement is often the initial therapy of choice for ectopic rhythms associated with digitalis toxicity. The serum potassium level should be maintained in the high normal range.[26] If potassium administration does not correct the arrhythmia, hypomagnesemia should be suspected.

Other Positive Inotropic Agents

Efforts to find another oral positive inotropic agent have been underway for years. Unfortunately, to date none have been found to be safe, effective, or able to decrease mortality. Therefore, the only positive inotropes used to treat CHF are IV medications.

Dopamine, dobutamine and amrinone are the three most commonly used inotropic agents. Table 16-4 details the dosage for each of these medications. As illustrated in the table, the primary action of dopamine will vary in accordance with the dose. Dopamine, a precursor of norepinephrine, as well as norepinephrine itself, may be used to increase myocardial contractility. Dopamine has both alpha and beta stimulation properties. The usefulness of these agents is limited by the other natural effect of catecholamines, which is peripheral arteriolar con-

TABLE 16–4

Inotropic Agents and Doses

DRUG	DOSE
Dopamine	1–5 μg/kg/min, renal dose
	5–10 μg/kg/min, inotropic dose
	>10 μg/kg/min, vasopressor dose
Dobutamine	1–20 μg/kg/min
Amrinone	0.75 mg/kg, loading dose, then 5–10 μg/kg/min

striction. This constriction increases afterload and thereby increases the workload of the heart.

Dobutamine is a synthetic catecholamine that increases myocardial contractility while limiting the side effects of tachycardia and elevation of arterial blood pressure. There is also a reduced left ventricular filling pressure and a decrease in heart size. Dopamine may be given simultaneously with dobutamine to cause renal artery vasodilation and increased renal blood flow, and to promote sodium and water excretion.

Dobutamine, as a beta stimulator, has the best chance of improving stroke volume in patients with simple contractility problems.[27] Dobutamine therapy is used most often in home care settings. Patients with contractility problems, such as those with end-stage cardiac disease or those awaiting heart transplantation, may be on low doses of dobutamine at home.

Amrinone is one of a new class of positive inotropic agents that act through a mechanism different from that of digitalis or the catecholamines. These medications inhibit phosphodiesterase type III, which increases the level of cyclic adenosine monophosphate (AMP). In turn, this enhances calcium entry into the myocardium and peripheral smooth muscle cells. The effect is an increase in CO and reduced left ventricular filling pressure without tachycardia or increased arterial pressure. There is also an arteriolar vasodilation that decreases afterload and, therefore, the workload of the heart.

DYSRHYTHMIAS IN HEART FAILURE

All types of dysrhythmias can occur in patients with heart failure. The relationship between dysrhythmias and heart failure is complex. Heart failure can cause dysrhythmia development. Pathological dysrhythmias can cause heart failure, or dysrhythmias may be a consequence of treatment strategies. At any rate, patients with advanced heart failure are prone to dysrhythmias that further alter their hemodynamic status. Alterations in heart rate can cause a decrease in CO and systemic blood pressure. Left untreated, some dysrhythmias are considered life-threatening and may predispose individuals to thromboembolic events or sudden cardiac death.

Dysrhythmias in heart failure can be due to the disease process itself. Ischemic heart disease, hypertension, valvular heart disease all have dysrhythmic complications. Unfortunately, dysrhythmias are poorly tolerated in patients with CHF.

Dysrhythmias can also be due to electrolyte disturbances. As discussed earlier, hypokalemia, hyperkalemia, and hypomagnesemia are electrolyte disturbances that may cause dysrhythmias. Hyperkalemia is not a common problem, but it may occur if renal insufficiency is present. Hyperkalemia may also occur secondary to the reduction in aldosterone seen with the use of ACE inhibitors.[28] Hypokalemia and hypomagnesemia are more frequent and are often side effects of diuretic therapy used to treat CHF.

Other drugs used to treat heart failure may also exhibit dysrhythmic side effects. Table 16-5 lists drugs used to treat heart failure that can cause dysrhythmias and potential dysrhythmic consequences.

Treatment

Antidysrhythmic therapy in patients with CHF requires an awareness of the effects that the heart failure may have on drug metabolism. Patients with renal or hepatic insufficiency secondary to heart failure are often at risk for altered metabolism and clearance. Drugs with the potential for negative inotropic effects should be used cautiously or avoided because they can lead to the worsening of heart failure.

Atrial fibrillation is one of the most common dysrhythmias seen in patients with CHF. It is particularly dangerous for those who already have some degree of ventricular dysfunction. Management of atrial fibrillation concentrates on the restoration of sinus rhythm and rate control. Restoration of sinus rhythm is difficult in this population because drugs such as quinidine possess negative inotropic properties and, therefore, may not be tolerated. Rate control is best achieved with digoxin. Small, frequent doses of a cardioselective beta-blocker, such as metoprolol, may also be appropriate.[29] When pharmacological therapy is ineffective, cardioversion may be considered. Patients with CHF and atrial fibrillation are also at risk for embolic events. Therefore, warfarin is recommended for patients with atrial fibrillation.

Ventricular dysrhythmias are also common in CHF. Table 16-6 lists conditions that increase the

TABLE 16–5

Possible Dysrhythmias Associated With Selected Drugs Used to Treat Heart Failure

DRUG	DYSRHYTHMIA/POSSIBLE CAUSE
Non-potassium-sparing diuretics: Furosemide Bumetanide Ethacrynic acid Hydrochlorothiazide Chlorothiazide	Atrial and ventricular ectopy due to hypokalemia and hypomagnesemia
Digoxin	First, second, or third-degree heart block due to slowed conduction through the AV node
	Atrial and/or ventricular fibrillation due to reduced refractory periods in atrial and ventricular tissue
	Atrial and/or ventricular ectopic beats due to effect of oscillatory membrane potentials

TABLE 16–6

List of Conditions That Increase the Risk for Ventricular Dysrhythmias in CHF

CONDITION	TREATMENT
Electrolyte imbalance: Hypokalemia Hypomagnesemia	Electrolyte supplementation, as needed
Acid–base imbalance	Correction of imbalance, including assessment of diuretic therapy
Myocardial ischemia	Anti-ischemic drug therapy and/or myocardial revascularization
Worsening heart failure	Additional therapy for CHF and removal of precipitating factor
Active myocarditis	Confirm by biopsy and consider immunosuppression
Increased catecholamines	Careful administration of beta-blockers
Digitalis intoxication	Decrease dosage or discontinue
Beta-agonist drugs	Discontinue or lower dose
Phosphodiesterase inhibitor	Discontinue and avoid use
Antiarrhythmic drugs	Avoid use/discontinue

From Deedwania P: Ventricular arrhythmias in heart failure: To treat or not to treat? Cardiol Clin 12:123, 1994; with permission.

risk for ventricular dysrhythmias in CHF. Treatment of ventricular ectopic beats begins with finding a precipitating cause, such as hypokalemia, intake of caffeinated beverages, or alcohol. Antidysrhythmic agents used to treat ventricular ectopy may include mexiletine or metoprolol.

Ventricular tachycardia seen in patients with heart failure is of relatively brief duration, polymorphic, and irregular.[30] Amiodarone is a very effective agent used to suppress ventricular dysrhythmias. The Congestive Heart Failure–Survival Trial of Antiarrhythmic Therapy is currently underway to investigate the efficacy of amiodarone in decreasing mortality in patients with heart failure.[31]

Heart block is also common in patients with heart failure. This may be due to the disease process itself, the effect of agents used to treat heart failure, or electrolyte disturbances. First- and second-degree heart block do not require treatment, other than perhaps an adjustment of therapy. Complete heart block is treated with pacing or isoproterenol. Long-term treatment may involve placement of a permanent pacemaker.

Heart failure patients who are prone to dysrhythmias may also benefit from insertion of an implantable cardioverter defibrillator. The use of these devices for prophylactic therapy in heart failure is currently being investigated. Other nonpharmacologic approaches to treatment of dysrhythmias include surgical correction of atrial fibrillation or ventricular tachycardia. Ablation therapy and cardiac transplantation are also alternatives available to some individuals.

Potassium and Magnesium Replacement

There are several recommendations for electrolyte supplementation in patients with CHF. Diuretic-induced hypokalemia is commonly associated with a metabolic alkalosis and a coexisting chloride deficit. Therefore, potassium chloride is the preferred supplementation. The dosage of potassium chloride is individualized, and dependent of the use of other medications, such as ACE inhibitors or concomitant diuretics.[32] (See Chapter 5 for specifics on treatment of hypokalemia.)

Hypomagnesemia is most often caused by chronic diuretic therapy, digitalis, or malnutrition in patients with severe chronic CHF. As stated earlier, there is a relationship between hypokalemia and hypomagnesemia; magnesium is a co-factor that ensures appropriate function of the Na-K-ATPase pump. Therefore, hypokalemia may persist until the magnesium deficiency is corrected.[33] Another potential problem of magnesium deficiency in patients with heart failure is the susceptibility to lethal dysrhythmias and sudden death. Patients with hypomagnesemia have been found to have more frequent premature ventricular contractions and episodes of ventricular tachycardia. When patients with hypomagnesemia were compared to patients with normal magnesium levels, patients with a low serum magnesium concentration had a poorer prognosis during follow-up, with 45% and 71% surviving for 1 year, respectively.[34]

In addition to increasing the incidence of dysrhythmias, hypomagnesemia increases peripheral resistance and decreases myocardial oxygenation.[35] Therefore, treatment should be aimed at prevention when applicable. It has been found that magnesium supplementation reduces the frequency of asymptomatic ventricular dysrhythmias (possibly due to secondary changes in potassium homeostasis) and produces a minor degree of vasodilation.[36] (See Chapter 7 for specifics on treatment of hypomagnesemia.)

PULMONARY EDEMA

Cardiogenic pulmonary edema is a result of excessive accumulation of lung water due to left ventricular failure or excessive administration of intravenous fluid. Pulmonary edema is an emergency situation. To deal with it, the patient should be quickly placed in a high Fowler's position to reduce venous pressure and preload. This position facilitates fluid gravitation to the pleural bases so that less dependent areas of the lung are better ventilated and the work of breathing is decreased. Humidified oxygen is best delivered by a face mask. In extreme cases, endotracheal intubation and mechanical ventilation may be needed. Positive end-expiratory pressure (PEEP) may be used but should be done with caution because an excessive increase in intrathoracic pressure compromises CO.

Intravenous administration of morphine sulfate may be used to achieve multiple effects:

1. Reducing preload through peripheral venous dilation and thereby decreasing venous return to the heart.
2. Reducing afterload by decreasing arterial blood pressure.
3. Reducing anxiety (and thereby decreasing sympathetic nervous system stimulation).

Diuretics may be given by intravenous push (IVP) to promote a rapid diuresis and thus decreased preload and pulmonary congestion. A vasodilator, such as nitroglycerin, may be given IV or sublingually to decrease preload. However, remember that an excessive drop in preload may abolish the stimulus for contractility caused by myocardial stretching. To monitor the patient's response and allow early detection of complications, measure arterial pressure, CO, and LVEDP at regular intervals. An inotropic agent, such as digitalis, may be given IV. Digitalis is most effective if the patient is experiencing a supraventricular tachycardia.

Patients with acute pulmonary edema may develop severe acid–base problems (respiratory acidosis and metabolic [lactic] acidosis). Reversal of the pulmonary edema is usually effective in restoring acid–base balance by improving gas exchange and allowing metabolism of excess lactate into bicarbonate. Alkali therapy should be used only for refractory and severe metabolic acidosis (pH <7.00–7.10).[37]

CARDIOGENIC SHOCK

Cardiogenic shock develops when the CO is insufficient to meet the metabolic demands of the body due to either an absolute decrease in cardiac output or a severe increase in metabolic demands. Acute myocardial infarction is the most common cause. Cardiogenic shock is characterized by left ventricular failure, low CO, arterial hypotension, and peripheral vasoconstriction. Most often the patient will have a systolic blood pressure less than 90 mmHg. When the mean arterial pressure falls below 75 to 85 mmHg, there is danger that coronary blood flow will be inadequate, leading to further damage to the myocardium. A urinary output of less than 20 mL/hr is also common, reflecting a decreased glomerular filtration rate. Mental status is impaired due to cerebral hypoxia. Poor skin perfusion secondary to peripheral vasoconstriction can cause cold, clammy skin.

Treatment of cardiogenic shock depends on the underlying cause. One basic problem that many patients will encounter is cellular hypoxia related to decreased CO. Oxygen may be given by a high-flow system such as a Venturi mask or endotracheal intubation. Atelectasis and retention of carbon dioxide must be prevented by initiating measures to mobilize secretions and then suctioning the patient as often as necessary. The goal of these interventions is to prevent or minimize acidosis, and to maintain a PaO_2 greater than 80 mmHg. When acidosis is pronounced (pH <7.2), myocardial contractility is reduced.

Inotropic agents, such as dopamine, dobutamine, norepinephrine, or amrinone, may be given to strengthen contractility, maintain adequate blood pressure, and redistribute blood flow to the vital organs. Arterial vasodilators, such as nitroprusside, may be given to decrease afterload in the presence of severe, persistent vasoconstriction.

Intravenous fluids should be given to correct hypovolemia, if present. However, fluids must be given cautiously to prevent overload and pulmonary congestion. Maintaining PCWP at 15 mmHg ensures adequate left ventricular filling.

An intraaortic balloon pump (IABP) may be used in the presence of severe cardiac injury when recovery is still possible. In this procedure, a catheter with a balloon is placed into the aorta. The pump is set so that the balloon inflates during ventricular diastole and deflates during systole. This cycle provides better coronary artery and systemic perfusion with no increase in peripheral resistance to left ventricular output.

ELECTROLYTES IN CARDIAC ARREST/RESUSCITATION

Cardiac arrest in patients with CHF may be the result of pulmonary edema, drug toxicity, electrolyte abnormalities, or dysrhythmias. Pathophysiologic changes in acid–base metabolism have been a subject of interest in recent studies.

SODIUM BICARBONATE

Recommendation and practice concerning pharmacological management of cardiopulmonary resuscitation (CPR) suggest a cautious use of sodium bicarbonate to manage acidosis. Because sodium bicarbonate has not been successful in improving intramyocardial pH or myocardial viability during early resuscitation, it is no longer recommended during the initial stages of CPR. Sodium bicarbonate is still recommended as appropriate therapy when CPR is prolonged.[38] Sodium bicarbonate can cause hyperosmolarity, hypernatremia, or metabolic alkalosis with resultant hypokalemia and hypocalcemia. The oxyhemoglobin curve may be shifted to the left so that there is a decreased release of oxygen to already hypoxic tissues. Also, concomitant administration of catecholamines and bicarbonate may result in inactivation of the catecholamines.

During cardiac arrest a significant increase in the arterial to tissue pH gradient develops. Arterial pH has been found to increase during CPR when compared to prearrest samples.[39] Venous pH, however, is markedly lower because anaerobic cellular metabolism produces carbon dioxide, which is not circulated to the lungs for excretion. Therefore, mixed venous blood most accurately reflects the acid–base status during CPR. Venous acidosis results in an intracellular hypercarbia and acidosis that is particularly deleterious to cardiac and cerebral function. Administration of sodium bicarbonate releases carbon dioxide, which can rapidly enter cells and aggravate the already existing hypercarbia.

Adequate ventilation and perfusion are now advocated as the best ways to prevent or treat acidosis early in cardiac arrest. If the arrest is prolonged, (ie, >10 min) and definitive treatment has been initiated, or if severe acidosis existed before the arrest, sodium bicarbonate may be given. When used, 1 mEq/kg should be given initially, with no more than half this dose given every 10 min thereafter.[40]

POTASSIUM

Extracellular potassium levels are often elevated during CPR. The energy-dependent sodium–potassium pump is impaired by cellular ischemia. This allows potassium to leak out of the cells and extracellular levels to rise.[41] One result of this can be myocardial electromechanical dissociation (EMD). When hyperkalemia is the cause, calcium chloride may be used if the QRS complexes are greater than 0.12 sec. Remember that calcium enhances the toxicity of digitalis and should not be given IV to the digitalized patient.

MAGNESIUM

Magnesium infusions can be given to correct selected life-threatening arrhythmias, especially torsade de pointes or dysrhythmias refractive to other agents. It can also be given prophylactically to patients with a myocardial infarction and hypomagnesemia. (See Chapter 7.) Magnesium ions are involved in keeping intracellular potassium, calcium, and phosphorus levels constant (which may explain the effectiveness of magnesium in reversing dysrhythmias).

CALCIUM

Hypocalcemia during cardiac arrest is due to the movement of calcium from the extracellular to the intracellular compartment. This is a sign of breakdown of basic cellular control mechanisms due to extreme cellular stress.[42] Currently, calcium is not recommended as part of the resuscitation protocol. The only time that the administration of IV calcium is recommended is for patients with severe cardiovascular compromise (hypotensive and in heart failure) refractory to other therapies.[43]

CASE STUDIES

16-1. Mr. H has chronic congestive heart failure and receives regular visits from a home health nurse. On a recent visit, the nurse notices that he is not quite his usual talkative self. In fact, he has trouble getting up from his chair to open the door, and tells the nurse to let herself in. At the previous visit his blood pressure was 118/68 mmHg and his pulse was 88 beats/min. Currently his blood pressure is 96/64 mmHg and his pulse is 110 beats/min.

COMMENTARY: A noninvasive assessment of this patient's cardiac output reveals that his systolic blood pressure is low and his heart rate is fast. This alerts you to the possibility that his cardiac output may be low. Remember that cardiac output is comprised of heart rate and stroke volume. Stroke volume is one of the three components of systolic blood pressure. Therefore, any rise in heart rate, or any drop in systolic blood pressure alerts you to the possibility that stroke volume has dropped. If stroke volume has dropped, cardiac output will be lower.

16-2. Mrs. S. is hospitalized on a coronary care step-down unit with newly diagnosed CHF. Her medications include furosemide and an ACE inhibitor. Her serum sodium level is 129 mmol/L.

COMMENTARY: Two concerns related to this patient's fluid and electrolyte balance include hypotension and hyperkalemia. Patients with serum sodium levels less than 130 mmol/L may be predisposed to an acute drop in blood pressure. In addition, loop diuretics administered with ACE inhibitors may result in excessive retention of potassium, and therefore, result in hyperkalemia. This would be one example of when a potassium-losing diuretic may be not be associated with hypokalemia.

16-3. Mr. D. is hospitalized in the cardiac surgical intensive care unit. He has a long-standing history of mitral valve disease and has had his mitral valve replaced with a prosthetic valve. His medications include furosemide and digoxin. ECG monitoring reveals that he is in atrial fibrillation with a rapid ventricular response.

COMMENTARY: Electrolyte disturbances that may be present include hypokalemia and hypomagnesemia. These would most likely be due to diuretic therapy and the use of digoxin. Checking both of these electrolyte levels would be warranted. Remember that dysrhythmias may be due to valvular heart disease, electrolyte disturbances, or drugs used to treat heart failure. Careful consideration of all these factors is warranted in this case.

REFERENCES

1. Leier C, Dei C, Metra M: Clinical relevance and management of the major electrolyte abnormalities in congestive heart failure. Am Heart J 128(3):564–574,1994
2. Ibid, p 566
3. Ibid, p 567
4. Ibid
5. Ibid
6. Ibid
7. Ibid, p 568
8. Ibid
9. Ibid, p 569
10. Ibid, p 570
11. Ibid, p 569
12. Ibid, p 572
13. Ibid
14. Ibid
15. Ibid, p 571
16. Parmley W: Pathophysiology and current therapy of congestive heart failure. J Am Coll Cardiol 13:771,1989
17. Barnet D, Pouler H, Francis G: The changing face of heart failure. In: Barnet D, Pouleur H, Francis G (eds): Congestive Cardiac Failure: Pathophysiology and Treatment, p 3. New York, Marcel Dekker, 1993
18. Woodley M, Whelan A: Manual of Medical Therapeutics, 27th ed, p 106. Boston, Little, Brown, 1992
19. Cohn J, et al: A comparison of enalapril with hydralazine-isosorbide dinitrate in the treatment of heart failure. N Engl J Med 325: 302–310,1991
20. Kayser S: Management of chronic congestive heart failure, Part II-Selection of treatment. Prog Cardiovasc Nurs 9:33–34,1994
21. The SOLVD Investigators. Effect of enalapril on survival in patients with reduced left ventricular ejection fractions and congestive heart failure. N Engl J Med 325:293–302,1991
22. Kayser, p 35
23. Shub C: Heart failure and abnormal ventricular function: Pathophysiology and clinical correlation (Part 2). Chest 96:906,1989
24. Uretsky B, et al: Randomized Study assessing the effect of digoxin withdrawal in patients with mild to moderate chronic congestive heart failure: Results of the PROVED trial. J Am Coll Cardiol 22:955–962,1993.
25. Weintraub N, Chaitman B: Newer concepts in the medical management of patients with congestive heart failure. Clin Cardiol 16:380–390,1993
26. Woodley, Whelan, p 110
27. Ahrens T: Treatment of low cardiac outputs, In: Ahrens T, Rutherford K (eds): Essentials of Oxygenation, p 157. Boston, Jones and Barlett, 1993
28. Kayser, p 36
29. Campbell R: Sudden death and arrhythmias. In: Barnet D, Pouleur H, Francis G (eds): Congestive Cardiac Failure: Pathophysiology and Treatment, p 343–371. New York, Marcel Dekker, 1993
30. Ibid, p 356
31. Kayser, p 36–37
32. Cody R, Pickworth K: Approaches to diuretic therapy and electrolyte imbalance in congestive heart failure. Cardiol Clin 12:37,1994

33. Ibid
34. Gottlieb S, Baruch L, Kukin ML, Bernstein J, Fisher M, Packer M: Prognostic importance of the serum magnesium concentration in patients with congestive heart failure. J Am Coll Cardiol 16:827–831,1990
35. Hix C: Magnesium in congestive heart failure, acute myocardial infarction and dysrhythmias. J Cardiovasc Nurs 8:22,1993
36. Bashir Y, Sneddon J, Stauton A, Haywood G, Simpson I, McKenna W, Camm A: Effects of long-term oral magnesium chloride replacement in congestive heart failure secondary to coronary artery disease. Am J Cardiol 72:1156,1993
37. Rose B: Clinical Physiology of Acid-Base and Electrolyte Disorders, 4th ed, p 472. New York, McGraw-Hill, 1994
38. Geheb M, Krus J, Haupt M, Desai T, Carlson R: Fluid and electrolyte abnormalities in critically ill patients. In: Naris R (ed): Maxwell and Kleeman's Clinical Disorders of Fluid and Electrolyte Metabolism, 5th ed, p 1479, New York, McGraw-Hill, 1994
39. Ibid, p 1473
40. Guidelines for cardiopulmonary resuscitation and emergency cardiac care. JAMA 268:2211,1992
41. Martin et al: Hyperkalemia during human cardiopulmonary resuscitation: Incidence and ramifications J Emerg Med 7:109,1989
42. Geheb et al, p 148
43. Ibid

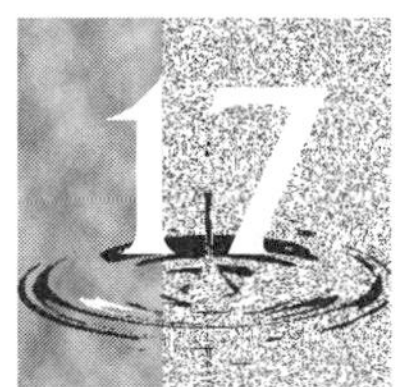

Renal Failure

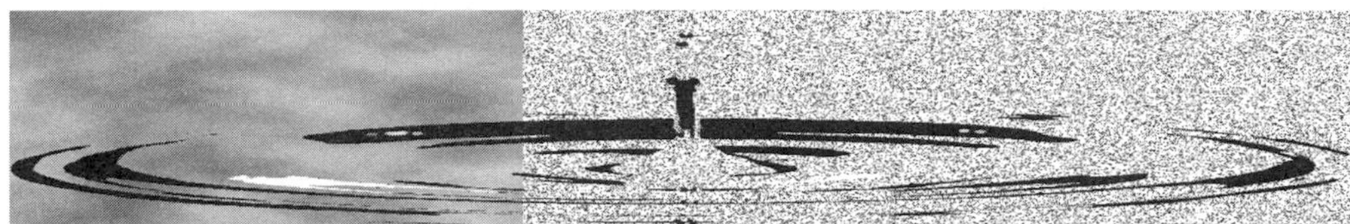

The renal system is the primary regulator of homeostasis of the body's internal environment. It performs its essential maintenance functions by participating in the following physiologic processes: (1) regulation of the volume, concentration, and pH of body fluids; (2) detoxification and elimination of waste products; (3) regulation of blood pressure; (4) regulation of erythropoiesis; (5) synthesis of prostaglandins; and (6) metabolism of vitamin D. Thus, when the renal system becomes dysfunctional, the result is an altered internal environment that is not compatible with life. Individuals who experience this dysfunction must rely on a complex set of therapeutic interventions that includes dietary and fluid restrictions, pharmacologic agents, and renal replacement therapies to sustain life. The biochemical and metabolic alterations that these individuals endure severely compromise their well-being and present a major challenge for clinicians. To assist the clinician in meeting this challenge, this chapter discusses the following: definitions of renal failure; differentiation between acute and chronic renal failure, particularly with regard to etiologies and clinical courses; overview of the systemic manifestations of renal failure; specific effects of renal failure on fluid, electrolyte, and acid–base balance; assessment of the patient experiencing renal failure; overview of the nursing diagnoses appropriate for delivering care to a patient experiencing renal dysfunction and the appropriate management therapies specific for those nursing diagnoses related to the fluid, electrolyte, and acid–base imbalances.

DEFINITION

Renal failure is the cessation of renal function, resulting in biochemical, metabolic, fluid, electrolyte, and acid–base derangements in the individual's internal environment that seriously threaten life. There are two types of renal failure, acute and chronic, that can be differentiated by their definitions, etiologies, and clinical courses, or disease progression.

ACUTE RENAL FAILURE

Acute renal failure is the abrupt, reversible cessation of renal function, rapidly accompanied by azotemia and uremia. The individual will usually present with oliguria; however, the urine volume can range from anuria to polyuria. Within the context of acute renal failure, the amounts of urine that comprise the continuum of volumes are defined as: (1) anuria, less than 100 mL/day; (2) oliguria, less than 400 mL/day; (3) nonoliguria, 400 to 1000 mL/day; and polyuria, 1000 to 2000 mL/day. Individuals with nonoliguric or polyuric acute renal failure may experience a shorter course of illness and/or have more therapeutic options available. However, despite their urine volume, they are still in acute renal failure. Thus, they cannot excrete the necessary solutes and are in a compromised state.

Various etiologies can produce acute renal failure and they can be categorized into three major types: prerenal, postrenal, and parenchymal. Prerenal etiologies are perfusion-related, whereas postrenal etiologies are associated with obstruction. The parenchymal, or intrinsic, renal etiologies reflect damage to functioning kidney tissue as a result of a prolonged or major cellular insult. Table 17-1 summarizes the three classifications of etiologies and delineates specific examples of frequently occurring clinical conditions that illustrate each category. In general, the prerenal and postrenal etiologies are reversible if corrective interventions are implemented rapidly enough. In the case of the prerenal etiologies, because perfusion is the primary problem, it is necessary to differentiate between prerenal oliguria and intrinsic acute renal failure to intervene appropriately. Thus, the clinician would evaluate the parameters included in Table 17-2 to determine the most appropriate interventions. Two of the parameters may need further explanations in terms of their calculations. The fractional excretion of sodium (FE_{Na}) is the percentage of filtered sodium that appears in the urine and it is calculated using the following formula:

$$\text{Fractional Excretion Na} = \frac{[\text{urine Na}] \times [\text{plasma creatinine}]}{[\text{plasma Na}] \times [\text{urine creatinine}]} \times 100$$

The renal failure index expresses the urinary sodium concentration as a function of the ratio of the urine/plasma creatinine concentration and is calculated using the following formula:

$$\text{Renal Failure Index} = \frac{[\text{urine Na}] \times [\text{plasma creatinine}]}{[\text{urine creatinine}]} \times 100$$

TABLE 17–1

Common Causes of Acute Renal Failure

CLASSIFICATION	EXAMPLES OF CLINICAL CONDITIONS
PRERENAL	
Hypovolemia	Vascular loss: hemorrhage Gastrointestinal loss: vomiting, diarrhea Renal loss: diuretic abuse, osmotic diuresis associated with diabetes Integumentary loss: burns, diaphoresis
Cardiovascular failure	Myocardial infarction Tamponade Vascular pooling: sepsis Vascular occlusion: thrombosis, embolism
POSTRENAL	
Obstruction	Ureteral: fibrosis, calculi, crystals, clots, accidental ligation Bladder: neoplasms Urethral: stricture, prostatic hypertrophy
PARENCHYMAL	
Glomerulonephritis	Acute poststreptococcal, systemic lupus erythematosus, Goodpasture's syndrome, bacterial endocarditis
Vasculitis	Periarteritis, hypersensitivity angiitis
Interstitial nephritis	Acute pyelonephritis, allergic nephritis, hypercalcemia, uric acid nephropathy, myeloma of the kidney
Renal vascular disease	Renal artery occlusion, renal vein thrombosis
Acute tubular necrosis	
Postischemia	Hypovolemia, cardiogenic shock, endotoxic shock
Nephrotoxins	Heavy metals, organic solvents, glycols, antibiotics, anesthetics, radiographic contrast media
Pigments	
Hemoglobin	Intravascular hemolysis: transfusion reactions, toxic hemolysis
Myoglobin	Rhabdomyolysis: trauma, muscle disease, seizures, severe exercise, prolonged coma

From Schoengrund L. Balzer P: Renal Problems in Critical Care. p 27. Albany, New York, Delmar Publishers, 1985, with permission.

TABLE 17–2

Selected Differential Assessment Parameters for Prerenal Oliguria and Intrinsic Acute Renal Failure

CLINICAL PARAMETER	PRERENAL	INTRINSIC ACUTE RENAL FAILURE
Creatinine clearance	15–80 mL/min	< 5 mL/min
Urine volume	>400 mL/24 hrs	<400 mL/24 hrs
Urine sodium	<20 mEq/L	>30 mEq/L
Urine specific gravity	>1.015	1.010
Urine osmolality	>500 mOsm/kgH_2O	<350 mOsm/kgH_2O
Serum BUN to creatinine ratio	>10	10
Urine to serum creatinine ratio	>20	<20
Urine to serum osmolality ratio	>1.2	<1.2
Fractional excretion of sodium	<1%	>1%
Renal failure index	<1%	>1%

The clinical course of acute renal failure is relatively short, lasting approximately 10 to 25 days, during which time the individual progresses through four phases of the pathophysiological process. The four phases are onset; oliguria or anuria; diuresis, both early and late; and convalescence. Technically, however, convalescence constitutes a separate phase because it actually occurs beyond the 10- to 25-day clinical course. A definition of each of these phases presents the clinician with an overview of the progression of the disease process.

ONSET PHASE

The onset phase extends from 0 to 2 days and is the period that elapses from the occurrence of the precipitating event until the beginning of the oliguria or anuria. During this phase, the patient's renal blood flow and oxygen consumption decrease to 25% of normal, urine volume decreases to about 20% of normal, and filtration clearance decreases to 10% of normal.

OLIGURIC–ANURIC PHASE

This phase is approximately 8 to 14 days in length and constitutes the period during which the patient's urine volume remains at less than 400 mL/day. Four hundred milliliters per day is the classic definition of an oliguric state. It should be noted that, although this phase is labeled oliguric–anuric, anuria rarely occurs in these patients. Indeed, the presence of anuria should lead the clinician to assess the patient further for indications of a urinary tract obstruction.

During this phase, the patient's renal blood flow and oxygen consumption remain at about 25% of normal, urine volume decreases further to an obligatory 5% of normal, and filtration clearance remains decreased at 10% of normal level. The longer the patient remains in this phase, the poorer the prognosis due to the additional opportunities for serious complications to occur as a result of excesses in fluids, electrolytes, and metabolic waste products.

DIURETIC PHASE

The diuretic phase lasts about 10 days and is comprised of two distinct segments, early and late diuresis. The early diuretic stage is the period from when the urine output is more than 400 mL/day until the serum laboratory values stop rising. The laboratory values do not begin to decrease during this stage but merely cease rising. During this stage of diuresis, the patient's renal blood flow and oxygen consumption increase slightly to about 30% of normal, urine volume soars to 150% of normal, and filtration clearance remains at 10% of normal. The increase in urine volume during this stage is usually more reflective of a change in renal perfusion and the presence of serum hyperosmolality than it is of a change in actual renal function. This is evident in the continuing low percentage of filtration clearance.

Late-stage diuresis occurs from the time the serum laboratory values begin to decrease until they stabilize at new, lower levels. Although lower, the new values remain somewhat elevated. The decrease and stabilization of the laboratory values at a higher than normal level is a reflection of the continuing improvement of renal blood flow and filtration clearance during this stage. Renal blood flow and oxygen consumption increase to about 50% of normal, urine volume peaks at about 200% of normal and then declines, and filtration clearance increases to 50% of normal. During this stage of the diuretic phase, the individual is vulnerable to developing fluid and electrolyte imbalances; at this time, however, these are likely to be deficits rather than excesses. These imbalances are easier to manage, and, although they still constitute a threat to the patient's well-being, they present much less of a hazard than the excesses that can occur during the oliguric–anuric phase. That these imbalances are less critical is related to the increased number of therapeutic options available because of the return of some renal function.

CONVALESCENT PHASE

The convalescent phase lasts from 4 to 6 months and is the period from the stabilization of the serum laboratory values until the patient attains either totally normal or optimal renal function. In some patients, particularly the elderly and those with a preexisting renal disease, the renal dysfunction will result in a 1% to 2% degree of residual impairment. Therefore, those particular patients may not regain 100% of their previous renal function. In most cases, however, the degree of residual impairment is clinically insignificant.

CHRONIC RENAL FAILURE

Chronic renal failure involves the slowly progressive, and often insidious, irreversible cessation of renal function accompanied by the sequential intensification of biochemical, metabolic, fluid, electrolyte, and acid–base imbalances. Many etiologies can result in chronic renal failure. Most can be classified as belonging to one of the following nine categories: glomerular diseases, tubular diseases, vascular diseases, infectious diseases, obstructive diseases, collagen diseases, metabolic renal diseases, congenital diseases, and neoplastic diseases. Table 17-3 summarizes these categories and gives some examples of clinical conditions that are illustrative of each category. The clinical conditions that occur most frequently appear to be chronic glomerulonephritis, hypertension, nodular glomerulosclerosis due to diabetes mellitus, and obstructive uropathy. In addition, many etiological categories can produce a broad pathological process called chronic interstitial nephritis, which also occurs frequently.

The clinical course of chronic renal failure progresses gradually, and the patient often is unaware of a problem until very late in the process. As the disease progresses, the patient goes through four phases of functional deterioration, including diminished renal reserve, renal insufficiency, renal failure, and the uremic syndrome. During the third phase, renal failure, the patient usually recognizes that there is a problem. The time from the onset of the renal dysfunction through the progressive deterioration phases is very specific to each patient and the pathological processes associated with the etiology. Thus, it is difficult to identify the precise time frames for each phase.

DIMINISHED RENAL RESERVE

The first phase of functional deterioration involves only a mild reduction in renal function. In this phase, the patient's creatinine clearance will decrease from an average normal level of 120 mL/min to approximately 50 mL/min, accompanied by an increase in the serum creatinine level from a normal range of 0.7 to 1.5 mg/100 mL to a range of 1.6 to 2.0 mg/100 mL. During this phase the patient still has about 50% of normal renal function and the kidney's primary regulatory, excretory, and metabolic functions remain intact. Consequently, there is little change in the individual's internal environment and no warning of what is to come.

TABLE 17–3

The Categories of Etiologies of Chronic Renal Failure

CATEGORY	EXAMPLES OF CLINICAL CONDITIONS
Glomerular diseases	Chronic glomerulonephritis Nephrotic syndrome Rapidly progressive glomerulonephritis
Tubular diseases	Renal tubular acidosis Chronic electrolyte imbalances • Hypercalcemic nephropathy • Hypokalemic nephropathy
Vascular diseases	Hypertension Arteriosclerosis Nodular glomerulosclerosis • Kimmelsteil-Wilson's syndrome
Infectious diseases	Pyelonephritis Tuberculosis
Obstructive diseases	Obstructive uropathy • Urethral strictures • Congenital deformities
Collagen diseases	Scleroderma Lupus nephritis Necrotizing vasculitis • Polyarteritis nodosa • Hypersensitivity angiitis
Metabolic renal diseases	Amyloidosis Hyperoxaluria
Congenital diseases	Polycystic kidney disease Medullary cystic disease Hypoplastic kidneys Hereditary nephritis • Alport's syndrome
Neoplastic diseases	Multiple myeloma Lymphoma

RENAL INSUFFICIENCY

As the functional deterioration continues, the patient experiences renal insufficiency. During this phase, creatinine clearance continues to decrease to about

10 mL/min and is accompanied by an increase in the serum creatinine level to a range of about 2.1 to 5.0 mg/100 mL. The patient experiences mild alterations in the internal environment that are usually not significant enough to seek health care interventions. If, however, the patient experiences additional physiological stress (such as an infection or dehydration) during this phase, the alterations in the internal environment will intensify and usually require therapeutic intervention.

RENAL FAILURE

During this phase of functional deterioration the patient usually realizes that a problem exists. There is now sufficient deterioration in renal function, usually a loss of more than 75% of normal function, to produce significant, constant alterations in the internal environment that threaten the patient's well-being. The patient now experiences clinical signs and symptoms that require management so that the activities of daily living can continue. During this phase, the individual's creatinine clearance has decreased to about 5 mL/min and the serum creatinine level is more than 8.0 mg per 100 mL.

THE UREMIC SYNDROME

The final phase of chronic renal failure is the onset of the uremic syndrome. At this point, the functional deterioration of the renal system is almost complete and the individual experiences clinical manifestations in every body system. The patient's creatinine clearance level is less than 5 mL/min and the serum creatinine level is more than 12 mg/100 mL and continues to rise.

THE SYSTEMIC MANIFESTATIONS OF RENAL FAILURE

The clinical signs and symptoms that manifest the presence of renal failure are collectively labeled the uremic syndrome. The uremic syndrome accompanies both acute and chronic renal failure. However, due to the relatively rapid resolution of acute renal failure, the syndrome may be less severe and may not evidence all components. For example, it is not likely that reproductive or chronic skeletal system alterations will be observed in a patient with acute renal failure, primarily due to the short duration of the renal dysfunction. Table 17-4 summarizes the clinical manifestations and their associated pathophysiological mechanisms according to body system. The fluid, electrolyte, and acid–base imbalances are so critical to caring for these patients that they require additional discussion.

FLUID VOLUME IMBALANCES

Fluid volume excess is usually evident in patients during either the oliguric–anuric phase of acute renal failure or in chronic renal failure. In both pathophysiological processes, the primary factor is the inability of the kidneys to excrete the appropriate amounts of fluid to maintain a homeostatic internal environment. The fluid volume excess may be a more serious problem in the oliguric–anuric phase of acute renal failure due to the rapidity of the onset of cessation of renal function. The rapid cessation of renal function does not allow time for the development of the adaptive mechanisms experienced by patients with chronic renal failure. Therefore, the patient in the oliguric–anuric phase of acute renal failure is much more vulnerable to fluid overload.

The fluid volume excess that accompanies the oliguric–anuric phase of acute renal failure results from several etiologies. Certainly a major factor is the decreased excretion of fluids due to a decreased glomerular filtration rate and tubular dysfunction. The following may also contribute: (1) excessive ingestion or administration of oral or intravenous (IV) fluids; (2) accumulation of water resulting from the metabolism of nutrients; and (3) accumulation of water that is released from injured or catabolized tissues.

As the patient progresses through the acute renal failure episode and enters the diuretic phase, the fluid imbalance is likely to shift to a deficit. During this phase the glomerular filtration rate and tubular functional capacities have improved sufficiently so that a marked increase in the volume of urine excreted is noted. The volume of urine that is excreted depends not only on the degree of functional improvement that has occurred but on the amount of excess water and solute that was retained by the individual since the onset of the disease process. Fortunately, because of the more aggressive dialysis therapy and other therapeutic interventions used recently, the degree of excess water and solute retention has been somewhat minimized. Thus, these individuals do not seem to

(text continues on page 301)

TABLE 17–4

The Systemic Manifestations of Renal Failure

SYSTEM	MANIFESTATION	PATHOPHYSIOLOGICAL MECHANISMS
Vascular	Fluid overload	Decreased excretion
	Electrolyte imbalances	Decreased excretion
	Metabolic acidosis	Decreased hydrogen ion secretion Decreased sodium ion reabsorption Decreased bicarbonate ion reabsorption and generation Decreased excretion of phosphate salts or titratable acids Decreased ammonia synthesis and ammonium excretion
	Hypertension	Fluid overload Increased sodium retention Inappropriate activation of the renin-angiotensin system
Cardiac	Congestive heart failure	Fluid overload Hypertension
	Dysrhythmias	Electrolyte imbalances, especially hyperkalemia, hypocalcemia and variations in sodium
	Pericarditis (more frequently seen in chronic renal failure patients)	Uremic toxins Increased pericardial membrane permeability
	Peripheral or systemic edema	Fluid overload and increased hydrostatic pressure (associated decrease in osmotic pressure would increase the degree of edema) Right ventricular dysfunction
Hematopoietic	Anemia	Decreased erythropoietin secretion Loss of red blood cells through the GI tract, mucous membranes, or dialysis Decreased red blood cell survival time due to uremic toxins Burr cells are produced by a hypertonic serum due to uremic toxins Uremic toxins interfere with folic acid action
	Alterations in coagulation	Platelet dysfunction due to uremic toxins Hypocalcemia could contribute but rarely does because of the metabolic acidosis
	Increased susceptibility to infection	Decreased neutrophil phagocytosis and chemotaxis due to uremic toxins
Respiratory	Pulmonary edema	Fluid overload Increased pulmonary capillary permeability Left ventricular dysfunction
	Pneumonia or pneumonitis	Thick, tenacious oral secretions due to decreased fluid intake Weak, lethargic patient with depressed cough reflex due to uremia Decreased pulmonary macrophage activity Fluid overload
	Kussmaul respirations	Increase in rate and depth of respirations to decrease the carbon dioxide in the body to compensate for metabolic acidosis

(continued)

TABLE 17-4 (cont.)

SYSTEM	MANIFESTATION	PATHOPHYSIOLOGICAL MECHANISMS
Gastrointestinal	Anorexia, nausea, and emesis	Uremic toxins Decomposition of urea in the GI tract releasing ammonia that irritates mucosa
	Stomatitis and uremic halitosis	Uremic toxins Decomposition of urea in the oral cavity releasing ammonia
	Gastritis and bleeding	Uremic toxins Decomposition of urea in the GI tract releasing ammonia that irritates GI mucosa, producing small ulcerations Increased capillary fragility
	Bowel problems Diarrhea	Uremic toxins Hypermotility due to electrolyte imbalances, especially hyperkalemia
	Constipation	Hypomotility due to electrolyte imbalances, decreased fluid intake, decreased activity, and decreased bulk in diet
Neuromuscular	Drowsiness, confusion, coma, and irritability	Uremic toxins produce uremic encephalopathy Metabolic acidosis
	Tremors, twitching, and convulsions	Electrolyte imbalances Uremic toxins produce uremic encephalopathy
	Peripheral neuropathy *Stage 1:* restless leg syndrome and paresthesias *Stage 2:* motor involvement leading to footdrop *Stage 3:* paraplegia (Stages 2 and 3 are rare in acute renal failure patients)	Decreased nerve conduction, both motor and sensory, due to uremic toxins
Psychosocial	Decreased mentation, decreased concentration, and altered perceptions (even to the point of frank psychoses)	Uremic toxins produce uremic encephalopathy Electrolyte imbalances Metabolic acidosis Tendency to develop cerebral edema
Integumentary	Pallor	Uremic anemia
	Yellow hue	Retained urochrome pigment is excreted through skin
	Dryness	Decreased secretions from oil and sweat glands due to uremic toxins
	Pruritus	Dry skin Calcium and/or phosphate deposits in the skin Uremic toxins' effects on nerve endings
	Purpura and ecchymoses	Increased capillary fragility Platelet dysfunction
	Uremic frost (seen only in terminal or severely critically ill patients)	Urea or urate crystals are excreted through the skin
Endocrine	Glucose intolerance (usually not clinically significant)	Peripheral insensitivity to insulin due to uremia Prolonged insulin half-life due to decreased renal metabolism

TABLE 17-4 (cont.)

The Systemic Manifestations of Renal Failure

SYSTEM	MANIFESTATION	PATHOPHYSIOLOGICAL MECHANISMS
Skeletal	Hypocalcemia	Hyperphosphatemia due to decreased renal excretion Decreased GI reabsorption due to decreased renal conversion of vitamin D
	Osteodystrophy	Increased osteoclastic activity in response to an increased secretion of parathormone
	Soft-tissue calcification	Deposition of calcium phosphate crystals in soft tissue and other structures
Reproductive	Infertility	Decreased sperm production and decreased ovulation due to uremia
	Decreased libido	Combination of the pathophysiological and psychological effects of uremia

From Schoengrund L, Baker P: Renal Problems in Critical Care, pp 29–31; New York, Delmar Publishers, 1985; with permission.

experience the massive fluid volume shifts and depletion characteristic of the diuretic phase in the past.

The patient with chronic renal failure usually experiences a fluid volume excess. In general, this fluid volume imbalance results primarily from the decreased glomerular filtration rate and decreased excretion of free water. In addition, it is enhanced by a dysfunctional concentrating and diluting mechanism and an increased solute load. The deficit in the concentrating mechanism probably occurs due to several pathophysiological alterations, including the following: (1) decreased medullary blood flow; (2) decreased response or resistance of the collecting tubules to the presence of vasopressin or antidiuretic hormone (ADH); (3) impaired sodium and chloride transport in the ascending limb of Henle's loop; (4) diminished urea gradient in the medullary interstitium due to dilution; (5) decreased physiological functioning of Henle's loop, distal convoluted tubules, and collecting tubules due to pathology and cellular injury; and (6) increased secretion or synthesis of vasoconstrictor substances, such as renin or prostaglandins to support glomerular blood flow, which further suppresses the response to ADH. The ultimate outcome of the decrease in concentrating ability is an increased solute load for the patient.

Patients with chronic renal failure also cannot dilute urine. The defect in the diluting mechanism probably results from the decreased glomerular filtration rate, the decreased number of functional nephrons due to pathology, and the increase in overall solute load. The result is an isosthenuria with a fixed osmolality that is similar to the plasma. Thus, the individual cannot dilute the urine and is unable to excrete excess free water.

ELECTROLYTE IMBALANCES

The patient with renal failure experiences deviations in almost every electrolyte. In general, the patient is hypernatremic (or dilutionally hyponatremic), hyperkalemic, hyperchloremic, hypocalcemic, hyperphosphatemic, and normomagnesemic (unless exogenous sources of magnesium are ingested or administered). Understanding the specific pathophysiological mechanisms that produce these imbalances during renal failure will assist the clinician in planning and implementing appropriate therapeutic measures to assist the individual in coping with these alterations in the internal environment.

Sodium

Patients with either acute or chronic renal failure often present initially with hyponatremia. This state, however, usually changes to hypernatremia during the progression and management of the disease process. The patient with acute renal failure tends to retain sodium due to a decreased glomerular filtration rate and tubular dysfunction. The increased sodium retention results in increased water retention and thus an extracellular fluid (ECF) volume expansion with a concomitant dilutional hyponatremia. Other factors that contribute to producing this almost "pseudo" hyponatremic state include increased ingestion or administration of free-water; increased accumulation of water resulting from increased metabolic processes; increased ECF volume resulting from cellular catabolism or injury; and intracellular shifts of sodium that occur as a result of the extracellular–intracellular exchanges among sodium, hydrogen, and potassium due to metabolic acidosis and hyperkalemia. Therefore, the patient often has a dilutional hyponatremia although there is a total body excess of sodium. A hypernatremic state may gradually appear if the patient's water intake is restricted. In some patients, however, the hypernatremia may never be evident because of the early, aggressive initiation of renal replacement therapy, usually in the form of hemodialysis.

As the individual with acute renal failure progresses to, and through, the late stage of diuresis, the possibility of a true hyponatremic state occurring becomes more distinct. The solute-induced diuresis, as well as the cellular shifts of electrolytes, is likely to create at least a transient sodium deficit. The imbalance will, however, usually resolve without therapeutic intervention as the diuresis decreases and more normal renal function occurs.

The sodium imbalances that accompany chronic renal failure usually shift from hyponatremia to hypernatremia as the renal function deteriorates to an end-stage level. The concept that sodium excretion decreases as the functional renal mass decreases certainly is valid. However, during the progressive deterioration in renal function, numerous adaptive mechanisms are stimulated that serve to maintain a certain degree of sodium balance. Those adaptive mechanisms appear to include the following: (1) extracellular fluid volume expansion as a result of sodium retention, which may increase the glomerular filtration rate; (2) sodium-potassium-adenosine triphosphatase (Na-K-ATPase) inhibition resulting in natriuresis; (3) increased circulating amounts of atrial natriuretic factor; (4) increased prostaglandin synthesis; (5) hypertrophy and hyperfiltration of the remaining nephrons; (6) tubular adaptation due to altered Starling forces at the peritubular membrane and an increased solute load; and (7) altered proximal tubule sodium reabsorption due to metabolic acidosis. These adaptive mechanisms appear to remain operative throughout the renal dysfunction but decrease in effectiveness as the disease process progresses to an end-stage level. Thus, as their effectiveness decreases, the occurrence of hypernatremia increases.

Potassium

Hyperkalemia is a significant electrolyte imbalance for patients with either acute or chronic renal failure. However, it is a greater threat to the patient with acute renal failure due to the rapidity of its onset and the patient's overall decreased capacity to activate appropriate adaptive mechanisms in response to the abrupt alteration. In fact, for patients with acute renal failure, hyperkalemia-induced complications are second only to sepsis as the leading cause of death.

The primary mechanisms present in acute renal failure that enhance the development and maintenance of a hyperkalemic state include (1) decreased glomerular filtration rate, loss of distal tubular function, and oliguria; (2) intracellular release of potassium from lysed, necrotic, or injured cells; (3) presence of acute metabolic acidosis; (4) cellular catabolism; and (5) inhibition of ATPase and a resulting defect in potassium transport mechanisms. In addition, any new stresses that occur, such as infection, fever, or gastrointestinal (GI) bleeding, will further compromise the patient and serve to enhance the hyperkalemia.

The patient with chronic renal failure uses adaptive mechanisms to handle the increased potassium load resulting from the decrease in renal function. These adaptive mechanisms remain intact and operative throughout the progression of the chronic renal failure until the patient becomes oliguric. Once oliguria is present, the adaptive mechanisms cease to be effective. Included among those adaptive mechanisms are (1) increased potassium per nephron excretion rate by the remaining intact nephrons; (2) increased potassium excretion by the large intestine; (3) increased renal Na-K-ATPase activity level; (4) increased tubular intraluminal flow rate; (5) increased peritubular potassium reabsorption; (6) increased potassium secretion by the collecting ducts; (7) increased distal tubular potassium secretion due to an increased aldosterone production; and (8) presence of chronic metabolic acidosis. Certainly if the patient with chronic renal failure experiences additional stressors that would further compromise the adaptive mechanisms, the hyperkalemic state could be exacerbated and rapidly become life-threatening. Such stressors might include volume depletion or catabolic events such as infection, GI bleeding, trauma, or surgery.

Chloride

Overall, chloride imbalance does not seem to be a significant problem for patients with either acute or chronic renal failure. Any imbalance that does occur reflects either the alterations in sodium, water, bicarbonate, and hydrogen ions or the presence of uremic manifestations or complications. Patients with acute renal failure are likely to have an actual increase in chloride as a result of the decreased glomerular filtration rate, tubular dysfunction, sodium retention, and bicarbonate deficit. The increase, however, may be masked by the dilutional effect of the excessive water that is retained.

Patients with chronic renal failure tend to remain normochloremic due to the adaptive mechanisms that are activated. Such balance appears to be evident throughout the progression of the chronic renal failure process, including during the uremic state. Although little is known regarding the adaptive mechanisms that can facilitate chloride balance maintenance during chronic renal failure, one hypothesis suggests that a chloruretic factor may be a primary contributor.

Calcium

Hypocalcemia is an imbalance frequently occurring in both acute and chronic renal failure. In acute renal failure, the decline in serum calcium levels can be noted as early as 48 hrs after the onset of oliguria. In most instances, the decrease will stabilize at approximately 6 mg/100 mL. In acute renal failure due to rhabdomyolysis, however, the levels may be much lower due to an exacerbated deficit of calcium as it shifts into the injured and necrotic tissues. The hypocalcemia that accompanies acute renal failure results from the following mechanisms: (1) phosphate retention due to a decreased glomerular filtration rate and tubular dysfunction; (2) exaggerated hyperphosphatemia due to the release of phosphate ions from injured tissues; (3) decreased 1,25-dihydroxycholecalciferol production by the kidneys and a concomitant decrease in the GI absorption of calcium; and (4) increased secretion of parathyroid hormone (PTH) in response to the hyperphosphatemia and suppressed serum calcium level. PTH acts directly on the bone to cause resorption of calcium and phosphate. Because the additional phosphate added to the bloodstream cannot be disposed of through the usual renal route, the serum calcium concentration cannot increase and remains a stimulus for increased PTH secretion. The clinical significance of hypocalcemia in patients with acute renal failure lies not so much in its ability to produce tetany as a result of altering neuron permeability, as in its potentiation of the effect of hyperkalemia on cardiac function. Indeed, the acute metabolic acidosis that is present in acute renal failure serves to modulate some of the effects of the hypocalcemia by increasing the proportional amount of ionized calcium that is available in the serum.

In chronic renal failure, the hypocalcemic imbalance has greater clinical significance. It often results in the following complications for the patient: renal osteodystrophy, soft tissue calcification, secondary hyperparathyroidism, and enhanced signs and symptoms of uremia. The mechanisms responsible for creating and maintaining the hypocalcemia include (1) excessive phosphate retention due to decreased renal parenchymal mass; (2) increased PTH production as a compensatory response; (3) impaired vitamin D metabolism by the kidneys; and (4) the physiologically depressive effects of the uremic toxins in the body. These mechanisms result in decreased GI calcium absorption, the formation of calcium–phosphate complexes, decreased bone mobilization of calcium due to a skeletal resistance to PTH, and suppression of the normal metabolic processes used to restore calcium to normal levels.

Initially, in chronic renal failure, an adaptive hypocalciuria occurs. Unfortunately, it is not sufficient to overcome the effects of the hyperphosphatemia and uremia producing the hypocalcemic state. Thus, the patient remains hypocalcemic, and the imbalance is accentuated as the chronic renal failure progresses to end-stage level.

Phosphorus

Patients with either acute or chronic renal failure experience hyperphosphatemia. In acute renal failure, the imbalance is created by (1) inadequate phosphate excretion due to a decreased glomerular filtration rate and tubular dysfunction; (2) intracellular shift of phosphate ions to the ECF due to catabolism, cellular injury, and tissue necrosis; and (3) acute metabolic acidosis that decreases glycolysis, resulting in the hydrolysis of intracellular sugar phosphates that increase the concentration of diffusible inorganic phosphate ions. Thus, this imbalance may be exaggerated in patients who are very catabolic.

Individuals with chronic renal failure do not experience hyperphosphatemia until renal function has deteriorated to a creatinine clearance level of 20 to 30 mL/min. At that point, not only are there reductions in the filtered load of phosphate due to a decreased glomerular filtration rate, but there is also impairment of the intrinsic tubular adaptive mechanisms that would normally decrease the reabsorption of phosphate in a hyperphosphatemic state. Increased PTH secretion is another adaptive mechanism that tends to blunt the severity of the hyperphosphatemic state. Unfortunately, the result of this compensatory response is secondary hyperparathyroidism that merely complicates the patient's clinical condition even more. Thus, the excess phosphate not only creates additional problems due to secondary hyperparathyroidism but also appears to (1) decrease the calcium mobilizing ability of PTH; (2) decrease GI calcium absorption; (3) inhibit the hydroxylation of vitamin D to 1,25-dihydroxycholecalciferol in the kidney; (4) facilitate the deposition of calcium in soft tissues; and (5) have a direct nephrotoxic effect.

Magnesium

Patients with either acute or chronic renal failure usually retain magnesium as a result of a decreased glomerular filtration rate and tubular dysfunction. In most instances, however, the hypermagnesemic state does not become clinically significant unless the patient ingests or receives additional magnesium from exogenous sources. The usual exogenous sources of magnesium include magnesium-based antacids and cathartics, pharmacologic agents, IV solutions, and hyperalimentation solutions.

During acute renal failure, the degree of magnesium retention in the oliguric–anuric phase is usually not sufficient to produce clinically significant alterations. Such clinical signs and symptoms are not frequently manifested until the serum magnesium level is in excess of 7 mEq/L. Fortunately, because acute renal failure is usually of short duration, the patient rarely experiences serum magnesium levels greater than 3 or 4 mEq/L unless an exogenous load of magnesium is provided. Thus, hypermagnesemia is present in patients with acute renal failure but usually, is not clinically apparent.

In chronic renal failure, the serum magnesium level remains within the normal range until the glomerular filtration rate decreases to less than 30 mL/min. As the disease progresses to end-stage level, adaptive mechanisms are initiated that tend to lessen the clinical impact of the continuing accumulation of magnesium due to decreased excretion. Those adaptive mechanisms include (1) increased fractional magnesium excretion due to the increased filtered magnesium load; (2) increased total volume of magnesium excreted as a result of natriuresis and the overall increased osmotic load; (3) increased magnesium excretion due to acidosis, which decreases magnesium tubular reabsorption; (4) decreased tubular response to PTH; (5) decreased intestinal absorption of magnesium due to uremia and the decreased production of 1,25-dihydroxycholecalciferol; and (6) increased deposition of magnesium in the bone and perhaps intracellularly. Eventually these adaptive mechanisms are unable to compensate for the excessive magnesium that is retained. As a result, the patient is more likely to accumulate magnesium, attain higher serum levels, and experience the clinical signs and symptoms associated with hypermagnesemia. Certainly the addition of any exogenous source of magnesium will exacerbate the imbalance and result in further clinical manifestations.

Acid–Base Disturbances

Metabolic acidosis is the predominant acid–base imbalance that accompanies both acute and chronic renal failure. In both disease processes, there is a retention of hydrogen ions due to a decreased glomerular filtration rate, tubular dysfunction, and an overall decrease in the number of functioning nephrons. The primary physiological alterations that contribute to producing the acidosis seem to be deficits in bicarbonate reabsorption and ammoniagenesis. The result is that the usual daily load of nonvolatile acids produced by the metabolism of dietary protein and the catabolism of endogenous tissue cannot be excreted. Thus, those acids, normally averaging about 1 mEq/kg/day of body weight, accumulate and result in metabolic acidosis.

Patients with acute renal failure usually experience more severe acid–base imbalances due to the rapid onset of the disease process and their catabolic state. The rapidity of the onset decreases the patient's ability to initiate complex adaptive mechanisms to modulate the effects of the imbalance. In addition, cellular catabolism releases anions (sulfate, phosphate, and organic ions) into the plasma that enhance the high anion gap metabolic acidosis (see Chapter 9). Because the patient rapidly uses the existing buffering substances and, due to renal dysfunction, cannot provide sufficient replacements, the acidosis persists. The respiratory compensatory mechanisms that are stimulated appear to ameliorate some of the negative effects of the acidosis, but the imbalance is usually too severe for those mechanisms to significantly affect the patient's overall situation.

In chronic renal failure, the metabolic acidosis appears to remain mild until renal function deteriorates below a creatinine clearance level of 25 mL/min. At that time, the acidosis intensifies and gradually becomes more severe. The imbalance is even more exaggerated because the usual renal adaptive mechanisms are insufficient to contribute significantly to modulating the adverse effects of the acidosis. Fortunately, however, there are other adaptive physiological mechanisms that are triggered by the acidosis which can substitute for the defective renal mechanisms. These mechanisms include (1) buffering by tissue alkali from the bone stores; (2) respiratory compensation, which seems to operate effectively until the bicarbonate level decreases to less than 18 mEq/L; and (3) intracellular shift of hydrogen ions. Unfortunately, these mechanisms are not sufficient to maintain any semblance of homeostasis in acid–base balance in the patient. Thus, patients with chronic renal failure almost always have some degree of metabolic acidosis. Even the combination of maintenance renal replacement therapies, pharmacologic agents, and dietary restrictions does not seem to restore or maintain a normal acid–base balance. Instead, the therapeutic management tends to decrease the hazardous effects of the imbalance and create a more stable internal environment for the patient.

CLINICAL ASSESSMENT

The clinical assessment of a patient experiencing renal dysfunction incorporates the following components: (1) documenting the patient's history; (2) inspection; (3) evaluation of vital signs; (4) palpation and percussion; (5) assessment of laboratory data; (6) noninvasive monitoring of the system; and (7) invasive monitoring of the system.

HISTORY

The individual's history contains four aspects that are very relevant to the renal system: (1) renal-related symptoms, (2) systemic diseases, (3) family history, and (4) pharmacologic history.

Renal-Related Symptoms

Exploring the symptoms a patient reports in relation to the renal system can provide essential information that will assist in structuring the assessment to obtain more relevant and specific data. For example, certain symptoms are more indicative of one or two specific pathological conditions than they are of others. Table 17-5 lists the most frequently reported renal-related symptoms and their correlated potential pathologies.

Systemic Diseases

Numerous systemic diseases can affect the renal system as part of their inherent pathological processes. These systemic diseases originate in another primary body system that has a direct effect on the renal system. Specific clinical examples of such diseases include cardiovascular diseases (hypertension and chronic congestive heart failure), respiratory diseases (Goodpasture's syndrome and tuberculosis), endocrine diseases (diabetes mellitus and hepatic dysfunction), and reproductive diseases (disseminated intravascular coagulation and hemolytic–uremic syndrome).

Family History

The family history information is important in the assessment process because it not only indicates those systemic diseases that the patient may be prone to develop, but also delineates specific hereditary or metabolic renal diseases that may already be present or be likely to develop in the future. Examples include hereditary pathologies such as hereditary glomerulonephritis, Alport's syndrome, polycystic disease, medullary cystic disease, and metabolic

TABLE 17–5

Selected Renal-Related Symptoms and Their Correlated Potential Pathologies

SYMPTOM	POTENTIAL PATHOLOGY	SYMPTOM	POTENTIAL PATHOLOGY
Anuria	Obstruction Acute renal failure (rare)	Nephralgia (cont.) Acute	 Calculi Infection Obstruction
Cystalgia	Infection Calculi Trauma	Nocturia	Infection Insufficiency Diabetes Prostatic enlargement
Dysuria	Infection	Oliguria	Insufficiency Neoplasms Failure Dysfunction
Dribbling	Prostatic enlargement Strictures	Pneumaturia	Fistula
Edema	Failure Nephrotic syndrome	Polyuria	Diabetes Some types of renal failure
Frequency	Infection Diabetes	Proteinuria	Glomerular membrane diseases Nephrotic syndrome
Hematuria	Trauma Glomerular membrane diseases Neoplasms Calculi Infection	Pyuria	Infection
Hesitancy	Prostatic enlargement Strictures	Renal colic	Calculi
Incontinence	Infection Neoplasms Prolapsed uterus	Secondary enuresis	Neurologic disease Aging
Nephralgia Dull	 Infection Trauma Neoplasms Ischemia	Urgency	Infection Prostatic disease

abnormalities such as calculi, amyloidosis, and hyperoxaluria.

Pharmacologic History

A medication history is important in assessing the renal system because the clinician not only documents and evaluates the currently prescribed and unprescribed medications ingested or administered but also specifically assesses for any drug use or abuse that might result in nephrotoxicity. Analgesic and antibiotic medications are primary offenders in this respect.

INSPECTION

Inspection is useful because many of the systemic manifestations of renal failure, which are reflected in almost every body system, are easily discernable visually. Table 17-6 depicts the various aspects and specific parameters that should be included when a clinician inspects a patient with renal dysfunction.

VITAL SIGNS

When assessing a patient's vital signs in relation to renal dysfunction, it is important for the clinician to recall the following: (1) patients with renal dys-

TABLE 17–6

Inspection Components for Clinically Assessing the Renal System

ASPECT	SPECIFIC PARAMETERS
General appearance	Posture General strength Motor functioning Affect and mental attitude General hygiene
Skin	Color Turgor and elasticity Odor Degree of intactness Texture Presence, severity, and location of edema
Mucous membranes	Color Characteristics of secretions Odor Intactness Hydration state
Eyes	Visual acuity Periorbital edema
Ears	Auditory acuity
Activity	Level or amount Gait Motor functioning
Muscle movement	Purposeful
Cognitive functioning	Orientation Level of consciousness Responses to various types of stimuli

function are usually hypertensive due to fluid and electrolyte imbalances and, possibly, hyperactivity of the renin-angiotensin system; (2) they usually exhibit a strong, irregular, and somewhat rapid pulse as a result of the fluid and electrolyte imbalances; (3) they often exhibit Kussmaul's respirations as a compensatory mechanism for their metabolic acidosis; and (4) they are usually hypothermic but may exhibit temperature elevations due to infection resulting from their increased susceptibility due to decreased phagocytic and chemotaxic mechanisms caused by uremia, as well as their overall debilitated state. Thus, a patient with renal dysfunction may exhibit vital signs comparable to the following: blood pressure, 160/98 mmHg; pulse, 104 beats/min and irregular; respirations, 30 breaths/min; and oral temperature, 37.2 °C (99 °F).

PALPATION AND PERCUSSION

The kidneys are palpated in the lower portions of the upper right and left quadrants of the abdomen. Normally, only the lower pole of the right kidney is palpable because other anatomical structures obscure the left kidney and the remaining portions of the right kidney. The primary purposes for palpating the kidneys are to determine size and to elicit pain if an infective process is present. The kidneys should be palpated both anteriorly and posteriorly, particularly in the flank area at the costovertebral angle.

Percussion of the kidneys is performed in the same areas that have been designated for palpation. The purposes of percussion are to determine size and to assess for the presence and degree of abnormally sequestered amounts of perinephric fluid.

LABORATORY DATA

Renal dysfunction is rapidly evident in the patient's serum laboratory values. Thus, these data should be assessed at least daily for patients with acute renal failure and at least weekly for those with chronic renal failure. Table 17-7 presents the biochemical substances that should be included in a laboratory data assessment and their variations associated with acute and chronic renal failure.

The urine laboratory values vary with the pathological processes and the progression of the acute or chronic renal failure. Therefore, they are less helpful overall but may be important for differentiating various aspects of the therapeutic interventions. For example, urine sodium is a significant parameter for differentiating between prerenal oliguria and the oliguria of intrinsic acute renal failure. In addition, urine values may assist in determining the dietary needs of patients with chronic renal failure. In general, however, the concept in renal failure is that substances are being retained in the serum and not excreted in the urine.

TABLE 17–7

Variations in Serum Laboratory Values Accompanying Acute and Chronic Renal Failure

BIOCHEMICAL SUBSTANCE	VARIATION IN ACUTE RENAL FAILURE	VARIATION IN CHRONIC RENAL FAILURE
Sodium	Increases or varies	Normal or varies
Potassium	Increases	Increases
Chloride	Increases or varies	Varies
Blood urea nitrogen	Increases	Increases
Creatinine	Increases	Increases
Calcium	Decreases	Decreases
Phosphorus	Increases	Increases
Uric acid	Increases	Increases
Carbon dioxide combining power	Decreases	Decreases
Magnesium	Increases or normal	Increases or normal
Osmolality	Increases or varies	Increases or varies
Hematocrit	Decreases	Decreases
Hemoglobin	Decreases	Decreases

The best measure of renal function is creatinine clearance. Unfortunately, in many clinical situations it is not pragmatic to measure creatinine clearance. Instead, serum creatinine and blood urea nitrogen (BUN) can be used to assess renal function. Significant increases in both of those serum values indicate renal dysfunction. Of the two values, however, BUN is the least reflective of renal function because it is easily influenced by other factors such as catabolism, internal bleeding, and dehydration. Also of note is the fact that the volume of urine output is not a good measure of renal function. Urine volume is more reflective of perfusion levels than of function. Thus, a decrease in urine volume may reflect perfusion deficits or renal pathology.

NONINVASIVE MONITORING

Noninvasive monitoring techniques include obtaining intake and output (I&O) measurements, obtaining daily weights, and consulting with the physician regarding existing radiographs. Intake and output measurements and daily weights provide some data regarding the patient's hydration state, but, as mentioned previously, they are not a valid measure of renal function. Of course, for these techniques to be useful, they must be accurate. Chapter 2 describes some frequently occurring errors associated with these measurements that the clinician may want to review.

The radiograph is one of the most frequently used techniques for obtaining gross assessment data regarding the renal system. A plain film of the abdomen, called a KUB (for kidneys, ureters, and bladder), is obtained for almost every patient before any invasive procedures. This radiograph provides data regarding the size, shape, position, and possible areas of calcification.

INVASIVE MONITORING

Invasive monitoring of the renal system includes several diagnostic procedures that provide essential information for the clinician. Any and all of the following procedures may be used with patients experiencing renal dysfunction: IV pyelography, com-

TABLE 17–8

Invasive Diagnostic Procedures for Assessing the Renal System

PROCEDURE	PURPOSE	POTENTIAL PROBLEMS
Intravenous pyelography	To visualize renal parenchyma, calyces, pelves, ureters, and bladder to obtain information regarding size, shape, position, and function of kidneys	Hypersensitivity reaction Acute renal failure Postinjection hematoma
Computerized axial tomography	To visualize renal parenchyma to obtain data regarding size, shape, and presence of lesions, cysts, masses, calculi, obstructions, congenital anomalies, and abnormal accumulations of fluid	Hypersensitivity reactions if a contrast medium is used Postinjection hematoma
Nephrosonography	To visualize renal parenchyma, calyces, pelves, ureters, and bladder to obtain data regarding size, shape, position, and internal structure of kidneys and perirenal tissue; to assess and localize urinary obstructions and abnormal accumulations of fluid	No potential problems currently identified
Nephrotomography	To visualize renal parenchyma, calyces, and pelves in layers to obtain information regarding tumors, cysts, lacerations, or areas of nonperfusion	Hypersensitivity reaction Postinjection hematoma
Renal angiography	To visualize arterial tree, capillaries, and venous drainage of kidneys to obtain data regarding presence of tumors, cysts, stenosis, infarction, aneurysms, hematomas, lacerations, and abscesses	Hypersensitivity reaction Hemorrhage at the catheter insertion site Acute renal failure
Renal scan	To determine renal function by visualizing appearance and disappearance of radioisotopes within kidney; also provides some anatomical information	Hypersensitivity reaction Postinjection hematoma
Renal biopsy	To obtain data for histological diagnosis to determine extent of pathology, appropriate therapy, and possible prognosis	Hemorrhage Postbiopsy hematoma Acute renal failure

puterized axial tomography, nephrosonography, nephrotomography, renal angiography, renal scan, and renal biopsy. Table 17-8 summarizes these diagnostic procedures, including their purposes and potential problems.

NURSING DIAGNOSES

The patient with acute or chronic renal failure experiences systemic manifestations that require nursing support to maintain life. The care that is planned and delivered to these patients is based on a comprehensive assessment of all the ramifications of the renal failure for the patient. In general, the care that is provided is based on the nursing diagnoses summarized in the Clinical Tip: Summary of Nursing Diagnoses Appropriate for Providing Care for Patients With Renal Failure. All the nursing diagnoses, except sexual dysfunction, apply equally to patients with acute or chronic renal failure.

MANAGEMENT THERAPIES

The primary therapeutic intervention for patients experiencing acute or chronic renal failure is renal replacement therapy. In patients with acute renal failure, aggressive renal replacement therapy is usually instituted early in the disease process in an attempt to keep the serum creatinine level at less than 10 mg/100 mL and the BUN at less than 100 mg/dL. The mainte-

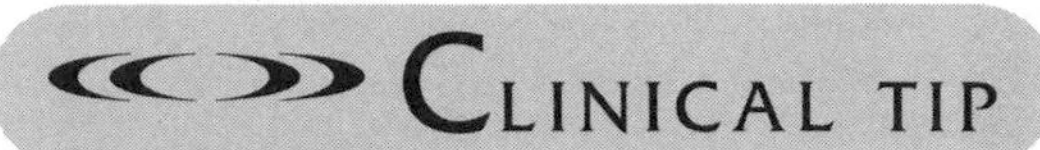

Summary of Nursing Diagnoses Appropriate for Providing Care for Patients With Renal Failure

NURSING DIAGNOSIS	RELATED TO
Alterations in fluid, electrolyte and acid–base balance Examples: • Alteration in potassium balance (hyperkalemia) related to decreased excretion • Fluid volume excess related to inability to excrete fluid • Alteration in acid–base balance (metabolic acidosis) related to retention of acid metabolites	Decreased excretion Catabolism Accumulation due to retention Intracellular–extracellular shifts Extracellular–intracellular shifts Excessive ingestion or administration Systemic effects of uremic toxins
Alterations in cardiac output	Fluid overload and hypertension Electrolyte imbalances Uremic toxins
Potential for infection	Uremic toxins Catabolism
Alterations in coagulation	Uremic toxins
Alterations in breathing patterns	Metabolic acidosis Fluid overload
Alterations in nutrition	Uremic toxins Decomposition of urea in the oral cavity and gastrointestinal tract Electrolyte imbalances Dietary restrictions
Alterations in bowel elimination	Electrolyte imbalances Decreased activity Fluid restrictions Decreased dietary bulk
Impaired physical mobility	Uremic toxins Anemia Electrolyte imbalances
Risk for injury	Uremic toxins Fluid, electrolyte, and acid–base imbalances
Sensory–perceptual alterations	Uremic toxins Uremic encephalopathy Fluid, electrolyte, and acid–base imbalances
Alterations in thought processes	Uremic toxins Uremic encephalopathy Fluid, electrolyte, and acid–base imbalances

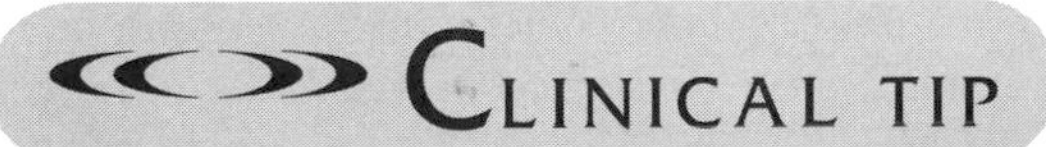

Summary of Nursing Diagnoses Appropriate for Providing Care for Patients With Renal Failure (cont.)

NURSING DIAGNOSIS	RELATED TO
Risk for impaired skin integrity	Uremic toxins Anemia Retained urochrome pigment Decreased sebaceous and sweat gland secretion Calcium phosphate deposition Increased capillary fragility Urea or urate crystal deposition
Altered oral mucous membranes	Uremic toxins Decomposition of urea in oral cavity Hyperosmolality Increased capillary fragility Fluid restrictions
Sexual dysfunction	Uremic toxins
Knowledge deficit	All facets of renal failure and renal replacement therapies

nance of serum values at the lower levels provides an internal biochemical environment that is more conducive to preventing many of the complications that usually accompany uremia. In addition, initiating early dialysis also broadens the scope of other therapeutic interventions that can be used in acute renal failure. The most effective and efficient renal replacement therapy for acute renal failure is hemodialysis. However, when an patient is sufficiently hemodynamically compromised that hemodialysis may pose an additional threat, one of the continuous renal replacement therapies may be instituted. Thus, the patient may receive continuous arteriovenous hemofiltration, continuous arteriovenous hemodialysis, continuous venovenous hemodialysis, or slow continuous ultrafiltration. In such cases, the nursing management of the fluid and electrolyte balances and imbalances becomes even more of a priority.

In patients with chronic renal failure, renal replacement therapies are not instituted until the disease progresses to end-stage level, usually characterized by a urinary creatinine clearance level of less than 5 mL/min. The renal replacement options for chronic renal failure include hemodialysis, continuous ambulatory peritoneal dialysis, and cyclical peritoneal dialysis.

In addition to renal replacement therapy, the patient will require dietary, pharmacologic, and other types of therapeutic support. The specific management therapies that are included in this discussion relate to the alterations in fluid, electrolyte, and acid–base balance.

HYPERVOLEMIA

In the oliguric phase of acute renal failure or the end stage of chronic renal failure, fluids are restricted to an amount sufficient to replace the fluids lost through insensible mechanisms, as well as through the urine. In most instances, the amount is 600 to 1000 mL plus the volume of urine from the previous 24 hrs. If the individual experiences unusual amounts of insensible losses due to hyperventilation or pyrexia, the fluid restriction is increased by an amount often based on changes in body weight.

Patients in the progressive stages of chronic renal failure before end stage, however, will not have fluid restrictions imposed until their creatinine clearance values and urine volumes decrease to levels that can no longer support the homeostasis of the internal environment. Instead, these patients are encouraged to ingest 2 to 3 L/day of fluid to support the fluid volume necessary for excreting waste products as effectively as possible by the remaining intact nephrons.

TOTAL BODY SODIUM EXCESS

Patients in the oliguric phase of acute renal failure and in the end-stage level of chronic renal failure have difficulty maintaining sodium balance and require dietary restrictions. The usual restrictions are 500 mg/day in acute renal failure and 1000 to 2000 mg/day in chronic renal failure. In the diuretic phase of acute renal failure and all other phases of chronic renal failure, the sodium intake must be individualized, usually in accordance with the amount excreted in the urine.

HYPERKALEMIA

Management of hyperkalemia is a primary therapeutic goal for patients with either acute or chronic renal failure. In oliguric acute renal failure and end-stage chronic renal failure, dietary restrictions are necessary. The usual dietary restriction is 40 mEq/day. (In contrast, a healthy adult typically consumes 50–100 mEq of potassium in the diet.) If the patient is severely catabolic, additional restrictions may be required. Table 17-9 summarizes the various therapeutic approaches, specific methods, and their efficacy in treating hyperkalemia. In general, the approaches that attempt to antagonize the membrane effect of hyperkalemia and shift the potassium intracellularly are used primarily as emergency measures.

When implementing measures to decrease both the total body and serum potassium levels, the clinician should (1) discourage the patient from using salt substitutes that are potassium-based; (2) avoid administering pharmacologic agents that contain potassium; and (3) avoid administering pharmacologic agents that are likely to exacerbate the potassium imbalance. Such pharmacologic agents include potassium-sparing diuretics, beta-adrenergic antagonists, and nonsteroidal antiinflammatory agents. In addition, recall the following facts regarding the use of the cation exchange resin Kayexalate: (1) sodium ions are exchanged for potassium ions in the intestine; thus, sodium is reabsorbed and potassium is excreted in the feces; (2) the exchange process is slow and requires hours and several repeated administrations to be maximally effective; (3) the exchange resin was designed to be given orally to maximize its contact with the surface area of the GI tract, but because many patients cannot ingest it orally due to nausea and regurgitation, it may be given rectally as a retention enema; (4) when the resin is administered as a retention enema it must be retained at least 20 to 30 min to be effective; (5) approximately 1 mEq of potassium is exchanged per gram of resin; and (6) the resin is usually mixed with a sorbitol solution to promote an osmotic diarrhea to facilitate excretory processes and prevent constipation.

HYPERCHLOREMIA

In most patients with renal failure, the chloride imbalance is clinically insignificant. If it is a problem, however, it is usually managed by dietary salt restriction, avoiding the administration of chloride-containing pharmacologic agents, and administering exogenous bicarbonate.

HYPOCALCEMIA

Therapeutic management of hypocalcemia that accompanies both acute and chronic renal failure requires a combined approach aimed at replacing the deficient calcium, controlling the excess phosphate, and slowly correcting the acid–base imbalance. The first component of this combined approach will be discussed here and the other components as the specific imbalances are addressed. Usually, pharmacologic replacement of 1 to 2 g/day of elemental calcium orally is sufficient to replace the deficit, particularly if it is augmented by the administration of 1,25-dihydroxycholecalciferol. The calcium replacement can take many forms, ranging from calcium carbonate to calcium gluconate or calcium gluceptate.

TABLE 17–9

Treatment Approaches for Hyperkalemia

APPROACH	METHODS	EFFICACY
Reduce the body potassium content	1. Decrease potassium intake to 40 mEq daily	May decrease plasma and total body potassium content over time
	2. Increase the fecal excretion of potassium using cation exchange resins such as Kayexelate 20 gm with 50 ml of 20% sorbitol orally	Takes 1–2 hours to be effective but will eventually decrease both plasma and total body potassium content; duration is 4–6 hours
	3. Increase the renal excretion of potassium by using mineralocorticoid agents (Fludrocortisone 0.1–0.2 mg), increasing salt intake, or using diuretic agents (furosemide 40–60 mg IV or PO)	Any of these would be effective in decreasing both plasma and total body potassium content if the individual has normal renal function—in renal failure they may have limited utility
	4. Dialysis	Decreases both plasma and total body potassium content within a 4- to 6-hour time frame
Shift the potassium intracellularly	1. Administer glucose 50 g and regular insulin 10 U intravenously	Decreases plasma potassium for about 2–4 hours, but has no effect on total body potassium content
	2. Administer an alkali such as sodium bicarbonate	Decreases plasma potassium for about 1 hour or less but has no effect on total body potassium content
	3. Administer albuterol sulfate 0.5 mg IV or 20 mg dissolved in 4 mL of saline and inhaled over 10 minutes	Decreases plasma potassium for 2–4 hours but has no effect on total body potassium content
Antagonize the membrane effect	1. Administer calcium salts (calcium gluconate 10 mL of a 10% solution at 2 mL/min)	Has no effect on either plasma or total body potassium content
	2. Administer hypertonic sodium salts	Has no effect on either plasma or total body potassium content

HYPERPHOSPHATEMIA

Hyperphosphatemia is an imbalance that occurs in patients with either acute or chronic renal failure. It is usually managed by restricting dietary intake and administering pharmacologic phosphate-binding agents. The dietary restriction is usually accomplished by limiting the daily phosphate intake to less than 700 mg and the daily protein intake to about 1 g/kg. Unfortunately, the dietary restrictions are often difficult to implement, and therefore the patient may not achieve the desired reduction in phosphate level by using dietary restrictions alone. Consequently, phosphate-binding agents, such as aluminum hydroxide gels or calcium-based antacids, are administered concurrently. These agents, usually administered within 20 min of meals, supply cations to the intestinal lumen that bind with the phosphate that is present to form an insoluble complex that is excreted in the feces. Use of these agents frequently results in constipation for the patient, and the aluminum-based binders may produce sufficiently high serum aluminum levels to interfere with bone mineralization.

HYPERMAGNESEMIA

Clinically insignificant elevations of serum magnesium levels are the norm in both acute and chronic renal failure. In most patients, dietary restrictions and avoiding pharmacologic agents that contain magnesium are adequate measures to prevent the retention of excessive amounts of magnesium. For patients who do experience clinically significant elevations of serum magnesium levels, dialysis is usually the therapeutic intervention of choice.

METABOLIC ACIDOSIS

The metabolic acidosis that accompanies oliguric acute renal failure usually develops rapidly, is severe, and necessitates early initiation of therapeutic measures. In fact, the daily acid production during catabolic oliguric acute renal failure may decrease the serum bicarbonate level by more than 15 mEq/L. Thus, replacement therapy is frequently a high therapeutic priority and is usually accomplished by sodium bicarbonate administration. In addition, because the metabolism of ingested exogenous protein will produce approximately 1 mEq/g of nonvolatile acid, dietary protein is usually restricted. Table 17-10 summarizes the general daily dietary restrictions and requirements for patients experiencing renal failure. These amounts are always adjusted upward or downward in accordance with the patient's specific physiological needs.

Patients with end-stage chronic renal failure usually experience approximately a 2 mEq/L/day decrease in serum bicarbonate. Therefore, they also require replacement therapy, often in the form of either sodium bicarbonate or sodium citrate and dietary protein restrictions. In addition, the management of metabolic acidosis in either acute or chronic renal failure also encompasses the following: (1) minimizing all catabolic processes, including infections and GI bleeding; (2) rapidly correcting any diarrhea that occurs; and (3) avoiding catabolic pharmacologic agents, such as corticosteroids.

The clinician should monitor the patient frequently for other fluid and electrolyte imbalances that might occur as a result of the therapeutic management of metabolic acidosis. The primary possibilities include hypervolemia, hypernatremia, more clinically significant hypocalcemia, an exaggerated hyperphosphatemia, and transient hypokalemia. With the exception of hypocalcemia, these imbalances are not usually clinically significant in most patients. The patient may, however, require additional IV or oral calcium supplement to manage the tetany and neuromuscular effects of the rapidly induced exaggerated hypocalcemia resulting from the overcorrection of the metabolic acidosis to an alkalotic state.

TABLE 17–10

Daily Dietary Requirements and Restrictions in Renal Failure

DIETARY COMPONENT*	DAILY AMOUNT IN ACUTE RENAL FAILURE	DAILY AMOUNT IN CHRONIC RENAL FAILURE
Water	400–600 mL plus the urine output	1000 mL or 600 mL plus the urine output
Calories	35–50 kcal/kg	35–50 kcal/kg
Protein	0.5–1.5 g/kg	1–1.2 g/kg
Sodium	500–1000 mg	2 g
Potassium	20–50 mEq	40–60 mEq
Phosphate	700 mg or less	700 mg or less
Calcium	800–1200 mg	1000–1200 mg
Carbohydrate	Unrestricted	Unrestricted
Fats	Variable	Variable

* Daily water-soluble vitamin supplements are also required in both acute and chronic renal failure.

Overall, it is clear that the patient who experiences either acute or chronic renal failure is in a very compromised state. Not only does the patient lack the ability to maintain a homeostatic internal environment compatible with life, but he or she also exhibits the clinical effects of the renal failure on all other body systems. Thus, many of the normal adaptive mechanisms are also dysfunctional. The result is a patient in jeopardy who must rely on external management therapies to sustain life. Such patients challenge clinicians not only to provide these therapeutic interventions competently and effectively, but also to anticipate and prevent other potential threats. This challenge demands that clinicians use their vast stores of intellectual resources to provide the requisite quality nursing care. It is hoped that this discussion has expanded those intellectual resources and increased the clinician's ability to meet the challenge presented by patients experiencing either acute or chronic renal failure.

CASE STUDIES

17-1. A 65-year-old man is admitted with a history of glomerulonephritis and a rising serum creatinine level over the past 2 months. Laboratory data include the following:

Total serum calcium = 6.0 mg/dL
Serum albumin = 1.5 g/dL
Serum creatinine = 6.0 mg/dL
Serum phosphate = 8.0 mg/dL

COMMENTARY Recall that approximately 0.8 mg of calcium binds to 1 g of albumin; therefore, a decrease in the serum albumin will result in a decrease in the total serum calcium level without affecting the ionized calcium level. The estimated corrected serum calcium level (accounting for the abnormal serum albumin level) can be obtained by subtracting the measured albumin level from the serum albumin's lower limit of normal

Corrected serum Ca = (3.5 − serum albumin) × 0.8 + serum calcium

Corrected serum Ca = (3.5 − 1.5) × 0.8 + 6.0 = 7.6 mg/dL

This is only an estimation as other factors (such as serum pH) can affect calcium ionization. It is better to obtain an ionized serum calcium level for a more accurate assessment of calcium stores.

It is thought that hyperphosphatemia associated with chronic renal failure (present in this patient) causes a reciprocal drop in the serum calcium concentration. Also, GI absorption of calcium is decreased in renal failure. The nephrotic syndrome itself may cause hypocalcemia because of loss of vitamin D-binding proteins in the urine.

17-2. A 25-year-old woman with a 10-year history of progressive renal failure has been admitted with mild hypertension. Laboratory data include:

Serum sodium = 139 mEq/L
Serum potassium = 5.9 mEq/L
Serum chloride = 105 mEq/L
Serum bicarbonate = 14 mEq/L
BUN = 80 mg/dL

COMMENTARY The low bicarbonate level indicates metabolic acidosis (the expected acid–base imbalance in a patient with chronic renal failure). In renal insufficiency, metabolic acidosis is due to the kidneys' inability to excrete the daily hydrogen load.

The anion gap (AG) is calculated by subtracting the sum of the serum bicarbonate and chloride levels from the serum sodium level.

$AG = Na - (HCO_3 + Cl)$

$AG = 139 - (14 + 105) = 20$ mEq/L

(Note that this is above the normally accepted range of approximately 12–15 mEq/L.) This is a high AG metabolic acidosis, indicating the retention of uremic toxins.

The patient's serum potassium level is above normal because renal failure causes poor renal excretion of potassium and metabolic acidosis favors shifting of cellular potassium into the plasma.

Oral bicarbonate replacement will likely keep the serum bicarbonate level at more than 15 to 18 mEq/L. Attention is given to avoiding overcorrection of the low serum bicarbonate level because alkalosis favors decreased calcium ionization. Of course, because hypocalcemia is a chronic problem in renal patients, it is important to avoid exacerbating symptoms by overcorrection of the metabolic acidosis.

BIBLIOGRAPHY

Allon M: Treatment and prevention of hyperkalemia in end-stage renal disease. Kidney Intern 43:1197–1209,1993

Baer CL: Acute renal failure. In: Kinney M, Packa D, Dunbar S (eds): AACN's Clinical Reference for Critical-Care Nursing, 3rd ed, pp 885–901, New York, McGraw-Hill, 1993

Baer CL: Acute renal failure. In: Hartshorn J, Lamborn M, Noll ML (eds): Introduction to Critical Care. Philadelphia, WB Saunders, 1993

Baer CL: Acute renal failure. Nursing 90 20(6):34–39, 1990

Baer CL: Regulation and assessment of fluid and electrolyte balance. In: Kinney M, Packa D, Dunbar S (eds): AACN's Clinical Reference for Critical Care Nursing, 3rd ed, pp 173–208, New York, McGraw-Hill, 1993

Baer CL: Regulation and assessment of acid–base balance. Ibid, pp 209–216

Baer CL: Renal Data Acquisition. Ibid, pp 873–883

Bergstrom J: Toxicity of uremia: physiopathology and clinical signs. Contrib Nephrol 71:1–9,1989

Brenner BM, Coe FL, Rector FC: Clinical Nephrology. Philadelphia, WB Saunders, 1987

Brenner BM, Lazarus JM: Acute Renal Failure. Philadelphia, WB Saunders, 1983

Butler BA: Nutritional management of catabolic acute renal failure requiring renal replacement therapy. ANNA J 18(3):247–254,257–259,1991

Eknoyan G, Knochel JP: The Systemic Consequences of Renal Failure. Orlando, FL, Grune & Stratton, 1984

Finn WF: Diagnosis and management of acute tubular necrosis. Med Clin North Am 74(4):873–891,1990

Franklin S, Klein K: Acute renal failure: Fluid and electrolyte and acid–base complications. In: Narin RG (ed): Maxwell & Kleeman's Clinical Disorders of Fluid and Electrolyte Metabolism, 5th ed, pp 1175–1194, New York, McGraw-Hill, 1994

Harper J: Rhabdomyolysis and myoglobinuric renal failure. Crit Care Nurse 10(3): 32–34,36,1990

Henry J: Clinical Diagnosis and Management by Laboratory Methods, 18th ed, p 130. Philadelphia, W.B. Saunders, 1991

Kee CC: Age-related changes in the renal system: causes, consequences and nursing implications. Geriatric Nursing 13(2):80–83,1992

Kupin WL, Narins G: The hyperkalemia of renal failure: pathophysiology, diagnosis and therapy. Contrib Nephrol 102:1–22,1993

Lancaster LE: Renal response to shock. Crit Care Clin North Am 2(2):221–233,1990

Lancaster LE: The Patient With End Stage Renal Disease, 2nd ed. New York, John Wiley & Sons, 1985

Lancaster LE, Baer CL: The pathophysiology of acute renal dysfunction. In: Schoengrund L, Balzer P (eds): Renal Problems in Critical Care, pp 21–46. New York, John Wiley & Sons, 1985

Lievaart A, Voerman HJ: Nursing management of continuous arteriovenous hemodialysis. Heart Lung 20(2):152–158, 1991

Mehta R: Therapeutic alternatives to renal replacement for critically ill patients in acute renal failure. Sem Nephrol 14(1):64–82, 1994

Mitch WE, Klahr S: Nutrition and the Kidney. Boston, Little, Brown, 1988

Porush JG: New concepts in acute renal failure. Am Fam Physician 33(3):109–118,1986

Price CA: Continuous renal replacement therapy: The treatment of choice for acute renal failure. ANNA J 18(3):239–244,1991

Schoengrund L: Nursing management of the patient with acute renal failure. In: Schoengrund L, Balzer P (eds): Renal Problems in Critical Care, pp 47–67. New York, John Wiley & Sons, 1985

Schrier RW: Renal and Electrolyte Disorders, 3rd ed. Boston, Little, Brown, 1986

Shenker D: Metabolic problems in acute renal failure and their treatment. Top Emerg Med 14(1):72–77, 1992

Strohschein BL, Caruso DM, Greene KA: Continuous venovenous hemodialysis. Am J Crit Care 3(2):92–99, 1994

Strupp TW: Post shock resuscitation of the trauma victim: Preventing and managing acute renal failure. Crit Care Nurs Quart 11(2):1–9,1988

Toto KH: Acute renal failure: A question of location. Am J Nurs 92(11):44–53,1992

Tuso PJ, Nissenson AR, Danovitch GM: Electrolyte disorders in chronic renal failure. In: Narin RG (ed): Maxwell & Kleeman's Clinical Disorders of Fluid and Electrolyte Metabolism, 5th ed, pp 1195–1211. New York, McGraw-Hill, 1994

Wilkins RG, Faragher EB: Acute renal failure in an intensive care unit: incidence, prediction, and outcome. Anaesthesia 7:628–624,1983

Wills MR: Effects of renal failure. Clin Biochem 23:55–60,1990

Wolfson M: Nutritional support in acute renal failure. Dial Transplant 16:493,496,1987

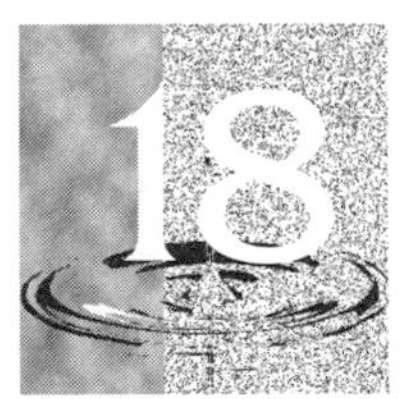

Diabetic Ketoacidosis and Hyperosmolar Syndrome

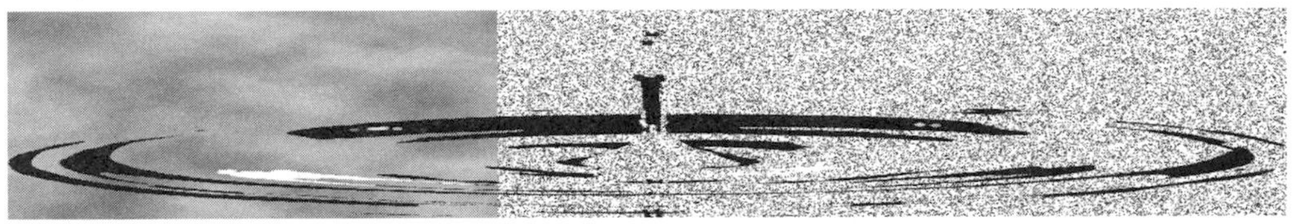

A relative or absolute insulin deficiency can result in severe hyperglycemia, which in turn leads either to diabetic ketoacidosis (DKA) or hyperosmolar hyperglycemic nonketotic syndrome (HHNS), depending on which type of diabetes mellitus is present. Diabetic ketoacidosis and HHNS can be viewed as opposite ends on the spectrum of metabolic derangements, and episodes of DKA and HHNS occurring simultaneously, rather than alone, have been reported.[1]

Type I, insulin-dependent diabetes mellitus (IDDM), can develop at any age, although most cases are diagnosed before age 30.[2] Persons with type I diabetes mellitus are insulinopenic and require exogenous insulin to prevent ketoacidosis and sustain life. An absolute deficiency of insulin, resulting from destruction of pancreatic beta cells, predisposes type I diabetics to ketosis. In 20% to 30% of cases, DKA may be the first manifestation of diabetes and is responsible for 2% to 14% of all hospitalizations attributable to diabetes.[3] Diabetic ketoacidosis is life-threatening and, despite treatment advances, mortality rates remain between 1% and 10%, depending on treatment circumstances and locale.[4]

Type II, noninsulin-dependent diabetes mellitus (NIDDM), usually begins in middle or later adulthood, is typically diagnosed after age 30, and accounts for approximately 90% of the known diabetic cases in the United States.[5] Persons with type II diabetes mellitus may have decreased, normal, or even increased serum insulin levels. The metabolic problems associated with type II diabetes mellitus are believed to result from peripheral insulin resistance, with decreased tissue sensitivity or responsiveness to exogenous or endogenous insulin.[6] Approximately 80% of type II diabetics are obese,[7] and many can be managed by dietary and weight control measures. In some cases, oral medications are required. Table 18-1 lists the oral medications currently used in the management of type II diabetes mellitus.

A percentage of type II diabetics may require some exogenous insulin for proper blood glucose control, at least initially or during times of stress (such as illness or surgery).[8] Persons with NIDDM are not as prone to ketosis; instead, they are at risk for HHNS when their hyperglycemia is severe, although in very rare cases, decompensated NIDDM can result in DKA.[9]

It is not fully understood why these individuals are ketosis-resistant. Although HHNS occurs less frequently than DKA, it is on the increase because of the rising population of elderly adults who have type II diabetes mellitus. It is a serious complication of many types of medical and surgical therapies in the elderly diabetic and has a higher mortality rate than DKA.[10]

Use of the term "coma" for these conditions is somewhat misleading because only a small percentage of patients are actually comatose when treatment is initiated.[11] However, both DKA and HHNS cause severe derangements of fluid and electrolyte balances, affecting almost all systems of the body; these emergency situations require expert and prompt intervention.

DIABETIC KETOACIDOSIS

HYPERGLYCEMIA AND HYPEROSMOLALITY

Diabetic ketoacidosis results from profound insulin deficiency and the effects of the counterregulatory hormones: glucagon, catecholamines, cortisol, and growth hormone. Underuse of glucose (most cells are relatively impermeable to glucose in the absence of insulin), excessive production of glucose from fats and amino acids by the liver (gluconeogenesis), and excessive production of glucose from glycogen (glycogenolysis) all lead to hyperglycemia. Glucagon appears to be the primary hormone responsible for stimulation of hepatic gluconeogenesis and the direct activation of glycogen breakdown.[12] Because of these processes, the blood glucose concentration rises markedly and increases plasma osmolality.

The following formula is used to calculate plasma osmolality, the normal range of which is 280 to 300 mOsm/L:

$$\begin{aligned} \text{pOsm} &= 2(\text{Na} + \text{K}) + \text{G}/18 + \text{BUN}/2.8 \\ &= 280\text{–}300 \text{ mOsm/kg} \end{aligned}$$

In the following example it is possible to see how hyperglycemia increases plasma osmolality:

Example: Patient with hyperglycemia:

Na^+	=	139 mEq/L
K^+	=	4 mEq/L
Serum glucose	=	1800 mg/dL
BUN	=	30 mg/dL
pOsm	=	2(139 + 4) + 1800/18 + 30/2.8
	=	397 mOsm/kg

TABLE 18–1

Oral Medications Used in Management of Type II Diabetes

GENERIC NAME	BRAND NAME	CLASSIFICATION
Tolbutamide	Orinase	First-generation sulfonylurea
Chlorpropamide	Diabenese	First-generation sulfonylurea
Acetohexamide	Dymelor	First-generation sulfonylurea
Tolazamide	Tolinase	First-generation sulfonylurea
Glyburide	DiaBeta Micronase Glynase Prestabs	Second-generation sulfonylurea*
Glipizide	Glucotrol Glucotrol XL	Second-generation sulfonylurea*
Metformin	Glucophage	Biguanide**

* Second generation agents are typically the medications of choice as they have fewer side effects, drug interactions, and alternate routes of excretion.

** Metformin was approved for use in the treatment of diabetes mellitus in 1995. It is an antihyperglycemic agent which increases glucose uptake in peripheral tissues.

This elevated osmolality of extracellular fluid (ECF) produces cellular dehydration as water shifts from the cells to the ECF.

Other researchers use the following formula (omitting the urea component) to calculate the effective osmolality, because urea diffuses freely across cell membranes and does not create an osmotic gradient between the intracellular and extracellular spaces:

$$\text{Effective pOsm} = 2(\text{Na} + \text{K}) + \text{Serum glucose}/18$$

These investigators reason that this equation can calculate a more clinically relevant value.[13–15]

OSMOTIC DIURESIS AND FLUID VOLUME DEFICIT

When the blood glucose level exceeds the renal threshold (normal, 180 mg/dL), glucose spills into the urine, taking water and electrolytes with it and increasing urine volume. Specific gravity (SG) of the urine is elevated due to the high glucose content. The polyuria eventually leads to fluid volume deficit (FVD). As the FVD worsens, glomerular filtration rate (GFR) decreases, as does renal blood flow, causing the patient to become oliguric or even anuric in spite of marked hyperglycemia. This FVD presents a danger of potential renal tubular damage with its resultant acute renal failure.

ELECTROLYTES

Potassium

Probably the most important electrolyte disturbance that occurs in DKA is the marked deficit in total body potassium. Causes of potassium depletion include:

1. Starvation effect with lean tissue breakdown
2. Depletion of tissue glycogen stores (potassium is normally deposited in the cells with glycogen)
3. Loss of intracellular potassium
4. Potassium-losing effect of aldosterone (aldosterone is stimulated by FVD)
5. Loss of potassium with osmotic diuresis
6. Severe anorexia (reducing intake) and vomiting (increasing loss of potassium)

Before treatment, the patient with DKA may have a normal or elevated serum potassium level, although there is a marked deficit of total body potassium. Factors that tend to elevate the serum potassium level in the untreated patient include:

- Plasma volume contraction with oliguria, which interferes with renal excretion of potassium.
- Metabolic acidosis (potassium shifts out of the cells into the extracellular compartment as hydrogen is buffered intracellularly).

This hyperkalemia is quickly alleviated by fluid replacement therapy and reestablishment of urine output. After treatment is begun, the serum potassium level decreases rapidly and usually reaches its lowest point within 1 to 4 hrs. Reasons for the decreased serum potassium level at this time include:

- Dilution by the intravenous (IV) fluids.
- Increased urinary potassium excretion due to plasma volume expansion.
- Formation of glycogen within the cells using potassium, glucose, and water from the ECF (a shift of potassium into the cells).
- Correction of acidosis with reentry of potassium into the cells.

Because insulin tends to lower serum potassium levels by enhancing its movement back into cells, it is believed that use of low-dose insulin therapy in the management of DKA is less likely to be associated with rapid decreases in serum potassium than is the use of high-dose insulin therapy.

Phosphorus

Hypophosphatemia almost invariably occurs during treatment in the patient with DKA, and for many of the same reasons that hypokalemia occurs. (Recall that both imbalances involve primarily cellular electrolytes.) One potentially serious consequence of phosphorus deficiency is decreased erythrocyte 2,3-DPG (diphosphoglycerate); a low level of 2,3-DPG may result in decreased peripheral oxygen delivery. Decreased myocardial function has also been observed when the serum phosphate concentration is less than 2 mg/dL.[16] When the serum phosphate concentration decreases to less than 0.5 mg/dL, serious disturbances in metabolism and neurologic abnormalities (both central and peripheral) may result; seizures, respiratory failure, impaired leukocyte and platelet function, abnormal skeletal muscle function, and gastrointestinal bleeding have been reported.[17]

Sodium

Plasma sodium concentration is usually below normal; this is partly due to hyperosmolality of the ECF. Accumulation of glucose in the ECF creates an osmotic gradient, causing water to be pulled out of the cells into the ECF and resulting in dilution of the plasma sodium level. If vomiting is present, the hyponatremia becomes more severe. Sodium also moves into the cells as they become depleted of potassium, further lowering the plasma sodium level.

KETOSIS

Insulin deficiency allows greater release of free fatty acids (FFA) from peripheral fat stores and activates ketogenic pathways in the liver; the excess fatty acids are converted by the liver to ketones, resulting in ketosis. The insulin deficiency also interferes with uptake of the ketones by peripheral tissues, further increasing the buildup of ketones in the bloodstream. The ketones (ketoacids) present in DKA are beta hydroxybutyrate and acetoacetate. Because ketones are strong acids, with one hydrogen ion created with each ion of beta hydroxybutyrate and acetoacetate, this overproduction and impaired metabolism soon overload the body's buffers, resulting in metabolic acidosis.[18] The anionic charge of bicarbonate is replaced by the negatively charged ketones.

The type of metabolic acidosis that occurs in DKA is manifested by a decrease in bicarbonate with a reciprocal increase in the anion gap (AG) as large amounts of unmeasured anions are produced. Calculate AG using the following formula:

$$\begin{aligned} AG &= Na^{+} - (HCO_3^{-} + Cl^{-}) \\ &= 12 - 15 \text{ mEq/L} \end{aligned}$$

Example: Patient with ketoacidosis:

$$\begin{aligned} Na^{+} &= 131 \text{ mEq/L} \\ Cl^{-} &= 95 \text{ mEq/L} \\ HCO_3^{-} &= 5 \text{ mEq/L} \\ AG &= 131 - (5 + 95) = 31 \text{ mEq/L} \end{aligned}$$

Calculation of AG is important in the assessment of acid–base disturbances in DKA because other findings may be misleading. For example, the vomiting that frequently accompanies DKA can superimpose a metabolic alkalosis on the preexisting ketoacidosis, making the plasma pH appear nearly normal. Measurement of AG will reveal the abnormal levels of ketone ions that are disrupting metabolism.

Excessive ketosis leads to ketonuria and even excretion of volatile acetone from the lungs (resulting in the classic "fruity" odor of the breath associated with DKA). It is not unusual for the plasma pH to drop to 7.25 or below and for the bicarbonate level to drop to 12 mEq/L or less. Possibly the greatest risks of prolonged uncorrected acidosis are decreased cardiac function, arrhythmia, and impaired hepatic handling of lactate.[19]

The body attempts to compensate for the metabolic acidosis associated with DKA by means of the kidneys and lungs. The kidneys eliminate hydrogen ions and conserve bicarbonate ions, resulting in decreased urinary pH. The lungs attempt to lighten the acid load by blowing off extra carbon dioxide, resulting in the deep, rapid breathing known as Kussmaul respiration. The expected decrease in arterial carbon dioxide pressure ($PaCO_2$) to compensate for metabolic acidosis can be calculated by the following formula:

$$\text{Expected } PaCO_2 \text{ (mmHg)} = 1.5\,(HCO_3) + 8 \pm 2$$

Example: The expected $PaCO_2$ in a patient with a bicarbonate level of 12 mEq/L would be between 24 and 28 mmHg:

$$PaCO_2 = 1.5\,(12) + 8 \pm 2 = 24\text{–}28 \text{ mmHg}$$

A decrease below the calculated amount indicates a superimposed respiratory alkalosis; failure of the $PaCO_2$ to decrease to the expected level indicates a complicating respiratory acidosis (a dangerous combination).

HYPEROSMOLAR HYPERGLYCEMIC NONKETOTIC SYNDROME

Hyperosmolar hyperglycemic nonketotic syndrome is a disorder that develops in middle-aged or elderly type II diabetics (sometimes not yet diagnosed), often as a result of stress caused by physical impairment such as renal or cardiovascular disease, infections, or effects of pharmacological therapy with drugs such as steroids or diuretics. Too rapid introduction of total parenteral nutrition (TPN) may also precipitate HHNS (see Chapter 11).[20] The condition develops more slowly than DKA; it is not uncommon for patients to experience polyuria, polydipsia, weight loss, and weakness for days and even weeks before seeking medical attention. Impaired thirst mechanism or impaired ability to replace fluids will exacerbate the tendency toward HHNS. Hyperglycemia may be extreme (>600 mg/dL and generally between 1000 and 2000 mg/dL), but without the ketosis of DKA.[21–23] The plasma pH is usually normal or only slightly low. The absence of ketoacidosis was formerly attributed to the higher residual insulin levels in these patients, but this explanation is no longer considered entirely adequate.[24,25]

Fluid volume deficit is profound in HHNS and may be life-threatening. Some sources report mortality rates as high as 50%, depending on the severity of the hyperosmolality and the occurrence of sequelae such as thromboembolic and respiratory complications.[26] Death from HHNS is associated with factors such as advanced age (>70 years), nursing home residency, hyperosmolality, and hypernatremia.[27]

Although there is a deficit of total body sodium, the serum sodium level may be normal or elevated because of a relatively greater loss of water. The plasma bicarbonate level is normal or slightly reduced. The BUN is usually more elevated than in DKA (60–90 mg/dL) and reflects the more severe FVD and the catabolic state. The serum creatinine is often elevated in HHNS, reflecting the common association of HHNS with underlying renal impairment. Potassium and phosphate depletion may occur, as they do in DKA.

RULING OUT HYPOGLYCEMIA AND OTHER CAUSES OF COMA

Hypoglycemia can often be seen in the individual treated with oral hypoglycemic agents as well as the insulin-requiring diabetic, and occurs as a result of a mismatch of nutrient intake, activity level, and insulin timing. Characteristically, signs and symptoms of hypoglycemia can be divided into two major categories, adrenergic and neuroglycopenic. The adrenergic symptoms are related to increasing epinephrine levels. The neuroglycopenic symptoms are associated with a lack of glucose availability to the brain with resultant cerebral dysfunction.[28]

Hypoglycemia can be divided into three levels: mild, moderate, and severe. Mild hypoglycemia is characterized by the presence of adrenergic symptoms such as tremors, palpitations, sweating, and excessive hunger. Moderate hypoglycemia is characterized by neuroglycopenic symptoms as well as some autonomic symptoms such as headache, mood changes, irritability, decreased attention, and drowsiness. Severe hypoglycemia is characterized by unresponsiveness, unconsciousness, or convulsions and always requires the assistance of another person for treatment.[29] With the advent of intensive therapy for the treatment of diabetes and prevention of the chronic complications, a two- to threefold increase in severe hypoglycemia has been seen.[30] Thus, the incidence of severe hypoglycemia occurring in the home setting or community may increase as more patients are practicing intensive therapy for glucose management.

In treating an unconscious diabetic patient, it should be determined whether hyperglycemia or hypoglycemia exists. When in doubt, in a hospital setting, an emergency room, or an environment with paramedical assistance it is best that IV glucose in the dose of 25 g be administered (one ampule of $D_{50}W$).[31] Outside of the hospital setting or when IV access is unavailable a 1-mg intramuscular injection of glucagon is the treatment of choice, although it has a slightly slower and less predictable recovery rate than IV glucose.[32] With either treatment, if hypoglycemia is the problem, the patient's condition will improve quickly; if DKA or HHNS is the problem, the small amount of dextrose or the mobilization of hepatic glycogen stores by glucagon will do no harm. Of course, a blood glucose determination should be made as quickly as possible.

Serum glucose measurement is an important first step in the evaluation of the diabetic patient with altered consciousness. A finding of hypoglycemia or hyperglycemia, however, may not fully explain the cause of the altered consciousness or coma. A thorough evaluation is needed so that other pathology, such as stroke, uremia, or drug intoxication, does not go untreated. Conversely, the signs and symptoms of hypoglycemia or hyperglycemia may mimic other conditions; for example, abdominal pain in patients with DKA may simulate an abdominal emergency. For this reason, even when there is no history of diabetes, serum glucose should be measured promptly in acutely ill patients. Recall that DKA or HHNS may be the first manifestation of diabetes in some individuals. Patients with alcoholic ketoacidosis may also occasionally have some degree of hyperglycemia, making differential diagnosis problematic.[33]

TREATMENT OF DKA AND HHNS

FLUID REPLACEMENT

Adequate and prompt rehydration is vital and must consider the patient's cardiovascular and renal status. Fluid replacement is usually begun with the administration of 1 to 3 L of isotonic saline (0.9% NaCl) infused at the rate of approximately 1 L/hr. Isotonic (normal) saline will expand the ECF and will begin to correct the hyperosmolality. In some cases of HHNS in which there is significant hypernatremia, hypertension, or risk for congestive heart failure, half-strength saline (0.45% NaCl) may be used. When there is a concern about the adequacy of the patient's cardiovascular status, central venous pressure or hemodynamic monitoring may be needed to help gauge the best rate of fluid replacement. Total fluid intake in 8 hrs should not exceed 5 L.[34]

After the initial infusion of normal saline, the IV fluid may be changed to half-strength saline to dilute the hyperosmolar plasma and provide free water for renal excretion. As fluid replacement continues, the rate and volume will be determined by the status of the patient. Patients with HHNS may need larger amounts of fluids to correct the FVD. When the plasma glucose levels decrease to the 250 to 300 mg/dL range, solutions containing 5% dextrose should be used to prevent hypoglycemia and other complications that might occur as a result of a too rapid fall in blood glucose level. As soon as oral intake is adequate, IV fluids can be discontinued.

INSULIN ADMINISTRATION

The aim of insulin therapy is to give enough rapid-acting (regular) insulin to correct the problem without subjecting the patient to the risk of hypoglycemia.

Regular insulin, which is a clear preparation, is the only insulin that may be used IV. Although it can also be given intramuscularly (IM) or subcutaneously (SQ), the continuous IV route is best for the very ill patient because absorption of insulin from poorly perfused muscle and fat depots may be erratic, especially if the patient is hypotensive.

Studies have demonstrated that large insulin doses are generally no more effective in correcting DKA than small doses. The low-dose regimen has been shown to lower blood sugar concentrations smoothly, improve ketosis, and repair acidosis at rates indistinguishable from those obtained by higher dose regimens. In addition, patients are less likely to develop hypoglycemia and hypokalemia than are patients receiving large doses.[35] Of course, when low doses do not achieve the desired effect, as in cases of insulin "resistance," larger doses must be given. Patients with HHNS will require somewhat less insulin than those with DKA.

The insulin dose for continuous IV infusion is usually 4 to 10 U/hr or 0.1 U/kg/hr. Sometimes an initial bolus of 5 to 10 units is given when therapy is initiated, although some studies have not documented any benefits from such a bolus.[36,37] The adsorption of insulin to IV containers and tubing has been documented, but there is disagreement about the extent to which it affects insulin delivery, particularly in low-dose therapy. To minimize the effect of adsorption, the infusion set should be flushed with the insulin solution to saturate the binding sites before connecting it to the patient. According to Peterson et al.,[38] the insulin-binding effect will be minimal if the solution contains a concentration of at least 25 units of insulin to 500 mL of saline, and 50 mL of the solution are flushed through the entire apparatus before patient infusion.

Of primary importance is the individualization of the dosage of insulin to the response of the patient, and adjustment of that dosage on the basis of ongoing blood glucose determinations. A too rapid drop in blood glucose level creates the risk of complications such as hypoglycemia and hypokalemia. There is also a risk that cerebral edema may occur from the osmotic gradient created between brain and serum osmolality by a too rapid decline in blood glucose concentration.[39] Although cerebral edema is an uncommon occurrence in adults, it can be fatal in children or lead to developmental disabilities for years after resolution of the DKA episode.[40] A controlled-rate infusion pump should be used to ensure accurate administration of the insulin. If one is not available, the solutions should be administered through a volume-controlled administration set. When the patient's condition is sufficiently stabilized, the insulin can be administered subcutaneously.

ELECTROLYTE REPLACEMENT

Potassium

Potassium is not added to the IV fluids until the first 2 or 3 L have been administered and adequate urinary output has been established, unless serum potassium levels have already decreased to normal or below. Potassium replacement is usually accomplished by adding 20 to 40 mEq of potassium to 1 L of half-normal saline (0.45% NaCl), infused at a rate appropriate to the status of the patient. Occasionally, larger amounts of potassium are needed if the hypokalemia is severe. Because the IV administration of potassium is always associated with risk of hyperkalemia, it is wise to monitor the serum potassium level at 1- or 2-hr intervals and to use serial electrocardiogram (ECG) tracings. (Rules for safe potassium administration are discussed in Chapter 5, Clinical Tip: Nursing Considerations in Administering Potassium Intravenously.) Oral potassium-containing fluids may be given when the patient is able to tolerate them.

Phosphorus

Because phosphate is lost during the osmotic diuresis of DKA and HHNS, some authorities favor replacing at least a part of the lost potassium with potassium phosphate. This can also reduce the risk of hyperchloremia associated with sole use of potassium chloride salts.[41] It is imperative, however, that significant renal failure be ruled out before phosphate is administered IV; serum phosphate levels should be monitored to prevent possible hyperphosphatemia. Administering too much phosphate can induce hypocalcemia; therefore, calcium levels should also be monitored if phosphate is administered. When oral intake is tolerated, skim milk is a good source of phosphorus. It is thought that phosphate replacement accelerates the recovery of reduced red blood cell 2,3-DPG levels, thereby decreasing hemoglobin–oxygen affinity and improving tissue oxygenation.

Bicarbonate

There has been controversy over the use of bicarbonate in the treatment of DKA. It is used for management of hyperkalemia, and is generally considered to be necessary in cases of severe acidosis (pH <7.1).[42] When bicarbonate is used to correct pH, it is not corrected above a level of 7.1; to normalize the pH could result in paradoxical central nervous system (CNS) acidosis.[43] Too rapid correction of acidosis can also induce hypokalemia (as potassium shifts into the cells). When bicarbonate is given, it should be infused with the IV fluids, not administered by bolus. Some authorities believe that bicarbonate replacement is unnecessary because insulin therapy reverses the biochemical abnormalities of DKA including the bicarbonate deficit.

Sodium

Isotonic saline that is administered initially supplies enough sodium to correct any sodium loss. Because the patient with DKA or HHNS may lose proportionately more water than sodium, a hypotonic solution (such as 0.45% NaCl) will be ordered after the 2 to 3 L of isotonic saline. Hypotonic solutions provide free water to correct cellular dehydration.

Other Electrolytes

Losses of calcium and magnesium may occur as a result of the osmotic diuresis. Often they are not considered of clinical consequence, but in some cases, magnesium is replaced if renal function is adequate.[44]

TREATMENT OF PRECIPITATING FACTORS

In addition to the above therapies, treatment will include identification and treatment of concurrent health problems, particularly those that might have been precipitating factors in the development of DKA or HHNS. Table 18-2 lists common precipitating factors for each condition.

USE OF THE NURSING PROCESS

NURSING ASSESSMENT

Nursing care of the patient with HHNS or DKA involves meticulous, ongoing assessment to detect significant changes. Tables 18-3 and 18-4 outline the clinical manifestations of DKA and HHNS. To achieve ongoing assessment, it is best to use a diabetic flow sheet, which often includes the following data:

1. Vital signs (blood pressure [BP], temperature, pulse, and respirations)
2. Weight
3. Fluid therapy (type, amount, and flow rate)
4. Insulin therapy (number of units per hour IV, IM, and SQ)
5. Hourly urine volume
6. ECG tracings
7. Level of consciousness
8. Deep-tendon reflexes
9. Relevant laboratory data, which may include:
   - Blood and urine glucose
   - Blood and urine ketones
   - Arterial blood gases (pH, $PaCO_2$, PaO_2, HCO_3)
   - Potassium
   - Magnesium
   - HCO_3
   - Sodium and chloride
   - Calcium and phosphorus
   - BUN and creatinine
   - White blood cell count
   - Hematocrit
10. Calculations:
    - Anion gap
    - Serum osmolality

Decisions as to which of the above parameters will be monitored, by whom, and at what intervals, will be made based on the patient's status and protocols related to the care setting (such as the emergency room, critical care unit, and nursing unit). Response to therapy must be observed and recorded carefully. This involves constant vigilance over the patient's clinical status so that critical judgments can be made to provide optimal therapy.

TABLE 18–2

Factors Contributing to Development of DKA or HHNS in Susceptible Patients

DIABETIC KETOACIDOSIS (DKA)	HYPEROSMOLAR HYPERGLYCEMIC NONKETOTIC SYNDROME (HHNS)
Infections, illness	Chronic renal disease
Physiological stresses (e.g., trauma, surgery, myocardial infarction, dehydration, pregnancy)	Chronic cardiovascular disease Acute illness, infection Surgery, burns, trauma
Psychological/emotional stress	Hyperalimentation, tube feedings
Omission/reduction of insulin	Peritoneal dialysis
Failure of insulin delivery system (pump)	Mannitol therapy
Excess alcohol intake	Pharmacological agents: • Chlorpromazine • Cimetidine • Diazoxide • Diuretics (thiazide, thiazide-related, and loop diuretics) • Glucocorticoids and immunosuppressive agents • L-asparaginase • Phenytoin • Propanolol

NURSING DIAGNOSES

Although there are many nursing diagnoses relevant to the diabetic patient, Clinical Tip: Examples of Nursing Diagnoses Related to Patients With Diabetic Ketoacidosis or Hyperosmolar Hyperglycemic Nonketotic Syndrome deals with diagnoses that relate primarily to fluid, electrolyte, and acid–base balance aspects of nursing care of patients with, or at risk for, DKA or HHNS. The listed etiologies and defining characteristics are those most likely to be applicable. In some situations, there may be others. See Chapters 3 through 9 for detailed descriptions of specific imbalances.

NURSING INTERVENTIONS

Nursing care of the patient with DKA or HHNS is complex and involves many traditional nursing actions plus sophisticated monitoring of the responses to medical therapy. The care plan includes many interventions that relate to the fluid and electrolyte status of the patient. Some of those most frequently used are outlined below:

1. Monitor degree of FVD and response to fluid replacement therapy.
   A. Assess BP (supine and sitting, if possible) and pulse. (A drop in systolic pressure by more than 10 to 15 mmHg on position change from lying to sitting is indicative of FVD. Remember that a severely volume-depleted patient will be hypotensive even in the supine position. The pulse will be rapid and of a weak volume as the heart pumps faster to compensate for the below-normal plasma volume.)
   B. Observe neck veins. (Collapse of the neck veins when the head is raised is a sign of FVD.)
   C. Check skin and tongue turgor and degree of moisture of mucous membranes.

(text continues on page 329)

TABLE 18–3

Clinical Signs of DKA and Their Probable Causes

CLINICAL SIGNS	PROBABLE CAUSES
Hyperglycemia (Normal blood glucose is 80–120 mg/dL. Elevations associated with DKA may be as high as 4000 mg/dL.)	Faulty glucose metabolism causes glucose to accumulate in the bloodstream (lack of insulin decreases glucose uptake by most cells and also increases gluconeogenesis in the liver)
Glucosuria	Blood glucose level exceeds renal threshold (normally 180 mg/dL, higher in the elderly) causing glucose to spill into the urine
Polyuria (initially) with high specific gravity	Osmotic diuretic effect of hyperglycemia, high renal solute load
Polydipsia	Thirst due to cellular dehydration (cells become dehydrated when water is drawn from them by the hypertonic ECF)
Anorexia, nausea, vomiting	Follows onset of DKA; interferes with fluid intake (hastening the development of fluid volume deficit)
Poor skin turgor, dry mucous membranes, poor tongue turgor	Fluid volume deficit
Acute weight loss	Fluid volume deficit (parallels degree of this imbalance)
Ketonemia and ketonuria	Excessive accumulation of ketones in the bloodstream causes them to spill out into the urine
Cherry red skin and mucous membranes	Marked peripheral vasodilatation associated with ketosis
Deep "air hunger" respirations (Kussmaul)	Compensatory mechanism to increase plasma pH by the elimination of large amounts of carbon dioxide
Acetone odor to breath (similar to that of overripe apples)	Acetone, a volatile ketone, is vaporized in the expired air (may be obscured by the odor of vomitus)
Abdominal pain (can simulate acute appendicitis, pancreatitis, or other acute abdominal problems)	Apparently due to the DKA per se (Note: Anorexia, nausea, and vomiting precede the abdominal pain when it is due to DKA; this is in contrast to most surgical emergencies in which the pain usually occurs first.)
Postural hypotension	Fluid volume deficit (eventually may be hypotensive even when supine)
Fatigue, muscular weakness	Lack of carbohydrate utilization, hypokalemia
Hypothermia or normal temperature	Fever is present only when there is a concurrent illness causing it
Blurred vision	Osmotic changes in lenses of eyes
Oliguria, anuria (late)	Fluid volume deficit causes decreased renal blood flow and decreased GFR. (Before assuming that urine formation is scanty, check for a distended, atonic bladder.)
Depressed sensorium (ranging from somnolence to frank coma)	Level of consciousness correlates best with level of hyperglycemia and plasma osmolality

TABLE 18–3 (cont.)

CLINICAL SIGNS	PROBABLE CAUSES
LABORATORY DATA:	
Hyperglycemia	Related to insulin lack (see above)
Elevated serum osmolality (normal; 280–295 mOsm/kg)	Related primarily to high glucose level; elevated BUN contributes to elevated level
Potassium variations	Serum potassium concentration may be elevated before treatment; later, however, may drop to seriously low levels (see explanation in text)
Hypophosphatemia	Osmotic diuresis
Increased BUN (often increased to 40 mg/dL; normal is 10–20 mg/dL)	Fluid volume deficit, decreased GFR, increased protein metabolism, increased hepatic production of urea (due to insulin lack)
Increased creatinine (normal is 0.7 to 1.5 mg/dL)	Prerenal azotemia due to FVD
Leukocytosis	Fluid volume deficit, acidosis, adrenocortical stimulation
Decreased serum bicarbonate (usually <15 mEq/L, may be extremely low; normal is 24 mEq/L)	Excessive ketonic anions in the bloodstream cause a compensatory drop in bicarbonate
Decreased arterial pH (usually <7.25; may be as low as 6.8 in severe cases; normal is 7.35–7.45)	Associated with the metabolic acidosis caused by ketosis
High anion gap (AG) acidosis (normal AG is <12–15 mEq/L)	Due to excessive ketones in the bloodstream
Increased hemoglobin, hematocrit, total protein	FVD (causes concentration of formed elements in blood)
Increased liver function tests	Does not necessarily reflect acute or chronic liver damage, as most often values return to normal in several weeks

BUN, blood urea nitrogen; DKA, diabetic ketoacidosis; ECF, extracellular fluid; GFR, glomerular filtration rate; FVD, fluid volume deficit.

TABLE 18–4

Summary of Hyperosmolar Hyperglycemic Nonketotic Syndrome

The typical patient at risk for HHNS has either undiagnosed diabetes or type II diabetes managed with oral diabetes medications, insulin, or diet alone; the typical patient at risk for DKA requires insulin for everyday management and to sustain life.

HHNS tends to occur in middle-aged or elderly Type II diabetics, often those suffering from underlying renal and cardiovascular impairment. In at-risk patients, the condition is often precipitated by the stress of an acute illness or by treatment with corticosteroids, diuretics, mannitol, phenytoin, and glucose solutions.

Onset of HHNS tends to be more gradual and insidious than that of DKA. (It is not uncommon for patients to experience polyuria, polydipsia, weight loss, and weakness for many days, and even weeks, before seeking medical attention.)

Hyperglycemia and related symptoms of hyperosmolality are often more pronounced in HHNS than in DKA. Abnormal neurological signs may occur, such as focal or generalized seizures. If water loss leads to hypernatremia, fever may occur.

HHNS is not associated with ketoacidosis; it has been postulated that in HHNS there is sufficient insulin to prevent ketosis but not enough to prevent hyperglycemia.

HHNS, hyperosmolar hyperglycemic nonketotic syndrome; DKA, diabetic ketoacidosis.

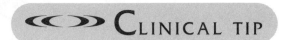

Examples of Nursing Diagnoses Related to Patients With Diabetic Ketoacidosis or Hyperosmolar Hyperglycemic Nonketotic Syndrome

NURSING DIAGNOSIS	ETIOLOGICAL FACTORS	DEFINING CHARACTERISTICS
Fluid volume deficit related to hyperosmotic diuresis	Hyperglycemia Hyperosmolality	Initially: Polyuria Later: Oliguria or anuria Other symptoms of FVD (see Ch 3)
Alteration in potassium balance (hypokalemia) related to increased potassium loss and insulin therapy (shift into cells)	Osmotic diuresis Dilution by IV fluids Increased excretion Reentry into cells	Drop in serum potassium for 1–4 hours after therapy (symptoms of hypokalemia in Ch 5)
Alteration in tissue perfusion: Renal, related to FVD	Severe FVD Decreased GFR Decreased renal blood flow	Oliguria or anuria symptoms of renal failure (see Ch17)
Risk for alteration in phosphorus balance (hypophosphatemia) and magnesium balance (hypomagnesemia) related to osmotic diuresis and insulin therapy	Osmotic diuresis Rapid fall in levels (especially phosphate) once fluid therapy is begun Reentry into cells	Symptoms of hypophosphatemia (see Ch 8) Symptoms of hypomagnesemia (see Ch 7)
Alteration in acid–base balance (metabolic acidosis) related to increased production and decreased use of ketones in DKA	Insulin deficiency in type I diabetes Increased activity of counterregulatory hormones Release of FFA from peripheral fat stores	Ketonemia Decreased plasma pH Ketonuria Decreased plasma HCO_3 Elevated anion gap Kussmaul respirations "Fruity" breath odor Clinical signs of acidosis (see Ch 9)
Alteration in nutrition: less than body requirements, related to insulin deficiency	Decreased glucose uptake and storage Decreased protein synthesis and fat assimilation Gastric retention Anorexia, nausea, and vomiting	Early: Weight loss and hunger in spite of adequate food intake; abdominal pain Later: Reduction in muscle mass and fat stores
Sensory-perceptual alteration related to effects of DKA and HHNS	Elevated serum osmolality FVD Severe elevated BUN Acidemia in DKA	Changes in level of consciousness Change in usual response to sensory stimuli
Risk for hypoglycemia related to insulin therapy	Insufficient dextrose in IV fluids Erratic absorption of insulin from peripheral sites Excess insulin	Rapid drop in blood glucose Negative urine glucose
Risk for uncontrolled diabetes related to inadequate management or stress factors	Insulin supply or use not adequate for metabolic needs Food intake excessive for exogenous or endogenous insulin supply Physiological or psychological stressors such as illness, surgery, personal crisis	Lack of adjustment of regimen during illness, infection, or severe emotional stress Decreased insulin dosage when food intake decreases Manipulation of insulin dose related to fear of hypoglycemic reaction Inadequate health care during periods of illness or severe crisis

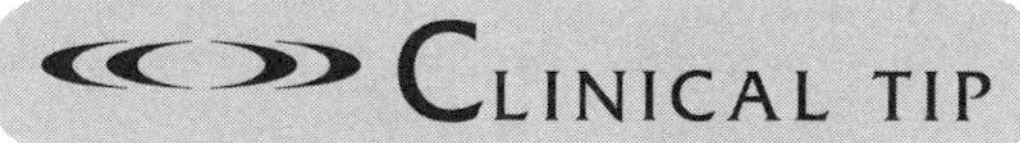

Examples of Nursing Diagnoses Related to Patients With Diabetic Ketoacidosis or Hyperosmolar Hyperglycemic Nonketotic Syndrome (cont.)

NURSING DIAGNOSIS	ETIOLOGICAL FACTORS	DEFINING CHARACTERISTICS
Potential for HHNS related to pharmacologic or other medical therapy	Type II elderly diabetic receiving drugs or therapies that can precipitate HHNS (see Table 18-2)	Hyperglycemia Polyuria Water intake inadequate to compensate for osmotic diuresis
Knowledge deficit of diabetic sick day management related to lack of exposure to diabetic sick day guidelines	No previous history of attending diabetic education program Poor understanding of diabetic sick day management	Does not follow sick day diet; does not monitor blood glucose levels; does not manipulate insulin dosage during illness
Ineffective management of therapeutic regimen related to complexity of diabetes regimen	Lack of understanding of diabetes regimen Patient's denial of the importance of the diabetes regimen	Does not take insulin or oral diabetes agents as prescribed; does not regularly self-monitor blood glucose levels; does not follow appropriate dietary recommendations.

FFA, free fatty acid; FVD, fluid volume deficit; DKA, diabetic ketoacidosis; HHNS, hyperosmolar hyperglycemic nonketotic syndrome; GFR, glomerular filtration rate.

D. Monitor urinary output.
   i. If patient is too stuporous to void, insert a retention catheter, using meticulous aseptic technique. (Recall that diabetic patients are very prone to urinary infections.) Remove the catheter as soon as the patient is able to empty the bladder by voiding.
   ii. Measure hourly urine volume in a device calibrated for accurate reading of small amounts (see Fig. 2-10). (Output should be at least 30–50 mL/hr. Oliguria related to FVD can lead to renal tubular damage and must be prevented. The hourly urinary output should increase if parenteral fluid replacement is adequate. Report a urine volume <30 mL/hr as well as failure of output to increase with fluid replacement.)
   iii. Measure SG of urine. (Urinary SG is elevated in FVD; if low with a scanty volume, renal damage may be present and should be reported. Heavy glucosuria invalidates SG readings; see Table 2-3.)
   iv. Compare the 8-hr and 24-hr intake and output as well as the total output. (During treatment, intake must exceed output until the FVD is corrected.)
   v. Monitor the BUN and creatinine levels. (An elevated BUN reflects FVD when elevated out of proportion to the serum creatinine level. See Table 2-2 for further discussion of these tests.)

E. Calculate the approximate degree of FVD.
   i. Weigh patient on admission and ascertain, if possible, the preillness weight. (A rapid loss of 1 kg [2.2 lb] of body weight is roughly equivalent to a loss of 1 L of

body fluid. Loss of weight from not eating may amount to 0.5 lb/day. Acute weight loss of 5% body weight constitutes a moderate FVD; 8% or greater is a severe FVD. Many cases have been reported in which as much as 10% to 20% of body weight has been lost acutely in patients with DKA and HHNS).

ii. Weigh patient each morning before breakfast. (Monitor for acute changes in body weight; anticipate that weight gain will parallel correction of the FVD.)

iii. If preillness weight cannot be determined, FVD may be calculated with a formula using the patient's plasma osmolality:

$$\text{FVD (L)} = \frac{(\text{Patient's pOsm} - \text{Normal osmolality})}{\text{Normal osmolality}} \times \text{liters of body fluid } (0.6 \times \text{Body wt in kg})$$

Example: Assume an adult patient has a plasma osmolality of 340 mOsm/kg and weighs 70 kg. (Use 280 mOsm/kg as the normal value.):

Liters of body fluid = 0.6 × 70 = 42
FVD (L) = (340 − 280)/280 × 42 = 9 L

F. Monitor neurological status. Look for depressed sensorium and focal neurological signs. A depressed sensorium results most often from hyperosmolality of body fluids and occurs to some degree in most cases of DKA and HHNS. Because of this it is necessary to consider the following points:

i. Maintain an adequate airway (a comatose patient with airway obstruction will require intubation).

ii. Insert nasogastric tube when indicated (gastric retention with regurgitation of contents is not uncommon).

G. Regulate fluid replacement rate and volume according to protocol and patient status. Consider the following facts:

i. After the initial infusion of saline solutions to rehydrate the patient, dextrose solutions are indicated to keep the serum glucose from falling too rapidly.

ii. Central venous pressure or hemodynamic monitoring may be needed in elderly patients and those with compromised cardiovascular or renal status.

iii. The patient with HHNS may need larger amounts of fluid than the patient with DKA because the degree of FVD is often worse in HHNS.

2. Monitor electrolyte status and response to replacement therapy.

A. Monitor potassium levels at frequent intervals (1–2 hrs) during the initial period of therapy. (The initial potassium level may be normal or elevated because of plasma volume contraction and shift from the intracellular fluid to the ECF; the potassium level drops rapidly with plasma dilution and reentry of potassium into the cells. Replacement therapy after the first 2 to 3 L of fluid should prevent a precipitous drop in serum potassium. Recall that potassium should not be administered to a patient with oliguria. See Chapter 5 for nursing considerations in the safe administration of potassium solutions.)

B. Use serial ECG tracings and other appropriate assessment parameters to detect effects of hypokalemia and to monitor responses to potassium infusion (see Chapter 5).

C. Promptly report abnormal laboratory levels of other electrolytes, such as a low phosphorus level. (Recall that decreased serum phosphorus levels often parallel those of low potassium. In fact, these electrolytes are often replaced together, in the form of potassium phosphate. See Chapter 8 for a description of hypophosphatemia.)

3. Monitor degree of hyperglycemia and response to insulin therapy.

A. Monitor blood sugar levels closely by use of capillary blood (finger stick) and a blood glucose meter plus regular laboratory determinations. Of course, a decrease in the plasma glucose level is the earliest sign of effective therapy.[45] (Recall that blood sugar determinations are much more accurate than urine glucose tests. Renal threshold varies among individuals, increases with age, and may be affected by renal disease.)

B. Monitor administration of insulin-containing IV infusions to prevent too rapid decrease in blood sugar level and serum osmolality. (*Cerebral edema* may occur with a too rapid drop in blood sugar levels. Blood glucose should decrease at an optimum rate of 50 to 100 mg/dL/hr.[46] At a blood glucose level of 250 mg/dL, IV solutions containing dextrose in saline should be used for both fluid replacement and insulin infusion to prevent the development of hypoglycemia.[47,48] As stated earlier, some clinicians recommend maintaining the serum glucose level at approximately 250 mg/dL for at least 24 hrs before allowing it to decrease to a normal level.)[49]

C. Observe the patient closely to prevent occurrence of hypoglycemia, and evaluate serum glucose measurements. (*Hypoglycemia* can be a major complication of therapy. A recent retrospective study indicated that 30% of patients hospitalized with DKA developed hypoglycemia during the first 14 days of treatment.[50] In the study, the risk of hypoglycemia was increased by the presence of fever, hepatic disease, renal disease, and "nothing by mouth" status.[51] When severe, hypoglycemia may have serious CNS effects and is potentially fatal. Of course, one should report a rapid drop in blood sugar level.)

4. Monitor altered acid–base balance (acidemia) and response to therapy, especially in type I diabetics with DKA.
   A. Monitor serum and urine ketones. (As a result of overproduction and decreased use, ketones build up in the blood and are excreted in the urine.)
   B. Observe rate and depth of respirations. (Extra carbon dioxide is blown off by Kussmaul respirations, which are stimulated by the acidemia and help to bring the arterial pH back toward normal. Be alert for a change from deep, rapid respirations to rapid, shallow, gasping breaths. This may indicate a severe drop in blood pH [<7] or impaired flow to the respiratory center because of FVD and circulatory collapse. The patient loses the compensatory action of Kussmaul breathing when this occurs and the acidosis becomes more severe.)
   C. Check for "fruity" breath odor. (This occurs as acetone is excreted from the lungs but may be masked by the odor of vomitus.)
   D. Observe for cherry-red color of skin and mucous membranes. (This is characteristic of DKA due to marked peripheral vasodilation; improvement of skin color indicates response to therapy.)
   E. Observe for signs of decreased cardiac function and arrhythmias. (This constitutes the greatest risk of prolonged, uncontrolled acidosis.)
   F. Monitor blood and urine pH and serum bicarbonate levels. (Plasma pH may fall to 7.25 or below and urine pH falls as kidneys eliminate hydrogen ions in an attempt to correct the acidosis. The serum HCO_3 may fall to 12 mEq/L or lower. An increase in serum bicarbonate to 15–20 mEq/L may be expected usually between 12 and 24 hrs after treatment has begun.)[52]
   G. Assess for presence and characteristics of abdominal pain. (Abdominal pain may occur in DKA and is preceded by nausea and vomiting. Other abdominal emergencies (e.g., pancreatitis and surgical abdomen) may coexist with or may have triggered DKA. In these conditions, the pain usually precedes other symptoms.

5. Use nursing measures to prevent and monitor for other complications that may occur with DKA or HHNS, such as:
   A. Respiratory or urinary tract infections, septic shock, adult respiratory distress syndrome (ARDS).
   B. Thromboembolic complications.
   C. CNS deterioration, prolonged coma.
   D. Gastrointestinal bleeding.
   (These complications have been responsible for deaths in some cases of DKA and HHNS.)

6. Use nursing measures to teach the recovering patient how to prevent recurrences of DKA and HHNS.
   A. Have the patient describe his or her daily routine and demonstrate methods used to carry out the diabetic regimen.[53] This enables one to assess the patient's understanding of the regimen and the degree of accuracy with which procedures such as glucose self-monitoring, meal planning, and insulin administration are being carried out. Some reteaching may be necessary and should be carefully evaluated for effectiveness.
   B. Review with the patient factors that could disrupt control of diabetes, leading to hyperglycemia and DKA or HHNS. (Many per-

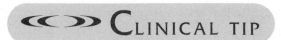

Sick Day Instructions

1. Contact your physician immediately if you have pain, fever, persistent diarrhea, or you are vomiting and cannot hold down food or liquid.
2. Always take your usual dose of insulin or oral diabetes medication. Never omit your medication even if you are unable to eat.
3. Test your blood glucose level every 3–4 hrs around the clock or a minimum of four times a day. It is essential that blood glucose levels be tested at least before each meal and at bedtime.
4. If you do not routinely check your blood glucose levels, buy a vial of 25 visual blood glucose strips, a finger lancet device, and lancets to use when you are ill. Check these supplies every six months to be sure they have not expired. Once the vial of strips has been opened, they will expire in 4 months.
5. If your blood glucose levels are greater than 240 mg/dL, test your urine for ketones. Ketone testing should also be done when you are ill from any cause. If ketones are present along with high serum glucose levels, you will need extra insulin. Regular (short-acting) insulin should be used. Consult your physician immediately to obtain guidelines for how much regular insulin you should use and how often to take it.
6. Drink a glassful of caffeine-free and alcohol-free liquid every hour. Fluids that are acceptable are water, caffeine-free tea, consomme, fruit juices, broth made from bouillon cubes, and regular or diet sodas. If your glucose levels are elevated, drink the diet variety. If your glucose levels are low and you are unable to eat, drink regular soda. If you are unable to take liquids because of nausea and vomiting, consult your physician immediately. A medication may be prescribed to stop the nausea and vomiting.
7. If you cannot follow your usual meal plan, refer to the food suggestions for sick days.
8. Over-the-counter and prescribed medications may contribute to hyperglycemia or hypoglycemia. Consult with your physician before taking any of these medications.
9. Allow friends and family to care for you. Rest and do not exercise.

Food Suggestions for Sick Days:

Food sources of carbohydrate that may be more easily digested during a period of illness include the following. Note that each portion provides approximately 15 grams of carbohydrate or 1 starch/bread exchange.

Food	Portion
Apple sauce (sweetened)	1/2 cup
Baked custard	1/2 cup
Cooked cereal	1/2 cup
Eggnog	1/2 cup
Fruit juices (unsweetened)	
Apple	1/2 cup
Cranberry	1/3 cup
Grape	1/2 cup
Orange	1/2 cup
Fruit yogurt	1/3 cup
Frozen yogurt on a stick	1 bar
Frozen yogurt from a container	1/3 cup
Gelatin	1/3 cup
Honey	3 tsp
Hershey's syrup	2 Tbs
Lifesavers	7
Milk (lowfat or skim)	1 cup
Popsicle (twin-pop)	1
Pudding (sweetened)	1/4 cup
Regular ice cream	1/2 cup
Regular jello	1/3 cup
Regular soda	3/4 cup (6 ounces)
Saltine crackers	6
Sherbet	1/4 cup
Soup (vegetable, noodle, or cream)	1 cup
Toast	1 slice
Tomato juice	1 1/2 cups
Vegetable juice	1 1/2 cups

Developed by Mary Kay Macheca, RN, MSN(R), CDE (11/94)

sons with diabetes are not aware of the less obvious precipitating factors [see Table 18-2]. The patient should be able to describe the factors and their effect on diabetes control.)

C. Discuss early symptoms of hyperglycemia with the patient. (Polyuria, polydipsia, polyphagia, fatigue, weakness, blurred vision, and headache should be discussed with the patient as commonly occurring symptoms of poor control.)

D. Assist the patient to learn a method of testing for elevated serum glucose and ketones. (Self-monitoring of serum glucose with a blood glucose meter is best, but testing with visual strips can also be effective. Ketones can be detected by the urine dipstick method. The patient should demonstrate testing methods in a simulated or real home setting and should interpret the results accurately.) Instruct the patient to monitor urine ketones anytime the blood glucose level is greater than 240 mg/dL or when illness occurs.

E. Provide the patient with realistic "sick day instructions" and identify different health care resources for daily routines, in emergencies, and when away from home. (See Clinical Tip: Sick Day Instructions. Stress the importance of keeping regular appointments with the health care provider to prevent loss of control. An "after-hours" telephone number to be used in serious or emergency situations should be provided when possible. Instruct the patient, when traveling, to seek help at emergency rooms of medical centers or community hospitals.)

F. Use careful and tactful assessment methods to identify cultural and socioeconomic factors that may interfere with maintaining the diabetes regimen.[54]

   i. Provide services of a social worker or counselor as indicated, especially in cases of recurrent DKA or HHNS.[55]
   ii. Review the meal plan with the client and suggest low-cost substitutes when possible.
   iii. Explore insurance reimbursement policies with the patient and identify less expensive sources of food, equipment, and supplies. (Economic factors such as low income, unemployment, lack of insurance coverage, or pressing family needs may prevent even the most committed patient from maintaining the proper regimen.)
   iv. Make sure the meal plan and exercise and medication schedules have been adjusted to the patient's lifestyle and work schedule. (Shift workers and others who have unusual schedules may experience difficulty maintaining control with a "typical" regimen.)
   v. Tailor instructional materials to the reading and learning level of the patient. (Functional illiteracy and perceptual learning disabilities are more widespread than is commonly recognized.)
   vi. When indicated, include family members or significant others in the education process. (When a family member has diabetes, the whole family must cope with it. Family conflict can interfere with good control. Some patients may need family assistance with certain aspects of the regimen.)

EVALUATION

This important step of the nursing process measures the effectiveness of nursing care for the patient with DKA or HHN. Evaluation is based on progress made toward short-term and long-term goals.

Short-term goal achievement is demonstrated by:

1. Return of blood sugar to desired levels without any episodes of hypoglycemia.
2. Correction of FVD with optimal cardiovascular function and urinary output.
3. Electrolyte levels approaching or within normal limits.
4. Prevention or correction of complications.
5. Prevention of immediate recurrence of DKA or HHNS.

Long-term goal achievement is demonstrated by:

1. Control of blood glucose levels within a range appropriate for the individual.

2. Prompt intervention when stressors are present that precipitate hyperglycemia.
3. Maintenance of general health, growth and development, and activity levels appropriate to the individual.

The importance of the nurse's role in the care of the diabetic patient cannot be overemphasized. Skillful use of the nursing process in the care of the patient with DKA or HHNS will contribute greatly to a successful outcome. Equally challenging is the nurse's role as a clinician and health care educator preparing the patient to maintain control of the diabetes in a way that will prevent recurrences of DKA or HHNS and will enable the best possible level of health.

CASE STUDY

18-1. Mrs. K, a 35-year-old insulin-dependent diabetic, developed viral gastroenteritis with nausea and vomiting. Two days before admission, she omitted her insulin because she was not eating. Her husband brought her to the Emergency Department because she was becoming increasingly lethargic.

Upon initial examination, she was found to have tachycardia (pulse rate, 140/min) and deep, rapid (Kussmaul) respirations. Her blood pressure lying flat was 98/70. She was able to void only a few milliliters; the urinary glucose and ketone levels were both 4+. Her skin and mucous membranes were dry and she had a fruity odor to her breath. The following laboratory data were obtained from venous blood:

Glucose = 940 mg/dL
Sodium = 130 mEq/L
Potassium = 6.8 mEq/L
Bicarbonate = 5 mEq/L
BUN = 45 mg/dL
Creatinine = 2.2 mg/dL
Arterial pH = 7.07
Bicarbonate = 2.6 mEq/L
$PaCO_2$ = 13 mm Hg

On the basis of the examination and the laboratory findings, a diagnosis of DKA was made. Mrs. K then was treated with 0.9% sodium chloride IV to correct the FVD and with low-dose regular insulin (5 U/hr). Over the course of the first 16 hrs of treatment, the laboratory data in Table 18-5 were recorded.

COMMENTARY: Diabetic ketoacidosis developed because the patient unwisely omitted her insulin during a time of increased need. The laboratory data indicate a severe high anion gap metabolic acidosis (pH 7.07). The anion gap is calculated by subtracting the sum of the bicarbonate and chloride levels from the serum sodium level (130 − [5 + 90] = 35 mEq/L). The calculated anion gap is 35 mEq/L, while the accepted normal range is approximately 12 to 15 mEq/L. This indicates an excess of about 20 mEq/L of ketones (flooding the bloodstream due to insulin lack). The deep rapid (Kussmaul) respirations were the body's attempt to compensate for the extremely low serum pH.

TABLE 18–5

TIME	BLOOD GLUCOSE (Mg/dL)	ARTERIAL pH	SODIUM (mEq/L)	POTASSIUM (mEq/L)	BICARBONATE (mEq/L)	CHLORIDE (mEq/L)	BUN/ CREATININE
5 PM	940	7.07	130	6.8	5	90	45/2.2
7 PM	520		132	6.6	7	100	43/1.9
9 PM	400	7.26	136	4.3	8	105	44/1.6
2 AM	325		140	4.5	16	115	30/1.4
9 AM	300		142	4.4	23	115	22/1.1

Signs of FVD included hypotension, tachycardia, dry skin and mucous membranes, low urinary output, and a high BUN to creatinine ratio. The serum sodium concentration was low initially because of the high serum glucose concentration (which pulled water out of the cells, thus diluting the serum sodium concentration). The serum potassium level was elevated initially due to the effect of starvation (release of potassium from the cells), acidosis (which also facilitates movement of cellular potassium to the bloodstream), and decreased renal excretion of potassium (due to the poor renal perfusion associated with FVD).

Notice how all of the abnormal parameters gradually corrected to normal (or near normal) during the course of the first 16 hrs of treatment. This was accomplished solely by the combination of low-dose insulin and fluid volume replacement with isotonic saline. These treatments allowed the metabolic defects to be corrected. For example, the formation of ketones was stopped by the insulin. The metabolic acidosis corrected itself as this occurred; no bicarbonate was administered. As the blood glucose level decreased, the serum sodium level increased. This correction of the dilutional hyponatremia occurred because water was no longer being pulled out of the cells to the intravascular space. In addition, isotonic saline contains a sizable amount of sodium and helped correct any sodium losses from vomiting. The potentially dangerous serum potassium level (6.8 mEq/L) decreased to normal as the starvation effect (due to insulin lack) and the metabolic acidosis were corrected by treatment with insulin and fluid resuscitation. The gradual drop in the BUN and serum creatinine levels reflected improved renal perfusion secondary to fluid resuscitation.

After stabilization, the patient received education about rules to be followed during sick days (see Clinical Tip: Sick Day Instructions).

REFERENCES

1. Wachtel T, Tetu-Mouradjian L, Goldman D, Ellis S, O'Sullivan P: Hyperosmolarity and acidosis in diabetes mellitus: A three-year experience in Rhode Island. J General Internal Medicine 6(November/December):501,1991
2. Santiago J, et al (eds): Diagnosis and Classification/Pathogenesis. Medical Management of Insulin-Dependent (Type I) Diabetes, 2nd ed, p 5. Alexandria, VA, American Diabetes Association, 1994
3. Moy C (ed): Diabetes complications. Diabetes 1993 Vital Statistics, p 32. Alexandria, VA, American Diabetes Association, 1993
4. Genuth S: Diabetic ketoacidosis and hyperosmolar hyperglycemic nonketotic syndrome in adults. In: Lebovitz H, et al. (eds): Therapy for Diabetes Mellitus and Related Disorders, 2nd ed, p 65. Alexandria, VA, American Diabetes Association, 1994
5. Raskin P, et al (eds): Diagnosis and classification. Medical Management of Non-Insulin-Dependent (Type II) Diabetes, 3rd ed, p 4. Alexandria, VA, American Diabetes Association, 1994
6. Ibid, p 16
7. Ibid, p 4
8. Quick W: Pathophysiology. In: Peragallo-Dittko V, Godley K, Meyer J (eds): A Core Curriculum for Diabetes Education, 2nd ed, p 114. Chicago, American Association of Diabetes Educators and the AADE Education and Research Foundation, 1993
9. Schwartz S: Hyperglycemia. In: Peragallo-Dittko V, Godley K, Meyer J (eds): A Core Curriculum for Diabetes Education, 2nd ed, p 305. Chicago, American Association of Diabetes Educators and the AADE Education and Research Foundation, 1993
10. Genuth, p 72
11. Carroll P, Matz R: Uncontrolled diabetes mellitus in adults: Experience in treating diabetic ketoacidosis and hyperosmolar nonketotic coma with low-dose insulin and a uniform treatment regimen. Diabetes Care 6:579,1983
12. Oster J, Kopyt N, Kleeman C, Dunfee T, Kreisberg R, Narins R: Diabetic acidosis and coma. In: Narins R (ed): Maxwell and Kleeman's Clinical Disorders of Fluid and Electrolyte Metabolism, 5th ed, p 828. New York, McGraw-Hill, 1994
13. Matz R: Hyperosmolar nonacidotic uncontrolled diabetes: Not a rare event. Clinical Diabetes 6:30,1988
14. Pope D, Dansky D: Hyperosmolar hyperglycemic nonketotic coma. Emerg Med Clin North Am 7:854, 1989
15. Siperstein M: Diabetic ketoacidosis and hyperosmolar coma. Endocrinol Metab Clin North Am 21:425,1992
16. Martin et al: Effect of hypophosphatemia on myocardial performance in man. N Engl J Med 297:901, 1977
17. Oster, p 840
18. Davidson J: Diabetic ketoacidosis and the hyperglycemic hyperosmolar state. In: Davidson J (ed): Clinical Diabetes: A Problem-Oriented Approach, 2nd ed, p 399. New York, Thieme Medical Publishers, 1991

19. Davidson, p 400
20. Sypniewski H, Mirtallo J, Schneider P: Hyperosmolar, hyperglycemic, nonketotic coma in a patient receiving home total parenteral nutrient therapy. Clin Pharm 6:69,1987
21. Wachtel T: The diabetic hyperosmolar state. Clin Geriatr Med 6:797,1990
22. White N, Henry D: Special issues in diabetes management. In: Haire-Joshu D (ed): Management of Diabetes Mellitus: Perspectives of Care Across the Life Span, p 256. St. Louis, Mosby Year Book, 1992
23. Raskin P, et al (eds): Detection and treatment of complications. Medical Management of Non-Insulin-Dependent (Type II) Diabetes, 3rd ed, p 79. Alexandria, VA, American Diabetes Association, 1994
24. Wachtel T: The diabetic hyperosmolar state. Clin Geriatr Med 6:798,1990
25. Oster, p 853
26. Wachtel T: The diabetic hyperosmolar state. Clin Geriatr Med 6:803,1990
27. Genuth, p 72
28. White, p 258
29. Macheca M: Diabetic hypoglycemia: How to keep the threat at bay. Am J Nurs 93(4):26,1993
30. The Diabetes Control and Complications Trial Research Group: The effect of intensive treatment of diabetes on the development and progression of long-term complications in insulin-dependent diabetes mellitus. N Engl J Med 329:982,1993
31. Cryer P, Fisher J, Shamoon H: Hypoglycemia. Diabetes Care 17:739,1994
32. Patrick A, Collier A, Hepburn D, Steedman D, Clarke B, Robertson C: Comparison of intramuscular glucagon and intravenous dextrose in the treatment of hypoglycemic coma in an accident and emergency department. Arch Emerg Med 7:76,1990
33. Davidson, p 403
34. Kitabchi A, Fisher J, Murphy M, Rumbak M: Diabetic ketoacidosis and the hyperglycemic, hyperosmolar, nonketotic state. In: Kahn C, Weir G (eds): Joslin's Diabetes Mellitus, 13th ed, p 760. Philadelphia, Lea and Febiger, 1994
35. Kitabchi A, Matteri R, Murphy M: Optimal insulin delivery in diabetic ketoacidosis (DKA) and hyperglycemic, hyperosmolar nonketotic coma (HHNK). Diabetes Care 5(1)(suppl):78,1982
36. Carroll, Matz, p 582
37. Lindsay R, Bolte R: The use of an insulin bolus in low-dose insulin infusion for pediatric diabetic ketoacidosis. Pediatr Emerg Care 5(2):78,1989
38. Peterson L, Caldwell J, Hoffman J: Insulin adsorbance to polyvinyl chloride surfaces with implications for constant infusion therapy. Diabetes 25:72,1976
39. Oster, p 858
40. Rogers B, Sills I, Cohen M, Seidel G: Diabetic ketoacidosis: Neurologic collapse during treatment followed by severe developmental morbidity. Clin Pediatr 29:456,1990
41. Oster, p 847
42. White N, Henry D, p 255
43. Oster, p 844
44. Davidson, p 410
45. Ibid, p 405
46. Ibid, p 405
47. White N, Henry D, p 255
48. Ellis E: Concepts of fluid therapy in diabetic ketoacidosis and hyperosmolar hyperglycemic nonketotic coma. Pediatr Clin North Am 37:316,1990
49. Santiago J, et al (eds): Diabetic ketoacidosis. Medical Management of Insulin-Dependent (Type I) Diabetes, 2nd ed, p 79. Alexandria, VA, American Diabetes Association, 1994
50. Malone M, Klos S, Gennis V, Goodwin J: Frequent hypoglycemic episodes in the treatment of patients with diabetic ketoacidosis. Arch Intern Med 152:2474,1992
51. Ibid
52. Schwartz S, p 322
53. Redman B: Teaching: Theory and interpersonal techniques. The Process of Patient Education, 7th ed, p 136. St. Louis, Mosby Year Book, 1993
54. Redman B: Assessment of motivation to learn and the need for patient education. The Process of Patient Education, 7th ed, p 24. St. Louis, Mosby Year Book, 1993
55. Henderson G: The psychosocial treatment of recurrent diabetic ketoacidosis: An interdisciplinary team approach. Diabetes Educator 17(2):122,1991

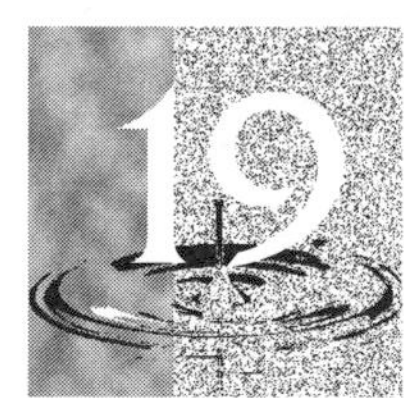

Fluid Balance in the Brain-Injured Patient

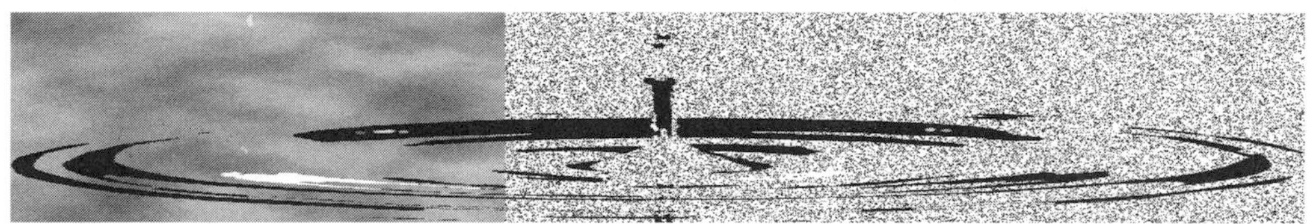

Traumatic and nontraumatic brain injury produce complications that compromise a patient's clinical course. Effective management of these complex injuries is aimed at reversing or reducing clinical deterioration. This chapter discusses nursing management of these disorders, emphasizing fluid and electrolyte imbalance, manifested by increased intracranial pressure (ICP) and disruptions in antidiuretic hormone (ADH) release.

PATHOPHYSIOLOGY

CEREBRAL EDEMA

The pathophysiology of brain injury varies according to etiology and severity, but the threat from cerebral edema is common. By definition, cerebral edema is an increase in brain volume caused by an increase in brain water.[1] Brain swelling that occurs most often in the immediate posttraumatic period is the result of vascular engorgement and impaired autoregulation. However, 24 to 48 hrs after impact, brain swelling is attributed to cerebral edema.[2] Untreated cerebral edema, despite the etiology, leads to elevated ICP.[3]

Classification

Cerebral edema can be classified into three different forms: (1) vasogenic, (2) cytotoxic (or cellular), and (3) interstitial (or hydrostatic). It is helpful to review briefly the features of these types of brain edema because therapeutic interventions for them can vary.

Vasogenic Edema

The most common form of brain edema is vasogenic edema; it occurs in cerebral mass lesions of any kind. Such conditions include brain tumor growths, abscess, hemorrhage, infarction, encephalitis, lead encephalopathy, and after brain radiation.[4] In this type of edema, the extracellular fluid (ECF) volume is increased with an elevation in plasma protein.[5] There is increased capillary permeability and a predilection for white matter. It is believed that white matter offers less resistance to the bulk flow than does gray matter.[6]

Cytotoxic (Cellular) Edema

In this type of edema, all the cellular elements of the brain (neurons, glia, and endothelial cells) may swell, with a consequent reduction in the brain's ECF space.[7] Most commonly associated with this form of edema are acute hypoosmolality (hyponatremia) and cerebral hypoxia (such as occurs after cardiac arrest or asphyxia). Cellular swelling is related to failure of the adenosine triphosphate (ATP)-dependent sodium pump within the cells, which causes sodium to accumulate rapidly within the cell and water to follow to maintain osmotic equilibrium.[8] However, patients with chronic hyponatremia do not suffer cerebral swelling (because the brain cells have had time to adapt by losing intracellular osmoles, mainly potassium). In this form of edema, both gray and white matter are affected.[9]

Current in vitro research suggests that free radicals (polyunsaturated fatty acids and excitatory amino acids) may induce brain cellular edema associated with ischemia and hyperosmolar states by inhibiting ($Na^+ + K^+$)-ATPase activity.[10] In response to this, new free oxygen radical scavengers, which are lipid-soluble and cross the blood–brain barrier, are being developed to treat and manage these untoward consequences.[11]

Interstitial Edema

As the name implies, interstitial or hydrostatic edema is characterized by an increase in the portion of the ECF surrounding the cells. It is related to blockage of cerebrospinal fluid absorption, most commonly by obstructive hydrocephalus.[12]

Disruption in Pressure and Volume Equilibrium

Cerebral edema represents a disruption in the pressure and volume equilibrium within the intracranial compartments. These compartments, encased in the inelastic cranial vault, contain brain tissue, blood, and cerebrospinal fluid (CSF). In adults, the pressure is maintained by an intracranial volume of approximately 1900 mL, of which about 80% represents brain volume, 10% blood volume, and 10% CSF volume.[13] When one compartment increases in volume, there must be a reciprocal compensatory change in one or both of the other components to maintain a constant total pressure. This is known as the Monro-Kellie doctrine. Because the brain is relatively incompressible, compensation occurs through shunting of CSF into the spinal dural sac, an increased CSF absorption, or a decreased cerebral blood volume. When the total volume of brain mass, blood, or spinal fluid exceeds the compensatory capacity, any additional increase in brain mass causes an exponential increase in ICP. Once ICP is raised to the stage of decompensation, intracranial hypertension results and the risk of brain displacement with herniation through the foramen magnum occurs.

CENTRAL DIABETES INSIPIDUS

Patients with neurologic injury are susceptible to abnormalities of sodium and water balance when central control mechanisms have been disrupted. As discussed in Chapter 4, diabetes insipidus is a disorder of water metabolism characterized by polyuria and polydipsia due to either insufficient production of ADH (central diabetes insipidus [CDI]), or renal unresponsiveness to ADH (nephrogenic diabetes insipidus).

Traumatic brain injury (head trauma) is a very frequent cause of CDI, usually as a result of temporary disruption in ADH release (secondary to postinjury brain swelling). As the brain swelling subsides, usually there is complete restoration of neurohypophyseal function. However, at times the diabetes insipidus may be permanent.

SYNDROME OF INAPPROPRIATE ANTIDIURETIC HORMONE SECRETION

When hyponatremia occurs in the presence of neurologic injury, the syndrome of inappropriate antidiuretic hormone secretion (SIADH) is often suspected. However, in some cases, recent evidence suggests that competing mechanisms (other than SIADH) may be responsible. As discussed in Chapter 4, a variety of central nervous system disorders may produce SIADH. Among these are head injury, encephalitis, meningitis, and brain tumors. The exact mechanisms by which SIADH is produced are unknown; presumably, relatively excessive vasopressin (ADH) is released from the neurohypophysis.[14] When hyponatremia occurs, despite adequate salt administration, it is believed to be attributable to excessive ADH secretion with resultant water retention.[15]

In addition, SIADH can cause cerebral edema due to cellular swelling (cytotoxic edema). For the most part, SIADH is self-limiting and subsides as the brain tissue heals; however, it can last for weeks or even months.

CEREBRAL SALT WASTING

In contrast, when hyponatremia develops in patients with subarachnoid hemorrhage (SAH), SIADH may not be responsible.[16–18] Sodium balance studies and direct measurements of blood volume have demonstrated volume depletion and renal sodium loss in SAH patients, which is inconsistent with ADH excess, and attributed to cerebral salt wasting.[19] Cerebral salt wasting is a syndrome characterized by hyponatremia, natriuresis, and extracellular (EC) volume contraction.[20] It has been reported most often in patients with SAH but also in patients with brain tumors, carcinomatous meningitis, and head trauma.[21] The pathophysiology of so-called cerebral salt wasting is unclear, but may include the release of an extra renal factor (atrial natriuretic factor [ANF]) which is responsible for disturbances of the central regulation of sodium homeostasis producing sodium loss.[22] ANF has been demonstrated to be released in the central nervous system possibly in response to increased ICP or blood in the diencephalic subarachnoid space.[23] This has led to an assumption that enhanced ANF activity may account, in part, for the observed salt wasting and volume depletion seen in SAH patients.[24]

ASSESSMENT

ELEVATED INTRACRANIAL PRESSURE

The most reliable data for assessing ICP are obtained through continuous ICP monitoring. Normal ICP is a mean pressure between 0 and 10 mmHg with normal fluctuations of up to 12 mmHg attributable to transient physiologic variations. Readings more than 15 mmHg are considered elevated.[25] However, absolute numbers of ICP must be evaluated within the context of the clinical condition being treated, as compliance varies.[26]

Several techniques exist for continuous ICP monitoring. These include intraventricular catheters, subarachnoid screws or bolts, epidural sensors, fiberoptic transducers, as well as the evolving development of telemetric ICP monitoring and ultrasonic transcranial Doppler.[27] Direct monitoring is highly valuable in assessing changes in ICP because it provides clinicians with visual pressure readings and waveforms. Neurosurgical centers use continuous ICP monitoring in all severely brain-injured patients to detect deterioration and guide therapeutic interventions.

When direct ICP monitoring is not available, clinical assessment becomes the primary method by which changes in ICP are determined. The symptoms of increased intracranial pressure are eventually the result of a reduction in cerebral blood flow and/or mass effect.[28] The classic signs and symptoms of elevated ICP include papilledema, headache, and vomiting. Unfortunately, these symptoms do not become evident until relatively late; therefore, interventions performed at this point are less helpful than when elevated ICP is in an earlier state of development. Earlier signs of elevated ICP can be detected by assessing for changes in the level of consciousness, motor and sensory function, pupil size and reactivity, vital signs, and other signs. Baseline assessment should be performed and compared with data obtained from subsequent assessments for early recognition of significant changes.

Deterioration in the Level of Consciousness

This is often the first sign of deterioration in the patient's condition because an increase in the ICP results in decreased cerebral oxygenation. The cells most sensitive to a reduction in oxygen supply are those of the cerebral cortex involved with higher intellectual functions, including thinking processes (such as memory and orientation). Changes in wakefulness should also be noted.[29]

Loss of Motor and Sensory Function

As the ICP rises, motor and sensory functions are compromised and focal changes may be observed. Motor loss progresses from hemiparesis to hemiplegia on the side of the body that is opposite the cerebral lesion. As the increase in ICP continues, the patient becomes progressively less responsive to light and deep touch, as well as to painful sensations. As the condition further deteriorates, decortication or decerebration may be observed either spontaneously or in response to painful stimuli.

Pupillary Changes

Change in pupil size usually occurs on the same side as the lesion (or pressure increase). The response to direct light in this pupil progresses from "equal and reactive" to "nonreactive." With continued deterioration, the patient reaches the terminal stage where pupils may become bilaterally nonreactive to light stimuli. The pupillary changes are all related to compression of the third (oculomotor) cranial nerve.

Alterations in Vital Signs

During the compensatory phase of increased ICP, there is an increase in systolic blood pressure to a level slightly higher than that of the CSF pressure (this response is known as the Cushing reflex and is due to brain ischemia). Blood pressure drops as the patient's condition continues to deteriorate and the decompensatory phase begins.

During the compensatory phase, the pulse rate drops to less than 60 beats/min. On palpation, the pulse is full and bounding. This change in rate and quality is related to an attempt by the heart to pump blood into vessels with increased resistance as a result of the increased ICP. During the decompensatory phase, the pulse rate becomes rapid and irregular, and the quality becomes thready.

Abnormalities in respiratory patterns vary according to the level of brain dysfunction. Cheyne-Stokes respiration is often the first irregular breathing pattern observed, although as brain dysfunction progresses, other abnormal breathing patterns become apparent.[30] Increased ICP can also result in acute neurogenic pulmonary edema, which further contributes to alterations in the respiratory pattern.[31]

During the compensatory phase of increased ICP, the body temperature usually remains within normal limits. In the decompensatory phase, however, it may rise very high as a result of hypothalamic dysfunction.

Papilledema

Papilledema is commonly seen in patients with chronic increased ICP; however, it is rarely seen in patients with head injury, even in the presence of raised ICP.[32] Usually by the time papilledema occurs, the ICP has reached markedly elevated levels. The aforementioned signs and symptoms, therefore, are more reliable indicators of the beginning stages of increased ICP.

Headache

Although not always present with increased ICP, headache represents pressure against those intracranial structures that are sensitive to pain. These structures include the middle meningeal arteries and branches, the large arteries at the base of the brain, the venous sinuses, and the dura at the base of the skull. When headache is present in the patient with increased ICP, it typically is worse on arising in the morning.

Vomiting

Vomiting is not always present with increased ICP. When it occurs, it is characteristically projectile in nature and indicates pressure against the vomiting center in the medulla.

CENTRAL DIABETES INSIPIDUS

As described in Chapter 4, central diabetes insipidus (CDI) is manifested by an abrupt onset of polyuria and polydipsia. The usual urine volume is 8 to 10 L/day.[33] Conscious patients usually exhibit extreme thirst and will drink large volumes of fluid, if able. For unknown reasons, there may be a preference for iced drinks. Because of the sustained polyuria, sleep deprivation can be a problem. Failure to consume enough fluids to adequately to match the large urine volume will produce profound volume depletion. Because the unconscious patient cannot experience thirst, or respond to it, there is a need to replace fluids by the parenteral route, titrated according to urine output and laboratory results. Classic laboratory findings include hypernatremia and slight serum hyperosmolality. Urine specific gravity is usually less than 1.005 and urine osmolality less than 200 mOsm/kg.

It should be noted that CDI may be triphasic in critically ill patients. That is, it may occur transiently for a few days after surgery or trauma and then resolve for a few days, only to reoccur.[34] Therefore, one should closely monitor urine output and laboratory values. Especially important are serum sodium and osmolality, as well as urine specific gravity or osmolality.

The reader is referred to Table 4-9 for a summary of clinical manifestations of diabetes insipidus and to Table 4-10 for a summary of assessments for this condition.

SYNDROME OF INAPPROPRIATE ANTIDIURETIC HORMONE SECRETION

The clinical criteria for SIADH includes hyponatremia, a high urine sodium concentration (>20 mmol/L), and a urine osmolality that exceeds serum osmolality.[35] The reader is referred to Table 4-4 for a detailed summary of clinical manifestations and laboratory findings in SIADH, and to Table 4-5 for a summary of nursing assessment for this condition.

CEREBRAL SALT WASTING

Differentiating cerebral salt wasting from SIADH is difficult, and routine laboratory tests are not very helpful. ADH is elevated in both syndromes; thus, careful assessment of the volume status is the most helpful feature. Weight loss of more than 1 kg/day (or other signs of hypovolemia) in the presence of worsening hyponatremia favors the conclusion of cerebral salt wasting.[36] The hyponatremia seen in cerebral salt wasting is attributed to true sodium loss as opposed to the dilutional effect associated with SIADH.

NURSING DIAGNOSES RELATED TO FLUID BALANCE

See Clinical Tip: Examples of Nursing Diagnoses Related to Fluid Balance in the Head-Injured Patient for a list of possible nursing diagnoses related to fluid and electrolyte problems in patients with brain injury. Interventions related to these nursing diagnoses are discussed below.

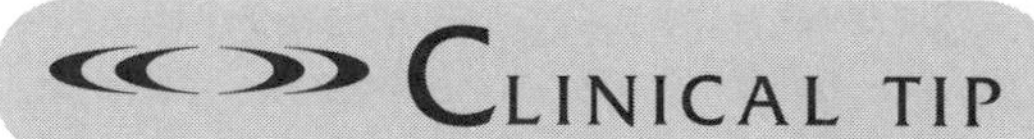

Interventions to Minimize Increased Intracranial Pressure

- Elevate the head of the bed to a 30° angle (as long as it does not interfere with cerebral perfusion).
- Keep the patient's head in a neutral (straight plane) position; avoid neck flexion and extension.
- Use a turn sheet to move the patient.
- Encourage the patient to exhale while turning or pushing self up in bed.
- Minimize noxious stimuli; use medications as indicated.
- Prevent constipation (straining for stools elevates ICP).
- Maintain a patent airway.
- Preoxygenate prior to suctioning; use intermittent brief suctioning, one or two passes for less than 10 seconds.
- If necessary, lidocaine may be used (with physician's order) during suctioning.[44]
- Maintain a quiet environment (noise can precipitate elevated ICP in a patient with an unstable ICP).
- Administer fluids cautiously to avoid accidental fluid overload.
- Monitor blood gases. Be alert for changes in PaO_2 and $PaCO_2$, be aware that the PaO_2 should be maintained at a suitable level (such as >70 mmHg) and the $PaCO_2$ should not be allowed to elevate above normal. (Indeed, the prescribed regimen frequently calls for decreasing it to below normal levels, such as 30–35 mmHg when ICP is elevated.)
- Monitor ICP readings and neurological signs. Implement prescribed medical regimen as appropriate.
- Monitor serum electrolytes and osmolality. Be particularly alert for hyponatremia since this condition tends to favor cerebral edema by promoting cellular swelling.
- Monitor temperature; administer antipyretics when appropriate.
- Use gentle tactile stimulation.[45]
- Use gentle auditory stimulation, calling the patient by name.[46]

ICP, intracranial pressure.

INTERVENTIONS

ELEVATED INTRACRANIAL PRESSURE

Management of the patient with elevated ICP is complex, evolving, and to some extent controversial. Nursing and medicine are both modifying protocols based on new research findings. However, basic to all interventions is ongoing neurological assessment. Depending on the patient's condition, the neurological and vital signs must be assessed every 15 min to every 4 hrs. The assessment should include mental status, level of consciousness, motor and sensory function, pupillary size, reaction to light, and eye movements. Results of each examination should be compared with those of previous assessments; significant changes should be promptly reported. Early subtle signs must be identified and acted on immediately because these signs can herald a change from a compensatory neurological status to one of irreversible decompensation.

In addition to continuing assessments, nursing interventions must be performed to meet the patient's basic needs. Nursing interventions for patients with elevated ICP have been the subject of much nursing research and, in some cases, have produced conflicting results. Some interventions have been shown to increase ICP (see Table 19-1). Activities that increase ICP should not be clustered together due to their cumulative effects.[41] For patients in whom *any* nursing interventions can precipitate dangerous levels of increased ICP, sedation may be required.[42] Potent analgesics (such as fentanyl and midazolam) may be required to control ICP.[43] In addition, efforts should be directed toward nursing interventions that prevent or minimize increased ICP (see Clinical Tip: Interventions to Minimize Increased Intracranial Pressure).

Standard therapeutic interventions that continue to be used in the management of increased ICP include hyperventilation, osmotic diuretics, fluid restriction, temperature control, and ventricular drainage.

TABLE 19–1

Nursing Activities That May Increase Intracranial Pressure[37–39]

- Suctioning the patient frequently (particularly when rotating the head to reach the mainstem bronchi)
- Turning the patient frequently
- Discussing the patient's condition or prognosis at the bedside*
- Placing the patient on the bedpan
- Rotating the patient's head
- Rapidly shifting the patient's position
- Range of motion exercises
- Applying noxious stimuli during nursing assessment

A recent study by Johnson et al.[40] indicated that neither an emotionally referenced conversation about the patient's condition nor any type of conversation significantly increased intracranial pressure over baseline.

Maintenance of Adequate Ventilation

If respiratory insufficiency is present as a result of brain injury, elevated levels of carbon dioxide (hypercapnia) and decreased levels of oxygen (hypoxemia) would be expected. Both hypercapnia and hypoxemia are potent vasodilating factors and thus contribute to increased ICP. Although hypercapnia and hypoxemia often occur together, hypercapnia alone will stimulate vasodilation.[47]

Recently, a method of detecting cerebral oxygenation by measuring oxygen saturation with a catheter in the jugular bulb (as it leaves the brain) has been introduced; this measure is know as the jugular venous oxygen saturation (SjO_2). A normal value should be between 60% and 80%. If the SjO_2 is between 50% and 55%, cerebral hypoxemia should be suspected. A low SjO_2 indicates rising oxygen demands and may be due to anemia, respiratory insufficiency, or low cardiac output.[48]

Because the effects of inadequate ventilation on ICP are so harmful, it is important to maintain respiratory function. Rate and quality of respirations should be assessed, and breath sounds should be auscultated at regular intervals. Interference with breathing related to complete or partial obstruction of the airway by mucus can be alleviated by periodic suctioning. For those patients who are intubated, guidelines have been developed to reduce the consequences of hypoxia and hypercapnea while suctioning the severely brain-injured patient. These include preoxygenating patients to prevent suction-induced hypoxia, limiting suctioning to less than 10 sec, and suction passes to only one or two. The use of suction at a negative pressure of more than 120 mmHg

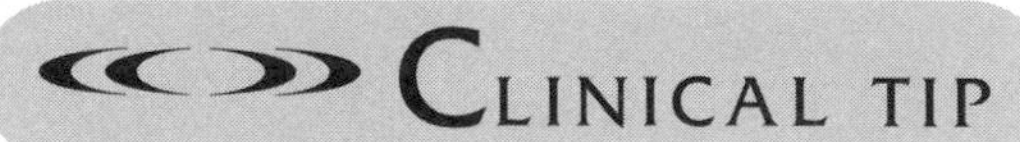

Examples of Nursing Diagnoses Related to Fluid Balance in the Head-Injured Patient

NURSING DIAGNOSIS	ETIOLOGICAL FACTORS	DEFINING CHARACTERISTICS
Alteration in cerebral perfusion related to cerebral edema	Interruption of cerebral venous and arterial blood flow	Decreased cognitive functioning, decreased level of consciousness
Hypervolemia related to early use of osmotic diuretic	Osmotic diuretic pulls fluid from cellular and interstitial spaces into bloodstream Decreased renal function (interferes with ability to excrete excess fluid)	Moist crackles Urine volume below level designated by physician (usually should be at least 30–50 mL/hr)
Alteration in sodium balance (hyponatremia) related to early use of mannitol, SIADH, or abnormal water gain or sodium loss (cerebral salt wasting)	Diffusion of water into bloodstream caused by early use of mannitol dilutes the serum Na^+ level Excessive secretion of ADH Excessive administration of free water in tube feedings or parenterally as D_5W	Serum Na^+ <135 mEq/L Serum osmolality <280 mOsm/kg ICP may increase because acute hyponatremia favors cellular swelling Neurological symptoms may worsen
Alteration in sodium balance (hypernatremia) with FVD related to prolonged use of osmotic diuretics or to diabetes insipidus	Osmotic diuretics (most often mannitol) cause a relatively greater loss of water than sodium (prolonged use can lead to an excess of sodium in the bloodstream) Deficiency of ADH leads to large renal water losses, causing serum Na^+ concentration to elevate	Serum Na^+ > 145 mEq/L Serum osmolality > 300 mOsm/kg Signs of FVD
Alteration in potassium balance (hypokalemia) related to use of osmotic and loop diuretics	Both osmotic and loop diuretics increase urinary K^+ losses	Serum K^+ <3.5 mEq/L Weakness, decreased bowel motility, arrhythmias
Potential for greater increase in ICP related to ineffective breathing	Respiratory insufficiency (due to cerebral edema) Obstruction of airway with mucus	PaO_2 <70 mmHg $PaCO_2$ >35 mmHg (or designated level) Decreased rate and depth of respirations Signs of increased ICP
Sensory-perceptual alteration (visual, auditory, gustatory, kinesthetic, tactile, olfactory) related to cerebral edema	Altered sensory perception, transmission, or integration	Disorientation, altered conceptualization, reported or measured changes in sensory acuity, changes in behavior pattern

ADH, antidiuretic hormone; FVD, fluid volume deficit; ICP, intracranial pressure; SIADH, syndrome of inappropriate antidiuretic hormone secretion.

and the use of catheters that occlude more than 50% of the endotracheal tube should be avoided.[49] The drainage of secretions pooled in the mouth can be facilitated by turning the patient from side to side at least every 2 hrs.

Clinical assessment of respiratory status must rely ultimately on arterial blood gas analyses to assess ventilation adequately. Findings from blood gas studies are crucial in planning measures to minimize increases in ICP. Some authorities recommend that the partial pressure of oxygen in arterial blood (PaO_2) be maintained at least at 70 mmHg (by intubation if necessary).[50] The partial pressure of carbon dioxide in arterial blood ($PaCO_2$) is often purposely lowered below normal as both a short- and long-term therapeutic measure for increased ICP.

Hyperventilation

The role of hyperventilation in managing ICP is somewhat controversial as the ability of the cerebrovascular vessels to respond may be compromised after a cerebral insult. Theoretically, lowering the arterial carbon dioxide pressure by inducing hyperventilation results in cerebral vasoconstriction and, therefore, prompt lowering of ICP by decreasing cerebral blood volume. (This works only in patients whose cerebrovascular vessels are able to respond by vasoconstricting.) Clinical studies indicate an acute reduction in arterial $PaCO_2$ of 5 to 10 mmHg lowers ICP approximately 25% to 50% in most patients.[51] The inability to lower ICP by hyperventilation is a grave prognostic indicator identifying a patient with a massive area of damaged brain.[52]

Hyperventilation reduces ICP by causing vasoconstriction of cerebral arterioles in response to lowered $PaCO_2$; a $PaCO_2$ of 30–35 mmHg is thought to be optimal, since lower levels may result in focal ischemia due to excessive vasoconstriction.[53] Care should be taken to avoid excessive decreasing of the $PaCO_2$ because severe vasoconstriction and decreased cerebral blood flow can occur. It is believed that the resulting ischemia causes vasodilatation (which contributes to cerebral edema), offsetting the effects of further hyperventilation.[54]

In severely head-injured patients, there is evidence that hyperventilation for more than 6 hrs may decrease the ability of cerebrovascular vessels to constrict in response to a lowered $PaCO_2$ level.[55] These patients experience an ischemic phase 12 to 24 hrs after injury; and, if hyperventilation is initiated too early (within the first 24 hrs), it may contribute to detrimental patient outcomes.[56]

Before administering high concentrations of oxygen during the hyperventilation process, the respiratory system should be assessed for lung pathology and, if present, specific guidelines for oxygen therapy must be provided by the physician.

Osmotic Agents and Other Diuretics

If treatments such as hyperventilation and head positioning in a straight plane at a 30° angle are not effective in lowering ICP, osmotic diuretics (such as mannitol) or loop diuretics (such as furosemide) may be indicated. In patients with vasogenic cerebral edema, osmotic diuretics reduce cerebral volume by pulling fluid out of healthy brain tissue into the bloodstream for subsequent excretion by the kidneys. Osmotherapy also reduces brain volume in patients with hypoosmolality, but is rarely useful in interstitial edema.[57] Furosemide has a diuretic effect on the renal tubules and possibly reduces CSF formation. Used in combination, mannitol and furosemide seem to have a synergistic effect in controlling elevated ICP.[58]

The primary osmotic diuretic is mannitol (Osmitrol). Mannitol has been shown to reduce ICP consistently and increase cerebral perfusion pressure within 10 to 20 min or less in head-injured patients with increased ICP.[59] Dosage varies and is calculated according to body weight. Before administering the drug, check the vital signs, urinary output, and body weight, and review the chart for serum electrolytes and renal function studies. Cardiac status should also be evaluated.

Hemodynamic Monitoring

Soon after administration of mannitol, the intravascular volume is expanded as fluid is pulled into the bloodstream from the tissues. Because of the potential for pulmonary edema, some authorities favor monitoring CVP, and even pulmonary wedge pressures, in patients with questionable cardiovascular function.

Assessment of Hydration

The status of hydration should be monitored closely. Measurement of fluid intake and output (I&O) is mandatory; frequency should be designated by the physician (such as every 15–30 min, or hourly). To facilitate accurate measurements, an indwelling urinary catheter is usually used for adults, and a pediatric collection device for children. At times it may be helpful to measure the urinary specific gravity to assess renal function and hydrational status. Vital signs should be monitored every 30 min or as ordered. The rate of infusion is usually adjusted to maintain a urine flow of at least 30 to 50 mL/hr.[60] A volume less than this amount (or an amount designated by the physician) should prompt discontinuance of mannitol to prevent fluid overload and fulminant congestive heart failure. (This is because the kidneys must be able to excrete the fluid being pulled into the bloodstream.) Serum creatinine and blood urea nitrogen (BUN) levels should be monitored to evaluate renal function and hydration status. (Osmotic diuretics are contraindicated in patients with significant renal disease because these individuals cannot effectively eliminate the excess fluid volume.) Variations in body weight should be monitored to detect excessive fluid retention or loss; an accurate in-bed scale is most useful. The serum osmolality should be measured at regular intervals. It should not exceed 320 mOsm/kg; the diuresis resulting from mannitol administration may exacerbate hypovolemia and hypotension.[61]

Assessment of Electrolyte Levels

Measurement of electrolytes, primarily sodium and potassium, is of vital importance in monitoring response to mannitol therapy. Be alert for imbalances in sodium and potassium and report their occurrence immediately. With mannitol use, there is initially an expansion of the plasma volume caused by diffusion of water into the bloodstream; therefore, hyponatremia is a possible complication. Later, as the fluid is excreted through the kidneys, hypernatremia may be observed (as relatively more water is excreted than sodium). Mannitol should not be administered if the serum sodium level exceeds 150 mEq/L.[62] Because the serum sodium level can be either decreased or increased with mannitol therapy, measured serum levels should be observed closely and abnormalities reported at once. Similarly, serum potassium levels may be variable. Hyperkalemia can occur when potassium levels build up in the bloodstream during presence of oliguria; conversely, hypokalemia can result when potassium is eliminated during the osmotic diuresis. See Chapters 4 and 5 for descriptions of sodium and potassium imbalances.

A potential problem associated with mannitol use (and other osmotic diuretics) is a rebound increase in ICP.[63] The rebound may result from retention of mannitol in the brain tissue as the blood mannitol level is dropping; this situation reverses the pressure gradient and allows water to diffuse back into the brain tissue, increasing ICP.

Corticosteroids

The efficacy of corticosteroids in the treatment of increased ICP is doubtful; however, they are effective in particular forms of cerebral edema. They are believed to be beneficial in vasogenic edema (as seen in brain tumor and abscess) but are not effective in cytotoxic edema (as in acute hyponatremia or hypoxia) and are of uncertain effectiveness in interstitial edema.[64] The most common corticosteroid given for control of increased ICP is dexamethasone (Decadron). When dexamethasone is administered, one should anticipate complications such as hyperglycemia, gastrointestinal (GI) bleeding, and increased incidence of infection. It is customary to monitor blood glucose levels during massive steroid therapy. Antacids are usually administered to patients receiving large doses of steroids, and H_2-receptor antagonists may be used to decrease gastric acidity.

Currently, clinical trials are evaluating the effectiveness of a new hydroxyl radical scavenger, known as 21-aminosteroid (tirilazad mesylate, U 74006 F). Therapeutic effects are believed to include scavenging free oxygen radicals, reducing cerebral edema, and enhancing cellular integrity. If results are favorable, these steroids may be part of the clinical protocol to manage increased ICP.[65]

High-Dosage Barbiturate Therapy

In recent years, barbiturates (most commonly pentobarbital) have been used to manage elevated ICP, primarily in patients who have not responded to more conventional methods. Barbiturates induce a significant decrease in cerebral blood flow and cerebral metabolism.[66] The subsequent effect is a lowering of cerebral blood volume and ICP. It is not known if the effects are sustained and if the eventual outcome is altered. With barbiturate therapy, continuous monitoring of ICP, arterial and preferably pulmonary capillary wedge pressures, and cardiac output is indicated.[67]

A major risk of barbiturate therapy is acute hypotension. This can profoundly affect the patient with a compromised myocardium. Hypothermia may also develop; however, core body temperature should not be allowed to drop below 34 °C (93.2 °F) because of the risk of cardiac instability.[68]

Certain components of the neurological assessment (such as level of consciousness and ability to follow commands) are, of course, negated by barbiturate therapy. However, pupillary dilatation as a result of brain stem compression will still occur at serum barbiturate levels of up to 3 or 4 mg %.[69] After achievement of a satisfactory ICP (<20 mmHg for 24–48 hrs), gradual reduction of the barbiturate dosage can begin.[70]

Fluid Restriction

In some patients, restriction of fluids from a half to two thirds of maintenance needs is all that is required to control ICP. Both the type and volume of fluids are important. Most clinicians avoid the administration of free water (such as 5% dextrose in water [D_5W]) in patients at risk for cerebral edema because a lowered serum sodium predisposes to this condition. Instead, half-strength normal saline (0.45% sodium chloride) is considered a suitable fluid.[71] For patients who are hyponatremic, or likely to become so, the physician may consider the use of 5% dextrose in normal saline (or its equivalent).[72] In those patients who require osmotic or other diuretic therapy, liberalization of iso-osmotic fluid intake to prevent dehydration is appropriate,[73] based on the following clinical parameters. These factors must be considered in determining fluid needs of patients at risk for cerebral edema:

- It is generally agreed that the desired amount of fluid to be administered should be based on the patient's serum osmolality, BUN, and electrolyte levels. Remember that the neurological patient is at risk for sodium imbalances in either direction.
- Of course, fluid therapy must also provide for any abnormal losses (such as occur from gastric suction, abdominal bleeding, or third-space fluid shifts related to major fractures). Care of the brain-injured patient with chest, abdominal, or orthopedic injuries is complicated. The clinician must judiciously balance fluid intake to maintain adequate circulating volume while not overloading the cerebral circulation.

Failure to maintain an adequate vascular volume interferes with cerebral perfusion pressure (CPP). The mechanism by which CPP and cerebral blood volume (CBV) remains constant is known as autoregulation. After a cerebral insult, the brain's ability to autoregulate may be disrupted. Recall that CPP equals mean arterial pressure (MAP) minus intracranial pressure (ICP). Thus, a low MAP associated with hypovolemia has serious implications for the cerebral perfusion pressure. The CPP should be maintained within a range of 60 to 70 mmHg.[74] Sustained low CPP readings have been directly associated with morbidity and mortality in neurologic patients. Care must be taken not to restrict fluids excessively in patients receiving dehydrating agents (such as osmotic or loop diuretics).

The amount of fluid to be administered to patients at risk for cerebral edema and elevated ICP requires careful consideration. Physician's orders should be specific and the patient's response to the fluids carefully monitored. Significant findings should be quickly communicated to the physician for necessary modifications in the fluid directives.

Temperature Control

Any elevation in body temperature must be controlled because this will increase the brain's need for oxygen, thereby increasing cerebral blood flow (and, in turn, ICP). Elevated temperature can be treated with antipyretic medications used alone or in conjunction with a cooling blanket.

Ventricular Drainage

In an attempt to control erratic increases in the ICP, a ventriculostomy may be performed in some patients. This involves the insertion of a drainage catheter into a cerebral ventricle for the purpose of draining off excess CSF. Because of the continual threat of infection, ventriculostomy patients are frequently given prophylactic antibiotics. Nursing responsibilities in caring for a patient with ventricular drainage include:

- Promoting absolute sterility of the equipment.
- Maintaining a sterile dry dressing at the catheter and incision site.
- Keeping the collection container adjusted to a level indicated by the physician.
- Observing the drainage system for kinks to assure patency of the tube.
- Observing and recording the amount of drainage in the collection container.

CENTRAL DIABETES INSIPIDUS

Patients with large urinary losses from CDI need water replacement. It may be given by mouth if the patient is conscious. If not, it may be given by the parenteral route in the form of D_5W or half-normal saline, depending on the patient's volume status and degree of water deficit.[75] To avoid producing cerebral edema, only half of the water deficit plus insensible water loss should be replaced in the first 24 hrs; the rest of the deficit can be replaced over the next 24 to 48 hrs.[76] Frequent assessment of neurological status is indicated to look for cerebral edema, a complication that can result from accumulation of intracellular solute during dehydration.[77] In addition to water, magnesium and potassium may be needed to replace losses of these electrolytes in the urine.

Acute diabetes insipidus after surgery or trauma may be treated with short-acting aqueous Pitressin. After a period, the treatment may be temporarily discontinued to determine if the diabetes insipidus is transient or permanent.

With administration of ADH substances, it is conceivable that the patient may become fluid overloaded if fluid intake (IV and oral) exceeds fluid output. Fluid overload may also result if third-space fluid from other injuries shifts back into the vascular space at the time ADH is being administered. Excessive water retention may cause the serum sodium level to drop below normal. Close assessment of neurological signs and laboratory data are required to maintain the delicate balance required with ADH replacement therapy in the patient with CDI.

SYNDROME OF INAPPROPRIATE ANTIDIURETIC HORMONE SECRETION

As is the case with all causes of SIADH, restriction of electrolyte-free water intake is indicated.[78] Adequate free water restriction will eventually increase the serum sodium concentration. In nonedematous patients in some situations, extra salt may be given in the diet or in the form of salt tablets in combination with mild fluid restriction.[79] However, if severe symptoms are present, it may be necessary to cautiously infuse a hypertonic saline solution (such as 3% of 5% NaCl). As discussed in Chapter 4, these solutions are extremely dangerous and should be handled with care. Hypertonic saline should be administered only in intensive care units under close observation. They are best administered in 100-mL containers to avoid an inadvertent excessive dosage. The reader is referred to Clinical Tip: Nursing Considerations in Administration of Hypertonic Saline Solutions in Chapter 4 for additional information regarding nursing considerations in administering hypertonic saline, and to Table 4-6 for a list of nursing interventions related to SIADH therapy.

CEREBRAL SALT WASTING

The concept of cerebral salt wasting has necessitated alternative therapy to manage susceptible neurological patients. Failure to correct severe hyponatremia may result in severe neurological deficits or even death. Although hyponatremia is present in both cerebral salt wasting and SIADH, opposite treatment strategies are recommended. True SIADH requires volume restriction and maintenance of adequate salt intake. Daily fluid intake is reduced allowing water losses to exceed intake and serum sodium concentration to rise. In contrast, treatment for the hyponatremia associated with SAH includes intravascular volume resuscitation and sodium replacement. Isotonic sodium solutions (such as 0.9% NaCl) or colloid (such as 5% albumin or fresh frozen plasma) may be used to expand the intravascular volume to reduce the stimulus for ADH secretion.[80] The regime for hypervolemia should be guided by a central venous pressure (CVP) of more than 10 cm H_2O or a pulmonary artery wedge pressure (PAWP) of more than 12 mmHg.[81] Fluid therapy, in conjunction with hypertensive therapy (a blood pressure of 10 mmHg more than normal value) and early administration of calcium entry blocking drugs (nimodipine) has been shown to reduce the incidence of brain infarction from vasospasm, a frequent complication of SAH.[82] This complex protocol (based on broad experience rather than prospective study)[83] requires the nurse to manage the deleterious effects of potential hypotension (associated with calcium channel blockers) with the effects of hypertensive hypervolemic therapy.

CASE STUDIES

19-1. A 35-year-old man was injured in a multiple vehicle accident and sustained a basilar skull fracture and multiple facial bruises. Upon admission to the Emergency Room, the patient was unconscious, with a Glasgow coma scale score of 7 and no focal neurologic abnormalities. A long bone fracture was discovered, and the patient received fluid resuscitation of large amounts of lactated Ringer's solution. Mannitol (100 mg) was given to treat his head injury. Twelve hours after the injury, the patient's urine output was noted to exceed 1 L/hr and the following laboratory data were available:

Serum sodium	=	175 mEq/L
Serum potassium	=	4.3 mEq/L
Serum chloride	=	134 mEq/L
Serum osmolality	=	365 mOsm/L
Urine sodium	=	10 mEq/L
Urine osmolality	=	80 mOsm/L

COMMENTARY The laboratory data are consistent with CDI. The serum sodium is markedly elevated, as is the serum osmolality. In contrast, the urine sodium and osmolality are low, reflecting large water loss in the urine. Basilar skull fracture is commonly associated with CDI.

After treatment with vasopressin, the urine volume should diminish and the serum sodium level should decrease.

Note that while a conscious patient with CDI would likely experience thirst and therefore drink extra fluids, an unconscious patient cannot make these responses. Thus, continued loss of large volumes of urine without adequate fluid replacement could result in severe hypovolemia.

19-2. A.J., a 30-year-old woman, presented in the emergency room with complaints of severe headache, vertigo, and stiff neck. She denied chest pain and had a normal electrocardiograph. Previously, she had been in good health and denied a history of hypertension or drug use. A head computed tomogram (CT) was done in the emergency room and showed an SAH.

Upon admission to the intensive care unit (ICU) she was lethargic, but opened her eyes when her name was called and responded appropriately to orientation questions before drifting back to sleep. A.J.'s pupils were 4/4 and brisk, her extraocular movements (EOM) were intact, her face was symmetrical, and her tongue was midline. She moved all extremities well; however, her left grasp was slightly weaker than the right.

A cerebral angiogram confirmed a right internal communicating artery aneurysm. A.J.'s heart rate (HR) was 80 to 110 beats/min, mean blood pressure (MBP) was 90 to 118 mmHg, respirations were 16 to 24 breaths/min, and her oxygen saturation was 94% to 98% on room air. A.J. was started on nimodipine (60 mg PO q4 hrs), Decadron (4 mg PO q6 hrs), Colace (100 mg PO bid), Dilantin (200 mg PO bid), Zantac (150 mg PO bid), Apresoline (5–20 mg IVP PRN), and morphine (1–2 mg IVP) for pain.

Twenty-four hours after her initial SAH, A.J. underwent a craniotomy for aneurysm clipping. Upon return to the ICU, she was alert and oriented to her name and could follow simple commands using all four extremities; her speech was clear but occasionally inappropriate. Her pupils were 2/2 brisk, her face was symmetrical, and her EOMs were intact. A left radial arterial line (A-line) was placed in the operating room to monitor her MBP; orders were received to maintain the pressure at more than 100 mmHg. In addition, a pulmonary artery catheter was placed in her right subclavian vein to monitor PAWP every hour and cardiac output readings every 2 hrs. Twenty hours after surgery, the patient's level of consciousness changed; she became lethargic and did not follow commands. No other neurologic deficits were apparent. Her MBP was 70 mmHg, CVP 2 mmHg, and the pulmonary capillary wedge pressure (PCWP) was 5 mmHg (all indicative of hypovolemia). At this time, her serum sodium level was found to be 130 mEq/L.

COMMENTARY: This patient was experiencing a cerebral vasospasm, a potential complication from SAH. Because of failure to administer intravenous fluids in sufficient volume to match her urinary sodium loss, she developed fluid volume deficit with hyponatremia (which in turn contributed to the cerebral vasospasm). Hyponatremia can signal either SIADH or cerebral salt wasting. In this case, because the hyponatremia coexisted with clinical signs of fluid volume deficit, it was more likely a problem of cerebral salt wasting (true sodium loss in the urine). The patient required additional administration of 0.9% sodium chloride to reduce the adverse effects of the cerebral vasospasm and hyponatremia.

REFERENCES

1. Williams MA, Razumovsky AY: Cerebrospinal fluid circulation, cerebral edema, and intracranial pressure. Curr Sci 6(6); 847,1993
2. Marshall et al: Neuroscience Critical Care: Pathophysiology and Patient Management, p 152. Philadelphia, WB Saunders, 1990
3. Chestnut RM, Marshall LF: Treatment of intracranial pressure. Neurosurg Clin North Am 2:269,1991
4. Hartman A, Stingele R, Schnitzer M. General treatment strategies for elevated intracranial pressure. In: Hacke W (ed): Neuro Critical Care, p 102. Berlin, Springer-Verlag, 1994
5. Ibid, p 102
6. Schmidley S: Cerebrospinal fluid, blood brain barrier and brain edema. In: Pearlman A, Collins R (eds): Neurological Pathophysiology, 4th ed, p 337. New York, Oxford Press, 1988
7. Ibid, p 340
8. Williams, Ibid, p 848
9. Kokko J, Tannen R: Fluids and Electrolytes, 2nd ed, p 169. Philadelphia, WB Saunders, 1990
10. Maxwell M, Kleeman C, Narins R: Clinical Disorders of Fluid and Electrolyte Metabolism, 4th ed, p 922. New York, McGraw-Hill, 1987
11. Furlan AJ, Busse O, Ringelstein EB, Hanley DF: Special aspects in the treatment of severe hemispheric brain infarction. In: Hacke W (ed.): Neuro Critical Care, 1st ed, p 590. Berlin, Springer-Verlag, 1994
12. Winston KR, Breeze R: Hydraulic regulation of brain parenchymal volume. Neurolog Res 13:December, p 251, 1992
13. Kantor MJ, Narayan RK: Intracranial monitoring. Neurosurg Clin North Am 2:258,1991
14. Hund EF, Bohrer H, Martin E, Hanley DF: Disturbances of water and electrolyte balance. In: Hacke W (ed): Neuro Critical Care, 1st ed, p 924. Berlin, Springer-Verlag, 1994
15. Ibid, p 924
16. Ibid, p 925
17. Archer DP, Shaw DA, Leblanc RL, Tranmer BI: Hemodynamic considerations in the management of patients with subarachnoid hemorrhage. Can J Anesthesiol 38(4):457,1991
18. Segatore M: Hyponatremia after aneurysmal subarachnoid hemorrhage. J Neurosci Nurs 25:92,1993
19. Archer et al, p 457
20. Hund et al, p 925
21. Ibid, p 925
22. Segatore, p 93
23. Ibid, p 93
24. Hund et al, p 925
25. Andrus C: Intracranial pressure dynamics and nursing management. J Neurosci Nurs 23:862,1991.
26. Chestnut, Marshall, p 270
27. Doyle PJ, Mark PW: Analysis of intracranial pressure. J Clin Monitor 5:81,1993
28. Hartman et al, p 105
29. Ibid, p 104
30. Ibid, p 107
31. Ibid, p 107
32. Ibid, p 107
33. Morrison G, Singer I: Hyperosmolal states. In: Narins R (ed): Maxwell and Kleemans, Clinical Disorders of Fluid and Electrolyte Metabolism, 5th ed, p 630. New York, McGraw Hill, 1994
34. Ibid, p 637
35. Hund et al, p 924
36. Ibid, p 925
37. Mitchell P, Mauss N: Relationship of patient–nurse activity to intracranial pressure variations. Nurs Res 27:4,1978
38. Boortz-Marx R: Factors affecting intracranial pressure: A descriptive study. J Neurosci Nurs 4:89,1985
39. Mitchell P, Ozuma J, Lipe H: Moving the patient in bed: Effects on intracranial pressure. Nurs Res 30:216,1980
40. Johnson S, Omery A, Nikas D: Effects of conversation on intracranial pressure in comatose patients. Heart Lung 18:56,1988
41. Parsons C, Smith A, Page M: The effects of hygiene interventions on the cerebrovascular status of severe closed head injured patients. Res Nurs Health 8:178,1985

42. Haitman et al, p 108
43. Kerr ME, Rudy EB, Brucia J, Stone KS: Head-injured adults: recommendations for endotracheal suctioning. J Neurosci Nurs 25:86,1993.
44. Greenberg J, Brawansky A: Cranial trauma. In: Hacke W(ed): Neuro Critical Care, p 696. Berlin, Springer-Verlag, 1994.
45. Walleck C: Controversies in the management of head-injured patients, Crit Care Nurs Clin North Am 1(1):72,1989
46. Pollack L, Goldsteen G: Lowering of intracranial pressure in Reye's syndrome by sensory stimulation. N Engl J Med 304:732,1981
47. Chestnut, Marshall, p 277
48. Ibid, p 193
49. Kerr, p 87
50. Chestnut, Marshall, p 277
51. Marshall, p 193
52. Ibid
53. Shoemaker W, Ayers S, Grenvik A, Holbrook P (eds): Textbook of Critical Care, 3rd ed, p 314. Philadelphia, W.B. Saunders, 1995
54. Ibid
55. Kerr ME, Brucia J: Hyperventilation in the head-injured patient: an effective treatment modality? Heart Lung 22(6):516,1993
56. Ibid, p 518
57. Chestnut, Marshall, p 277–278
58. Ibid, p 278
59. Ibid
60. Marshall, p 195
61. Shoemaker et al, p 1534
62. Ibid
63. Chestnut, Marshall, p 278
64. Hartman, p 108
65. Furlan, p 590
66. Marshall, p 199
67. Ibid
68. Ibid
69. Ibid, p 200
70. Ibid
71. Hund, p 924
72. Ibid, p 925
73. Ibid
74. Chestnut, Marshall, p 269
75. Kokko, Tannen, p 835
76. Ibid
77. Ibid
78. Ibid, p 172
79. Ibid
80. Adams HP: Prevention of brain ischemia after aneurysmal subarachnoid hemorrhage. Neurol Clin 10(1):251–268,1992
81. Ibid
82. Steiner H, Fink M, Kremer P, Diringer M: Subarachnoid hemorrhage. In: Hacke W (ed): Neuro Critical Care, p 648. Berlin, Springer-Verlag, 1994
83. Alvisi C, Giulioni M, Ursino M: The control mechanism involved in post-subarachnoid hemorrhage vasospasm. J Neurosurg Sci 35(1):1–8,1991

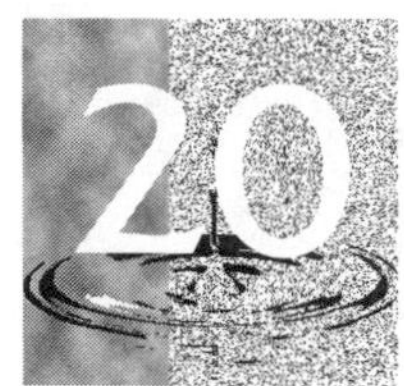

Acute Pancreatitis

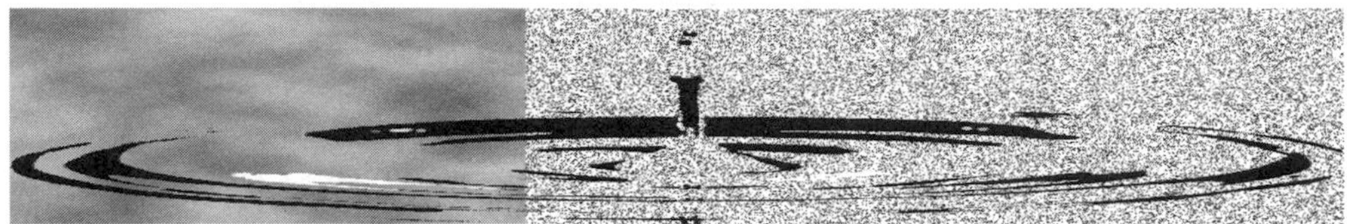

PATHOPHYSIOLOGY

Acute pancreatitis is a nonbacterial inflammation of the pancreas caused by digestion of the gland by its own enzymes.[1] The pancreas becomes edematous and may pull enough fluid into itself to produce hypovolemia; swelling may be severe enough to compress the vascular bed and cause ischemia and necrosis. In addition, severe pancreatitis can produce irritation of the peritoneal surface (measuring 1.0–1.5 m^2) and cause the transudation of substantial volumes of protein-rich fluid.[2]

Tissue changes are characterized by pancreatic and peripancreatic edema and fat necrosis; this form of the disease is sometimes referred to as edematous pancreatitis. [3] A more severe form involves extensive pancreatic and peripancreatic fat necrosis, and hemorrhage into and around the pancreas (referred to hemorrhagic or necrotizing pancreatitis).[4]

ETIOLOGICAL ASSOCIATIONS

Acute pancreatitis is a common disorder.[5] Collectively, biliary tract stone disease and alcohol abuse account for 60% to 80% of the cases of pancreatitis.[6] Among other possible causes are trauma and operation and certain drugs (such as steroids and thiazide diuretics); sometimes the cause is unknown and is labeled idiopathic.

FLUID AND ELECTROLYTE DERANGEMENTS

HYPOVOLEMIA

In acute pancreatitis, pancreatic inflammation and autodigestion lead to peripancreatic edema and loss of edema fluid and/or blood into the retroperitoneal tissue. Release of digestive enzymes from the inflamed pancreas can cause a peritoneal burn that, when severe, equals a burn covering up to a third of the body's surface.[7] The resulting fluid shifts from the extracellular space may produce profound hypovolemia. This hypovolemia's severity depends on the extent of fluid and blood lost in the retroperitoneum and peritoneal cavity; the volume of fluid sequestered in the bowel during adynamic ileus; and the volume of vomitus or fluid loss from nasogastric suction. Acute renal failure may follow untreated severe intravascular volume depletion; in this case, both the blood urea nitrogen and the serum creatinine levels will increase. The hematocrit may be elevated in edematous pancreatitis because of plasma loss from the vascular space (causing the red blood cells to be suspended in a smaller blood volume), or low in hemorrhagic pancreatitis as a result of blood loss.

Note in Table 20-1 that the estimated amount of fluid sequestered in the abdomen after the onset of pancreatitis is one of the prognostic signs for risk of complications, as is the extent to which the hematocrit is decreased (reflecting the amount of blood loss in hemorrhagic pancreatitis).

HYPOCALCEMIA

Hypocalcemia has been reported to occur in 40% to 75% of patients with acute pancreatitis.[8] In part, the drop in the total serum calcium level (sum of the ionized and bound fractions) is related to the concurrent hypoalbuminemia predictably associated with the leakage of protein-rich fluid into the peritoneal cavity. (Recall that when hypoalbuminemia is present, the total serum calcium appears lower than it actually is.) However, there also is a true decrease in ionized calcium.[9] Calcium supplementation may be indicated to prevent cardiac dysrhythmias.

Several hypotheses have been proposed to explain the hypocalcemia of acute pancreatitis. For example, discovery of calcium ions deposited in areas of fat necrosis in the pancreas led to the proposal that calcium soap formation was the main cause of hypocalcemia in pancreatitis.[10,11] However, if this were the only cause, it would be difficult to explain why parathyroid hormone (PTH) does not quickly stimulate the release of calcium stored in the bones. Recently, it has been shown that decreased secretion of PTH contributes to the hypocalcemia.[12–14] The exact etiology of hypocalcemia is not certain.[15,16]

The extent of hypocalcemia is often used as an indicator of risk for complications in the patient with acute pancreatitis (see Table 20-1).

TABLE 20–1

Prognostic Signs Used to Estimate Risk of Major Complications or Death From Acute Pancreatitis

At time of admission or diagnosis:
- Age >55 years
- WBC >16,000/mm^3
- Blood glucose >200 mg/dL
- SGOT >250 Sigma Frankel Units %

During initial 48 hrs:
- Ht decrease >10 percentage points
- BUN increase >5 mg/dL
- Serum calcium <8 mg/dL
- PaO_2 <60 mmHg
- Base deficit >4 mEq/L
- Estimated fluid sequestration >6000 mL

Information from Ranson J: Etiological and prognostic factors in human acute pancreatitis: A review. Am J Gastroenterol 77(9):633–638,1982.

HYPOMAGNESEMIA

Mild hypomagnesemia may occur during acute pancreatitis. As is the case with hypocalcemia, at least in part, hypomagnesemia has been attributed to precipitation of magnesium ions in the inflamed tissues in and around the pancreas as insoluble magnesium soaps.[17] Also, like with hypocalcemia, hypomagnesemia is often at least partially related to hypoalbuminemia (meaning that much of the change may be in bound rather than in ionized magnesium). Of course, contributing to the hypomagnesemia may be a direct loss by means of vomiting, gastric suction, and diarrhea. If the pancreatitis is due to alcoholism, the hypomagnesemia is likely to be more severe (because of the multiple magnesium-lowering effects of alcohol). A recent study concluded that patients with acute pancreatitis and hypocalcemia commonly have intracellular magnesium deficiency despite normal serum magnesium concentrations, and that magnesium deficiency may play a significant role in the pathogenesis of hypocalcemia.[18]

HYPOPHOSPHATEMIA

Hypophosphatemia may occur in patients with acute pancreatitis and is usually associated with respiratory alkalosis.[19] It has also been reported in patients with acute pancreatitis in the absence of respiratory alkalosis. Possible reasons for the association include increased catecholamine production, alterations in circulating insulin or glucagon, or the intravenous (IV) administration of glucose.[20] See Chapter 8 for a more thorough discussion of hypophosphatemia.

ACID–BASE DISTURBANCES

Acid–base disturbances may vary widely, depending on clinical circumstances. For example, metabolic alkalosis may result from the frequent vomiting associated with acute pancreatitis, as well as from the gastric suction used during treatment to put the pancreas "at rest" and to alleviate an adynamic ileus. On the other hand, a high anion gap metabolic acidosis is likely in the presence of poor tissue perfusion; a normal anion gap metabolic acidosis may be seen with acute renal failure.

The pulmonary complications to which patients with pancreatitis are predisposed (such as pneumonia, pleural effusions, pulmonary edema, pulmonary emboli, and atelectasis) may cause respiratory acid–base problems (either acidosis or alkalosis). Severe pain may stimulate ventilation and cause respiratory alkalosis.

DIAGNOSIS/PROGNOSTIC INDICATORS

The patient with acute pancreatitis usually presents with severe epigastric pain that radiates to the back, causing abdominal guarding and inability to find a comfortable position. Other common symptoms include nausea and vomiting, mild fever, tachycardia, and tachypnea. Among conditions to consider in differential diagnosis are peptic ulcer (with or without perforation), biliary colic, and small bowel obstruction and infarction.[21]

Heavily relied on in the diagnosis of acute pancreatitis is increased serum amylase activity. A serum amylase level two to three times normal, coupled with abdominal pain, is most often indicative of acute pancreatitis.[22] A number of investigators have studied commonly used combinations of clinical and laboratory data that can indicate the severity of pancreatitis within the first 48 hrs after hospital admission,[23–25] Those listed by Ranson[26] are summarized in Table 20-1. When fewer than three criteria are present, the mortality is predicted to be 1%; when three or four are present, 15%; when five or six are present, 40%; and when seven criteria or more are present, 100%. Awareness of prognostic indicators is helpful in planning the degree of aggressiveness required in therapy for acute pancreatitis. The criteria differ slightly according to the cause of pancreatitis (gallstone-related versus nongallstone-related). It has been noted that these criteria are most useful when applied to groups of patients rather than to individuals; that is, they are ideal for comparing series of patients treated in various ways.[27] Other investigators have applied the APACHE II criteria to pancreatitis patients; an advantage of this set of criteria is that it can be used at any point in the patient's illness (not just the first 48 hrs).[28]

A diagnostic peritoneal tap can be helpful in differentiating between pancreatitis and other intraabdominal conditions. A sterile, straw- to prunish-colored peritoneal fluid with a high amylase content may accompany acute pancreatitis, whereas a dark prune-colored fluid is suggestive of severe hemorrhagic pancreatitis. In contrast, foul-smelling fluid containing bacteria may suggest a perforated viscus.[29]

COMPLICATIONS

Nearly 25% of all attacks of pancreatitis are severe and lead to complications; the mortality rate approaches 9%.[30] Severe disease can be associated with both local and systemic complications. Among the local complications are necrosis, pseudocysts, abscesses, fistulas, and gastrointestinal (GI) hemorrhage. The two most common systemic complications of acute pancreatitis are renal and respiratory failure.[31]

In a study of 267 consecutive patients admitted with acute pancreatitis, 63 (24%) developed multiple organ system failure (defined as two or more organ systems).[32] Most common in this patient population were renal, respiratory, and cardiovascular failure. Depressed myocardial function may be related to the release from the inflamed pancreas of phospholipase A_2 (the so-called myocardial depressant factor).[33] To some extent, the multiple organ system failure may be caused by secondary pancreatic infections.

ACUTE RENAL FAILURE

In the above mentioned study of 267 consecutive patients with acute pancreatitis, renal failure occurred in 16%; overall mortality from acute renal failure was 81%.[34] For the most part, acute renal failure is explained on the basis of hypovolemia and hypotension.[35] In fact, renal failure from inadequate fluid replacement is a frequent finding in patients who die from pancreatitis.[36] The need for adequate fluid resuscitation to prevent this complication is obvious. Sufficient fluid replacement should be given to maintain adequate circulatory blood volume and urine output.

RESPIRATORY FAILURE

Respiratory complications (such as atelectasis, pleural effusions, pneumonia, and adult respiratory distress syndrome [ARDS]) are among the more frequent life-threatening features of patients with acute pancreatitis. Frequently there is evidence of basilar atelectasis resulting from abdominal distention and splinting of the diaphragm, as well as pleural effusions (most notable on the left side).[37] About 30% of patients with acute pancreatitis develop arterial hypoxemia (partial pressure of oxygen in arterial blood [PaO_2] <70 mmHg) and require supplemental oxygen by mask.[38] Because the onset of hypoxemia is often insidious, in most patients it is prudent to determine arterial blood gases every 12 hrs for the first several days after admission.[39]

Factors contributing to respiratory complications may include the following:

- Immobility and retained secretions
- Release of pancreatic enzymes into the systemic circulation, which may cause damage to pulmonary tissues
- Pleural effusions, more prominent on the left side (a result of inflammation from pancreatic enzymes and extravasation of fluids)

- Ascites (which interferes with respiratory excursions)
- Overzealous fluid replacement therapy

In most cases, the respiratory failure usually improves as the acute attack of pancreatitis subsides; however, some patients progress to a more severe form of respiratory failure similar in all respects to ARDS.[40] Marked hypoxemia can occur and mandate mechanical ventilation, an ominous prognostic sign.

In a laboratory study performed on rats with experimentally induced pancreatitis, it was reported that initial manifestations of pancreatitis-associated lung injury revealed a pronounced clustering of polymorphonuclear leukocytes in pulmonary microvessels, followed by severe damage of alveolar endothelial cells.[41] The increase in vascular permeability of the lung resulted in interstitial edema formation. Structural changes were maximal after 12 hrs and reversed completely after 84 hrs. The structural appearance of pulmonary injury in the laboratory animals was similar to that reported in the early stages of ARDS.

It has also been suggested that pancreatitis-associated ARDS may result from degradation of surfactant by circulating enzymes (such as phospholipase) released from the inflamed pancreas.[42] Other investigators believe that most patients with pancreatitis-associated ARDS develop the complication on a nonspecific basis as the result of uncontrolled infradiaphragmatic inflammation.[43]

TREATMENT

The treatment of acute pancreatitis is primarily supportive and includes vigorous IV fluid replacement, elimination of oral intake, possible use of nasogastric suction, adequate parenteral analgesics for pain relief, correction of electrolyte and glucose abnormalities, and renal and respiratory support as needed.

FLUID REPLACEMENT

Maintenance of an adequate circulating blood volume is of paramount importance in the patient with acute pancreatitis. The need for restoring volume cannot be overemphasized because the death rate from this disease in the acute stage is directly correlated with the adequacy of fluid resuscitation. Not only does hypovolemia predispose to acute renal failure, pancreatitis itself may be made worse by the hypovolemic shock state because of impaired pancreatic perfusion.[44]

Fluid losses through fluid pooling in the abdomen and retroperitoneal area, as well as from nasogastric suction, vomiting, and diaphoresis, must be considered and replaced. As a rule, crystalloid solutions (such as lactated Ringer's solution) will suffice because the fluid lost into the retroperitoneum has the composition of the extracellular fluid (ECF). However, in severe cases of hemorrhagic pancreatitis, blood products and colloid solutions may be needed.

Close monitoring of vital signs and urine output is mandatory in guiding fluid replacement therapy (see section on Nursing Assessment). A Swan-Ganz catheter may be needed to monitor central filling pressures, an indwelling arterial line to monitor arterial oxygen tension, and a urinary catheter to follow urinary output.[45]

ELECTROLYTE REPLACEMENT

Because hypocalcemia and hypomagnesemia are frequently present in acute pancreatitis, it may be necessary to administer these electrolytes by the parenteral route. Ionized fractions (Ca^{2+} and Mg^{2+}) should be measured when possible because they are significant in physiological functioning. When evaluating total calcium or magnesium levels, the effect of hypoalbuminemia should be considered. Hypokalemia is frequently a problem that must be dealt with by potassium replacement.

PAIN MANAGEMENT

The pain of pancreatitis is caused by edema and distention of the pancreatic capsule, obstruction of the biliary tree, and peritoneal irritation caused by pancreatic products. Pain is usually sudden in onset and precedes the development of nausea and vomiting. The pain of acute pancreatitis is usually located in the epigastrium, but may be felt anywhere in the abdomen or lower chest area.[46] A constant, knife-like, boring pain radiating to the mid back is commonly reported and is partially relieved by sitting and leaning forward or by lying on the side with the knees drawn upward.

Large doses of narcotic medications may be needed to control the severe pain often associated with acute pancreatitis. Some researchers state there is no reason to believe that any one opiate is more or less likely to cause spasm of the sphincter of Oddi, and therefore no reason to choose one opiate over another.[47] However, meperidine is often recommended by others because it presumably has no significant effect on the sphincter of Oddi.[48] No oral feedings should be given until the patient is painfree; premature introduction of food can exacerbate a severe recurrence.

NASOGASTRIC SUCTION

Nasogastric (NG) suction is used for most patients with acute pancreatitis, unless the disease is mild and not associated with significant vomiting or pain.[49] It is definitely needed in patients with protracted nausea and vomiting.[50] A benefit of NG suction is relief from the intestinal ileus so frequently present in acute pancreatitis. Also, theoretically, this therapy helps to "put the pancreas at rest" by stopping the secretin–pancreozymin stimulus to pancreatic secretion. Although this therapy is advocated by many, its ability to shorten or reduce the severity of an acute attack of pancreatitis has not been demonstrated. Several clinical studies have failed to prove the beneficial effects from NG suction in patients with pancreatitis, unless vomiting is a problem.[51,52]

RESPIRATORY CARE

Supportive respiratory care should be given during the course of acute pancreatitis. As stated earlier, a number of respiratory complications have been described in patients with acute pancreatitis (including diaphragmatic elevation, fleeting infiltrates, pleural effusions, atelectasis, and arterial hypoxemia).[53] For this reason, blood gases should be monitored in acutely ill patients and respiratory support provided when indicated (such as humidified oxygen, intratracheal intubation, and assisted ventilation). Nursing management is discussed in the section on Nursing Interventions.

NUTRITIONAL SUPPORT

The patient is not allowed anything by mouth until the ileus and pain have resolved because oral consumption of nutrients stimulates pancreatic secretion.[54,55] Still, patients are often hypercatabolic because of the severity of their illness. The problem becomes one of deciding how to supply nutrients in adequate amounts. The choice is essentially between total parenteral nutrition (TPN) or enteral feeding of an elemental formula into the jejunum. The decision as to which is indicated must be made on an individual basis.

IV administration of glucose, amino acids, and fat stimulates little if any pancreatic output.[56] Thus, many patients with pancreatitis have traditionally been fed by TPN because TPN provides nutritional support and can "rest" the pancreas. Unfortunately, there are no data to indicate that TPN favorably alters the course of acute pancreatitis.[57] For example, in a retrospective study of 46 patients with acute pancreatitis, Goodgame and Fischer[58] concluded that parenteral nutrition had little effect on disease pathophysiology as judged by mortality and morbidity; disturbingly, TPN was associated with a higher incidence of catheter-related sepsis. Other studies have drawn similar conclusions (that is, no advantage of TPN as well as an increased rate of catheter-related sepsis).[59,60]

Enteral nutrition is cited by some investigators as the preferred method for initial nutritional support of patients with pancreatitis.[61] Feeding into the jejunum causes less pancreatic stimulation than does feeding into the duodenum or stomach. Also, elemental (amino acid, low-fat) diets have been found to cause less stimulation of pancreatic exocrine secretion than do complex diets. Therefore, infusion of elemental diets into the proximal portion of the jejunum by feeding tube is a recommended method for feeding patients with mild disease.[62] Several reports have indicated that small-bowel feedings are tolerated by patients with acute pancreatitis.[63–65] However, it may be difficult to achieve adequate levels of calories and protein because the feeding must be introduced slowly and the rate reduced if intolerance develops. For more seriously ill patients, enteral feeding may be precluded by ileus or other GI malfunctions. It may be necessary to start with TPN and then gradually convert to enteral feeding as tolerance allows.

PERITONEAL LAVAGE

Peritoneal lavage is sometimes used to remove toxins and various metabolites from the peritoneal cavity during attacks of acute pancreatitis; theoretically, this minimizes their systemic absorption.[66] Although in theory this treatment should improve the acutely ill patient's chance for recovery, two controlled studies of peritoneal lavage indicated that it did not affect the morbidity or mortality associated with severe pancreatitis.[67,68] Another study indicated that selected patients (those with more than five risk factors according to the Ranson criteria) who received long-term lavage (7 days), as compared to those who received short-term lavage (2 days), had a decreased mortality rate due to pancreatic abscess formation.[69]

Peritoneal lavage requires the insertion of a peritoneal lavage catheter and the infusion and withdrawal of lactated Ringer's solution (1 to 2 L/hr) for several days or longer.[70] A response, if it occurs, is most likely in the first 6 to 8 hrs.[71]

INSULIN ADMINISTRATION

Small doses of regular insulin may be needed to treat the transient hyperglycemia that may occur in patients with acute pancreatitis. Apparently this is caused by damage to the beta cells (thus decreasing insulin secretion) and increased glucagon release from the alpha cells (elevating the blood sugar level). In some patients, permanent diabetes may follow.

NURSING ASSESSMENT

Nursing care of the patient with acute pancreatitis is complex and requires sophisticated monitoring for complications and response to medical therapy. The following steps are necessary to detect changes in the patient's often rapidly fluctuating status:

1. Carefully measure and record fluid intake and output (I&O) from all routes. Fluid replacement is partially based on fluid losses that are directly measurable (for example, vomiting and gastric suction). Because of third-space fluid shifts into the retroperitoneum and abdomen, not all of the fluid loss can be measured directly. Therefore, in the early phase of the third-space fluid shift, it is often necessary to give more fluid than would be indicated by measured losses. Fluid replacement is primarily guided by hourly urine outputs, vital signs, and invasive hemodynamic monitoring (such as central venous pressure [CVP] and pulmonary capillary wedge pressures [PCWP]).
2. Monitor for the following signs of hypovolemia due to excessive fluid loss:
   - Decreased skin turgor
   - Dry mucous membranes
   - Initially, postural hypotension; later, decreased systolic pressure in all positions
   - Tachycardia (pulse rate >100/min)
   - Urinary output less than 30 mL/hr in adults. Low urine volume may be a function of insufficient fluid replacement or may indicate renal failure (acute tubular necrosis).
   - Blood urea nitrogen (BUN) elevated out of proportion to serum creatinine level
   - Low CVP
   - Low pulmonary artery capillary pressure
   - Low cardiac output
   - Hematocrit may be elevated (red cells are suspended in less plasma as intravascular fluid is shifted into third space)

   Because of sequestering of fluid into the abdominal and retroperitoneal areas plus vomiting and NG suction, fluid loss may be severe enough to induce serious hypovolemia. This situation must be detected before perfusion to vital organs is compromised, leading to permanent renal or cerebral damage. As stated above, monitoring I&O alone is not sufficient to guide fluid replacement therapy. With adequate fluid replacement, the above parameters will remain within or return to normal limits.
3. Monitor for the following signs of hemorrhagic shock if the patient has necrotizing hemorrhagic pancreatitis:
   - Hypotension
   - Tachycardia
   - Anxiety
   - Oliguria
   - Cool, clammy skin
   - Falling hematocrit
   - Low central venous pressure
   - Low PCWP

   Blood loss can be significant in necrotizing hemorrhagic pancreatitis and must be detected before serious perfusion problems develop.

Although this condition resembles simple fluid volume deficit, it tends to occur more rapidly and is associated with a decreased rather than an elevated hematocrit.

4. Monitor response to fluid replacement therapy. Fluid replacement therapy should be aggressive enough to keep the vital signs and hourly urine volume within normal limits. If the patient has underlying cardiovascular problems, it may be necessary to monitor the CVP and PCWP. A close working relationship between the nurse and physician is necessary if the correct volume of fluid replacement is to be achieved.
5. Monitor for respiratory distress or infection:
   - Hypoxemia (as evidenced by a low PaO_2)
   - Breath sounds indicating the presence of infiltrates
   - Tachypnea and labored respirations
   - Cyanosis
   - Temperature elevation

   Patients with pancreatitis are predisposed to pulmonary complications, such as ARDS, fleeting infiltrates, pleural effusions, and atelectasis.
6. Monitor for hypocalcemia:
   - Monitor serum calcium levels (consider albumin level and pH if total calcium is measured).
   - Note complaints of numbness or tingling in the extremities or circumoral region
   - Look for latent tetany as indicated by Trousseau's and Chvostek's signs (see Chapter 2)
   - Expect dysrhythmias to be more frequent if hypocalcemia is present

   See Chapter 6 for further discussion on hypocalcemia.
7. Monitor for hypomagnesemia:
   - Check laboratory reports for lowered serum magnesium levels. Magnesium deficiency is most likely to be present in patients who were previously malnourished or alcoholic. Note that this imbalance looks a lot like hypocalcemia. Unfortunately, magnesium is not an ingredient in commonly used IV fluids; for that matter, neither is calcium (except for the small amount in lactated Ringer's solution). Magnesium is available for parenteral use and is discussed in Chapter 7.
   - Look for tremors, confusion, hallucinations, tachycardia, and positive Chvostek's and Trousseau's signs. See Chapter 7 for a more thorough discussion of assessment for hypomagnesemia.
8. Monitor for hypokalemia:
   - Check laboratory reports for decreased serum potassium levels
   - Look for arrhythmias, weakness, GI hypomotility, and paresthesias. See Chapter 5 for further a more thorough discussion of assessment for hypokalemia.
9. Assess for infection by monitoring for pain and elevated body temperature. Consider the location, severity, and duration of pain. Be aware that subtle changes in the nature and frequency of pain may be indicative of pancreatic abscess. Also, be aware that a temperature above the usual low-grade fever associated with acute pancreatitis may signal a complicating infection. Septic complications of acute pancreatitis include pancreatic abscess, infected pancreatic necrosis, and infected pseudocyst.[72]
10. Monitor serum glucose levels to detect hyperglycemia. Serum glucose levels (determined by capillary "sticks") are more valid than urinary glucose levels. Once the renal threshold for glucose has been determined to be normal, one can rely on urine glucose measurements.
11. Assess bowel sounds and abdominal girth at regular intervals to monitor degree of adynamic ileus.

NURSING DIAGNOSES

Alterations associated with acute pancreatitis involve rapidly changing derangements in fluid, electrolyte, and perhaps acid–base balance. Because of these changes, a number of physiological nursing diagnoses may be appropriate. Clinical Tip: Examples of Nursing Diagnoses Related to Acute Pancreatitis lists examples of several physiological nursing diagnoses related to the care of patients with acute pancreatitis.

NURSING INTERVENTIONS

Much of what the nurse does in caring for the critically ill patient with acute pancreatitis revolves around monitoring the current clinical status and working collaboratively with the physician to provide supportive care. The following interventions are often needed:

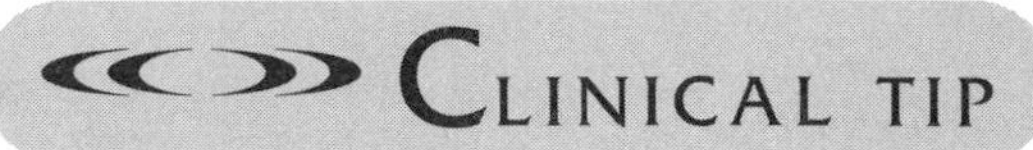

Examples of Nursing Diagnoses Related to Acute Pancreatitus

NURSING DIAGNOSIS	ETIOLOGICAL FACTORS	DEFINING CHARACTERISTICS
FVD related to third-spacing of fluid and gastric loss by vomiting and suction	Escape of secretions into abdomen and retroperitoneum, vomiting, and nasogastric suction (aggravated by fever and diaphoresis)	Tachycardia, hypotension, urine output <30 mL/hr, concentrated urine, BUN elevated out of proportion to creatinine, poor skin turgor (see Chapter 3)
Ineffective breathing pattern related to immobility, pain, and pleural effusions	Immobility, retained secretions, and pleural effusions (result of inflammation from pancreatic enzymes and extravasation of fluid), aggravated by overzealous fluid administration	Dyspnea, shortness of breath, tachypnea, cyanosis, cough, nasal flaring, decreased arterial oxygenation

FVD, fluid volume deficit; BUN, blood urea nitrogen.

1. Collaborate with the physician to safely administer fluids and electrolytes based on physiological indices. If desired responses are not achieved, consult with the physician to revise fluid orders (see section on Nursing Assessment).
2. Maintain correct position and patency of the NG tube to alleviate nausea and vomiting and relieve distention.
   - The tip of the tube should be well into the stomach (near the pylorus); if the tip rests high in the stomach, hydrochloric acid (HCl) may escape through the duodenum and theoretically stimulate secretions.
   - Once the tube has been correctly positioned, mark the exterior portion and make every effort to maintain the position.
   - Maintain patency of the tube by irrigating with approximately 20 mL of isotonic saline every 2 hrs. Viscous gastric secretions may necessitate more frequent irrigations.
   - Check suction apparatus periodically to be sure it is working correctly.
3. Implement measures to relieve pain.
   - Administer prescribed analgesics as frequently as indicated. Pain can be quite severe and should be treated with regular analgesic injections. Medical directives frequently call for meperidine. If pain persists despite analgesics, discuss problem with physician. In addition to promoting comfort, pain relief from analgesics decreases restlessness and anxiety, which probably also decreases pancreatic secretions.
   - Assist the patient to achieve a position of comfort. Pain relief may sometimes be partially attained by sitting up or lying curled on the right or left side. Patients with peritoneal irritation are likely to remain very still. (This may present a problem in terms of retained respiratory secretions.)
4. Attempt to prevent or minimize respiratory complications.
   - Turn patient at regular intervals to foster drainage of secretions.
   - Encourage deep breathing at regular intervals.
   - If necessary, suction retained secretions to keep airway open.

- Monitor rate of fluid replacement to avoid overloading the circulatory system and predisposing to pulmonary edema.

The physician may prescribe humidified oxygen to help support the patient. In severe situations, intubation and mechanical ventilation will be indicated. It should be noted that impaired pulmonary function may occur in all patients with pancreatitis (regardless of severity of illness).

5. Administer insulin per medical directives as indicated, based on capillary blood sugars, to control hyperglycemia.
6. Provide patient with periods of rest between nursing activities and attempt to minimize anxiety-producing situations.
7. Consider the patient's need for nutrients.
   - Administer TPN or jejunal feedings if prescribed. (See section on nutritional support under Treatment.)
   - Be aware that after NG suction is discontinued, the patient is usually maintained without oral feedings for at least 24 to 48 hrs before a low-fat diet is gradually introduced. Great care must be taken to avoid feeding too quickly as this can exacerbate another episode of acute pancreatitis.
   - When the acute phase subsides and clear liquids are allowed by mouth, monitor bowel sounds and watch for recurring pain and nausea.
   - Keep a record of the patient's nutrient intake so that deficiencies can be brought to the attention of the physician and dietitian.

CASE STUDY

20-1. A 50-year-old intoxicated man with a long history of alcoholism was admitted to the hospital for evaluation of epigastric pain that radiated through to the mid-back. The only way the patient could find relief was to sit in bed with his knees drawn to his chest. He stated he was nauseated and had been vomiting intermittently since the abdominal pain started 2 days earlier.

His vital signs were as follows:

Blood pressure = 108/64 mmHg
Pulse rate = 120/min
respiratory rate = 26/min
temperature = 38.5 °C

On examination, his abdomen was found to be diffusely tender to palpation. A chest x-ray revealed a large effusion at the right lung base.

Laboratory results from a venous blood sample were as follows:

Sodium = 143 mEq/L
Potassium = 3.3 mEq/L
Chloride = 92 mEq/L
CO_2 content = 22 mEq/L
Total calcium = 8.2 mg/dL
Magnesium = 1.2 mg/dL
BUN = 48 mg/dL
Creatinine = 1.2 mg/dL
Amylase = 900 IU
Glucose = 200 mg/dL
White blood cell count = 13,400 mm^3

Laboratory results from an arterial sample for blood gases were as follows:

pH = 7.28
$PaCO_2$ = 41 mmHg
PaO_2 = 56 mmHg
HCO_3 = 19 mEq/L

Laboratory results from a urinalysis were as follows:

3+ ketones

On the basis of the above findings, a diagnosis of acute pancreatitis was made. The patient was treated with NG suction, IV fluid replacement, and parenteral analgesia. Within the next few days, the abdominal pain, fever, and nausea subsided.

COMMENTARY Hypotension and tachycardia indicate a low blood volume, as does an elevated BUN (reflective of decreased renal perfusion). A number of potential problems could be present in this patient. For example:

- Hypoxemia (PaO_2, 54 mmHg) could cause lactic acidosis, a form of high anion gap metabolic acidosis.
- Absence of food intake (common in alcoholics during heavy drinking spells) and ethanol intoxication could cause alcoholic ketoacidosis, a form of high anion gap metabolic acidosis (note that patient had 3+ ketones in the urine).

- Loss of gastric acid by vomiting and NG suction could cause metabolic alkalosis and a lower than normal serum potassium (note that the patient's potassium is slightly lower than normal).
- The below normal pH indicates acidosis. The lower than normal bicarbonate level indicates *metabolic acidosis*; calculation of the anion gap indicates that this is a high anion gap metabolic acidosis due to excessive lactic acid production for hypoxemia (see Chapter 9). The bicarbonate level would have been even lower if vomiting had not been present to cause a predisposition to metabolic alkalosis (and thus an increase in bicarbonate concentration).
- *Respiratory acidosis* is also present. This imbalance can be determined by calculating the expected $PaCO_2$ and comparing that value to the actual reading. Using Winter's formula:

$$\begin{aligned} \text{Expected } PaCO_2 &= 1.5\,(HCO_3) + 8 \pm 2 \\ &= 1.5\,(19) + 8 \pm 2 \\ &= 34.5 \text{ to } 38.5 \text{ mmHg} \end{aligned}$$

Thus, the expected $PaCO_2$ should range between 34.5 to 38.5 mmHg. Instead, it is 41 mmHg (indicating a slight degree of carbon dioxide retention in addition to the expected compensatory change).

Note that the patient has a pleural effusion that could be interfering with ventilation, as can abdominal distention and splinting of the diaphragm. It is also thought that release of pancreatic enzymes into the systemic circulation may cause damage to pulmonary tissues.

As noted in Table 20-1, a serum calcium level of less than 8 mg/dL is one indicator of poor outcome after the onset of pancreatitis. Although this patient's serum calcium level is not less than 8 mg/dL, it is below normal. Calcium supplementation may be indicated to prevent cardiac dysrhythmias. Because the patient is acidotic, a greater proportion of calcium exists in the ionized form (making adverse effects of hypocalcemia less prominent).

Like hypocalcemia, hypomagnesemia has at least in part been attributed to precipitation of magnesium ions in the inflamed tissues in and around the pancreas as insoluble magnesium soaps. Losses from vomiting, gastric suction, and diarrhea intensify hypomagnesemia. Because this patient has a history of alcoholism, hypomagnesemia may also be related to the multiple magnesium-lowering effects of alcohol.

REFERENCES

1. Schwartz S, Shires T, Spencer F: Principles of Surgery, 6th ed, p 1406. Baltimore, Williams & Wilkins, 1994
2. Shoemaker et al (eds): Textbook of Critical Care, 2nd ed, p 734. Philadelphia, WB Saunders, 1989
3. Schwartz, p 1406
4. Ibid
5. Steinberg W, Tenner S: Acute pancreatitis. N Engl J Med 330(17):1198–1210,1994
6. Yamada T, Alpers D, Owyang C, Powell D, Silvestein F (eds): Textbook of Gastroenterology, Philadelphia, JB Lippincott, 1991
7. Shoemaker et al, p 734
8. Narins R (ed): Clinical Disorders of Fluid and Electrolyte Metabolism, 5th ed, p 1026. New York, McGraw-Hill, 1994
9. Kokko J, Tannen R: Fluids and Electrolytes, 2nd ed, p 938. Philadelphia, WB Saunders, 1990
10. Pemberton L, Pemberton D: Treatment of Water, Electrolyte and Acid–Base Disorders in the Surgical Patient, p 208. New York, McGraw-Hill, 1994
11. Narins, p 1484
12. Pemberton, Pemberton, p 208
13. Narins, p 1026
14. Robertson G, et al: Inadequate parathyroid response in acute pancreatitis. N Engl J Med 294:512,1976
15. Chernow B (ed): The Pharmacologic Approach to the Critically Ill Patient, 3rd ed, p 782. Baltimore, Williams & Wilkins, 1994
16. Yamada et al, p 1866
17. Narins, p 2202
18. Ryzen E, Rude R: Low intracellular magnesium in patients with acute pancreatitis and hypocalcemia. West J Med 152:145,1990
19. Narins, p 1053
20. Lachter et al: Hypophosphatemia and idiopathic pancreatitis. N Engl J Med 81:1221,1986
21. Wyngaarden J, Smith L, Bennett J: Textbook of Medicine, 19th ed, p 723. Philadelphia, WB Saunders, 1992
22. Ibid
23. Ranson J, Rifkind K, Roses D, et al: Prognostic signs and the role of operative management in acute pancreatitis. Surg Gynecol Obstet 139:69–81,1974
24. Ranson J: Etiological and prognostic factors in human acute pancreatitis: A review. Am J Gastroenterol 77(9):633–638,1982
25. Blamey et al: Prognostic factors in acute pancreati-

tis, Gut 25:1340–1346,1984
26. Ranson, p 637
27. Yamada, p 1866
28. Wilson et al: Prediction of outcome in acute pancreatitis: A comparative study of APACHE II, clinical assessment and multiple factor scoring systems. Br J Surg 77:1260–1264,1990
29. Wyngaarden et al, p 723
30. Steinberg, Tenner, p 1204
31. Yamada et al, p 1871
32. Tran et al: Prevalence and prediction of multiple organ system failure and mortality in acute pancreatitis. J Crit Care 8(3):145–153,1993
33. Schwartz, p 1412
34. Tran et al: Acute renal failure in patients with acute pancreatitis: Prevalence, risk factors, and outcome. Nephrol Dialysis Transplant 8(10):1079–1084,1993
35. Agarwal N, Pitchumoni C: Acute pancreatitis: A multisystem disease, Gastroenterol 1(2):115–128,1993
36. Schwartz, p 1411
37. Yamada et al, p 1863
38. Schwartz, p 1411
39. Ibid
40. Yamada et al, p 1871
41. Willemer et al: Lung injury in acute experimental pancreatitis in rats. Intern J Pancreatol 8(4):305–321,1994
42. Agarwal, Pitchumoni, p 121
43. Yamada et al, p 1872
44. Schwartz, p 1411
45. Yamada et al, 1866
46. Ibid, p 1863
47. Ibid, p 1866
48. Woodley M, Whelan A (eds): Manual of Medical Therapeutics, 27th ed, p 306. Boston, Little, Brown, 1992
49. Schwartz, p 1411
50. Woodley, Whelan, p 306
51. Fuller R, Loveland J, Frankel M: An evaluation of the efficacy of nasogastric suction treatment in alcoholic pancreatitis. Am J Gastroenterol 75:349,1981
52. Switz D: Acute alcoholic pancreatitis: Effect of clinical presentation and therapies on outcome at a VA hospital. Ann Intern Med 78:816,1973
53. Toledo-Pereyra L: The Pancreas: Principles of Medical and Surgical Practice, p 184. New York, John Wiley & Sons, 1985
54. Schwartz, p 1411
55. Woodley, Whelan, p 306
56. Zaloga G (ed): Nutrition in Critical Care. St. Louis, CV Mosby, 1994
57. Ibid
58. Goodgame J, Fischer J: Parenteral nutrition in the treatment of acute pancreatitis: Effect on complications and mortality. Ann Surg 186:651–658,1977
59. Kalfarentzos F, Karavias D, Karatzas T, et al: Total parenteral nutrition in severe acute pancreatitis. J Am Coll Nutr 10:156–162,1991
60. Sax H, et al: Early total parenteral nutrition in acute pancreatitis: Lack of beneficial effects. Am J Surg 153:117–127,1987
61. Zaloga, p 316
62. Rombeau J, Caldwell M (eds): Clinical Nutrition: Enteral and Tube Feeding, 2nd ed. Philadelphia, WB Saunders, 1990
63. Kudsk K, et al: Postoperative jejunal feedings following complicated pancreatitis. Nutr Clin Pract 5:14–17,1990
64. Voitk K, et al: Use of an elemental diet in the treatment of complicated pancreatitis. Am J Surg 125:223–227,1973
65. McArdle A, Echave W, Brown R, et al: Effect of elemental diet on pancreatic secretion. Am J Surg 128:690–692,1974
66. Schwartz, p 1411
67. Ihse I, et al: Influence of peritoneal lavage on objective prognostic signs in acute pancreatitis. Ann Surg 204:122–127,1986
68. Mayer A, et al: Controlled clinical trials of peritoneal lavage for the treatment of severe pancreatitis. N Engl J Med 312:399–404,1985
69. Ranson J, Berman R: Long peritoneal lavage decreases pancreatic sepsis in acute pancreatitis. Ann Surg 211:708–716,1990
70. Schwartz, p 1411
71. Ibid
72. Krumberger J: Acute pancreatitis. Crit Care Clin North Am 5(1):185–202,1993

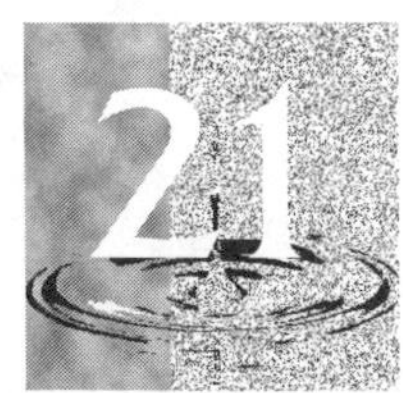

Cirrhosis With Ascites

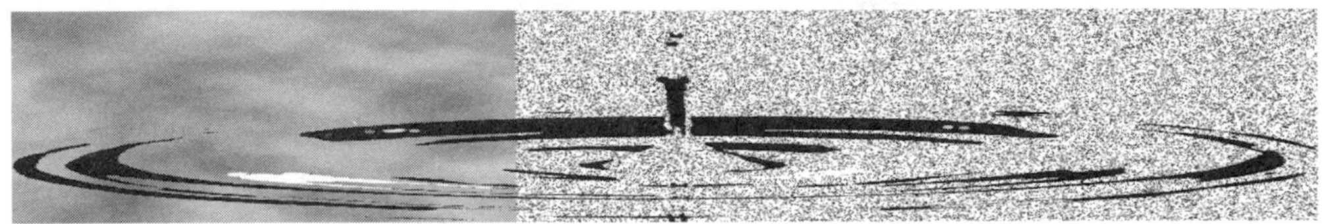

PATHOPHYSIOLOGY

Cirrhosis is characterized by an extensive increase of fibrous tissue within the liver structure. As blood, lymph, and biliary channels become compressed by fibrotic changes, intrahepatic pressure increases, reducing the liver's capacity to fulfill its functions. At first the liver is enlarged with fatty tissue; later, it becomes small, hard, and nodular.

ASCITES FORMATION

Ascites is not a disease but rather a symptom of a disease, such as cirrhosis, in which a collection of serum-like fluid forms within the peritoneal cavity. In cirrhosis, ascitic fluid accumulates as venous outflow is impeded through the fibrotic liver, and then seeps from the surface of the liver into the peritoneal cavity to produce ascites. Because of the fluid's high protein content, it pulls additional fluid from the surfaces of the gut and mesentery by osmosis.

Exact mechanisms in the development of ascites remain unclear; however, several theories have been proposed, including "overfilling" and "underfilling." Recently, an "integrated" theory has been developed. Early on, intrahepatic hypertension activates a hepatic baroreceptor reflex that enhances renal sodium retention and increases plasma volume. As the cirrhotic disease progresses, this overflow spills into the peritoneal cavity as ascites. The fluid shift from the vascular system into the peritoneal space causes underfilling, which eventually dominates the clinical picture. Stimulation of the renin-angiotensin system increases renal sodium retention and therefore plasma volume.[1]

Decreased Effective Arterial Volume

Decreased effective arterial volume refers to a state in which the total extracellular fluid (ECF) volume is normal or even expanded, although the kidneys respond as if they were underperfused.[2] They do so by retaining sodium and producing a concentrated urine. Presumably, this is what occurs in the patient with cirrhosis and ascites formation.

Hypoalbuminemia

Severe *hypoalbuminemia* may also contribute to ascites formation. Causes of low serum albumin levels in cirrhotic patients include decreased synthesis of protein by the diseased liver, dilutional effect (due to salt and water retention), and a shift of protein from the vascular space to the peritoneal cavity. The protein content of ascitic fluid may be as high as half that of serum.[3] Because the serum albumin level is below normal, plasma oncotic pressure is reduced, an effect that favors shifting of fluid from the vascular space into the peritoneal cavity.

However, hypoalbuminemia is not nearly as important in ascites formation as is the increased pressure generated by the hepatic postsinusoidal obstruction.[4] Relief from ascites has been reported when portal hypertension is corrected by surgical shunting procedures.

EDEMA

Edema formation in cirrhotic patients has several causes. Increased pressure in the vena cava (secondary to ascitic fluid and enlarged liver size) interferes with venous drainage of the lower extremities. Contributing to edema formation is the hypoalbuminemia that is frequently present in patients with advanced liver disease. By lowering the plasma oncotic pressure, hypoalbuminemia promotes shifting of fluid from the intravascular to the interstitial space.

At first, edema appears in dependent areas; later on, it spreads to nondependent areas, varying in severity with the degree of sodium intake.[5] The edema associated with liver disease is of the "pitting" variety (see Fig. 2-3).

FLUID AND ELECTROLYTE DISTURBANCES

The common disorders of fluid, electrolyte, and acid–base metabolism observed in patients with hepatic cirrhosis are fluid volume excess with edema and ascites, hyponatremia, hypokalemia, respiratory alkalosis, and metabolic acidosis.[6]

Fluid Volume Excess

The patient with advanced cirrhotic disease has a complex fluid balance problem. Although there is an excess of total body fluid with an accumulation in the peritoneal cavity (ascites) and in the interstitial space (edema), there is also a problem of decreased effective arterial blood volume. Because of this, the kidneys strive to build up the intravascular volume by retaining sodium and water (although the blood volume may actually be normal or even above normal). Plasma aldosterone levels are often above normal due to increased adrenal secretion and inability of the liver to deactivate this hormone (of course, aldosterone causes sodium and water retention). Nonsteroidal antiinflammatory drugs (NSAID) should be avoided because they may cause deterioration in renal function (with further fluid retention) if given in sufficient doses to patients with ascites due to liver disease.[7]

Hyponatremia

Hyponatremia is common in patients with advanced hepatic cirrhosis and is usually caused by impaired ability to excrete water. Experimental and clinical evidence suggests that the impaired water excretion is related to persistent release of antidiuretic hormone (ADH).[8] A derangement in renal hemodynamics may also contribute to this effect. This hyponatremia occurs in addition to fluid volume excess. That is, although there is abnormal retention of both sodium and water, a relatively greater degree of water retention occurs. As such, the serum sodium level is diluted below normal although the total body sodium is excessive (see Fig. 4-2A). Other factors that can contribute to hyponatremia are sodium loss through frequent paracentesis or excessive diuretic use or too stringent sodium restriction.

Hypokalemia

Hypokalemia is common in patients with chronic liver disease.[9] Among the causes of hypokalemia are low dietary intake and renal loss of potassium caused by hyperaldosteronism and diuretics, as well as losses from the gastrointestinal (GI) tract.[10] One of the most common causes is diuretic use. In one study, almost two thirds of the cirrhotic patients developed a serum potassium level less than 3.1 mEq/L.[11] It has been suggested that potassium depletion can induce hepatic encephalopathy.[12] Additional adverse effects of hypokalemia include ileus, muscle weakness, myocardial irritability, and decreased renal concentrating ability.

Although less common than hypokalemia, *hyper*kalemia is occasionally seen in patients with chronic liver disease. Most often, it is associated with the use of potassium-sparing diuretics (such as spironolactone, amiloride, and triamterene). Potassium supplements and potassium-sparing diuretics should be stopped when serum potassium levels exceed 5.5 mEq/L.[13]

Acid–Base Imbalances

All four acid–base imbalances may be encountered in patients with liver disease. The most frequent is respiratory alkalosis.[14] In a study of 91 patients with portal cirrhosis, 64% had respiratory alkalosis.[15] As a rule, the degree of respiratory alkalosis increases as the severity of the hepatic disease increases.[16] It has been postulated that elevated blood ammonia levels stimulate hyperventilation and resultant respiratory alkalosis; however, it is unlikely that increased blood ammonia is the sole factor.[17] Another possible cause is an elevated progesterone level; this hormone (normally degraded by the liver) is a respiratory stimulant.[18]

Metabolic alkalosis occurs in many patients with hepatic disease and is usually associated with use of potassium-losing diuretics. It can also be caused by vomiting or nasogastric (NG) suction, or alkali loading from sources such as antacids or citrate from blood transfusions.[19]

High anion gap metabolic acidosis has been observed in 10% to 20% of patients with chronic liver disease.[20] The percentage increases as the severity of disease increases. It has been suggested that patients with liver disease are more susceptible to lactic acidosis because of the decreased ability of their diseased livers to remove lactic acid from the circulation. Also, they are susceptible to increased lactic acid production (as may occur with hypotension secondary to GI hemorrhage).[21]

Other Imbalances

Additional possible fluid and electrolyte disturbances related to cirrhosis of the liver are listed in Table 21-1, along with probable etiological associations.

EFFECTS ON BODY SYSTEMS

Cirrhosis of the liver has an insidious onset and affects most body systems. Brief discussions of the effects on various body systems follow.

TABLE 21–1

Possible Water and Electrolyte Disturbances in Patients With Advanced Cirrhosis and Ascites

DISTURBANCE	ETIOLOGY
Increased total ECF volume but decreased effective arterial volume	Enhanced renal tubular reabsorption of sodium Increased plasma aldosterone level due to increased adrenal secretion (in response to decreased effective arterial volume) and decreased degradation of this hormone by the diseased liver
Increased water retention, causing dilutional hyponatremia	Impaired renal water excretion related to excess ADH secretion (in response to decreased effective arterial volume)
Hypokalemia	Direct loss in vomiting or diarrhea Decreased intake due to anorexia Excessive use of potassium-losing diuretics (Note that hypokalemia is especially harmful to patients with hepatic failure because it increases ammonia formation and can induce hepatic coma.)
Hyperkalemia	Excessive use of potassium-sparing diuretics, especially when renal insufficiency is present or potassium-containing salt substitutes are used to make the low- sodium diet more palatable
Elevated serum ammonia level	Under normal circumstances, the large amounts of ammonia formed in the intestines by bacterial action are absorbed into the bloodstream and carried to the liver to be converted to urea for renal excretion. However, in cirrhosis, the liver cannot convert the ammonia to urea; thus, the blood ammonia level increases.
Hypomagnesemia	Loss of magnesium in vomiting and diarrhea, poor dietary intake, and renal wasting of magnesium in patients with cirrhosis due to alcoholism
Hypocalcemia	Possibly a result of inadequate storage of vitamin D by diseased liver; also associated with hypoalbuminemia
Hyperventilation with respiratory alkalosis	May be related to hyperammonemia (high ammonia level may act as a respiratory stimulant)
Respiratory acidosis	May occur if ascites is severe enough to compromise diaphragmatic movement
Metabolic alkalosis	Common in patients treated with potassium-losing diuretics such as furosemide, thiazides, and ethacrynic acid
Mild metabolic acidosis	May occur in patients treated with spironolactone (Aldactone) alone (due to interference by spironolactone with sodium/hydrogen ion exchange in the distal tubules)

ECF, extracellular fluid; ADH, antidiuretic hormone.

Gastrointestinal System

Development of esophageal varices is the most serious complication associated with hepatic failure and portal hypertension. Severity of bleeding from varices is intensified by coagulopathies associated with liver failure. Enlarged abdominal veins and internal hemorrhoids may also be caused by portal hypertension.

Malnutrition is common in patients with hepatic failure because the frequently associated anorexia, nausea, and vomiting preclude the recommended dietary intake. Many GI symptoms are related to venous engorgement of the GI organs. Muscle wasting and weight loss may be masked by fluid retention. Fetor hepaticus is often noted.

Cardiovascular System

Right ventricular heart failure often occurs in patients with hepatic failure secondary to high pressure in the portal system. Contributing to cardiac problems is the hypokalemia commonly found in cirrhotic patients as a result of the use of potassium-losing diuretics. Potassium deficiency predisposes to ventricular arrhythmias. Of course, arrhythmias may also result from hyperkalemia, which can occur in patients treated with potassium-sparing diuretics, particularly if renal disease is present.

Renal System

Hepatorenal syndrome (HRS) encompasses a type of renal failure that occurs in patients with hepatic failure. In recent years, we have begun to develop an understanding of the mechanisms that lead to its evolution. Even so, it is an ominous occurrence associated with a high mortality rate. Although patients with hepatic failure demonstrate extremely low systemic vascular resistance, intrarenal resistance is increased. In progressing hepatic disease, renal vasoconstrictors, such as leukotrienes and endothelins, are activated. Under normal circumstances, a balance is maintained with the production of vasodilating prostaglandins and kallikreins. When vasoconstrictors overpower vasodilators, HRS develops.[22] Although our understanding of HRS is expanding, effective treatment options continue to be elusive. Low-dose dopamine, a potent renal vasodilator, is often used in an attempt to increase renal perfusion and slow the development of HRS. Although HRS often precedes death, the cause in most patients is due to hepatic, rather that renal, insufficiency. Death usually occurs before uremia develops.[23] Hepatorenal syndrome is manifested by oliguria, increased serum creatinine (usually >10 mg/dL), increased blood urea nitrogen (BUN), low urinary sodium output, and maintained ability of the kidneys to concentrate urine until the last stages of the syndrome. Evidently the abnormality is functional rather than structural because few or no histological changes are demonstrated. This latter statement is substantiated by reports that the kidney from a patient with HRS may be transplanted into a patient with normal liver function.[24] Also, when liver transplants are performed on patients with HRS, renal function may normalize.[25]

Neurological System

Portal systemic encephalopathy (PSE) refers to the syndrome of disordered consciousness and altered neuromuscular activity seen in patients with hepatic failure. In the presence of hepatic failure, a variety of toxins bypass the liver (where they would normally be destroyed) and enter the systemic circulation in abnormal concentrations. Although the exact toxins are not defined, ammonia is one of the implicated substances. Recall that the normal liver converts ammonia into urea for renal excretion. When this process is altered by a diseased liver, the serum ammonia level may rise sharply. However, the degree of serum ammonia elevation is not always predictive of the severity of PSE. Whatever the precise biochemical trigger of PSE, interference with cerebral metabolism and neurotransmission appears to be the basic underlying mechanism. Symptoms may range from mild (sleep-wake disturbances and ataxia) to severe (coma and seizures).

Precipitating causes of PSE episodes include fluid volume depletion from overzealous use of diuretics, high-protein diet, digestion of blood from GI bleeding, constipation, infection, progressive liver dysfunction, and hypokalemia with alkalosis. Inability of the liver to convert the end products of protein metabolism to urea results in an elevated serum ammonia level. Constipation increases the systemic absorption of toxins from the colon. Hypokalemia increases ammonia production and alkalosis promotes movement of ammonia and other toxins into the brain.

In hepatic failure patients not all neurological symptoms are due to PSE. They may be related to sodium derangements, especially hyponatremia. For this reason, even mild hyponatremia may be treated aggressively. Another cause of neurological symptoms may be severe malnutrition, which often accompanies hepatic failure. For example, deficiencies of B vitamins can lead to paresthesias, sensory disturbances, peripheral nerve degeneration, palsy of the sixth cranial nerve, and ptosis.

Respiratory System

The primary respiratory complication associated with hepatic failure is decreased lung expansion secondary to upward pressure on the diaphragm from ascites. Lung capacity may also be reduced due to hydrothorax when ascitic fluid leaks through the diaphragm into the pleural cavity. Also, pulmonary hypertension is sometimes associated with uncontrolled portal hypertension. Hypoxemia and hypercarbia may result in all of the above circumstances. However, if a high serum ammonia level is present, hyperventilation with respiratory alkalosis may occur due to stimulation of the respiratory center.

Immune System

The patient with chronic hepatic failure has an increased risk for infection because the liver is no longer able to filter bacteria effectively from the blood. In addition, associated hypersplenism causes a decreased white blood cell count. Infection, particularly full-blown sepsis, places the patient at increased risk for fluid and electrolyte disturbances.

Dermatological System

There are dermatological signs of liver failure, including varying degrees of jaundice, palmar erythema, hair changes, and spider angiomas. Spider angiomas are small dilated superficial vessels resembling bluish-red spiders that may appear in the skin of the face, forearms, and hands. They may represent a large shunting of blood and can bleed profusely.

Hematological System

Anemia may occur in hepatic failure because the hypersplenism caused by portal hypertension increases the rate of red blood cell destruction. Also, the malnutrition that commonly accompanies hepatic failure decreases the rate of red blood cell formation.

Increased bleeding tendencies due to vitamin K deficiency and decreased prothrombin formation leave the patient at risk for excessive bleeding from menses, nosebleeds, gingivitis, GI mucosal changes, and even bruising. Recall that as bleeding in the GI tract is increased, buildup of ammonia secondary to digestion of blood (a protein-containing substance) is increased. Blood transfusions increase the chance of the patient with hepatic failure to develop hyperammoniemia if aged whole blood is used (see Chapter 10).

TREATMENT

Treatment of advanced cirrhotic patients is in part directed at controlling the excess fluid in the peritoneal cavity (ascites) and interstitial space (edema). Among the therapies for these problems are sodium restriction, bedrest, diuretics, water restriction (when hyponatremia is a problem), paracentesis, albumin administration, and peritoneovenous shunts. Other therapeutic interventions for patients with advanced hepatic disease are directed at preventing hepatic coma. Among these are dietary protein restriction and administration of lactulose, bowel-sterilizing antibiotics, and laxatives or enemas.

SODIUM RESTRICTION

Patients with ascites are first treated with sodium-restricted diets. Dietary sodium restriction varies according to need, but daily limitations of 500 mg are usually necessary initially.[26] A more liberal sodium intake (1500–2000 mg/day) may be allowed when a diuresis is effected.[27] Low-sodium diets are discussed in Chapter 3.

BEDREST

Patients with new-onset ascites should be managed with bedrest and moderate sodium restriction.[28] Unless life-threatening complications of ascites are present, patients should be given a trial of 3 to 4 days of bedrest and sodium restriction.[29] After diuresis has been initiated, a gradual increase in activity can be allowed.

DIURETICS

Diuretics should be considered for patients who do not respond to salt restriction and bedrest.[30] The amount of ascites that can be mobilized through the peritoneal capillaries is limited to approximately 700 to 900 mL/day in most patients; therefore, diuretic dosage should be determined cautiously.[31] Overvigorous use of diuretics may result in severe contraction of the intravascular fluid volume causing azotemia and worsening of hepatic encephalopathy. Of course, in edematous patients, diuretics promote fluid loss from the tissue space as well as from the pool of ascites. It is generally accepted that the goal of diuretic therapy is a daily weight loss of 0.5 to 1.0 kg in edematous patients with ascites and approximately 0.25 kg in those having ascites but no edema.[32] These figures are consistent with findings from the classic study reported by Shear and associates in 1970.[33] A more recent study reported that cirrhotic patients without peripheral edema could safely undergo diuresis of 0.75 kg/day as compared to more than 2 kg/day for those with peripheral edema.[34]

Spironolactone (an aldosterone-blocking agent) is usually the first diuretic prescribed when conservative measures (sodium restriction and bedrest) fail to induce an adequate diuresis. Loop diuretics (furosemide, bumetanide, or ethacrynic acid) may be added to spironolactone in patients who fail to respond to spironolactone alone. Because loop diuretics are potassium-losing agents, hypokalemia must be avoided because this imbalance can contribute to the development of hepatic encephalopathy. A frequently advocated method to avoid hypokalemia is the concomitant administration of a potassium-sparing agent, such as spironolactone, with a potassium-losing agent. This not only helps avoid hypokalemia but provides two agents to eliminate excess body sodium.

WATER RESTRICTION

Water restriction is not indicated for all patients. However, if dilutional hyponatremia occurs, a fluid restriction to 1000 to 1500 mL/day will usually suffice.[35] For severe hyponatremia, fluid restriction to the amount necessary to replace insensible loss plus urine output may be needed.

PARACENTESIS

Eventually, patients with ascites may become refractory to diuretics and require paracentesis to relieve respiratory distress and symptoms of marked intraabdominal pressure. Ultrasound has become an effective tool to determine the presence and volume of ascitic fluid in the abdomen.[36] Several studies suggested that paracentesis in patients with massive ascites results in a shorter hospital stay and a decreased incidence of fluid and electrolyte disturbances when compared with treatment with diuretics alone.[37–39] In a related study, it was reported that the intravenous (IV) administration of 40 g of albumin after each large-volume paracentesis appeared to minimize the risk of intravascular volume depletion due to rapid reaccumulation of ascites.[40]

The desired rate for removing ascites is somewhat unclear. Removing more than 1.5 to 2.0 L/day from patients with ascites but no peripheral edema may lead to a reduction in cardiac output, particularly if albumin infusions are withheld.[41] Patients with ascites who also have peripheral edema may be treated with daily 4 to 6 L paracenteses.[42] In some patients large-volume paracentesis has been reported to lead to circulatory collapse, encephalopathy, or renal failure. When paracenteses are performed regularly, the state of tissue perfusion must be monitored. This can be simply estimated by monitoring the BUN and plasma creatinine concentration; stable levels indicate that renal perfusion and, presumably, that of other organs is well maintained and paracentesis can be safely continued.[43]

ALBUMIN ADMINISTRATION

Although 25% albumin is sometimes administered IV to ascitic patients to help correct intravascular volume depletion, it is expensive and appears to offer little advantage over crystalloid solutions for volume expansion.[44] A study conducted in 1949 reported that albumin administered IV passed into the ascites pool in significant quantities, causing the researchers to conclude that albumin was not markedly beneficial in the management of the underlying liver disorder.[45] However, recent studies indicated that albumin infusion is helpful in preventing fluid volume complications when repeated large-volume paracenteses are performed on patients with massive ascites.[46]

PERITONEOVENOUS SHUNTS

Peritoneovenous shunts (such as the LeVeen or Denver shunt) are sometimes used for the 5% to 10% of patients with ascites who do not respond to sodium restriction, diuretics, or other types of medical therapy.[47] The *LaVeen shunt* consists of a long tube (with openings along the sides) inserted into the abdominal cavity, running through the subcutaneous tissue into the jugular vein. With the shunt in place, reinfusion of ascitic fluid into the venous system is allowed (a one-way valve prevents backflow of blood). Pressure changes of respiration permit the shunt to operate. An average weight loss of 10 kg during the first week after shunt placement is not unusual.[48] To achieve adequate post-shunt diuresis, diuretics are essential; the response is markedly improved after shunt placement.[49] Although the shunt may be effective in controlling ascites, its use is associated with a number of serious complications, which include episodes of disseminated intravascular coagulation (due to entry into the bloodstream of endotoxin or other procoagulant material in the ascitic fluid), frequent shunt thrombosis, sepsis, and hemodilution. Shunts should not be used in patients with recent variceal hemorrhage because of the risk of further bleeding, which is increased by the volume expansion as the ascitic fluid is drained into the venous system. Other contraindications are coagulopathies or bacteria in the ascitic fluid. Shunt failure reportedly occurs in one-third of cases.[50] Mortality may approach 25% in the first month.[51]

DIETARY PROTEIN RESTRICTION

Impending hepatic coma is an indication to eliminate protein temporarily from the diet. A reduced protein intake decreases ammonia formation and thus the likelihood for hepatic encephalopathy. Adequate nonprotein calories (25–30 cal/kg) must be supplied by the enteral or parenteral route.[52] It appears that vegetable proteins are better tolerated by patients with portal-systemic encephalopathy than diets containing meat proteins.[53] As the patient improves, more protein can be added in small increments every few days as tolerated. Specialized enteral and parenteral formulas are commercially available for malnourished patients with hepatic failure and concomitant hepatic encephalopathy; these formulas are designed to correct the abnormal amino acid profile associated with hepatic encephalopathy. They contain low quantities of aromatic amino acids and methionine and high quantities of branch-chain amino acids.[54]

BOWEL-STERILIZING ANTIBIOTICS

Bowel-sterilizing antibiotics, such as neomycin, can reduce ammonia formation caused by excessive bacterial growth in the bowel. Recall that neomycin (given orally, by nasogastric tube, or by enema) kills urease-producing bacteria, causing less urease to be produced, and hence, less urea to be broken down into ammonia. There is a risk of nephrotoxicity and ototoxicity when neomycin is used, particularly in patients with renal impairment. Metronidazole is an agent that is useful for short-term therapy when neomycin is unavailable or poorly tolerated.[55]

LACTULOSE AS LAXATIVE

Constipation should be prevented because the systemic absorption of toxic nitrogenous substances from the intestinal lumen is more likely when constipation is allowed to occur. Lactulose is a poorly absorbed substance used to promote more frequent stools and prevent or treat PSE. About 97% of the lactulose taken orally reaches the colon unabsorbed. The mechanisms by which it reduces PSE are unclear, but three actions have been suggested. First, through the conversion of lactulose to organic acids (such as lactic acid) the pH of colonic contents decreases, inhibiting the diffusion of ammonia (NH_3) from the colon into the blood. Second, because the pH of the bowel vasculature is relatively higher than the contents of the colon under treatment with lactulose, ammonia is converted into ammonium (NH_4), preventing its absorption. Due to this same pH gradient, absorption of amines (also implicated in PSE) from the colon to the bloodstream is reduced. Third, lactulose has a cathartic effect caused by an osmotic effect, which increases the water contents of stool.

By monitoring the pH of stool (with regular pH paper) and adjusting lactulose accordingly, it is possible to reach more precisely a desired pH level of 5.[56] Oral dosage begins at 20 to 30 g three or four times a day for 1 or 2 days; the dosage is then adjusted so that two or three soft stools are produced daily.[57]

Lactulose can be administered rectally when it is not tolerated orally or when pulmonary aspiration is a great risk. (Two hundred grams can be diluted in 700 mL of water or saline, depending on risk of sodium absorption and current serum levels.)[58] The solution is given through a rectal balloon catheter and retained for 30 to 60 min. If not retained, it can be repeated immediately. The process should be repeated every 4 to 6 hrs until symptoms of PSE begin to reverse and oral administration can be started. Soapsuds or other enemas with alkalinizing agents are to be avoided because their use can reverse the effects of lactulose.

BENZODIAZAPINE ANTAGONISTS

Patients with symptoms of PSE should have all sedation withheld. If benzodiazapines have been administered, a trial of the antagonist flumazenil may be useful. After as little as 1 mg, patients have awakened immediately after injection of this medication. Because it has an extremely short half-life and some benzodiazapines have very long half-lives, it may be necessary to repeat it frequently or administer it as a continuous infusion.[59]

NURSING ASSESSMENT

Nursing assessment of cirrhotic patients with ascites focuses largely on fluid balance parameters, such as fluid gains and losses (as measured by input and output [I&O] records, body weights, and abdominal girth). More specifically, the nurse is responsible for monitoring responses to therapy and for changes indicating metabolic abnormalities. Listed below are some of the more important nursing assessments with a brief discussion of rationales.

1. Monitor response to diuretics and sodium restriction by the following assessments:
   A. Determine abdominal girth on a serial basis, measuring the abdomen at the same place each time. To ensure accurate placement of the measuring tape, it is helpful to draw lines above and below the tape on each side of the abdomen. Be sure the tape is not kinked under the patient's body. Measurements should be made with the patient in the same position each time (Fig. 21-1).
   B. Measure I&O; expect to see output exceed intake during effective diuresis. Be aware of the danger of excessive diuresis (see Rationale below).
   C. Monitor vital signs at least twice daily. Be alert for hypotension and tachycardia, indications of excessive diuresis and decreased circulating blood volume.
   D. Monitor for dependent pitting edema. This is helpful in assessing the degree of sodium and water retention.
   E. Measure body weight daily. Weights are most accurate when measured in the early morning before breakfast and after voiding, using the same scale each time. Compare the expected therapeutic weight loss with the actual weight loss (see Rationale below).

Rationale: With adequate sodium restriction and diuretic use, a decrease in abdominal girth, a urinary output relatively greater than the intake during period of diuresis, a decrease in peripheral edema, and a decrease in body weight should be anticipated. The desired weight loss with treatment varies with the patient's clinical status. However, as discussed in the section on treatment, an ascitic patient without peripheral edema might be expected to lose 0.25 kg (1/2 lb) per day, whereas an ascitic patient with peripheral edema might be expected to lose 0.5 to 1.0 kg (approximately 1–2 lb) per day. Also, as mentioned in the treatment section, one study suggested that weight loss might safely occur more rapidly (e.g., 0.75 kg/day in ascitic patients without peripheral edema and >2 kg/day in those with peripheral edema).[60] Because of differences among patients and treatment plans to induce fluid

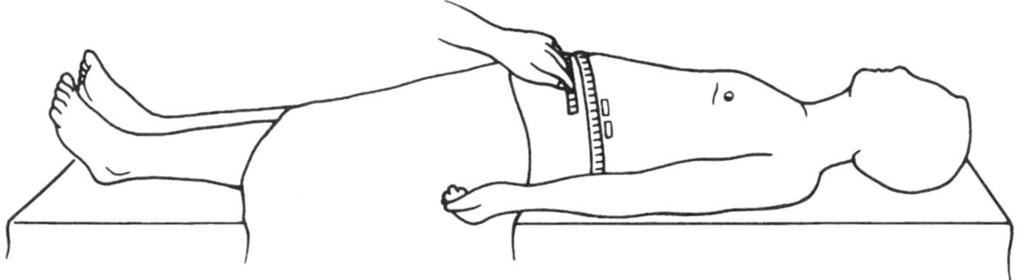

Figure 21–1. Measurement of abdominal girth.

diuresis, the need for careful clinical observations (such as vital sign variations) is evident. The treatment of ascites and edema must be undertaken cautiously. Although the fluid retained as ascites and edema is uncomfortable and cosmetically unpleasing, it is seldom life-threatening. However, overly aggressive therapy can lead to hepatic encephalopathy and compromised renal function.

2. Monitor patients undergoing paracentesis carefully for the following adverse effects:
   - Circulatory collapse (e.g., pallor; weak, rapid pulse; hypotension; fall in central venous pressure)
   - Decline in renal function (oliguria, rise in BUN, serum creatinine)
   - Worsening of neurological function (lethargy, confusion, slurred speech)

Rationale: Hypovolemia is most likely to result when too much fluid is removed at one time. The mechanism involves a rapid reaccumulation of ascitic fluid resulting from flow of sodium and plasma volume. As indicated in the treatment section, the removal of as little as 1500 mL may precipitate hypotension in some patients, particularly in those without peripheral edema. However, some sources state that as much as 5 L may be safely removed in edematous patients, provided the fluid is removed slowly (over 30–90 min) and a fluid restriction is initiated to avoid hyponatremia.[61] Excessive fluid removal with paracentesis or diuresis can precipitate the hepatorenal syndrome (manifested by oliguria or rise in serum creatinine and BUN) or portal-systemic encephalopathy (manifested by lethargy, confusion, and slurred speech). As discussed earlier, some investigators report that the administration of albumin helps prevent fluid balance problems after massive paracentesis.[62]

3. Monitor patients receiving diuretics for disturbances in potassium balance.

Rationale: Patients receiving potassium-losing diuretics (such as furosemide and thiazides) are at risk for hypokalemia. Symptoms include fatigue, muscle weakness, leg cramps, decreased bowel motility, paresthesias, electrocardiographic (ECG) changes (flat T waves and depressed ST segments), arrhythmias, and increased sensitivity to digitalis. On the other hand, patients taking potassium-conserving diuretics (such as spironolactone, Dyrenium, and amiloride) are at risk for hyperkalemia. Symptoms include weakness, paresthesias, ECG changes (tented T waves), and arrhythmias. See Chapter 5 for a review or nursing responsibilities related to potassium imbalances.

4. Monitor patients receiving neomycin for hearing difficulty.

Rationale: Large doses of neomycin can damage both the kidneys and the ears; deafness may occur, particularly when neomycin is administered with furosemide (Lasix) or ethacrynic acid (Edecrin).

5. Monitor patients for symptoms of PSE.

Rationale: This disturbance is particularly likely to occur in individuals who are bleeding into the intestinal tract. Symptoms include lethargy, loss of memory, slurred speech, personality change, and disorientation. Convulsive seizures and coma may follow untreated or refractory PSE.

6. Monitor patients for hyponatremia.

Rationale: This imbalance must be detected early so that fluid restriction can be initiated before the imbalance becomes severe. Symptoms are primarily those of cerebral swelling (lethargy and somnolence), making this imbalance difficult to distinguish from other disturbances affecting the neurological status.

NURSING DIAGNOSES

Examples of nursing diagnoses related to fluid and electrolyte balance in patients with cirrhosis are listed in Clinical Tip: Examples of Nursing Diagnoses Related to Fluid and Electrolyte Problems in Patients With Cirrhosis, along with etiologies and defining characteristics. Nursing interventions and rationales are discussed below.

NURSING INTERVENTIONS

Nursing interventions are directed at promoting adaptation and minimizing ill effects of the disease process.

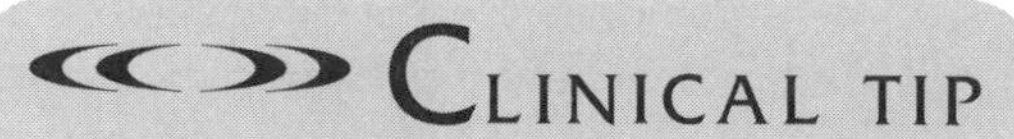

Examples of Nursing Diagnoses Related to Fluid and Electrolyte Problems in Patients With Cirrhosis

NURSING DIAGNOSIS	ETIOLOGICAL FACTORS	DEFINING CHARACTERISTICS
ECF volume excess (total body sodium and water increased), but decreased effective arterial volume, related to pathophysiological changes of cirrhosis	Despite increased total ECF volume due to renal retention of sodium and water, body responds as if arterial volume is diminished (decreased effective arterial volume)	Ascites Peripheral edema first noted in lower extremities and later becoming generalized (dependent on sodium intake)
Risk for hypovolemia related to rapid reaccumulation of ascitic fluid after large volume paracentesis	Ascites may reaccumulate rapidly (particularly when albumin is not administered after paracentesis) following the removal of large volumes of ascites	Reduced cardiac output Decreased blood pressure Increased pulse rate
Alterations in thought processes related to increased toxins (such as ammonia)	Elevated serum ammonia level (results when liver is unable to convert ammonia formed in intestines to urea) Bleeding into GI tract increases protein metabolism Excessive diuresis contracts plasma volume and increases concentration of toxins	Slowed response, memory loss, sleep disturbances, confusion, disorientation, personality change, stupor, coma, seizures
Alteration in thought processes related to dilutional hyponatremia	Increased ADH secretion due to decrease in ineffective arterial volume	Lethargy, somnolence, personality change, serum sodium <135 mEq/L (see Chapter 4)
Alteration in potassium balance (hypokalemia) related to use of potassium-losing diuretics	Potassium-losing diuretics (such as furosemide or bumetanide)	Fatigue, muscle weakness, leg cramps, decreased bowel motility, arrhythmias, ECG changes (see Chapter 5)
Risk for impaired gas exchange related to decreased lung expansion	Large accumulation of ascites causes diaphragm to press upward on lungs, causing decreased respirations. Condition is aggravated by generalized weakness, lethargy, and immobility	Decreased respiratory depth Increased $PaCO_2$

ECF, extracellular fluid; ADH, antidiuretic hormone.

1. Continue ongoing assessment of fluid balance status as the basis for collaborative interaction with the physician in regulation of therapy (see section on Nursing Assessment).
2. Prevent constipation by administering lactulose as prescribed and indicated (goal is to produce two or three soft stools per day).
   - Attempt to minimize the unpleasant sweet taste of lactulose by diluting it with fruit juice, water, or milk or administering it in foods (such as desserts).
   - If lactulose is given through a GI tube, it should be well diluted to prevent vomiting and the risk of pulmonary aspiration.
   - If aspiration is likely, it may be necessary to administer the lactulose by retention enema.
   - Monitor for excessive loose stools because severe fluid and electrolyte depletion could occur.
     Rationale: Constipation should be prevented because it contributes to the accumulation of ammonia. Bleeding in the GI tract increases ammonia formation (due to digestion of blood proteins) and may precipitate hepatic coma. Bowel evacuation removes blood from the intestine and therefore decreases a source of urea and other false neurotransmitters. Use of lactulose (orally and by enema) is described further in the section on Treatment.
3. Encourage rest periods in which the patient lies down.
   Rationale: Assumption of the supine position is often associated with a spontaneous diuresis, resulting in significant weight loss with mobilization of peripheral edema fluid and ascitic fluid. The diuresis induced by bedrest results from improvement in cardiac output and effective circulating blood volume. The patient with severe ascites is usually better able to tolerate the lateral recumbent position.
4. Maintain a safe environment for the patient with the potential for, or actual presence of, PSE.
   - When deemed necessary, remove potential sources of harm (such as matches or sharp objects) from the immediate environment.
   - Caution significant others that the patient's ability to drive or perform usual activities (such as cooking) should be closely monitored. Driver's licenses are often restricted or revoked for this group of patients making it necessary for significant others to assume many additional responsibilities for home-bound patients (e.g., cooking and transportation to treatment facilities).
   Rationale: Because episodes of encephalopathy may interfere with thought and reasoning processes, physical safety of the patient and others must be considered.
5. Initiate patient instruction in self-care.
   A. Teach home-bound patients how to monitor their fluid I&O and body weights, and when to seek intervention from the health care provider.
   B. Instruct patient or significant other in how to manage a sodium-restricted diet at home; written information that can be taken home is advantageous, as is accessibility of a dietary consultant when questions arise.
   C. Promote the patient's understanding of his or her diuretic therapy. For example, the patient should be able to name the diuretic as well as its purpose and common side effects. The desirability of taking the diuretic in the morning to avoid disturbing sleep at night should be emphasized.
   D. Promote the patient's understanding or that of significant others of potassium supplements when they are required. The patient or caregiver should be able to name the agent, its dosage, the reason for taking it, and possible side effects. Because some potassium supplements can be unpleasant, the reason for taking the substance should be emphasized (recall that hypokalemia associated with metabolic alkalosis can lead to the development of portal systemic encephalopathy).
   E. Promote the patient's understanding of salt substitutes, if used. For example, the patient should be able to name acceptable agents. Instruct patients receiving a combination potassium-conserving, potassium-losing diuretic (such as Aldactazide or Dyazide) that salt substitutes should be used sparingly, if at all. When only a potassium-conserving diuretic is used, the danger of hyperkalemia is present; for such patients, salt substitutes are generally not recommended.

Recall that most salt substitutes contain sizable amounts of potassium (see Table 5-2).

Rationale: Understanding dietary and pharmacological regimens will promote adherence to these treatment modalities and promote optimal wellness.

CASE STUDY

21-1. Mrs. N, a 50-year-old woman with a long history of alcoholism and cirrhosis with ascites, was admitted with complaints of difficulty breathing and a weight gain of 13 lbs over the past 2 weeks. On questioning, she stated she had omitted her diuretic (spironolactone) and failed to adhere to her sodium-restricted dietary regimen over this same period of time.

On physical examination, her abdomen was found to be largely distended with ascites. Her lower extremities were edematous and she had jugular venous distention. Vital signs were: temperature, 98.6 °F; pulse rate, 100/min; respiratory rate, 20/min; and blood pressure, 170/98 mmHg. Laboratory results indicated that all serum electrolytes were within normal limits (serum sodium, 137 mEq/L).

COMMENTARY The signs of excessive sodium and water retention included acute weight gain, lower extremity edema, ascites, hypertension, and jugular venous distention. Increasing ascitic fluid accumulation placed pressure on the diaphragm and made it difficult for her to breath normally. Because she gained 13 lbs over this relatively short period of time, it can be concluded that Mrs. N retained about 6 L of fluid. (One liter of fluid = 2.2 lbs.) The increased ascitic fluid accumulation that occurred over the 2-week period did not produce a deficit in the vascular space because it developed relatively slowly, allowing time for sodium and water to be retained by the kidneys to replace fluid shifted from the vascular space to the ascitic pool. Treatment includes diuretics and a sodium-restricted diet. The peritoneum limits the transfer of ascitic fluid into the vascular space to about 750 mL/day. Because Mrs. N. also had peripheral edema, she could be expected to diurese edema fluid in addition to the ascitic fluid (perhaps allowing her to excrete up to 1 L of fluid per day initially without compromising her intravascular volume). Patients with ascites often are treated with spironolactone (a potassium-sparing diuretic) because it is an aldosterone antagonist that reduces sodium reabsorption by the kidney. It does not cause potassium depletion; this is an important consideration in a cirrhotic patient because hypokalemia increases ammonia production and predisposes to hepatic encephalopathy.

REFERENCES

1. Schrier et al: Peripheral arterial vasodilation hypothesis: A proposal for the initiation of renal sodium and water retention in cirrhosis. Hepatology 8:1151,1993
2. Herrera JL: Current medical management of cirrhotic ascites. Am J Med Sci 302:31,1991
3. Runyon BA: Ascites. In: Schiff L, Schiff E (eds): Diseases of the Liver, 7th ed, p 992. Philadelphia, JB Lippincott, 1993
4. Ibid
5. Ibid
6. Kinouchi T: Fluid, electrolyte, and acid–base disorders in liver cirrhosis. Nippon Rinsho-Japanese J Clin Med 52(1):124–131,1994
7. Porayko MK, Wiesner RH: Management of ascites in patients with cirrhosis. Postgrad Med 92(2):194,1993
8. Longmire-Cook SJ: Pathophysiologic factors and management of ascites. Surg Gynecol Obstet 176(2):194,1993
9. Narins R (ed): Clinical Disorders of Fluid and Electrolyte Metabolism, 5th ed, p 1160. New York, McGraw-Hill, 1994
10. Narins, p 1159
11. Sherlock S: Ascites formation and its management. Scand J Gastroenterol 7(Suppl):9,1970
12. Narins, p 1160
13. Ibid, p 1161
14. Ibid, p 1163
15. Ibid
16. Ibid
17. Ibid, p 1164
18. Ibid
19. Ibid, p 1165
20. Ibid
21. Ibid
22. Badalamenti S, et al: Hepatorenal syndrome: New perspectives in pathogenesis and treatment. Arch Intern Med 153:1960,1993
23. Kokko J, Tannen R: Fluids and Electrolytes, 2nd ed, p 672. Philadelphia, WB Saunders, 1990

24. Badalamenti, p 1965
25. Ibid
26. Epstein M: Renal complications of liver disease. In: Schiff L, Schiff E (eds): Diseases of the Liver, 7th ed, p 1023. Philadelphia, JB Lippincott, 1991
27. Herrera, p 34
28. Ibid, p 33
29. Chiou SS, Changchien CS: Management of end-stage liver disease. Transplant Proceed 25:2948,1993
30. White HM: Hepatic diseases. In: Woodley M, Whelan A (eds): Manual of Medical Therapeutics, 27th ed, p 321. Boston, Little, Brown, 1992
31. Epstein, p 1023
32. Porayko, Weisner, p 162
33. Shear L, et al: Compartmentalization of ascites and edema in patients with hepatic cirrhosis. N Engl J Med 282:1391,1970
34. Porayko, p 158
35. Herrera, p 34
36. Ibid, p 32
37. Porayko, Weisner, p 162
38. Kellerman PS, Linas SL: Large-volume paracentesis in the treatment of ascites. Ann Intern Med 11:889,1990
39. Reynolds TB: Renaissance of paracentesis in the treatment of ascites. Adv Intern Med 35:365–373,1990
40. Gines et al: Randomized comparative study of therapeutic paracentesis with and without intravenous albumin in cirrhosis. Gastroenterol 94:1493,1988
41. Reynolds, p 370
42. Porayko, Weisner, p 162
43. Reynolds, p 368
44. Arroyo et al: Treatment of ascites in cirrhosis. Gastroenterol Clin North Am 21(1):251,1992
45. Faloon et al: An evaluation of human serum albumin in the treatment of cirrhosis of the liver. J Clin Invest 28:583,1949
46. Gines, p 1493
47. Epstein M: Peritoneovenous shunt in the management of ascites and the hepatorenal syndrome. Gastroenterol 82:790,1982
48. Wapnick S: Randomized prospective matched pair study comparing peritoneovenous shunt and conventional therapy in massive ascites. Br J Surg 66:667,1979
49. Maskovitz M: The peritoneovenous shunt: expectations vs reality. Am J Gastroenterol 85:917,1990
50. Longmire-Cook, p 199
51. Maskovitz, p 919
52. Wagner et al: Pathophysiology and clinical basis of prevention and treatment of complications of chronic liver disease. Gastroenterol Hepatol 69:113,1991
53. Chiou, Changchien, p 2950
54. Rombeau J, Caldwell M: Clinical Nutrition: Enteral and Tube Feeding, 2nd ed, p 300. Philadelphia, WB Saunders, 1990
55. White, p 320
56. Bircher J, Sommer W: Portal systemic encephalopathy. In: Prieto et al (eds): Hepatobiliary Diseases, p 424. New York, Springer-Verlag, 1992
57. Bircher, Sommer, p 423
58. Knauer CM: Liver, biliary and pancreas. In: Tierney LM et al (eds): Current Medical Diagnosis and Treatment, p 517. Norwalk, Appleton & Lange, 1993
59. Bircher, Sommer, p 423
60. Herrera, p 34
61. Reynolds, p 369
62. Gines, p 1493

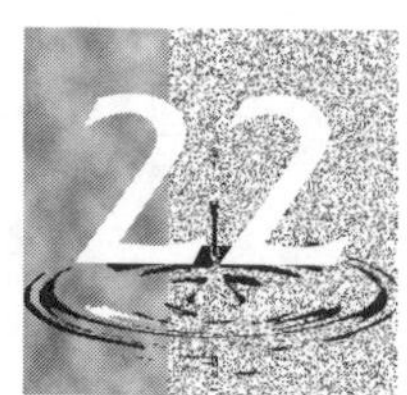

Oncologic Conditions

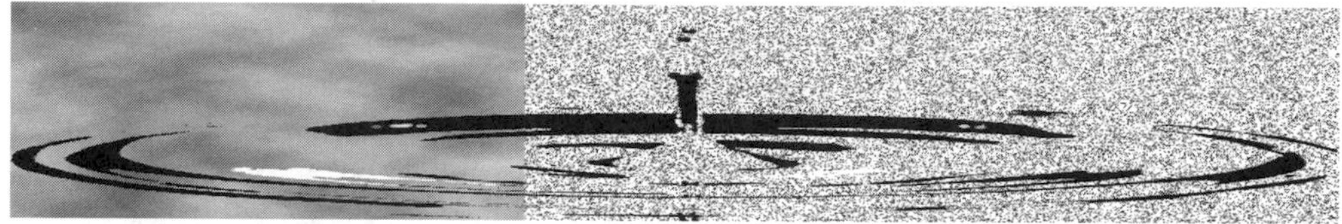

Maintaining fluid and electrolyte balance is often difficult in patients with cancer. In some situations, fluid and electrolyte problems are the initial symptoms that cause the individual to see the physician. At other times, these problems are related to the development of metastatic disease. Unfortunately, they may often be the *consequence* of aggressive therapy. A majority of oncology patients will experience a problem with fluid and electrolyte regulation during the course of their illness. Often various fluid and electrolyte disturbances exist simultaneously.[1] The treatment of electrolyte disorders needs to be monitored closely as the correction of one imbalance can lead to the appearance of another imbalance (e.g., the treatment of hypercalcemia can lead to hypokalemia and hypomagnesemia). Patients with cancer may also suffer from other unrelated health conditions that can cause fluid and electrolyte imbalances; among these are congestive heart failure, hypertension, renal diseases, and gastrointestinal (GI) disorders. The complete picture of the cancer patient needs to be considered when evaluating fluid and electrolyte imbalances. These problems can be acute or chronic and vary significantly in the degree of severity.

CAUSES OF FLUID AND ELECTROLYTE PROBLEMS IN CANCER PATIENTS

Among the causes of fluid and electrolyte imbalances in cancer patients are excessive loss or decreased intake of electrolytes; another is faulty hormonal regulation of water and electrolyte balance (see Table 22-1.)

FAULTY REGULATION OR AVAILABILITY OF ELECTROLYTES

Fluid and electrolyte problems associated with cancer are most commonly related to faulty regulation or availability of one of the following substances:

- Calcium
- Uric acid
- Sodium
- Potassium
- Phosphate
- Magnesium

ALTERED HORMONAL REGULATORY MECHANISMS

Electrolyte imbalance in oncology patients is frequently due to alterations in various hormonal regulatory mechanisms caused by a variety of tumors. These malignant tumors produce ectopic polypeptide hormones or pseudohormone substances that interfere with water and electrolyte balance. Involved hormones (or hormone-like substances) include the following:

- Antidiuretic hormone (ADH)
- Parathyroid hormone (PTH)
- Calcitonin
- Factors possessing osteoclastic-activating activity including interleukin-1, tumor necrosis factors alpha and beta, and prostaglandins
- Growth factors including transforming growth factor-alpha
- Adrenocorticotrophic hormone (ACTH)

Production of these hormones is not regulated by normal suppression feedback loops; as a consequence, the ectopic hormone continues to be released by the tumor, often causing life-threatening electrolyte imbalances. The generally accepted theory that accounts for the production of ectopic hormones is faulty genetic regulation by the malignant tumor itself.[2,3]

THIRD-SPACE FLUID ACCUMULATION

Cancer patients frequently develop third-space fluid accumulations; these may be due to the following:

- Malignant effusions into the peritoneal, pericardial, or pleural compartments. Direct tumor involvement of the cavity's serous surface appears to be the most frequent cause of effusions in cancer patients. However, peritoneal effusions also known as ascites commonly occur with liver disease secondary to malignancy.
- Edema. This is trapping of excess fluid in the interstitial fluid space due to obstruction of lymphatic drainage or venous return secondary to tumor pressure. Protein seepage through the capillary bed in the edematous site pulls fluid with it, making the edema more severe. Low serum oncotic pressure (due to hypoalbuminemia)

(text continues on page 382

TABLE 22–1

Fluid and Electrolyte Imbalances in Cancer Patients

ELECTROLYTE IMBALANCE	PHYSIOLOGICAL PROCESS	UNDERLYING CAUSE/MALIGNANCY
Hypercalcemia	Increased osteolytic activity of tumor	Breast cancer Kidney cancer Non-small-cell lung cancer Colon cancer Ovarian cancer
	Ectopic PTH production or PTH-related protein	Epidermoid lung cancer Renal adenocarcinoma Oral cavity squamous cancer
	Increased osteoclastic-activating activity related to one or more of the following: • Interleukin-1 • Tumor necrosis factors (alpha and beta) • Vitamin D-like sterols • Lymphotoxin • Transforming growth factor alpha	Leukemia Lymphoma Multiple myeloma Treatment with: • Estrogens • Progestins • Androgens • Antiestrogens
*Hypocalcemia	Increased calcium use	"Hungry bone syndrome" Metastases from prostate or breast cancer treated with hormonal therapy Rapid healing of bony lesions
	Decreased calcium intake	Starvation Hyperalimentation with inadequate calcium supplementation
	Decreased calcium absorption	Fistulae (with loss of fluid before absorption can occur) Lymphoma of small bowel
	Decreased serum albumin	Starvation Transudation of protein into third-space fluid accumulation
*Hyperuricemia	Increase in uric acid precursors	Polycythemia vera Chronic granulocytic leukemia
	Rapid tumor dissolution with increased nucleic acid release	Induction therapy for leukemia Radiosensitive/chemotherapy-sensitive lymphomas or bulky solid tumors
Hyponatremia	Loss of sodium	Fistulas Prolonged vomiting and/or diarrhea Prolonged nasogastric suction Hyperproteinemic states can produce "pseudohyponatremia"

TABLE 22–1 (cont.)

ELECTROLYTE IMBALANCE	PHYSIOLOGICAL PROCESS	UNDERLYING CAUSE/MALIGNANCY
Hyponatremia (cont.)	Ectopic ADH production (SIADH)	Small-cell lung cancer Lymphoma Thymoma Drug-induced: • High-dose cyclophosphamide • Vincristine (Oncovin) • Vinblastine (Velban) • Cisplatin • High-dose Melphalan • Narcotics
Hypernatremia	Increased water loss	Renal damage associated with multiple myeloma
*Hyperkalemia	Increased release of potassium from cellular breakdown	Induction therapy for acute leukemia Radiosensitive/chemotherapy-sensitive lymphomas or bulky tumors
	Acute renal failure	Renal cancer Untreated hyperuricemia Nephrotoxic antineoplastic drugs or anti-infective agents
Hypokalemia	Decreased intake	Anorexia or nausea secondary to pain, tumor obstruction, depression, or chemotherapy/radiation therapy
	Increased GI loss of potassium	Prolonged mechanical GI suction, fistulae drainage Prolonged vomiting secondary to obstruction or chemotherapy/radiation therapy treatments Prolonged diarrhea secondary to malignancies, infectious agents in the GI tract, radiation/chemotherapy treatments, bone marrow transplant induced graft versus host disease
	Increased renal tubular loss	Tubular damage secondary to chemotherapy for leukemia Nonabsorbable ions present in certain antibiotics including penicillin, ampicillin, carbenicillin, and ticarcillin Nephrotoxic antibiotics including the aminoglycosides Nephrotoxic anti-fungal agent—amphotericin B

(continued)

TABLE 22–1 (cont.)

ELECTROLYTE IMBALANCE	PHYSIOLOGICAL PROCESS	UNDERLYING CAUSE/MALIGNANCY
Hypokalemia (cont.)	Increased renal tubular loss (cont'd.)	Nephrotoxic chemotherapeutic agents including cisplatin, carboplatin, and high-dose methotrexate
	Ectopic ACTH production	Small-cell lung cancer Thymoma Islet cell pancreatic cancer Bronchial carcinoid
Hypophosphatemia	Increased urinary loss	Multiple myeloma
	Respiratory alkalosis	Sepsis (Recall that fever causes hyperventilation, which in turn causes respiratory alkalosis.)
	Decreased intake	Starvation, hyperalimentation with inadequate phosphate
	Consumption of phosphate by tumor cells	Acute leukemia
*Hyperphosphatemia	Increased cellular release	Acute leukemia Sensitive lymphomas and bulky tumors
Hypomagnesemia	Increased loss	Renal magnesium wasting from therapy with cisplatin and aminoglycoside antibiotics Chronic diarrhea
	Decreased intake	Prolonged inadequate dietary intake or inadequate supplementation intravenously
	Mechanism not understood	Cyclosporine and amphotericin B

ACTH, adrenocorticotrophic hormone; PTH, parathyroid hormone; SIADH, syndrome of inappropriate antidiuretic hormone secretion; GI, gastrointestinal.

*Components of tumor lysis syndrome.

along with extremity dependence contributes to ankle and leg swelling in oncology patients who sit for long periods.

Major shifts of water and electrolytes into potential fluid spaces result in extracellular fluid volume deficit (FVD). This condition is manifested by decreased urinary output, increased urinary specific gravity, and postural hypotension. Body weight does not decrease (as it does with actual fluid loss) because fluid is trapped inside the body; in fact, weight may increase with parenteral fluid replacement (given to correct intravascular fluid volume depletion). Unfortunately, administration of intravenous (IV) fluids to correct the FVD also allows an increase in the fluid volume trapped in the third space, which only adds to the patient's discomfort.

In the case of peritoneal effusions, a paracentesis can be performed to drain the fluid for comfort measures; however, replacement of the fluid, electrolytes, and albumin lost during this procedure must be considered. (Refer to Chapter 21 for a discussion of paracentesis for ascites.)

For a long-term resolution of third-space fluid accumulation, the *cause* of the fluid shift must be corrected. This can only be accomplished if the malignant process producing the third-space fluid accumulation responds to treatment.

TREATMENT-RELATED IMBALANCES

The treatment of malignancies can *create* fluid and electrolyte imbalances. Examples of treatment-induced imbalances include the following:

- Hypercalcemia associated with hormonal (tamoxifen) treatment of breast cancer
- Hyponatremia, hypokalemia, and hypomagnesemia occasionally caused by chemotherapy-induced nausea and vomiting (uncontrolled by antiemetics)
- Hyponatremia (water intoxication) associated with the use of certain chemotherapeutic drugs (such as vincristine [Oncovin] and cyclophosphamide [Cytoxan]).
- Hypokalemia and hypomagnesemia associated with diarrhea caused by certain chemotherapy and/or radiation treatments
- Hypomagnesemia associated with hypocalcemia that is nonresponsive to calcium replacement therapy
- Hyperuricemia associated with cell destruction and release of pools of nucleic acids that are metabolized to uric acid (seen in patients with acute leukemia, Burkitt's lymphoma, diffuse histiocytic lymphoma, and preexisting renal disease)
- Release of large amounts of intracellular electrolytes (phosphate and potassium) into the serum due to destruction of rapidly growing neoplasms (tumor lysis syndrome). Also, high levels of free phosphate radicals combine with ionized serum calcium creating hypocalcemia (see Clinical Tip: Management of Tumor Lysis Syndrome).[4,5]

FLUID AND ELECTROLYTE DISTURBANCES

Mechanisms responsible for fluid and electrolyte imbalances in cancer patients, as well as the tumors (or associated problems) causing the imbalances are described in this section (see Table 22-1).

Treatment to correct common electrolyte imbalances is also described in this section. Note that treatment of tumor-related fluid and electrolyte problems initially is directed at relieving immediate life-threatening problems and later at controlling the underlying tumor causing the imbalance. It is essential that the treatment for the malignancy be successful for a permanent resolution of the imbalance.

HYPERCALCEMIA

One of the more common problems of malignant disease is hypercalcemia. About 10% to 20% of all persons with cancer will develop an elevated serum calcium level during the course of their illness. The incidence increases to 40% to 50% in patients with metastatic breast cancer and multiple myeloma.[6,7] Hypercalcemia is associated with virtually any type of malignancy, from solid tumors with or without bony metastases to hematological malignancies, and may include the following:

1. Solid tumors with bony metastases:
   - Breast
   - Lung
   - Renal
   - Colon
   - Ovary
   - Epidermoid cancers of the head and neck
2. Solid tumors without bony metastases:
   - Lung
   - Head and neck
   - Renal
   - Ovary
3. Hematological malignancies:
   - Lymphoma
   - Leukemia
   - Multiple myeloma

Since the late 1980s researchers and clinicians have greatly increased their understanding of the pathogenesis of hypercalcemia.[8] Hypercalcemia of malignancy was initially thought to result from significant malignant tumor invasion of bone either by direct extension or through metastasis. This older explanation was known to be incomplete because bony metastases do not consistently cause hypercalcemia; furthermore, patients with limited amounts of bony metastases or with hematological malignancies may develop hypercalcemia. Clinicians also discussed a process called humoral-mediated hypercalcemia;

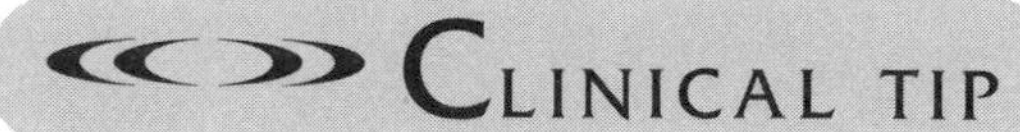

Management of Tumor Lysis Syndrome

Prevention:

- Assessment of patients at risk:
  Those with leukemia, diffuse histiocytic lymphoma, Burkitt's lymphoma, and potentially any patient with bulky tumors or with tumors that have rapid cell growth.
- Pretreatment intravenous hydration (3000 mL/m^2) over 24 hours for 1 to 2 days prior to chemotherapy treatment:
  Carefully monitor kidney function and for potential fluid overload. Check vital signs and lung sounds, look for edema, and monitor fluid intake and output. Foley catheters may be recommended for accurate monitoring of urine output in certain situations.
- Urinary alkalinization with 50–100 mEq sodium bicarbonate added to intravenous fluid to maintain urinary pH ≥ 7
  When monitoring urinary output, observe for any signs of solute precipitation in the urine.
- Administration of allopurinol (200–500 mg/m^2)
  Initial dose is often divided into BID schedule; observe for potential side effects (such as fever, rash, eosinophilia, and hypersensitivity reactions).
- Monitor serum electrolytes, using baseline levels for comparison.
  - Assess serum potassium, calcium, phosphorus, creatinine and BUN q 6 hrs. Inform physician immediately of any variation from normal.
  - Assess for symptoms of hyperkalemia, hypocalcemia, hyperuricemia, and hyperphosphatemia.

Treatment:

- Treatment of hyperkalemia, hypocalcemia, hyperuricemia, and hyperphosphatemia if these electrolyte imbalances occur
- Treatment of fluid volume overload if needed
- Hemodialysis if renal failure occurs

BUN, blood urea nitrogen.

this was thought to involve the secretion of ectopic PTH by a variety of solid tumors. In the 1990s, investigators are attempting to determine the presence of other factors (sometimes called humoral factors) that may be involved in the humoral-mediated hypercalcemia process. The following brief review suggests a variety of pathways other than osseous metastases as a basis for hypercalcemia of malignant disease.

Mechanisms

Regardless of the type of malignancy, the basic mechanism responsible for an elevated serum calcium level is an increase in calcium release from bone that exceeds calcium excretion from the renal tubules. The following physiological mechanisms may be responsible for the increase of calcium release from bone in neoplastic states:

1. Tumor-related mechanisms

Direct

- Lysis of bone

Indirect (humoral hypercalcemia of malignancy [HHM])

- Prostaglandin activity, specifically prostaglandin E series
- Tumor release of PTH or PTH-related protein
- Cytokines with osteoclastic-activating activity including interleukin-1 and tumor necrosis factors alpha and beta
- Growth factors including transforming growth factor alpha
- Tumor release of vitamin D-like sterols

2. Treatment-related mechanisms
   - Use of androgens, estrogens, progestins, or anti-estrogens
3. Non–tumor-related mechanisms
   - Coincidental primary hyperparathyroidism

Presence of malignant tumor cells in bony spaces has been demonstrated to cause an increased release of calcium from bone and a loss of skeletal integrity. In women with breast cancer with bony metastasis this is the most common mechanism for hypercalcemia. In addition to the direct resorption of bone by tumor cells, prostaglandin action has been proposed as a mechanism for increased calcium release from the bone.[9] Animal models have shown that prostaglandins have osteolytic activities.[10] It is not known if this animal model principle can be transferred to humans. The source and exact action of prostaglandins (specifically of the E series) remain under intense investigation. Other factors that potentially interact with prostaglandin and PTH-related protein include the transforming growth factors.

Solid tumors without bony metastases have been associated with hypercalcemia states, as documented in patients with squamous cell carcinoma of the head and neck and carcinomas of the lung and kidney. Further investigation is needed to demonstrate the actual mechanisms responsible for hypercalcemic clinical syndromes in patients with radiographically negative skeletal series. In these cases, PTH-related protein, transforming growth factor alpha, interleukin-1, tumor necrosis factor, and possibly prostaglandins may all be influential factors.[11,12]

Hypercalcemia is less commonly associated with hematological malignancies than are other cancers. Although not clearly understood, Mundy[13] notes that hypercalcemia may be associated with the presence of a vitamin D-like sterol and PTH-related protein in the patient with lymphoma. Some evidence indicates a bone-resorbing lymphotoxin (a type of cytokine that possesses osteoclastic-activating activity) and interleukin-1 may also be linked to this electrolyte imbalance in the multiple myeloma patient.[14]

The only treatment-related cause of hypercalcemia is associated with the use of hormonal therapy (androgens, estrogens, anti-estrogens, and progestins). Metabolic alterations associated with use of these agents cause calcium release from bone into the serum. Obviously, patients should have their serum calcium levels monitored closely. Any marked increase in the calcium level warrants discontinuation of therapy. Usually no additional treatment is required once hormonal therapy is stopped.

Clinical Presentation

The cancer patient often suffers from malnutrition and therefore a decrease in serum albumin. This decrease in serum albumin concentration has an effect on the total serum calcium level reported by the laboratory. That is, the total serum calcium concentration decreases by 0.8 mg/dL for every 1-g/dL decrease in serum albumin below normal. For example, a patient with a total serum calcium level of 10 mg/dL and a normal serum albumin level actually has a calcium concentration of 10 mg/dL. In contrast, a patient with a total serum calcium level of 10 mg/dL and a serum albumin level of 1.5 g/dL actually has mild hypercalcemia (11.6 mg/dL).

It is helpful at this point to recall that the total serum calcium level is the sum of the amount of calcium bound to albumin (approximately 50%) and the amount in ionized form (also about 50%). In the presence of a low serum albumin concentration, there is less bound calcium and the amount of free ionized calcium remains normal. If the laboratory measures the total serum calcium level in a hypoalbuminemic patient, the nurse needs to be aware that the reported level will be deceptively low. Although most laboratories have the capability of measuring ionized calcium levels, they usually measure the total serum calcium concentration (making it necessary to apply the formula to calculate the actual calcium level) (see Clinical Tip: Formula for Correction of Total Serum Calcium When Hypoalbuminemia Is Present).

The symptoms of hypercalcemia are directly related to its severity and rate of development (and are modified by the patient's age, underlying disease process, and the presence of other imbalances). In review, symptoms of hypercalcemia may include anorexia, nausea and vomiting, constipation, muscular weakness and hyporeflexia, disturbance in behavior, confusion, psychosis, tremor, and lethargy. Differential diagnosis in a cancer patient with hypercalcemia should include primary hyperparathyroidism. A detailed review of symptoms of hypercalcemia is presented in Chapter 6.

Treatment

Treatment for tumor-related hypercalcemia is similar to that of other causes of elevated serum calcium levels (see Chapter 6). Therapies discussed in this section are those most commonly used in the oncology patient population. The treatment of choice often depends on the severity of the hypercalcemic state, the significance of the side effects for the particular patient, and the clinician's preference. Isotonic saline (0.9% NaCl) administration facilitates renal excretion of calcium by increasing the glomerular filtration rate. However, before the initiation of any large fluid infusion, renal function needs to be evaluated. Furosemide (Lasix) may also be helpful because it selectively inhibits resorption of calcium and facilitates the diuresis. Usually serum calcium levels will decrease 24 to 48 hrs after initiation of saline therapy.

Synthetic calcitonin may be used to treat hypercalcemia as it promotes calcium excretion by the kidneys (even in patients with compromised renal function). Although calcitonin may cause the serum calcium level to decrease 9 to 12 hrs after the initial dose, the reduction is generally small and is sometimes

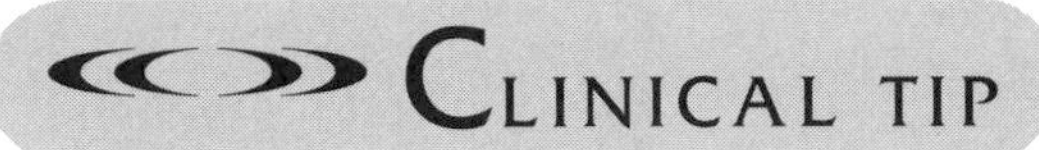

Formula for Correction of Total Serum Calcium When Hypoalbuminemia Is Present

Equation

Measured calcium + (3.5 – patient's albumin level g/dL) x 0.8

Equation Directions

The measured calcium is added to the difference between the patient's serum albumin level and the midrange of normal for serum albumin level. This sum is multiplied by 0.8, which is the correction factor. Remember that 0.8 mg/dL is added for every 1 g/dL of serum albumin that is less than 3.5 g/dL.

Example

Serum albumin = 2.0 g/dL
Total serum calcium = 13.0 mg/dL

13 + [(3.5 – 2.0)] x 0.8 = 13 + (1.5 x 0.8) = (the multiplication is done first, then the addition)

13 + 1.2 = 14.2 mg/dL

The corrected calcium is 14.2 mg/dL and demonstrates a value higher than the measured total calcium value. This information is vital in the management of a cancer patient who presents with a low albumin level since the patient may also be presenting with hypercalcemia.

not sustained for longer than 24 hrs. Repeated doses of calcitonin may be given but results of this treatment are also limited.[15] Glucocorticoids, often used along with calcitonin, are helpful in the treatment of hypercalcemia secondary to osteolytic processes.

Plicamycin (Mithramycin), an antineoplastic antibiotic, lowers the serum calcium level by inhibiting osteoclastic activity; however, its action does not begin until 12 to 24 hrs after administration, with maximal results seen usually in 36 to 72 hrs. Unfortunately, plicamycin may cause a precipitous drop in the platelet count. This is particularly problematic for the patient who has received previous chemotherapy and is already thrombocytopenic.

Gallium nitrate, an agent that inhibits osteoclastic function, has also been used in the treatment of hypercalcemia. Intravenous therapy continues for 5 to 7 days; the serum calcium begins to fall 24 to 72 hrs after the initiation of the infusion and the peak effect is achieved in 5 to 10 days.[16]

If other therapy is required, the diphosphonates (also called biphosphonates) are considered to be strong antihypercalcemic agents. Drugs, such as etidronate (Didronel) and pamidronate (Aredia), inhibit osteoclastic-induced resorption of bone. A third drug in this category called clodronate is available only in Europe. Etidronate is available in intravenous and oral forms. Intravenous therapy is given for 3 to 7 days, followed by daily oral doses for maintenance. Pamidronate has become more popular because treatment regimens include a one-time intravenous dose administered over 24 hrs. Onset of action begins 24 to 72 hrs after administration with peak effect in 4 to 9 days. Duration of response rate for pamidronate ranges from 1 to 10 weeks, with an average of 2 to 3 weeks. This drug was approved by the U.S. Food and Drug Administration in 1992, and many clinicians have found it successful in the treatment of hypercalcemia.[17,18] Recent guidelines from the manufacturer suggest safe administration for certain dosages with more rapid infusion rates of at least 4 hrs.[19]

A more thorough discussion of the treatment of hypercalcemia is given in Chapter 6. In addition to the immediate control of symptoms, long-term therapy for the cancer patient with tumor-induced hypercalcemia must be considered. Although hypercalcemic cancer patients may respond rapidly to emergency treatment, it is important to remember that the serum calcium level may return to an elevated state and remain a chronic management problem unless the malignancy is controlled with antineoplastic therapy. Dietary restrictions of calcium food products is not well supported by scientific research and therefore is not recommended. The mechanisms involved in hypercalcemia are due to calcium resorption from the bones and are not related to the GI absorption of calcium.[20]

HYPOCALCEMIA

Malnutrition with a resultant decrease in the serum albumin level is a major cause of below-normal serum calcium values reported by the laboratory when the total serum calcium level is measured. (The reader is referred to Clinical Tips: Formula for Correction of Total Serum Calcium When Hypoalbuminemia Is Present.) True hypocalcemia is uncommon in cancer patients; when it occurs, it is usually secondary to:

- Production of calcitonin by medullary carcinomas
- Malabsorption due to extensive bowel resection or loss of small bowel absorptive surface secondary to tumor size
- Magnesium depletion
- Tumor lysis syndrome (causing the sudden release of free phosphates from the destroyed cells, which then causes a reciprocal drop in the serum calcium concentration)

Symptoms of hypocalcemia include weakness, fatigue, irritability, progressive paresthesia, carpopedal spasms, and tetany. Treatment of hypocalcemia consists of oral or intravenous calcium gluconate administration (using serial calcium levels to guide dosages until normal states are achieved.[21]

HYPERURICEMIA

Hyperuricemia with hyperuricosuria is a significant problem for patients with myeloproliferative disorders, lymphomas, myeloma, or leukemia.[22] It is not usually a problem for patients with solid tumors. The serum uric acid elevation that occurs is usually related to the following:

- Overproduction of uric acid precursors by the tumor (most commonly noted in patients with polycythemia vera and chronic granulocytic leukemia)
- Certain rapidly proliferating neoplasms with a high nucleic acid turnover (may present with hyperuricemia even in the absence of previous chemotherapy)
- Rapid release of nucleic acids due to tumor cell lysis as a result of radiation therapy or chemotherapy (most commonly noted in patients with lymphoma or leukemia)

Malignant tumors with high cell mass and growth rates release excessive amounts of nucleic acids when treated. Consequently, metabolism of these nucleic acids leads to elevated serum uric acid levels. Diagnosis of hyperuricemia is established by measurement of uric acid in serum and urine. The normal excretory rate for uric acid is 300 to 500 mg/day.

Untreated serum uric acid levels may reach 20 mg/dL (normal, 3.0–9.0 mg/dL). The patient may exhibit ureteral colic, oliguria, and azotemia. Hemodialysis should be considered in patients with urate nephropathy.[23]

Prevention of hyperuricemia is the cornerstone of management. Prophylactic treatment of hyperuricemia consists of the following:

- Vigorous hydration
- Administration of allopurinol
- Alkalinization of the urine

Hyperuricemia must be viewed as a preventable complication rather than as an emergent condition. Hyperuricemia is found most often in conjunction with tumor lysis syndrome rather than as an isolated imbalance. Therefore, careful assessment is performed to determine the presence of hyperkalemia, hyperphosphatemia, and hypocalcemia, along with hyperuricemia. Treatment is then directed toward correcting all of these imbalances (see Table 22-1).

HYPONATREMIA

Hyponatremia has been associated with a variety of cancer sites, including the lung, pancreas, duodenum, larynx, brain, esophagus, and ovary; it may also be seen in patients with leukemia, Hodgkin's disease, lymphosarcoma, and multiple myeloma.[24] The main reasons cited for decreased serum sodium levels in cancer patients include the following:

- Ectopic release of an antidiuretic hormone-like substance from certain tumors, especially small-cell bronchogenic cancer
- Inappropriate release of ADH induced by certain antineoplastic agents and narcotics
- Salt loss from the GI tract (as occurs in vomiting, diarrhea, or fistulous drainage)
- Hyperproteinemic states, including multiple myeloma and hyperglobulinemia (induce an artifactual decrease in serum sodium or "pseudohyponatremia")
- Presence of edema and ascites in cancer patients with liver metastasis[25]

Secretion of inappropriate antidiuretic hormone (SIADH) may occur in persons with certain malignancies. Although most commonly seen with small-cell bronchogenic cancer, other cancers that may present with SIADH include tumors of the pancreas and duodenum, ureter, nasopharynx, leukemia, Hodgkin's disease, and thymoma. Normally, ADH is produced by the hypothalamus in response to hypovolemia or hyperosmolal states. The antidiuretic hormone acts on the kidney to decrease water excretion and to produce sodium excretion and is controlled by a feedback mechanism. However, in certain tumors, an ectopic ADH-like substance is produced in excess (uncontrolled by any feedback mechanism), resulting in the presence of decreasing serum sodium levels and serum osmolality.[26] The serum sodium level falls dangerously low and creates a myriad of clinical manifestations. Table 4-4 details the characteristics of hyponatremia. In some cases, these clinical symptoms may alert the clinician to investigate the possibility of a cancer diagnosis (e.g., in a patient with a history of smoking who has no obvious respiratory disorder).

Antitumor agents associated with SIADH include cyclophosphamide (Cytoxan), vincristine sulfate (Oncovin), vinblastine sulfate (Velban), cisplatin, and high-dose melphalan (Alkeran).[27,28] Patients receiving high-dose cyclophosphamide should be monitored for water intoxication. Cisplatin can cause the release of ADH from the posterior pituitary and can cause SIADH. Because vigorous hydration and perhaps diuretic administration are important components with this nephrotoxic treatment, the problem of water retention is accentuated. Hyponatremia associated with vincristine and vinblastine administration is usually accompanied by other signs of toxicity associated with the drug. The most common of these are ileus and peripheral neuropathy. Because cisplatin, cyclophosphamide, vincristine, and vinblastine are agents commonly used to treat lung cancer, the patient is at even greater risk for developing hyponatremia and should be assessed carefully.

Some cancer patients are treated with narcotics for pain control. Narcotics have also been associated with SIADH. All drugs prescribed to cancer patients should be evaluated for their potential to contribute to hyponatremia as problems may arise from a cumulative effect of this significant side effect.

In patients with multiple myeloma, or any state of hyperproteinemia, more non-sodium solids and less water will be present, leading to pseudohyponatremia. Patients with extensive liver metastasis who present with hyponatremia also sometimes have elevated plasma concentrations of ADH and aldosterone and low plasma albumin levels.[29]

Successful treatment of the tumor is the most direct treatment of SIADH. Chemotherapy, radiation therapy, or surgery may be used, depending on the malignancy involved. In the majority of patients chemotherapy for small-cell bronchogenic cancer successfully resolves the hyponatremia. Clinicians who administer any antineoplastic drugs known to induce hyponatremia should closely monitor serum sodium levels and serum osmolality. In the case of drug-induced hyponatremia, discontinuation of the drug usually causes a resolution of the disorder.

Other standard measures to control water excess and restore normal serum sodium concentrations are described in Chapter 4. On a short-term basis, fluid intake is restricted to the extent that negative water balance is induced; this may require restriction to as little as 400 to 700 mL/day. Administration of furosemide plus salt replacement has accomplished an increase in the serum sodium concentration. Use of demeclocycline (Declomycin) for long-term control of hyponatremia may be indicated, particularly in patients with uncontrolled malignancies; this agent inhibits the action of ADH on the kidneys, allowing increased urinary output and an increase in serum sodium. Long-term restriction of water is not commonly used as a treatment modality because many patients find this extremely unpleasant.

HYPERKALEMIA

An increased serum potassium level can result from acute renal failure (as may occur in untreated hyperuricemia, use of nephrotoxic or antineoplastic drugs, or renal malignancy). However, most often hyperkalemia is seen as a component of the tumor lysis syndrome, which may present during or after the successful treatment of leukemias and lymphomas. The rapid cell destruction from the treatment may cause a precipitous release of cellular potassium and an increase in the serum potassium level. This large amount of potassium in the extracellular fluid surpasses the kidney's potassium excretion ability.[30] Again, assessment must include monitoring for other electrolyte imbalances such as hyperphosphatemia, hypocalcemia, and hyperuricemia. Treatment is directed at the correction of all known imbalances. Treatment for hyperkalemia is outlined in Chapter 5.

A falsely high serum potassium level may be reported in the presence of a high white blood cell count. (Increased leukocyte fragility and lysis of cells after venous sampling may falsify the level in the clotted serum sample.) Validation of a supposed hyperkalemic state with the expected electrocardiographic changes and other clinical signs of hyperkalemia is needed to determine whether the serum potassium level is truly elevated in a patient with a high white blood cell count due to a leukemic process.

HYPOKALEMIA

Hypokalemia in patients with cancer may be associated with decreased intake or excessive loss of potassium ions. Excessive loss of potassium may occur from renal or extrarenal routes. A decrease in serum potassium related to decreased intake may be commonly associated with anorexia or nausea related to cancer pain, depression, tumor obstruction, chemotherapy, or radiation therapy. Administration of potassium-free IV fluids for treatment of dehydration only exaggerates the potassium reduction.

Extrarenal loss of potassium can be associated with excessive vomiting, fistula drainage, diarrhea, and prolonged mechanical GI suction. Vomiting may be associated with chemotherapy and radiation therapy or GI obstruction secondary to the malignancy.

In cancer patients diarrhea may be caused by a variety of factors. A number of malignancies (including villous adenoma of the colon, pancreatic carcinoma, carcinoid syndrome, medullary carcinoma of the thyroid, and small or large intestinal cancers) have been associated with diarrhea. Diarrhea may also be present as a result of antibiotic therapy, infectious agents in the GI tract (such as *Clostridium difficile* and candidiasis), radiation therapy to the bowel, bone marrow transplant-induced graft versus host disease, and certain antineoplastic drugs.[31] Diarrhea secondary to chemotherapy has been most commonly associated with cytarabine (cytosine arabinoside) and other antimetabolites including fluorouracil (5-fluorouracil) in combination with levamisole (ergamisol), or leucovorin calcium (leucovorin).[32] Vomiting and diarrhea can also lead to a state of volume depletion. When this occurs, aldosterone production is increased, causing renal potassium loss.

Renal loss of potassium may be due to renal tubular damage, the presence of excess aldosterone secondary to ectopic ACTH production, serum sodium concentration, serum magnesium concentration, drug interactions with potassium ions, and diuretic therapy.[33] Excessive loss of potassium (due to renal tubular damage) occurs in many patients during induction therapy for acute nonlymphocytic leukemia. Renal tubular damage in this patient population is attributed to two processes:

- Acute tubular necrosis due to antineoplastic drugs, anti-infective therapy, or antifungal therapy with amphotericin B
- Elevated lysozymuria due to cellular breakdown[34]

Both of these mechanisms for increased potassium loss revert to normal after the patient recovers from induction therapy.

Certain malignancies produce a decreased serum potassium level due to an ACTH-like substance released by cancer cells. These malignancies include the following:

- Small-cell carcinoma of the lung
- Thymoma
- Tumors of the adrenal cortex
- Medullary carcinoma of the thyroid
- Carcinoid tumors of the bronchus[35,36]

Patients with ACTH-like tumor-related hypokalemia do not usually exhibit clinical signs associated with Cushing's disease. The main manifestations of ectopic ACTH tumor release include such things as elevated urinary 17-hydroxycorticosteroid content, decreased serum potassium, edema, and the presence of ACTH in the tumor extract. High ACTH levels stimulate gluconeogenesis, which results in hyperglycemia. As with ectopic ACTH production, normal feedback regulatory inhibition does not occur; thus, normal-dose dexamethasone suppression is not successful. Only high-dose dexamethasone administration will depress ACTH levels due to ectopic tumor production. Surgical removal of the tumor is warranted to control the production of the ectopic ACTH. If this is not possible, surgical adrenalectomy or treatment with aminoglutethimide may be indicated.

ACTH stimulates the adrenal cortex to produce glucocorticoids and aldosterone (a mineralocorticoid). Aldosterone has a significant effect on the excretion of potassium and the retention of sodium, whereas glucocorticoids have a lesser effect on these electrolytes. The administration of large doses of prednisone and prednisolone, two drugs that have a mineralocorticoid effect, can result in hypokalemia. These steroids are often used in the treatment of hematological malignancies, spinal cord compression, and sepsis.

Nonabsorbable anions present in certain antibiotics bind to the potassium ion and increase potassium excretion. These antibiotics include penicillin, ampicillin, carbenicillin, and ticarcillin, drugs commonly used in the treatment of infections in cancer patients.[37,38]

Treatment

Potassium losses can be replaced with oral supplements, sometimes requiring titration of potassium doses up to 120 mEq/day. Most often the emergent nature of hypokalemia necessitates intravenous potassium supplementation initially. Although the mechanism is not clearly understood, magnesium depletion affects potassium absorption. When hypokalemia is present, the magnesium level needs to be assessed; if decreased, it needs to be corrected before or concurrently with the correction of hypokalemia. Chapter 5 further describes treatment of hypokalemia.

HYPERPHOSPHATEMIA

Massive tumor breakdown due to treatment releases large amounts of uric acid, potassium, and phosphate, creating the tumor lysis syndrome. The elevated serum phosphate level may not occur until 1 or 2 days after treatment is initiated; levels as high as 20 mg/dL may persist for several days afterward. Hyperphosphatemia usually occurs along with hyperuricemia, hyperkalemia, and hypocalcemia. An elevated phosphate level alone does not cause symptoms.

Renal damage (perhaps even acute renal failure) may be a serious problem resulting from the precipitation of calcium phosphate in the kidneys. If the patient's ionized calcium concentration is markedly reduced, tetany may develop. High phosphate levels must be reduced rapidly to prevent or to correct renal damage. Treatment of tumor lysis syndrome most often corrects hyperphosphatemia (see Clinical Tip: Management of Tumor Lysis Syndrome).

HYPOPHOSPHATEMIA

Hypophosphatemia may be associated with some untreated rapidly proliferating malignancies (e.g., acute leukemia), presumably due to the consumption of phosphate by the tumor cells. Severe hypophosphatemia (<1 mg/dL) can result in hemolysis and subsequent hemolytic anemia.[39] Although uncommon, hypophosphatemia can be caused by the use of androgens and large doses of estrogens for the treatment of prostate cancer.[40] Hypophosphatemia associated with malignant disease occurs subsequent to nutritional deprivation and cachexia. Prolonged hyperalimentation, without appropriate phosphate additives, and respiratory alkalosis, which is associated with the septicemic episodes of neutropenic patients, may also result in hypophosphatemia. Therapy consists of phosphate replacement by either the oral or the IV route. IV replacement is indicated in severe cases (see Chapter 8).

HYPOMAGNESEMIA

Hypomagnesemia may present as a single electrolyte imbalance or in combination with other disorders seen in the cancer patient, such as hypokalemia, hypophosphatemia, hypocalcemia, and SIADH. Although hypomagnesemia is a common clinical problem for patients in general, certain patients are at increased risk. These include those with tumors of the head and neck, ovary, cervix, testicle, lung, and intestine (as well as hematological malignancies such as leukemia).[41] This population of cancer patients represents a group of persons exposed to pharmacological agents associated with hypomagnesemia.

Cisplatin is a potentially nephrotoxic agent used to treat tumors occurring in a variety of sites (such as the lung, bladder, stomach, and ovary) as well as sarcomas and lymphomas. Cisplatin causes renal magnesium wasting in a dose-related manner. The cause of the renal magnesium wasting is not clear; among the possible causes are a direct effect of cisplatin on the renal absorption of magnesium and interstitial nephritis due to the drug (causing damage to Henle's loop and reduction in magnesium absorption).[42]

Cyclosporine is commonly used for the prevention of transplant rejection in the bone marrow transplant population. Several clinical studies have found a correlation between hypomagnesemia and the use of cyclosporine, although the exact cause is unclear. In addition, amphotericin B (a common agent used in the treatment of fungal infections in the immunocompromised patient) has been associated with hypomagnesemia.[43]

Many cancer patients with various diagnoses develop Gram-negative sepsis during the course of their treatment. Drugs used to treat this infection have been associated with hypomagnesemia. These antibiotics include the aminoglycosides. The renal wasting process caused by these drugs is thought to involve an inhibition of magnesium transport by the proximal tubule, leading to increased magnesium delivery to the loop of Henle. The absorptive power of the loop of Henle is exceeded by the magnesium load, causing increased magnesium excretion in the urine.

Other causes of hypomagnesemia are those that can occur in any patient (e.g., magnesium loss in chronic diarrhea or prolonged diuretic use, and inadequate magnesium supplementation during hyperalimentation). The reader is referred to Chapter 7 for a discussion of other causes of hypomagnesemia as well as its treatment.

SUMMARY OF TREATMENT

Traditionally, many fluid and electrolyte problems experienced by oncology patients are managed with replacement or restrictive treatment. However, the underlying cause of the electrolyte problem must be considered or a chronic problem will develop. Tumor elimination or control is a primary consideration. Careful, continued observation of the patient is indicated to effectively control the malignancy and its associated fluid and electrolyte problems.

When patients are diagnosed with a malignancy, the nurse's teaching session should include information regarding the fluid and electrolyte imbalances that pose the greatest risk to the particular patient. Patients and family members or caregivers should then be instructed regarding the signs and symptoms of fluid and electrolyte imbalances and the importance of seeking immediate attention from the health care team if symptoms appear. Patients and family members also need to be instructed regarding the importance of continuing mineral supplementation and follow-up laboratory appointments when a disorder has been diagnosed. In some cases, the recurrence of a fluid and electrolyte disorder is the first sign of recurrence of the malignancy; therefore, it is essential that patients and family members understand the critical nature of reporting this information to the health care team. In situations where patients have received significant doses of nephrotoxic chemotherapeutic agents, mineral supplementation may be necessary for the rest of their lives. The chronic nature of this situation must be made clear to both the patient and family. The reader is referred to Chapter 2 for a review of assessment for fluid and electrolyte problems, and Chapters 3 through 9 for information dealing with specific imbalances.

CASE STUDIES

Normal serum laboratory values for reference:

Sodium	=	135–145 mEq/L
Potassium	=	3.5–5.0 mEq/L
Chloride	=	97–110 mEq/L
Carbon dioxide combining power	=	22–31 mEq/L
Blood urea nitrogen (BUN)	=	8–25 mg/dL
Creatinine	=	0.6–1.5 mg/dL
Uric acid	=	3.0–9.0 mg/dL
Phosphorus	=	2.5–4.5 mg/dL
Albumin	=	3.5–4.5 mg/dL
Calcium	=	8.9–10.3 mg/dL
Magnesium	=	1.3–2.1 mEq/L

22-1. Mrs. J is a 61-year-old woman who was initially diagnosed with lymphoma several years ago, and was diagnosed with recurrent lymphoma last month. She presented with anxiety, decreased appetite, dehydration, and feelings of fatigue. Laboratory results included:

Sodium	=	133 mEq/L
Potassium	=	3.0 mEq/L
Chloride	=	95 mEq/L
CO_2 combining power	=	21 mEq/L
BUN	=	14 mg/dL
Creatinine	=	0.9 mg/dL
Uric acid	=	3.0 mg/dL
Albumin	=	3.8 g/dL
Total calcium	=	8.8 mg/dL
Magnesium	=	0.5 mEq/L

Although she had decreased intake for several days, she had no symptoms of vomiting, diarrhea, or fistula drainage. She also had no obvious signs and symptoms of hypokalemia or hypomagnesemia. She had received cisplatin (Platinol), etoposide (VePesid) and cytarabine (cytosine arabinoside) 3 days previously. She was treated with 100 mEq of potassium and 1 g of magnesium via the IV route. She then received 100 to 120 mEq of potassium orally for 3 days. The day of discharge, her serum potassium and magnesium levels had returned to normal. Discharge medications included: 40 mEq of oral potassium (TID), and 400 mg of magnesium oxide (TID). She was given an appointment to return to the clinic for laboratory evaluation of serum electrolytes in 3 days. A detailed instruction sheet was given to her regarding the administration of her medications. She also received a written list of signs of hyper/hypokalemia and of hyper/hypomagnesemia and was instructed to report any signs described in the list to the clinic staff. In addition to being told of the importance of continuing the medications as prescribed, she was instructed to call the clinic staff if she had any difficulty taking the medications.

COMMENTARY: This case involves a lymphoma patient 3 days after chemotherapy treatment but does not include the expected picture of tumor lysis syndrome. Instead, the electrolyte disorders of hypokalemia and hypomagnesemia are seen and are probably related to the side effects of cisplatin. Again, the relationship between hypomagnesemia and hypokalemia is not clearly understood, but magnesium levels must be adequate for the potassium replacement to be effective. Therefore, magnesium supplementation was given in conjunction with potassium.

Because the discharge medications involve significant doses of replacement potassium and magnesium, the patient needs to observe for signs of hyperkalemia and hypermagnesemia. This is because the effect of cisplatin on renal excretion of potassium and magnesium usually reverses a short time after treatment. Thus, although chronic replacement may be necessary, the doses for long-term maintenance may need to be lower than those used at discharge. Repeated laboratory tests are critical in monitoring electrolyte imbalances. Instructing the patient about the signs and symptoms of hypokalemia and hypomagnesemia is important in the event that this situation occurs again after the next chemotherapy treatment. Also, the patient needs to have detailed instructions about taking these medications and about not discontinuing them without direction from the clinic staff.

22-2. A 68-year-old newly diagnosed patient with acute myelogenous leukemia was admitted to the hospital for induction therapy scheduled to begin the next day. Intravenous hydration was begun with 0.9% sodium chloride and added sodium bicarbonate at the rate of 150 mL/hr. Allopurinol (300 mL orally) was ordered to begin the day of admission and to continue daily. All admission blood work was within normal ranges (serum albumin, 4.0 g/dL). The next day, chemotherapy was begun with cytarabine (cytosine arabinoside) by continuous infusion over 7 days and idamycin (idarubicin hydrochloride) once daily for 3 days. On the third day of treatment, the laboratory results from venous blood were as follows:

Potassium = 6.0 mEq/L
Phosphorus = 14.9 mg/dL
Uric acid = 10.3 mg/dL
Calcium = 7.5 mg/dL

Although all of these values were outside the normal range, the patient displayed no symptoms of electrolyte abnormalities. At this time, hydration with 0.9% sodium chloride (with added sodium bicarbonate) was increased to 300 mL/hr. On the fourth day, the following serum values were reported by the laboratory:

Potassium = 4.1 mEq/L
Phosphorus = 10.0 mg/dL
Uric acid = 8.5 mg/dL
Calcium = 8.0 mg/dL

All laboratory results returned to within normal ranges on the final day of treatment (5 days after chemotherapy was begun).

COMMENTARY: This patient experienced tumor lysis syndrome secondary to the large amounts of potassium and phosphate ions that shifted from the intracellular space into the serum. This is a common occurrence in a patient with the diagnosis of leukemia undergoing induction therapy. To prevent renal complications of hyperuricemia, large-volume IV hydration (along with sodium bicarbonate to keep the urine alkaline) was given. Allopurinol was given to reduce the production of uric acid (accomplished by inhibiting the chemical reactions that occur immediately preceding its formation). When the patient's laboratory results were abnormal (hyperkalemia, hyperphosphatemia, hyperuricemia, and hypocalcemia), treatment was initiated to correct these imbalances. The basic treatment consisted of increased hydration (preceded by assessment of renal function). Amphogel was also given to bind phosphate for excretion through the intestinal tract. The patient had no existing cardiac abnormality and had no symptoms from the hyperkalemia; therefore, no specific treatment of hyperkalemia was initiated. If the laboratory findings on the fourth day did not demonstrate an improvement in the tumor lysis syndrome, additional therapy to correct the hyperkalemia and the hypocalcemia might have been initiated. Although this syndrome can continue for several days after therapy has been completed, this patient had no further problems during this hospitalization.

REFERENCES

1. McDermott K, et al: The diagnosis and management of hypomagnesmia: A unique treatment approach and case report. Oncol Nurs Forum 18:1149,1991
2. Lind J: Ectopic hormonal production: Nursing implications. Sem Oncol Nurs 1(4):251,1985
3. Odell W: Endocrine complications of cancer. In: Calabresi P, Schein P (eds): Medical Oncology, 2nd ed, p 177. New York, McGraw-Hill, 1993
4. Stucky L: Acute tumor lysis syndrome: Assessment and nursing implications. Oncol Nurs Forum 20:49,1993
5. Cunningham E: Fluid and electrolyte disturbances associated with cancer and its treatment. Nurs Clin North Am 17(4):579,1982
6. Warrell R: Metabolic emergencies. In: DeVita et al (eds): Cancer Principles and Practices of Oncology, 4th ed, p 2128. Philadelphia, JB Lippincott, 1993
7. Chernecky C, Ramsey P: Critical Nursing Care of the Client with Cancer, p 1. East Norwalk, Connecticut, Appleton-Century-Crofts, 1984
8. Kaplan M: Hypercalcemia of malignancy: A review of advances in pathophysiology. Oncol Nurs Forum 21(6):1041,1994
9. Singer F, Fernandez M: Therapy of hypercalcemia and malignancy. Am J Med 82:2A,1987
10. Bockman R: Hypercalcemia in malignancy. Clin Endocrinol Metab 9(2):317,1980
11. Kaplan, p 1041
12. Mundy G: Pathophysiology of cancer-associated hypercalcemia. Sem Oncol 17:2(suppl 5):12,1990
13. Mundy, p 13–14
14. Lang-Kummer J: Hypercalcemia. In: Groenwald S, et al (Eds): Cancer Nursing: Principles and Practice, 3rd ed, p 656. Boston, Jones & Bartlett, 1993
15. Dorr R, VonHoff D: Cancer Chemotherapy Handbook, 2nd ed, p 43. Norwalk, Connecticut, Appleton & Lange, 1994
16. Ibid, p 45–46
17. Ibid, p 47–50
18. Lange-Kummer, p 658
19. Physician's Desk Reference, p 878. Montvale, NJ, Medical Economics Data Production, 1995
20. Coward D: Cancer-induced hypercalcemia. Cancer Nurs 9(3):125,1986
21. Lowitz B: Paraneoplastic syndromes. In: Haskell C (ed): Cancer Treatment, 3rd ed, p 844. Philadelphia, WB Saunders, 1990
22. Ibid, p 844
23. Ibid, p 845
24. Chernecky, p 14
25. Narins R (ed): Clinical Disorders of Fluid and Electrolyte Metabolism, 5th ed, p 591. New York, McGraw-Hill, 1994
26. Cunningham, p 581
27. Lowitz, p 846
28. Moore J: Syndrome of inappropriate antidiuretic hormone secretion (SIADH). In: Gross J, Johnson B (eds): Handbook of Oncology Nursing, 2nd ed, p 702. Boston, MA, Jones & Bartlett, 1994
29. Narins, p 595
30. Stucky, p 49
31. Grant M, Ropka M: Alterations in nutrition. In: Baird S, McCorkel R, Grant M (eds): Cancer Nursing, pp 737–738. Philadelphia, WB Saunders, 1991
32. Tenebaum L, Leshin D: Gastrointestinal system alterations. In: Tenebaum L (ed): Cancer Chemotherapy and Biotherapy—A Reference Guide, 2nd ed, p 249–250. Philadelphia, WB Saunders, 1994
33. Narins, p 670
34. Ibid, p 680
35. Lind, p 252
36. Odell, p 178
37. Gill M, et al: Hypokalemic, metabolic alkalosis induced by high-dose ampicillin sodium. Am J Hosp Pharm 34:528,1977
38. Klastersky J, et al: Carbenicillin and hypokalemia. Ann Intern Med 78:774,1973
39. Narins, p 1046
40. Nanji A: Drug-induced electrolyte disorders. Drug Intelligence Clin Pharm 17:181,1983
41. McDermott, p 1149
42. Lam M, Adelstein D: Hypomagnesemia and renal magnesium wasting in patients treated with cisplatin. Am J Kidney Dis 8:164,1986
43. Narins, p 1103

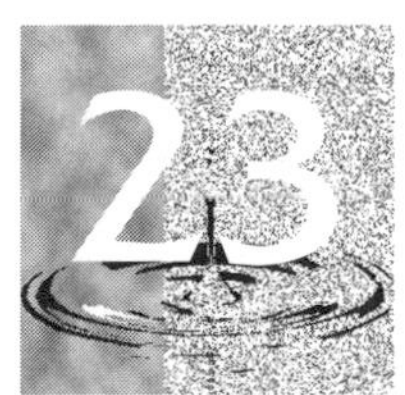

Pregnancy

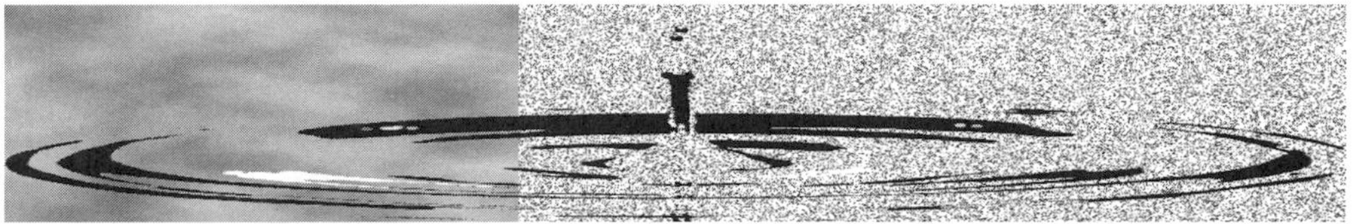

Although physiologically normal in pregnancy, changes in fluid retention and blood volume expansion and alterations in acid–base and electrolyte balance would be considered abnormal in the nonpregnant woman or in men. These changes are temporary and necessary adaptations to provide for the growing fetus and for maternal health needs during pregnancy. Despite alterations in water and electrolyte balance, pregnancy is considered a wellness state because the changes serve a useful function.

Changes in body water and electrolyte balance in normal pregnancy will be explored in this chapter, as will some abnormal disease or treatment states that directly affect fluid and electrolyte balances.

NORMAL PHYSIOLOGICAL WATER AND ELECTROLYTE CHANGES

INCREASED BLOOD VOLUME

In a woman pregnant with one fetus, a 30% to 50% blood volume increase may be expected; an even greater increase occurs in a woman pregnant with twins.[1–3] Although both plasma and red blood cell volumes are increased, plasma volume increases disproportionally to red blood cell mass, resulting in the so-called "physiological anemia of pregnancy" or "pseudoanemia." A hematocrit of 33% to 38% and a hemoglobin of 11 to 12 g/100 mL may be observed. During pregnancy, however, true anemia exists if the hemoglobin is less than 10 g/100 mL and the hematocrit is less than 30%.[4] When iron stores are adequate, the decline in blood values is usually minimal. It has been noted that the increase in maternal plasma volume may be beneficial to fetal outcome as significant correlations have been found between maternal plasma volume expansion and birth weight.[5]

SODIUM AND WATER RETENTION

To meet her own needs and those of her growing fetus, the pregnant woman must retain additional fluid and electrolytes. To accomplish this, renal excretory responses are modified resulting in new balances of fluid and electrolytes. The regulation of sodium and water homeostasis involves the hormones arginine vasopressin or antidiuretic hormone (ADH) and the renin-angiotensin-aldosterone system. These systems must also be altered to respond appropriately to this new equilibrium occurring during pregnancy.

In normal pregnancy, retention of approximately 950 mEq (3–6 mEq/day) of sodium and 6 to 8 L of water is expected.[6,7] Approximately 60% of the sodium is used by the fetus and placenta, and the rest is distributed in the maternal blood and extracellular fluid. Most of the sodium retention occurs during the last 8 weeks of pregnancy.[8] Increased amounts of body water in the extracellular spaces accounts for 70% to 75% of the maternal weight gain. Interstitial fluid volume increases 1.5 to 5 L with the greatest accumulation during the second half of pregnancy.[9] Accumulation of more than 1.5 L of interstitial fluid is associated with edema.

In the past, diuretics and salt restriction were used at the first sign of edema in pregnant women.[10] However, at present diuretics are not routinely used because it is understood that diuretics can cause a number of problems during pregnancy (e.g., electrolyte imbalance, hyperglycemia, and hyperuricemia). The body's demand for sodium actually *increases* during pregnancy due to the normal increased fluid retention.[11] It is now generally agreed that dietary sodium intake should not be restricted during normal pregnancy, although excessive use should be avoided because of the relationship of sodium to the development of hypertension in those at risk for this problem. During pregnancy, it is wise to limit salt intake to a moderate level (such as 5 g/day), but no less than 2 to 3 g of sodium should be consumed on a daily basis.[12] Because sodium represents about 40% of the weight of salt (sodium chloride), 1 g of sodium chloride is equivalent to 0.4 g of sodium. Thus, 5 g of salt is equivalent to 2 g of sodium. See Chapter 3 for a discussion of low-salt diets.

Edema

By definition, *edema* refers to an expansion of the interstitial fluid volume. Redistribution of fluid between the intracellular and extracellular compartments secondary to sodium retention is associated with the "physiologic" edema of many normal pregnancies.[13,14] In fact, 35% to 80% of healthy normotensive women develop edema at some time during pregnancy.[15,16]

Edema can be dependent or generalized. Dependent edema of the ankles frequently occurs when the pregnant woman assumes an upright position and is of little physiological significance. Several factors predispose to dependent edema; most significant is venous pressure. Impingement of blood flow through the inferior vena cava by the pregnant uterus causes stagnation of blood in the lower extremities. Increased permeability of the capillary walls may also influence the rate of filtration. Generalized edema is manifested by rapid weight gain and edema of the hands and upper half of the body. This type of edema can also occur in normal pregnancy. However, when generalized edema is accompanied by a rise in blood pressure and proteinuria, it is considered a disease process.[17]

In summary, sodium and water retention of normal pregnancy commonly causes mild peripheral edema, particularly in the third trimester when pressure on the inferior vena cava by the enlarged uterus has a contributory effect.[18] When the pregnant woman elevates her legs or lies on her side, the hydrostatic pressure is partially overcome and interstitial fluid is returned to the circulation. Immersion of the pregnant woman in water has also been suggested as an effective treatment in forcing the edema fluid back into the vascular space.[19,20]

The dependent edema associated with normal pregnancy can be quite annoying. Clinical Tip: Example of Nursing Diagnosis and Nursing Process in Care of Patient With Pedal Edema gives an example of the application of the nursing process to deal with this problem.

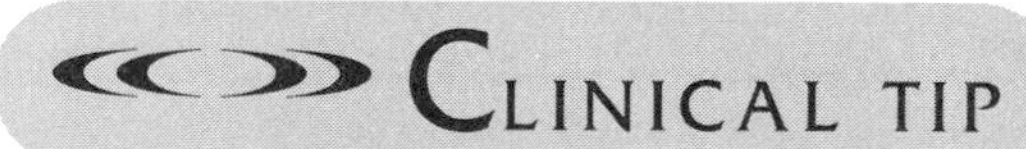

Example of Nursing Diagnosis and Nursing Process in Care of Patient With Pedal Edema
Problem: Discomfort Related to Pedal Edema

ASSESSMENT	INTERVENTIONS	EXPECTED OUTCOME
28-year-old sales clerk in last trimester of pregnancy complains of ankle swelling after standing for a few hours at work Pedal edema present; no edema in face or hands BP, 120/82 No proteinuria	1. Advise client to avoid constrictive garments around the legs 2. Recommend use of support hose 3. Advise against prolonged standing; suggest that she obtain a stool to sit on periodically during time at work 4. Instruct client regarding passive exercises to improve circulation 5. Advise frequent rest periods when feasible in which lateral position can be assumed (with legs slightly elevated to reduce venous pressure) 6. Advise ample fluid intake (8 to 10 glasses of water/day) 7. Encourage client to report increase in pedal edema or appearance of edema in face, hands, or other parts of body	Client will use self-care measures to increase comfort and decrease edema Client will verbalize decrease in discomfort Dependent edema will diminish or become no worse Client will be knowledgeable of possible abnormal developments

Plasma Sodium Concentration

Plasma sodium concentration decreases approximately 5 mEq/L in almost all pregnant women during late pregnancy, and plasma osmolality decreases approximately 10 mOsm/kg in spite of the normal ability of the pregnant woman to dilute the urine.[21] These responses are partly due to increased release of ADH (which in turn causes water retention) and the increased thirst common in pregnant women.[22] The lowered plasma sodium level quickly returns to normal after delivery.

CALCIUM BALANCE

Calcium is a particularly important element during pregnancy. Total serum calcium concentration begins to decrease during the second or third month of pregnancy and reaches its lowest point during the third trimester.[23] In large part, this is caused by the fetal demands for calcium as well as decreased calcium binding.[24]

The current recommended daily allowance (RDA) for calcium during pregnancy is 1.2 g, 33% higher than for nonpregnant women.[25] Therefore, under normal circumstances calcium balance in pregnancy is easily maintained by dietary intake. Approximately 25 to 30 g of calcium are accumulated during pregnancy; most of this is required for fetal skeletal calcification.[26] Needed calcium is acquired during pregnancy through an increase in intestinal calcium absorption and increased rate of maternal bone turnover. Calcium absorption and bone turnover are enhanced by alterations in certain hormones during pregnancy, including estrogen, parathyroid hormone, and glucocorticoids.[27] It has been suggested that calcium supplementation during pregnancy may have positive effects on the incidence of gestational hypertension and preterm delivery; however, the value of calcium supplementation in reducing the incidence of pregnancy-induced hypertension is controversial.[28,29]

MAGNESIUM BALANCE

The serum magnesium levels decrease by about 6% to 9% in pregnancy.[30] However, rather than reflecting actual hypomagnesemia, this small decrease probably represents the effects of plasma volume expansion and decreased protein binding associated with mild hypoalbuminemia.[31] Of course, actual magnesium deficiency may develop if dietary intake is inadequate. In pregnancy, formation of new tissues requires that dietary magnesium be higher than in nonpregnant women of the same age.[32]

POTASSIUM BALANCE

A cumulative retention of approximately 350 mEq of potassium occurs during pregnancy.[33] The retained potassium is stored in the fetus, uterus, breasts, and red blood cells.[34] This retention occurs in spite of increased circulating levels of mineralcorticoids and increased delivery of sodium to the distal nephron resulting from the increased glomerular filtration rate.[35] Concentration of potassium in the maternal plasma either remains at a prepregnancy level or is slightly decreased. Prolonged nausea and vomiting or the use of diuretics may lead to hypokalemia and metabolic alkalosis.

ACID–BASE CHANGES

Pregnancy is associated with a compensated respiratory alkalosis, which begins early and continues until delivery. The cause is hyperventilation, secondary to the potent stimulating effect of progesterone on the medullary respiratory center.[36] As a result of hyperventilation, the partial pressure of carbon dioxide (PCO_2) decreases from the normal 40 mmHg to approximately 30 mmHg during gestation, causing an arterial pH of 7.44 $\pm$ 0.003 compared with the normal measurement of 7.40.[37]

As with any form of chronic respiratory alkalosis, the one associated with pregnancy is compensated for by changes in the serum bicarbonate concentration. This metabolic compensation causes the bicarbonate level to drop to approximately 20 mEq/L by the third trimester (compared with the normal bicarbonate level of 24 mEq/L).[38] Because the total buffering capacity is reduced by renal compensation, pregnant women are more likely to develop severe acidosis when conditions causing either ketoacidosis or lactic acidosis are present. If the serum bicarbonate level is normal or elevated in late pregnancy, the possibility of a second imbalance (metabolic alkalosis) should be investigated. Possible causes of the latter could be persistent vomiting or excessive use of potassium-losing diuretics.

RESEARCH FINDINGS

Hormonal changes associated with the menstrual cycle and pregnancy might be expected to alter the activity of the cell membrane Na^+-K^+ pump. A study was recently reported in which venous blood was drawn from 26 women: 10 in both the luteal and follicular phases of their menstrual cycles; 8 pregnant women; and 8 age-matched non-pregnant women (studied at random times in the menstrual cycle).[39] Intracellular erythrocyte and plasma sodium and potassium concentrations were measured by flame photometry. Findings indicate that erythrocyte sodium decreases during pregnancy, possibly due to the increased activity of the Na^+-K^+ pump as well as to the increased secretion of aldosterone during pregnancy. The researchers concluded that altered activity of the cell membrane Na^+-K^+ pump can produce some of the physiological changes associated with pregnancy.

ABNORMAL CONDITIONS AFFECTING OR AFFECTED BY FLUIDS AND ELECTROLYTES

PREGNANCY-INDUCED HYPERTENSION

Pregnancy-induced hypertension (PIH) is a disease unique to pregnancy, which is characterized by progressive hypertension, pathologic edema, and proteinuria. This disorder may have mild, moderate, or severe symptoms. The terms *preeclampsia* and *eclampsia* are used to refer to the nature and degree of the symptoms involved in PIH. Preeclampsia is characterized by hypertension with proteinuria, edema, or both, and usually occurs after 20 weeks of gestation. If the pregnant woman develops convulsions, the term eclampsia is used. The term "preeclampsia" is used synonymously with "pregnancy-induced hypertension."[40]

Pregnancy-induced hypertension occurs in 5% to 7% of all pregnancies and is the third leading cause of maternal death in the United States. It is primarily a disease of the nullipara, usually involving women younger than 20 years or older than 35 years. It develops after the 20th week of gestation and has its highest incidence among women who have a strong predisposition to hypertension. There is a strong familial predisposition to the development of preeclampsia. Preeclampsia occurs more frequently in black women and is associated with multiple pregnancy, polyhydramnios, vascular disease, trophoblastic disease, and abruptio placentae.[41]

The pathogenesis of PIH is unknown; in fact, this condition has long been known as the "disease of theories." Evidently it is somehow related to the physiological changes of pregnancy as the condition improves and the disease apparently disappears after the termination of pregnancy. It has been conjectured that immunological changes, among other factors, have a pathogenetic role. The pathological changes associated with preeclampsia indicate that poor perfusion secondary to vasospasm is a major factor leading to the derangement of maternal physiological functions and increased perinatal morbidity.[42,43]

Sodium Retention and Fluid Distribution Changes

As discussed earlier, sodium retention is expected with normal pregnancy; however, the retention that occurs with preeclampsia may be pathological. Although rapid weight gain and sodium retention are characteristic of preeclampsia, they are not universally present or, as indicated earlier, unique to preeclampsia. At most, these signs are a reason for closer observation of blood pressure and monitoring of urinary protein. The primary indicators of preeclampsia are hypertension and proteinuria.

Paradoxically, the plasma volume is often diminished in women with preeclampsia, despite the increase in total body sodium. The intense vasoconstriction that is characteristic of preeclampsia may result in a shift of the retained sodium and water from the vascular space into the interstitial space, causing a reduced plasma volume (reflected by a rising hematocrit) and increased interstitial fluid volume.[44]

Clinical Indicators

Hypertension in the pregnant woman is defined as a blood pressure reading of more than 140/90 mmHg or a reading that represents an increase over baseline readings of 30 mmHg systolic or 15 mmHg diastolic.[45] Two abnormal blood pressure readings taken at least 6 hrs apart are required. Note that the typically accepted level of 140/90 mmHg may be inaccurate in a patient who normally has a low blood pressure. For example, in a woman with a normal baseline blood pressure of 90/50 mmHg, a reading of 130/80 mmHg may well represent hypertension. Proteinuria is often the most valid clinical indicator of preeclampsia. Because proteinuria tends to be a late change, PIH *may* be diagnosed without the presence of proteinuria.[46] Significant proteinuria approximates a 2+ urinary protein. The definitive evaluation of the degree of proteinuria is a quantitative analysis of a 24-hr urine collection. (A level of 300 mg is accepted as the upper limit of normal in pregnancy.[47]) (See Table 23-1 for a summary of suggested nursing assessment parameters for abnormal fluid balance changes associated with preeclampsia and eclampsia.)

Therapeutic Measures

Diuretics are not generally used except in the presence of heart failure. This is because plasma volume is already decreased in preeclamptic women and the natriuresis associated with diuretic use may be counterproductive.[48] Also, some preeclamptic women have insidious sodium losses or are in negative sodium balance because of dietary manipulations. In these women, administration of diuretics may cause severe hyponatremia.[49] Similarly, strict sodium restriction has no role in the prevention or therapy of preeclampsia and may actually be counterproductive (again because of the decreased plasma volume in preeclamptic women).[50] However, moderate sodium restriction may minimize the discomfort of women with significant edema.[51]

Antihypertensive therapy (usually hydralazine) is generally reserved for women with severe hypertension that could lead to intracranial bleeding or left ventricular failure.[52,53] When antihypertensive therapy of preeclampsia is directed at reduction of peripheral vascular resistance, a shift of excess sodium and water from the interstitial into the intravascular space may occur. As a result, excessive expansion of the intravascular space may cause an inadequate response to antihypertensive therapy. To monitor the volume status of seriously ill preeclamptic or eclamptic patients, it may be necessary to use a Swan-Ganz catheter to identify those patients with elevated wedge pressures who might benefit from the judicious use of diuretics.[54]

Preeclamptic women may develop oliguria, either because of a diminished intravascular volume or renal problems.[55] Fluid administration in the presence of oliguria must be undertaken cautiously because if the oliguria is renal in origin, fluid overloading is likely to result. Although oliguria due to hypovolemia may be corrected by fluid infusion, excessive fluid administration can lead to congestive heart failure. Also, excessive fluid administration can lead to cerebral edema if the serum sodium level is very low. To avoid lowering the plasma osmolality, hypotonic fluids should not be used (particularly if oxytocin is being administered). Either isotonic electrolyte or colloid-containing fluids may be considered. For the woman with seriously decreased colloid oncotic pressure secondary to hypoalbuminemia, colloid-containing fluids may be indicated. The rate of fluid administration must be closely titrated to urine output and other clinical indicators such as central venous or, preferably, pulmonary wedge pressure.[56]

Magnesium Sulfate as an Anticonvulsant

The therapeutic use of magnesium sulfate in preeclampsia–eclampsia is due to its pharmacological effects on the central nervous system through depression and vasodilatation. More specifically, magnesium ions block nerve transmission by presynaptic inhibition, decreasing smooth muscle contractility, and depressing central nervous system irritability.[57] Also, magnesium tends to block catecholamine release from the adrenal medulla and may cause peripheral vasodilatation.

Magnesium sulfate can be given intramuscularly (IM) or intravenously (IV); however, because the IM administration of large volumes of magnesium sulfate is painful and the rate of absorption cannot be controlled, this route of administration is seldom used. Magnesium sulfate is commonly given IV with an initial bolus followed by a continuous slow infusion, titrating the rate of administration against maternal deep tendon reflexes.[58] The desired dosage of magnesium sulfate varies depending on renal status and the patient's response to the drug. Intravenous administration of magnesium at doses up to 2 g/hr appears to be safe for the patient with normal renal function.[59] However, doses exceeding this level require that serum magnesium concentrations be monitored at least every 2 hrs until a steady state has been achieved.

Most authorities agree that magnesium sulfate ($MgSO_4 7H_2O$) is a safe and efficient agent to prevent convulsions. Eclamptic convulsions are usually prevented if plasma magnesium levels are maintained at 4 to 7.5 mEq/L.[60] (Recall that the normal plasma magnesium concentration is 1.3–2.1 mEq/L).

The loss of deep tendon reflexes is the first sign of toxicity; therefore, the presence of deep tendon reflexes indicates that the serum magnesium concentration is not dangerously high[61] (see Summary of Hypermagnesemia in Chapter 7). However, in addition to monitoring patellar reflexes, rate and depth of respirations should be observed regularly as respiratory paralysis and cardiac arrest can result if serum magnesium levels increase too high. Because magnesium is primarily eliminated by the kidneys, the adequacy of renal function must be monitored during its administration. It is generally agreed that urine output should total at least 100 mL every 4 hrs. If toxic symptoms occur from magnesium overdosage, calcium gluconate may be prescribed as an antidote. A commonly recommended dose is 1 g (10 mL of a 10% solution) given slowly over 3 min.[62] Mechanical respiratory support may also be needed if respirations are severely depressed.

A major advantage of magnesium sulfate therapy is that at effective anticonvulsant doses it is very safe for the fetus and neonate. Neonatal serum magnesium concentrations are nearly identical to those of the mother. Although amniotic fluid magnesium concentrations increase with prolonged infusion due to fetal renal excretion of magnesium, fetal serum magnesium levels do not increase and there is no evidence of cumulative effects of prolonged magnesium administration on the neonate.[63]

Magnesium sulfate is not a perfect anticonvulsant; some women have convulsions even with high serum magnesium levels. Other anticonvulsants are being studied in clinical trials to assess their efficacy in the care of pregnant women. Specifically, phenytoin has been described as equally effective for the treatment and prophylaxis of eclamptic seizures and could be a reasonable alternative in settings in which magnesium would be best avoided (e.g., markedly compromised renal function, myasthenia gravis).[64]

Nursing Interventions

Home care for high-risk obstetric patients by qualified perinatal nurses is increasing.[65] If the preeclampsia is mild and fetal growth retardation is not a problem, management can be accomplished in the home. Home therapy includes two to three weekly medical and nursing assessments, encouraging the patient to participate in the care, dietary modifications, and bedrest.[66]

Of importance is teaching the patient self-assessment of weight, edema, fluid intake and urine output, and assessment of proteinuria as well as recognition of central nervous system (CNS) symptomatology (e.g., blurred vision, headaches, nausea, and vomiting). An essential part of home management for preeclampsia, home blood pressure monitoring is now less complicated and more reliable as a result of technological advances.[67,68]

Although research indicates that antepartum hospitalization is a significant stressor for high-risk pregnant women, appropriate management for severe preeclampsia and eclampsia can only be accomplished when the woman is hospitalized.[69] The following interventions are often indicated for patients with severe preeclampsia and eclampsia:

1. Maintain bedrest with patient in the lateral recumbent position. (Bedrest in this position increases renal perfusion and, thus, urinary output. Placental perfusion is also increased.)
2. Monitor changes in blood pressure, degree of edema, and degree of proteinuria (see Table 23-1). Frequency of these observations depends on the severity of the patient's condition; for example, they may be needed hourly if the condition is advanced.
3. Provide a quiet, nonstimulating environment (preferably a private room.)
4. Monitor closely for development of labor; monitor fetal status (use fetal monitor).
5. Keep artificial oral airway device at bedside and maintain seizure precautions. Have emergency tray immediately accessible.
6. Monitor for hyperreflexia.

TABLE 23–1

Summary of Nursing Assessment Parameters for Abnormal Fluid Balance Changes Associated with Preeclampsia

ASSESSMENT PARAMETER	COMMENTS
Weight changes	Weigh on same scale each time, after voiding, and with same amount of clothing (Normal weight curve is a 10-lb weight gain at 20 weeks with a 0.5-lb/wk gain until 40 weeks. In patients with PIH, weight gain is usually greater than 30 lbs by the third trimester)
BP changes	Establish baseline BP in early pregnancy Assess BP with client in same position and in same arm each visit; use cuff of appropriate size Although 140/90 serves as a rough baseline for hyepertension, it is better to look for a degree of elevation over baseline. • As a rough rule of thumb, consider BP abnormal if systolic elevates >30 mmHg or diastolic elevates >15 mmHg. • Two abnormal readings taken at least 6 hours apart are required for a diagnosis of hypertension.
Edema*	+1 edema: minimal edema of lower extremities +2 edema: marked edema of lower extremities (as evidenced by inability to wear usual shoes) +3 edema: edema of lower extremities, face, and hands (as in inability to wear rings) +4 edema: generalized massive edema including the abdomen and face (puffy eyelids and blunted facial features)
Proteinuria	Obtain clean-catch voided specimen, avoid contamination with vaginal secretions (causes false positive) • Significant if 1+ or 2+ on two or more occasions or if greater than 500 mg in a 24-hr urine collection

*Edema without other clinical indicators of preeclampsia can occur in normal pregnancy (see text).
PIH, pregnancy-induced hypertension; BP, blood pressure.

7. Inquire about subjective symptoms such as headaches, epigastric pain, visual disturbances. Record results of daily funduscopic examinations; edema of the retina reflects retinal ischemia and is a serious development.
8. If prescribed, administer magnesium sulfate according to facility protocol. The goal is to prevent convulsions without creating generalized CNS depression. To prevent overdose of magnesium, it is necessary to do the following:
   A. Check patellar reflexes at regular intervals (if depressed, notify physician).
   B. Check respirations (12 or less per minute is cause to notify physician).
   C. Monitor urine output (notify physician if <30 mL/hr).
   D. Monitor serum magnesium levels, reporting elevations above the therapeutic range designated by physician. The reader is referred to the Clinical Tip in Chapter 7 for nursing considerations in administering IV magnesium and to the Summary of Hypermagnesemia in Chapter 7 for a list of indicators of hypermagnesemia.
9. Administer oxygen if needed after convulsion. Monitor breath sounds for signs of pulmonary edema.

Research Findings

Since the association between eclampsia and hypertension was first recognized, the measurement of blood pressure during pregnancy has been an essential part of good antenatal care. A study was recently conducted to investigate the clinical and psychological outcome of blood pressure monitoring using a telemetry system at home.[70] Fifty-three previously normotensive women found to have significant hypertension during a routine antenatal visit participated in the study. These women would normally have been hospitalized; however, for purposes of the study, they were allowed to return home and use a telemetry system, which provided regular and accurate monitoring of their blood pressure. Results indicated that home telemetry is a highly acceptable method of managing moderate hypertension in pregnancy. Most frequently the women commented that use of the telemetry system avoided hospital admission and enabled them to remain at home where they were more comfortable and relaxed. Women with young children were particularly positive about the system. Negative responses were mainly associated with the few technical problems that arose with the transmission of blood pressure readings.

HYPONATREMIA AS A COMPLICATION OF OXYTOCIN ADMINISTRATION

Labor induction with oxytocin delivered in an appreciable amount of an aqueous solutions (such as 5% dextrose in water [D_5W]) can lead to water retention, severe hyponatremia, and seizures in both the mother and fetus.[71] Recall that the pharmacological action of oxytocin includes a potent antidiuretic effect causing increased water retention. Although the plasma sodium concentration may return to normal after the water diuresis that follows discontinuance of the infusion, permanent neurological sequelae or even death may occur.[72]

Symptoms of water intoxication (dilutional hyponatremia) include lethargy, headache, blurred vision, twitching, convulsions, and coma. See Chapter 4 for a more complete discussion of this topic. This complication can be prevented by using an electrolyte solution instead of dextrose and water as a vehicle for oxytocin administration, limiting the amount of fluid intake, and monitoring serum electrolytes.[73] Oxytocin should not be infused by gravity as the rate of flow by this method is too erratic to assure a steady delivery of the drug. Instead, it should be administered by a continuous infusion pump (such as a Harvard pump or a peristaltic-type pump). For induction of labor, the standard dilution is 1 mL (10 units) of oxytocin in 1 L of lactated Ringer's solution or 0.9% sodium chloride.[74] Initial dose is usually 1 to 2 mU/min; the maximum dose rarely exceeds 20 mU/min.[75]

HYPEREMESIS GRAVIDARUM

Hyperemesis gravidarum is defined as severe vomiting occurring before the 20th week of gestation.[76] Although nausea and vomiting are symptoms encountered in 50% to 90% of pregnancies, the incidence of hyperemesis gravidarum varies from 0.3% to 1%.[77] Excessive vomiting causes fluid volume deficit (FVD), starvational ketoacidosis, and, at times, metabolic alkalosis with hypokalemia. (These imbalances are commonly seen with excessive vomiting; see Chapter 13 for a discussion of fluid and electrolyte disturbances associated with gastric fluid loss.) Significant weight loss may occur and reflects fluid as well as lean tissue loss. Also indicative of FVD is decreased urinary output with a high specific gravity and a high blood urea nitrogen (BUN) level. Ketonuria can occur and is reflective of starvation; excessive ketones in the bloodstream cause metabolic acidosis. As stated above, metabolic alkalosis is also a possibility with the loss of gastric acid.

The cause of hyperemesis gravidarum is unknown. It has been postulated that it is related to several factors; among these are vitamin B_6 deficiency, impaired function of the adrenal cortex, hyperthyroidism and excess human chorionic gonadotropin (hCG) secretion, change in gastrointestinal (GI) physiology, poor nutrition, and emotional state.[78]

Prognosis is good if proper management is instituted. Treatment usually includes hospitalization; however, IV therapy may be initiated in an outpatient setting to correct mild to moderate dehydration. In severe cases, parenteral nutrition is provided until vomiting ceases, oral intake can be initiated, and serum electrolytes return to normal. At times, total parenteral nutrition may be indicated to achieve adequate nutrient intake and allow the GI tract to rest. Careful use of antiemetics or mild sedatives may also be indicated for some patients. Attention should be given to handling any psychological component of the patient's illness. Monitoring needs of patients with hyperemesis gravidarum include daily weights, fluid intake and output, vital signs, and laboratory measures of electrolytes and general metabolic status (including potassium, sodium, BUN, glucose, and serum creatinine levels).

FLUID AND ELECTROLYTE DISTURBANCES ASSOCIATED WITH TOCOLYTIC THERAPY

The most widely used drugs for tocolysis or treatment of preterm uterine contractions are the betamimetics (i.e., ritodrine hydrochloride and terbutaline sulfate) and magnesium sulfate. Tocolytic agents are usually *initially* administered intravenously. For example, ritodrine is initially administered intravenously at 50 to 100 mcg/min increasing by 50 mcg/min every 10 min until uterine contractions stop. The usual maintenance dose of ritodrine is 150 to 350 mcg/min, continued for 12 hrs after contractions have stopped. Oral administration of ritodrine is initiated 30 min before discontinuing the IV infusion.[79] Beta-mimetic treatment is associated with sodium and fluid retention.[80] To avoid this risk, the total amount of intravenous hydration should be limited to 1500 to 2500 mL/24 hrs; however, excess fluid volume may result in spite of limiting IV fluid intake. Beta-adrenergic drugs also induce a fall in plasma potassium levels.[81] Electrolytes should be monitored before and after 24 hrs of treatment with beta-adrenergic agents.

Home management of preterm labor may include the oral administration of either ritodrine or terbutaline.[82] The subcutaneous administration of small doses of terbutaline through a terbutaline pump may also be included in home management of preterm labor (Fig. 23-1) with the frequency of administration determined by uterine activity and maternal pulse. (Tachycardia is a side effect of betamimetic drugs).

Magnesium sulfate is known to decrease uterine activity and is currently being evaluated for its use as a tocolytic agent. As was previously mentioned, magnesium sulfate is usually administered IV, but may be given IM and orally. Therapeutic maternal serum levels of magnesium range between 4 and 8 mg/dL.[83] Nursing interventions are the same as for the woman receiving magnesium sulfate for severe preeclampsia.

CASE STUDIES

➤ 23-1. During her prenatal visit, a 19-year-old primigravida is hospitalized for the treatment of severe preeclampsia. Physical examination reveals that her blood pressure is 164/110 mmHg, her urine is +2 for protein, her deep tendon reflexes are 3+ without clonus, and she

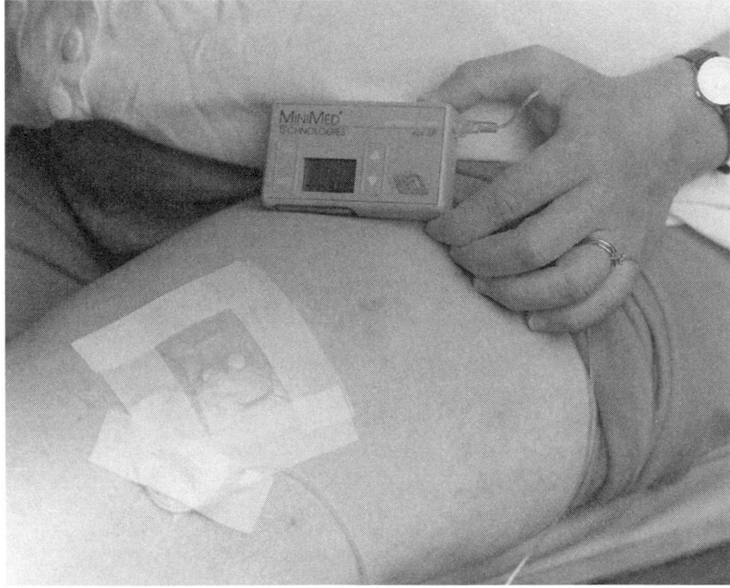

Figure 23–1. Subcutaneous administration of a tocolytic agent in the home management of preterm labor.

has 3+ edema. She is treated with $MgSO_4$ to decrease blood pressure and prevent convulsions. On the second day of $MgSO_4$ administration, nursing assessment reveals absent patellar reflexes.

COMMENTARY: The absence of deep tendon reflexes is a clear sign of magnesium toxicity. The $MgSO_4$ should be discontinued immediately. Magnesium toxicity *could* even result in respiratory or cardiac arrest. Calcium gluconate, the antidote for magnesium sulfate toxicity, should always be kept at the bedside of any patient receiving $MgSO_4$.

23-2. A 26-year-old gravida 2, 30 weeks gestation, is being treated for preterm labor. The physician orders an IV infusion of ritodrine hydrochloride, increasing the infusion rate every 10 to 30 min depending upon uterine response; the IV rate is *not* to exceed 125 mL/hr. Intake and output is to be strictly measured. Vital signs are to be taken every 15 min until stable and then follow hospital protocol. In particular, the patient's pulse rate, regularity, and quality are to be noted. A serum potassium level is to be determined before initiation of the ritodrine infusion and again in 24 hrs.

COMMENTARY: Because a common side effect of beta-mimetic agents is water retention, adherence to strict guidelines for IV fluid administration and recording of intake and output are important nursing functions. Tachycardia may also be an adverse effect of ritodrine administration. Electrolyte levels should be monitored before initiating the medication to obtain a baseline level and after 24 hrs to determine the effect on the patient's potassium level as beta-mimetic agents also induce a decrease in plasma potassium.

REFERENCES

1. Arias F: Practical Guide to High-Risk Pregnancy and Delivery, 2nd ed, p 2 14. St. Louis, Mosby Year Book, 1993
2. Guyton A: Textbook of Medical Physiology, 8th ed, p 922. Philadelphia, WB Saunders, 1991
3. Creasy R, Resnik R: Maternal-Fetal Medicine: Principles and Practice, 3rd ed, p 758. Philadelphia, WB Saunders, 1994
4. Arias, p 245
5. Theunissen I, Parer J: Fluid and electrolytes in pregnancy. Clin Obstet Gynecol 37(1):6,1994
6. Creasy, Resnik, p 764–765
7. Blackburn S, Loper D: Maternal, Fetal, & Neonatal Physiology: A Clinical Perspective, pp 342, 344. Philadelphia, WB Saunders, 1992
8. Ibid, p 342
9. Ibid, p 344
10. Worthington-Roberts B, Williams S: Nutrition in Pregnancy and Lactation, 5th ed, p 153. St. Louis, Mosby, 1993
11. Ibid
12. Ibid, p 156
13. Theunissen, Parer, p 3
14. Creasy, Resnik, p 806
15. Theunissen, Parer, p 4
16. Blackburn, Loper, p 346
17. Gilbert E, Harmon J: High Risk Pregnancy & Delivery, p 383. St. Louis, Mosby, 1993
18. Blackburn, Loper, p 346
19. Theunissen, Parer, p 4
20. Katz et al: A comparison of bed rest and immersion for treating the edema of pregnancy. Obstet Gynecol 75(2):147,1990
21. Paller M, Ferris T: Fluid and electrolyte metabolism during pregnancy. In: Narins G (ed): Maxwell & Kleeman's Clinical Disorders of Fluid and Electrolyte Metabolism, 5th ed, p 1128. New York: McGraw-Hill, 1994
22. Ibid
23. Creasy, Resnik, p 1020
24. Repke J: Calcium homeostasis in pregnancy. Clin Obstet Gynecol 37(1):62,1994
25. Worthington-Roberts, Williams, p 144
26. Repke, p 62
27. Ibid
28. Ibid
29. Worthington-Roberts, Williams, p 144
30. Paller, Ferris, p 1132
31. Ibid
32. Worthington-Roberts, Williams, p 147
33. Paller, Ferris, p 1128
34. Ibid
35. Ibid
36. Ibid, p 1132
37. Ibid
38. Ibid
39. Webb B, et al: Changes in sodium transport during the human menstrual cycle and pregnancy. Clin Sci 84:401,1993
40. Krening, C: Perinatal hypertensive crisis. NAACOG's Clinical Issues in Perinatal and Women's Health Nursing 3(3):413, 1992
41. Creasy, Resnik, p 807
42. Ibid, p 806
43. Arias, p 186
44. Ibid
45. Ibid, p 183

46. Gilbert, Harmon, p 383
47. Arias, p 185
48. Gilbert, Harmon, p 388
49. Arias, p 199
50. Creasy, Resnik, p 828
51. Ibid
52. Ibid, p 831
53. Arias, p 194
54. Creasy, Resnik, p 828
55. Krening, p 415
56. Creasy, Resnik, p 832
57. Ibid, p 829
58. Arias, p 193
59. Gilbert, Harmon, p 397
60. Ibid, p 398
61. Ibid
62. Creasy, Resnik, p 830
63. Ibid, p 831
64. Ibid
65. Harmon J, Barry M: Antenatal testing, mobile outpatient monitoring service. J Obstet Gynecol Neonatal Nurs 18(1):21,1989
66. Bobak I, Jensen M: Maternity & Gynecologic Care, 5th ed, p 828. St. Louis, Mosby Year Book, 1993
67. Smith C, Selig C, Rayburn W, Yi P: Reliability of compact electronic blood pressure monitors for hypertensive pregnant women. J Reprod Med 35(4):399,1990
68. Mooney P, Dalton K, Swindells H, Rushant S, Cartwright W, Juett D: Blood pressure measured telemetrically from home throughout pregnancy. Am J Obstet Gynecol 163(1):30,1990
69. Heaman M: Stressful life events, social support, and mood disturbance in hospitalized and non-hospitalized women with pregnancy-induced hypertension. Can J Nurs Res 24(1):23,1992
70. Cartwright W, et al: Home measurement of pregnancy hypertension. Prof Care Mother Child 3:8,1993
71. Rayburn W, Zuspan F: Drug Therapy in Obstetrics and Gynecology, 3rd ed, p 237. St. Louis, Mosby Year Book, 1992
72. Lillien A: Oxytocin induced water intoxication: A report of maternal death. Obstet Gynecol 32:171,1968
73. Cherry S, Merkatz I: Complications of Pregnancy: Medical, Surgical, Gynecologic, Psychosocial, and Perinatal, 4th ed, p 774. Baltimore, Williams & Wilkins, 1991
74. Rayburn, Zuspan, p 235
75. Deglin J, Vallerand A, Russin M: Davis's Drug Manual for Nurses, 2nd ed, p 852. Philadelphia, FA Davis
76. Long P, Russell L: Hyperemesis gravidarum. J Perinatal Neonatal Nurs 6(4):22,1993
77. Theunissen, Parer, p 9
78. Long, Russell, p 23
79. Deglin, Vallerand, Russin, p 1021
80. Theunissen, Parer, p 9
81. Ibid, p 10
82. Bobak, Jensen, p 1074
83. Mandeville L, Troiano N: High-Risk Intrapartum Nursing, p 67. Philadelphia, JB Lippincott, 1992

V

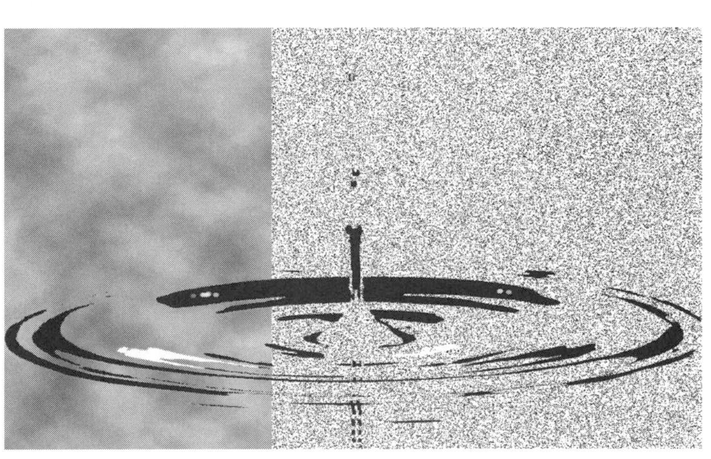

Special Considerations in Children and the Elderly

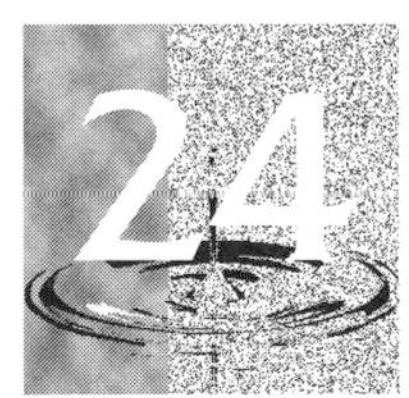

Fluid Balance in Infants and Children

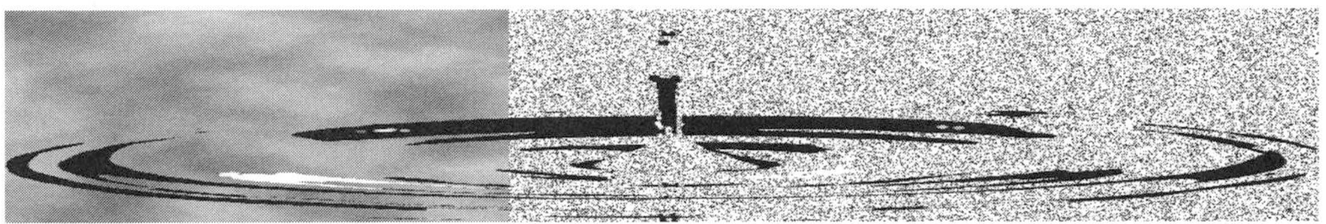

An obvious difference between young children and adults is size. However, children are not merely miniature adults; the child's body composition and homeostatic controls differ from those of the adult. The younger the child, the greater the differences. It is helpful to compare the child's body composition with that of the adult and review the salient characteristics of the child's homeostatic and metabolic functioning.

DIFFERENCES IN WATER AND ELECTROLYTE BALANCE IN INFANTS, CHILDREN, AND ADULTS

BODY WATER CONTENT

The premature infant's body is approximately 90% water; the newborn infant's body, 70% to 80%; the adult's body about 60%. Infants have proportionately more water in the extracellular compartment than do adults. For example, 40% of the newborn infant's body water is in the extracellular compartment, as compared with less than 20% in the case of the adult.

As the infant becomes older, the ratio of extracellular to intracellular fluid volume decreases. Loss of extracellular fluid (ECF) is attributed to the growth of cellular tissue and the decreasing rate of growth of collagen relative to muscle growth during the early months of life.[1] The decrease is particularly rapid during the first few days of life, but continues throughout the first 6 months. After the first year, the total body water is about 64% (34% in the cellular compartment and 30% in the ECF compartment). By the end of the second year, the total body water approaches the adult percentage of approximately 60% (36% in the cellular compartment and 24% in the ECF compartment). At puberty, the adult body water composition is attained.

DAILY BODY WATER TURNOVER IN INFANTS AND ADULTS

The fact that infants have a relatively greater total body water content does not protect them from excessive fluid loss. On the contrary, infants are *more* vulnerable to fluid volume deficit (FVD) because they ingest and excrete a relatively greater daily water volume than adults. Infants may exchange half of their daily ECF, whereas the adult may exchange only one-sixth during the same period. Therefore proportionately, the infant has a smaller reserve of body fluid than does the adult.

The daily fluid exchange is relatively greater in infants, in part because their metabolic rate is two times higher per unit of weight than that of adults. Infants expend 100 kcal/kg of body weight, whereas adults expend only 40 kcal/kg. Owing to the high metabolic rate, the infant has a large amount of metabolic wastes to excrete. Because water is needed by the kidneys to excrete these wastes, a large urinary volume is formed each day. Contributing to this volume is the inability of the infant's immature kidneys to concentrate urine efficiently. In addition, relatively greater fluid loss occurs through the infant's skin because of the proportionately greater body surface area.

HOMEOSTATIC DIFFERENCES BETWEEN CHILDREN AND ADULTS

Young children have immature homeostatic regulating mechanisms that must be considered when planning water and electrolyte replacement.

Renal Function

The newborn's renal function is not yet completely developed. If infant and adult renal functions are compared on the basis of total body water, the infant's kidneys appear to become mature by the end of the first month of life. However, if body surface area is used as the criterion for comparison, the child's kidneys appear immature for the first 2 years of life. Because the infant's kidneys have a limited concentrating ability and require more water to excrete a given amount of solute, the infant has difficulty conserving body water when it is needed. Also, the infant has difficulty excreting an excess fluid volume.[2] Thus, infants are less able to adapt to too little, or too much, fluid. Although adults may be able to tolerate fluid imbalances for days, infants may tolerate similar disturbances for only hours before the situation becomes acute.

Acid–Base Homeostasis

Newborn and premature infants have less homeostatic buffering capacity than do older children. They have a tendency toward metabolic acidosis, with pH averages slightly lower (7.30–7.35) than normal.[3] The mild metabolic acidosis (base bicarbonate deficit) is believed to be related to high metabolic acid production and to renal immaturity. Because cow's milk has higher phosphate and sulfate concentrations than breast milk, newborns fed cow's milk have a lower pH than do breast-fed babies.

Body Surface Area Differences

The skin represents an important route of fluid loss, especially in illness. This is an important concept when considering fluid balance in infants and young children because their body surface area is greater than that of older children and adults. For example, compared with the older child and adults, the premature infant has approximately five times as much body surface area in relation to weight, and the newborn, three times. Therefore, any condition causing a pronounced decrease in intake or increase in output of water and electrolytes threatens the body fluid economy of the infant. Because the gastrointestinal (GI) membranes are essentially an extension of the body surface area, their area is also relatively greater in the young infant than in the older child and adult. Hence, relatively greater losses occur from the GI tract in the sick infant than in the older child and adult. In comparing fluid losses in infants with those in adults, one might regard the baby's body as a smaller vessel with a larger spout.

Calcium–Phosphorus Regulation

Newborn infants are vulnerable to hypocalcemic tetany because of a transient physiologic hypoparathyroidism. Serum calcium levels are known to correlate with gestational age; therefore, the incidence of hypocalcemia in premature infants is extremely high.[4] Other factors that increase the risk of hypocalcemia include low birth weight, intrauterine growth retardation, and cow's milk feedings.

Cow's milk is a high-phosphate food. A young infant who is fed cow's milk can develop hypocalcemia because of an elevated serum phosphate level. During infancy, there is a relatively high renal tubular reabsorption of phosphate and a low glomerular filtration rate.[5] If the infant's parathyroid glands are not able to produce sufficient parathyroid hormone, the level of serum calcium will continue to decrease. Clinical manifestations of hypocalcemic tetany progress from tremors, irritability, and muscular twitching, eventually to convulsions. Carpopedal spasms are not seen in infants. Because human milk is low in phosphorus, breast-fed infants are not likely to develop hypocalcemic tetany.

Electrolyte Concentrations

Plasma electrolyte concentrations do not vary strikingly among infants, small children, and adults. The plasma sodium concentration changes little from birth to adulthood. The potassium concentration is higher in the first few months of life than at any other time, as is the plasma chloride concentration. Magnesium and calcium are both low in the first 24 hrs after birth. As stated above, the inability of the premature infant to regulate calcium ion concentration can bring on hypocalcemic tetany.

NURSING ASSESSMENT

Initial assessment of the infant or child with a suspected or potential fluid and electrolyte imbalance includes a review of the history and laboratory data as well as systematic observation and physical inspection. An infant or child who is ill appears flaccid and the eyes lack their usual brightness and sparkle.

A history from the parents will usually reveal that the child has a decreased appetite, is less active, and is more irritable than usual. Additional information may reveal large losses of fluid through diarrhea or vomiting, and an inability to "get anything" into the child. The history should include the frequency and amount of voiding as well as the number and consistency of stools before admission. All this information should be carefully recorded in the child's record.

Additional objective assessments should be obtained and include the child's weight and vital signs. A blood pressure reading in a young child is not a reliable sign of fluid volume status because the elasticity of the blood vessels may keep the blood pressure stable initially even when volume is diminished.[6] See Chapter 2 for a review of a systematic approach to assessment of fluid balance status. The following discussion is specific to children.

TISSUE TURGOR

Tissue turgor in the child is best palpated in the abdominal areas and on the medial aspects of the thighs (see Fig. 24-1). In a normal situation, pinched skin will fall back to its normal configuration when released. In a patient with FVD, the skin may remain slightly raised for a few seconds. Skin turgor begins to decrease after 3% to 5% of the body weight is lost as fluid. Severe malnutrition, particularly in infants, can cause depressed skin turgor even in the absence of fluid depletion.

Obese infants with FVD often have skin turgor that is deceptively normal in appearance. An infant with water loss and excess of sodium loss (hypernatremia, or sodium excess) has a firm, thick-feeling skin. This same phenomenon is observed in the child who has sodium excess owing to an excessive sodium intake such as occurs in salt poisoning. The thickened turgor is believed to be associated with pulling of water from the cells into the hypertonic interstitial fluid.

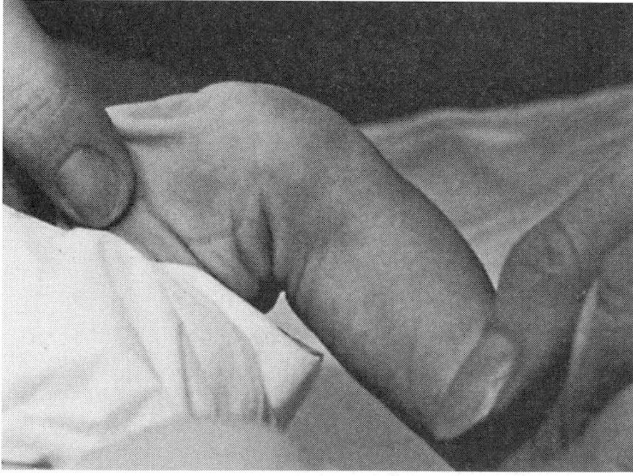

Figure 24–1. Poor skin turgor in infant.

MUCOUS MEMBRANES

Dry mouth may be due to FVD or to mouth breathing. When in doubt, the nurse should run a finger along the oral cavity to feel the mucous membrane where the cheek and gums meet. Dryness in this area indicates a true FVD. The tongue of the fluid-depleted child is smaller than normal. Mucous membranes in the child with sodium excess are dry and sticky. The absence of tearing and salivation is a sign of FVD that becomes obvious with a fluid loss of 5% of the total body weight.

BODY TEMPERATURE

Fluid volume deficit is often associated with a subnormal temperature because of reduced energy output. Depending on the underlying disease, however, fever can accompany FVD. If fever is present, its height should be recorded frequently. The rate of insensible water loss is greatly increased with fever. The amount of water loss depends on the degree and duration of the fever. Fever may indicate excessive water loss from the body with resultant sodium excess, or it may indicate an infection. The extremities are cold to the touch in severe FVD, even when fever is present; this is due to decreased peripheral blood flow.

URINE VOLUME AND CONCENTRATION

When possible, all urine should be collected and measured in the child with a real or potential body fluid disturbance. Unfortunately, this is often difficult to do in infants and small children. In this situation, at least the frequency of voiding should be noted. In addition, the nurse should estimate the portion of the diaper saturated with urine. One would do well to weigh a dry diaper occasionally and compare its weight with that of the same diaper after the child has voided. The urine's concentration, as revealed by its color, should also be noted. When necessary, urinary specific gravity can be measured with a refractometer; fortunately, this device requires only a drop of urine for the test.

Hourly urinary output reflects the adequacy of hemodynamics and hydration. It will be zero if there is no perfusing pressure (<70–80 mmHg systolic) and less than normal when there is an FVD of 20% or more of the blood volume.[7] As a general rule, normal urinary output is about 1 mL/kg of body weight per hour.[8] Because urine flow rates in sick newborns may vary considerably from hour to hour, the average output should be calculated every 6 hrs. The urine output should average at least 5 mL/kg in each 6-hr period.[9]

When an accurate hourly recording of urine output is indicated, the nurse must devise a method to collect all the urine passed. A number of devices are available. Regardless of the type used, check frequently for leakage and provide good skin care to prevent irritation of the genitalia.

A child with FVD has a decreased urinary output and an increased urinary specific gravity. If the FVD is severe, a child may go as long as 18 to 24 hrs without voiding and still not have a distended bladder. If a child with a known FVD excretes large amounts of dilute urine, renal damage probably exists. If renal concentrating ability is impaired or if the child is receiving a high-solute diet, the urine volume will be somewhat above normal to clear all the metabolic wastes. The same is true if a hypercatabolic state (such as fever or infection, or both) is present.

WEIGHT CHANGES

If possible, the child's weight before the onset of the illness should be obtained from the parents or from the family physician, who may have a record of the normal weight from a recent office visit.

Weight loss can be caused by loss of fluid or by catabolism of body tissues. The weight loss associated with FVD occurs more rapidly than that caused by starvation. A mild FVD in an infant or child entails a loss of 3% to 5% of the normal body weight; a moderate FVD, from 5% to 9%; a severe FVD, 10% or more. (An acute loss of 15% of the body weight will likely cause hypovolemic shock.)

If weighing is not performed accurately, it is useless. Even a minor error is important when the patient is small. The child should be weighed at the same time each day, before eating, and after having voided. The same scales should be used each time. The child should be undressed and covered with a light blanket to protect against chilling while being weighed. (The same blanket should be used each time for consistency.)

OTHER CONSIDERATIONS

Additional assessment parameters pertaining to evaluation of fluid balance status are presented in other sections of the text. For example, evaluation of laboratory data is presented in Chapter 2; findings expected in specific imbalances are described in Chapters 3 through 9.

CONDITIONS IN CHILDREN PREDISPOSING TO FLUID AND ELECTROLYTE DISTURBANCES

See Chapters 10 through 23 for discussion of specific entities; although these chapters are primarily concerned with the care of adults, some information is also applicable to children. The discussion below concerns specific fluid and electrolyte problems occurring in a pediatric population.

CRITICAL ILLNESS OR INJURY

The resuscitation of an infant or child in severe hypovolemic shock or cardiac arrest requires immediate vascular access for the administration of medicines, blood, and fluids. Intravenous access is extremely difficult because of peripheral circulatory collapse, and precious minutes may be wasted in trying to access a peripheral vein.[10] The use of the intraosseous route for parenteral infusions in such emergency situations may be life-saving.[11] Pediatric Advanced Life Support programs provide training in the technique of intraosseous infusion for the emergency treatment of infants and children. See the section on the intraosseous route for parenteral infusions later in this chapter.

PYLORIC STENOSIS

Pyloric stenosis is a condition in which the circular muscle of the pylorus is elongated and hypertrophic. The condition produces progressive narrowing of the lumen of the outlet from the stomach to the duodenum and results in vomiting after feedings. The condition becomes evident in the first few weeks of life as vomiting becomes progressive and eventually projectile in nature. The condition affects approximately 1 in every 150 male infants and 1 in every 750 female infants.

Because of the repeated vomiting, the infants are poorly nourished. Although this condition can be corrected surgically, preoperative correction of the water and electrolyte disturbances caused by the prolonged vomiting is mandatory.[12]

Vomiting causes the same imbalances in children as it does in adults. These include metabolic alkalosis, potassium deficit, sodium deficit, and FVD. See Chapter 13 for a discussion of imbalances associated with vomiting.

The infant with hypertonic pyloric stenosis has the following symptoms:

- Difficulty in retaining feedings, which becomes progressively worse during the first few weeks of life; eventually, projectile vomiting follows each feeding
- Signs of malnutrition
- Signs of FVD (see Chapter 3)
- Constipation
- Decreased respiration (compensatory action of lungs to retain carbon dioxide and thus help counteract metabolic alkalosis)
- Tetany accompanying alkalosis (owing to decreased calcium ionization in an alkaline pH)
- Palpable pyloric mass
- Ketoacidosis (may appear if starvation is prolonged)

Once the infant's fluid and electrolyte balance is restored, surgical correction of the pyloric obstruction can be accomplished and oral feedings resumed.

DIARRHEA

Fluid and Electrolyte Disorders

Diarrhea is a common cause of water and electrolyte disturbances in infants and small children. In the United States the rotavirus is the pathogen that is responsible for the vast majority of cases. The virus attacks the absorptive cells of the small bowel, which results in watery diarrhea.[13] A large loss of liquid stools can rapidly deplete the young child's ECF volume, especially when it is combined with vomiting. Usually water and electrolytes are lost in isotonic proportions (FVD or "isotonic dehydration"). However, water can be lost in excess of electrolytes (FVD with sodium excess or "hypertonic dehydration"), and electrolytes can be lost in excess of water (FVD with sodium deficit or "hypotonic dehydration"). Because sodium is the chief extracellular ion, its excess or deficit is of primary importance in producing symptoms.

Isotonic Dehydration (FVD)

Approximately 70% of patients with severe diarrhea undergo a proportionate loss of water and electrolytes. Symptoms of FVD due to infantile diarrhea include the following:

- History of large quantities of liquid stools
- Acute weight loss
- Dry skin with poor turgor (see Fig. 24-1)
- Diminished tearing
- Soft eyeballs with a sunken appearance (resulting from decreased intraocular pressure)
- Skin ashen or gray in color and extremities cold (owing to inadequate peripheral perfusion)
- Depressed body temperature, unless infection is present
- Lethargy
- Weak, rapid pulse
- Oliguria, increased specific gravity
- Serum sodium concentration between 130 and 150 mEq/L

Hypertonic Dehydration (FVD With Hypernatremia)

Approximately 20% of patients with severe diarrhea have suffered a relatively greater loss of water than of electrolytes. If the infant has ingested a high-solute-containing formula during illness or has been inadvertently given an overly concentrated electrolyte mixture, the resultant increased renal water loss will intensify the sodium excess already present. Recall that the infant cannot concentrate urine efficiently and therefore, needs a relatively large water intake to excrete solutes. The infant's need for water is further intensified by a large body surface area and resultant increased insensible water loss.

Symptoms of FVD and sodium excess (hypertonic dehydration) caused by diarrhea include the following:

- History of large quantities of liquid stools associated with a low water intake, high solute intake, poor renal function, or all three
- Weight loss
- Serum sodium greater than 150 mEq/L
- Thickened, firm-feeling skin (caused by fluid being pulled from cells into interstitial space)
- Avid thirst (hypertonic ECF draws water from cells producing cellular dehydration)
- Irritability when disturbed; otherwise behavior is lethargic
- Tremors and convulsions
- Muscle rigidity
- Nuchal rigidity
- Pronounced signs of hypernatremia; signs of FVD are variable
- Brain injury (Hypernatremia causes the brain tissue to shrink; if the imbalance is severe and occurs rapidly, small blood vessels may rupture. See Chapter 4 for further discussions of hypernatremia.)

Hypotonic Dehydration (FVD With Hyponatremia)

Approximately 10% of patients with severe diarrhea experience a relatively greater loss of electrolytes than water in the stool. Bacillary dysentery and cholera are two diseases that may result in hypotonic dehydration because the concentration of sodium in the stool rises with the increasing volume of the stool.[14] Viral infections are not associated with such severe losses of sodium. However, hyponatremia can occur in children with viral enteritis if they are given electrolyte-free fluids to replace their losses. See the next sections for a discussion of oral rehydration therapy and the consequences of excessive water intake.

Symptoms in hypotonic dehydration are due to decreased ECF volume and sodium deficit. Symptoms include the following:

- Gray pallor
- Cold, clammy skin with poor turgor
- Slightly moist mucous membranes
- Sunken eyes
- Rapid pulse
- Lethargy that may advance to coma
- Serum sodium less than 130 mEq/L

Metabolic Acidosis

Metabolic acidosis usually accompanies frequent liquid stools. (Recall that the intestinal secretions are alkaline because of their high bicarbonate content; therefore, loss of alkaline secretions in diarrheal stools results in metabolic acidosis.) Decreased dietary intake contributes to metabolic acidosis. In the absence of adequate food intake, the body uses its own fats for energy purposes. The metabolism of these fats causes the accumulation of acidic ketone bodies in the blood, further contributing to the metabolic acidosis caused by bicarbonate loss.

A major symptom of metabolic acidosis is increased depth of respiration, a compensatory mechanism that blows off carbon dioxide, thus reducing the carbonic acid content of the blood and influencing the carbonic acid–base bicarbonate balance in the direction of an increased pH. If ketosis of starvation is present, an acetone odor may be noted on the breath.

Other Electrolyte Imbalances

Deficits of potassium and magnesium are also common disturbances with prolonged diarrhea. These imbalances are discussed in Chapters 5 and 7, respectively.

Treatment—Oral Rehydration

The dehydration that results from diarrhea in infants and children can be treated by the oral administration of a balanced glucose–electrolyte solution. In many parts of the world, oral rehydration therapy is the only form of treatment available, and it has been shown to reduce significantly the mortality rate from acute diarrhea.[15] The oral rehydration solution (ORS) recommended by the Diarrhea Disease Control Program of the World Health Organization contains sodium, potassium, chloride, base, glucose, and water. The glucose in the solution functions to facilitate the transport of sodium across the bowel wall.[16]

TABLE 24–1

Oral Electrolyte Solutions: Concentration When Diluted

PRODUCT	Na (mEq/L)	K (mEq/L)	Cl (mEq/L)	Base (mEq/L)	Glucose (g/L)
Rehydration					
ORS (WHO)	90	20	80	30	20
Rehydralyte (Ross)	75	20	65	30	25
Maintenance					
Pedialyte (Ross)	45	20	35	30	25
Ricelyte (Mead Johnson)	50	25	45	34	30*

*Rice syrup solids.

Table 24-1 presents the composition of ORS and several other products that are available in grocery and drug stores throughout the United States. The commercial products are sold with directions for administration. Recommended amounts to use are calculated on the basis of weight, both in pounds and kilograms, and stool frequency.

Because there is a high sodium concentration in ORS, there also is a risk of inducing hypernatremia. To prevent hypernatremia, the full-strength solution should be used for rehydration only. Breast feeding should be continued during rehydration with infants who are breast-fed; plain water should be encouraged with infants who are formula-fed.[17] Once rehydration has been achieved, a maintenance solution with a sodium concentration of 30 to 50 mEq/L should be used. Children (including infants who have started on solids) should be fed during maintenance therapy beginning with bland, starchy foods such as rice, cereal, and bananas.[18]

Modifications in the original ORS composition have been studied in an effort to find an ideal rehydration solution that would reduce the severity and duration of diarrhea symptoms.[19] Complex carbohydrates such as cereal and rice have been used in place of glucose. Results of clinical trials to compare these solutions with ORS have been variable. Feeding an infant or child a rice-based diet after ORS rehydration appears to decrease the duration of diarrhea symptoms.[20] The administration of a rice-based electrolyte solution at the onset of diarrhea symptoms may prevent the development of dehydration and also decrease stool volume.[21]

Oral rehydration solutions can be offered by bottle, spoon, or cup. Vomiting is not necessarily a contraindication to oral rehydration therapy.[22] Spoon-feeding appears to minimize vomiting. Throughout the rehydration phase, the solution should be offered in small amounts at frequent intervals. Skin turgor, body weight, and behavioral responses should be assessed frequently to evaluate the child's progress. Nursing strategies for administering oral fluids to infants and young children are discussed later in this chapter.

Treatment—Parenteral Fluid Therapy

Infants and children with diarrhea who are in impending hypovolemic shock, or who are unable to drink because of lethargy or persistent vomiting, must have parenteral fluid therapy to replace their losses and restore their fluid and electrolyte homeostasis. See section on Principles of Parenteral Fluid Replacement in Children later in this chapter.

CONSTIPATION

Undesirable effects of enemas for the treatment of constipation in infants and young children are discussed in Chapter 13. Serious electrolyte complications (primarily hyperphosphatemia, hypocalcemia, and hypernatremia) have been reported with the use of sodium phosphate (Fleet) enemas in young children. As indicated below, excessive absorption of

TABLE 24–2

Range of Average Water Requirements of Children at Different Ages Under Ordinary Conditions

AGE	AVERAGE BODY WEIGHT (kg)	TOTAL WATER IN 24 HOURS (mL)	WATER PER kg BODY WT IN 24 HOURS (mL)
3 days	3.0	250–300	80–100
10 days	3.2	400–500	125–150
3 mo	5.4	750–850	140–160
6 mo	7.3	950–1100	130–155
9 mo	8.6	1100–1250	125–145
1 yr	9.5	1150–1300	120–135
2 yr	11.8	1350–1500	115–125
4 yr	16.2	1600–1800	100–110
6 yr	20.0	1800–2000	90–100
10 yr	28.7	2000–2500	70–85
14 yr	45.0	2200–2700	50–60

Adapted from Behrman RE: Nelson Textbook of Pediatrics, 14th ed, p 107. Philadelphia, WB Saunders, 1992.

water from tap water enemas can lead to hyponatremia. When a young child needs an enema, an isotonic saline (0.9% NaCl) solution should be used. The solution can be made in the home by dissolving one teaspoon of table salt in one pint of tap water.

EXCESSIVE WATER INTAKE

Healthy older children and adults can tolerate large increases in free water intake, but infants cannot. Because the urinary diluting capacity of infants is limited by a low rate of glomerular filtration,[23] excess water cannot be excreted efficiently. The accumulation of free water in the extracellular space produces acute dilutional hyponatremia (water intoxication), which is a very serious fluid and electrolyte problem.

Acute dilutional hyponatremia can develop in infants who are fed excessively diluted formula[24] or who swallow large amounts of water during swimming lessons.[25] The condition also can occur in infants who are given tap water enemas because excessive water may be absorbed from the large intestine.[26] The inappropriate use of glucose solutions in water, either as oral or parenteral therapy, to treat infants with dehydration can result in acute dilutional hyponatremia.[27]

As the extracellular sodium dilutes, water shifts to the intracellular space, pulmonary and cerebral edema develop, and intracranial pressure increases. Signs of acute dilutional hyponatremia include the following:

- Lethargy and irritability
- Subnormal temperature
- Focal or generalized seizures
- Respiratory distress

Treatment is directed toward restricting free water intake and carefully increasing the serum sodium level.[28] With skilled medical and nursing care, the prognosis is good. In a report of 29 infants with acute dilutional hyponatremia, all of whom experienced seizures and six of whom required endotracheal intubation, all recovered without apparent sequelae.[29]

PRINCIPLES OF PARENTERAL FLUID REPLACEMENT IN CHILDREN

DAILY REQUIREMENTS

Daily requirements for water are related to both caloric consumption and expenditure. The normal water requirements per kilogram of body weight for healthy infants and children are listed in Table 24-2.

Infants and children who cannot tolerate oral feedings, particularly when abnormal losses are occurring, must receive parenteral fluid therapy to meet maintenance and replacement needs. Maintenance requirements can be computed in several ways. One common method is based on total body weight and uses the following formula:

100 mL/kg of body weight for the first 10 kg
50 mL/kg of body weight for the second 10 kg up to 20 kg
20 mL/kg of body weight for each kg above 20 kg

Another method for calculating maintenance fluid requirements is based on total body surface area in square meters (m^2) and the formula of 1500 $mL/m^2/day$. Body surface area (BSA) can be determined by plotting the child's height and weight on a nomogram (Fig. 24-2).

Maintenance requirements calculated by either of these formulas may have to be modified on the

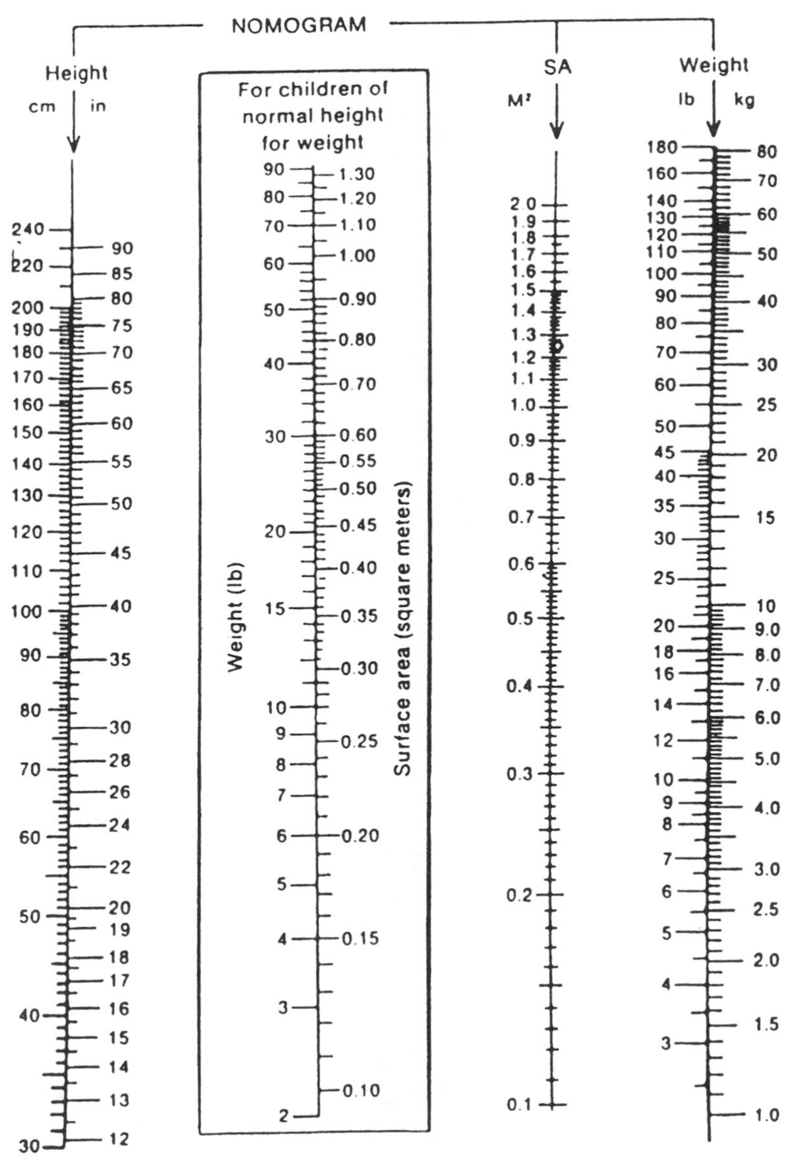

Figure 24–2. West Nomogram for Estimating Surface Area of Infants and Young Children. The surface area is indicated where a straight line connecting the child's height and weight intersects the surface area (SA) column or, if the child appears to be of normal proportion, from the weight alone (enclosed area). Nomogram modified from data of E. Boyd by CD West. In: Behrman RE: Nelson Textbook of Pediatrics, 14th ed, p 1827. Philadelphia, WB Saunders, 1992; with permission.

basis of assessment data. Factors such as an extremely humid environment or the ability to take in and retain some oral fluids will reduce the amount of maintenance fluids to be delivered parenterally. Factors such as hyperventilation, an extremely dry environment, or a high body temperature will require an increase in the amount of maintenance fluids.

In addition to the rough guidelines described above, fluid volume replacement must be based on the history, on clinical assessment of circulatory impairment or changes in skin elasticity (discussed earlier), and on laboratory values such as serum electrolytes and osmolality. See Chapter 2 for a discussion of laboratory tests and Chapter 10 for a discussion of water and electrolyte solutions and nursing considerations in their administration. In summary, the amount and type of parenteral fluid to be administered must be based on the degree and type of dehydration (isotonic, hypertonic, or hypotonic), serum electrolyte levels, and the nature of acid–base balance.

CORRECTION OF ISOTONIC DEHYDRATION (FVD)

Isotonic constriction of body fluids is observable by dry skin and mucous membranes as well as tachycardia when about 5% of the body weight has been lost during a 24-hr period. Marked circulatory impairment evidenced by mottled, cool, inelastic skin and sunken eyes occurs when the child has lost 10% of the body weight over a 1- to 2-day period. Losses of 15% of the body weight over this time period can produce a moribund or near-moribund state.[30]

When the degree of fluid and electrolyte imbalance has been determined, therapy is administered in phases. The objective of the first phase (the emergency period) is to restore circulation by rapid expansion of the ECF volume, either to treat shock or prevent its occurrence. The repletion period lasts 6 to 8 hrs and replaces ECF losses with half the estimated volume deficit. During the next 16 of the first 24 hrs, the concern is with cellular fluid restoration, and the second half of the day's estimate plus any additional disease-related losses is administered.

CORRECTION OF HYPERTONIC DEHYDRATION (FVD WITH HYPERNATREMIA)

Recall that in this type of fluid loss, water loss has exceeded sodium loss. The child will likely have central nervous system involvement, evidenced by irritability, lethargy, nuchal rigidity, and seizures. The principle of therapy is *very gradual* replacement of water over time so that the brain does not swell. A dilute sodium solution (e.g., 20–30 mEq of sodium/L) to replace gradually the estimated water deficit over a 48-hr or longer period is sometimes recommended. To control seizures, practitioners may administer 3 to 5 mL/kg of a 0.3% NaCl solution.[31] (See Chapter 4 for a discussion of safe correction of hypernatremia.)

Potassium losses may be extreme; replacement is gradual over a 3- to 4-day period. Potassium replacement is an important factor in restoring water to cells.

CORRECTION OF HYPOTONIC DEHYDRATION (FVD WITH HYPONATREMIA)

This condition tends to occur in patients with fluid loss replaced primarily with water; in such instances, the serum sodium level decreases below normal. Management of this condition depends on how low the serum sodium level becomes. If it is extremely low and neurological symptoms are present, it may be necessary to administer, with caution, a small volume of hypertonic sodium solution. Half the calculated amount is usually given and then the clinical situation (including serum sodium measurement) is reevaluated. If results are as expected, the second half is given. See Chapter 4 for a discussion of treatment of hyponatremia, including principles for administering hypertonic sodium solutions.

Once the ECF volume has been restored, the child is managed in the same manner as one with isotonic body fluid constriction. Potassium deficits should be considered and replaced as indicated. Nursing considerations in potassium administration are discussed in Chapter 5.

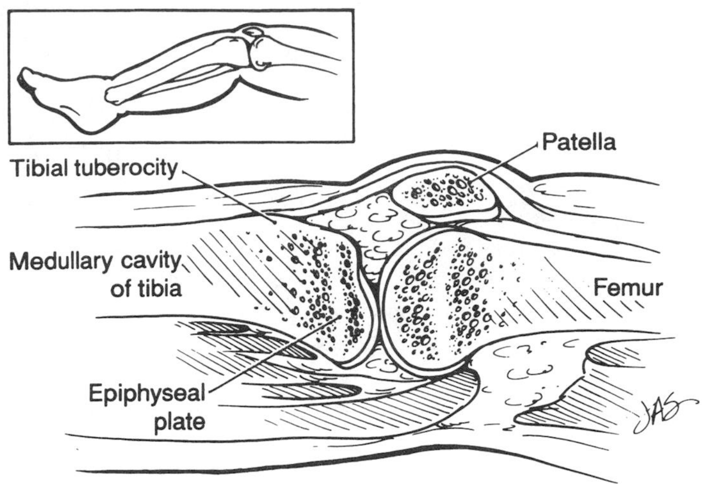

Figure 24–3. Structure of the proximal tibia and medullary cavity for intraosseous infusions.

THE INTRAOSSEOUS ROUTE FOR PARENTERAL INFUSIONS

The emergency care of infants and children who experience hypovolemic shock or cardiac arrest requires immediate access to the vascular system. The intraosseous route provides an avenue to the rich vascular network within the medullary cavity of long bones.[32] The medial aspect of the proximal tibia is the preferred location in treating infants and children (see Fig. 24-3). The technique requires the use of a rigid needle with an inner stylet, either a bone marrow needle or one specifically designed for pediatric intraosseous infusions (see Fig. 24-4). The insertion site should be cleansed thoroughly, and a local anesthetic agent should be used if the child is responsive to painful stimuli. The needle is inserted through the bone cortex into the medullary space, and placement is confirmed by the aspiration of bone marrow. After the needle is flushed with heparinized saline, medicines and volume expanders can be infused. The transfer of medicines and fluids from the medullary cavity to the general circulation is very rapid. Dosages of medicines are the same as for intravenous administration; likewise, the rate of flow for infusing volume expanders is the same.

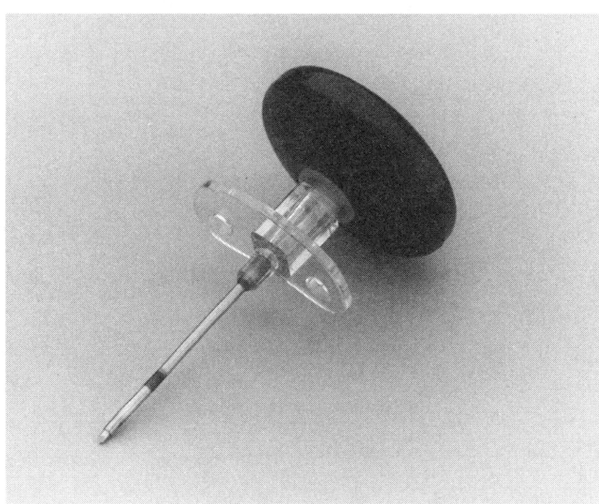

Figure 24–4. A Cook Disposable Intraosseous Infusion Needle. Available in lengths of 2.5, 3.0, and 4.0 cm. Photograph courtesy of Cook Critical Care, A Division of Cook Incorporated, Bloomington, IN.

The infusion site should be observed frequently for signs of infiltration, as with an intravenous line. Infiltration is evident in swelling of the medial or lateral area of the proximal tibia and indicates that the needle is not placed properly. Either the needle is too superficial or it has pierced through the bone.

Complications from intraosseous infusion are uncommon. Osteomyelitis is the greatest concern and appears to be related to the length of time that an infusion line is left in place.[33] Once adequate circulation has been restored and an intravenous line has been established, the intraosseous line should be discontinued.

NURSING CONSIDERATIONS IN INTRAVENOUS FLUID REPLACEMENT

Emotional Preparation

Because children regard intravenous (IV) fluid replacement procedures as intrusive and threatening, they should be given adequate time to develop coping mechanisms. This will be facilitated if the procedure is explained at the child's cognitive level, if the child is given an opportunity to handle the equipment, and if opportunities are provided for play to reduce stress. The IV should be initiated in a quiet, private setting. The child should be encouraged to "hold still" during insertion; however, an adequate number of people must be available to help restrain the child if necessary. The parents should be offered the opportunity to remain with the child to provide emotional support if they so choose. Children feel more in control when they can sit up during the insertion procedure.

The most common sites for infusing fluids are the superficial veins located in the arm, wrist, and scalp (see Fig. 24-5). Ability to immobilize the area is an important consideration in children. The older child should be allowed site selection, when possible, to promote feelings of control and lessen interference with activities such as writing or coloring with the preferred hand. For the infant, scalp veins are convenient and accessible; because there are no valves in these veins, the IV can be infused in either direction. However, the head must be partially shaved for access to the site and the parents must be prepared for this alteration in the infant's appearance. The nurse also should make certain the parents understand that the fluid to be administered will not damage the infant's brain. Some parents might not have any knowledge of the circulatory system in the region of the scalp.

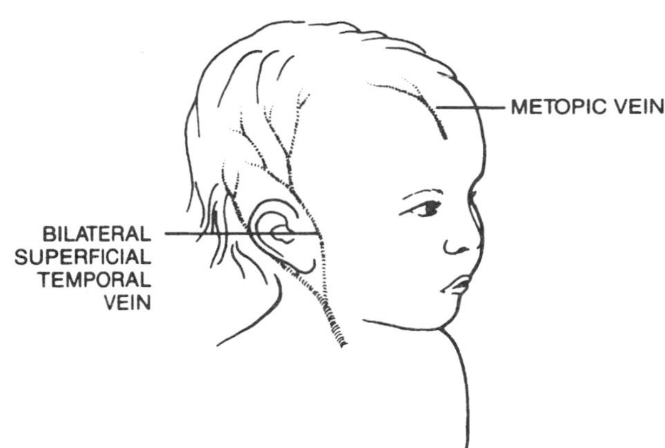

Figure 24–5. Scalp veins in infant.

Equipment to Deliver Fluids Safely

Special equipment is used for infusing fluids into children as it is necessary to avoid overloading the smaller system with too large a volume at too rapid a rate. The danger of administering an excessive fluid volume must be a real consideration in all age groups. Infants and small children face special dangers simply because of their small size and the fact that fluids tend to be supplied in adult-sized containers. Children are more susceptible to pulmonary edema from excessive fluid overload than are adults because they have greater difficulty excreting excessive fluid volume. In fact, pneumonia from overhydration is believed to be one of the most common treatment-related diseases of hospitalized children.

One method to promote safety with gravity flow is to use a microdrip delivery set with a calibrated volume-control chamber that limits the amount of fluid that can be infused. The microdrip delivers a reduced-size drop (60 microdrops/mL) that is one-fourth the size of a macrodrop (usually 15 macrodrops/mL). The calculation for infusion is simplified because the number of prescribed milliliters per hour equals the number of microdrips per minute; for example, 15 mL/hr equals a rate of 15 microdrops/min. Volume-controlled sets are favored to limit the amount of fluid available for administration in the event of an accident. Infusion pumps that can be set at a prescribed rate per hour are an additional safety feature for infants and young children. It has been recommended that quantities exceeding 150 mL not be connected to children younger than 2 years, no more than 250 mL to children younger than 5, and no more than 500 mL to children younger than 10 years.

Monitoring Flow Rate and Infusion Site

Although drop size adaptors, small containers, and infusion pumps are used to reduce the possibility of error, the nurse must still keep a close vigil on the flow rate as well as on the patient's response to the fluids. The flow rate should be counted at frequent intervals and adjusted as necessary. A pediatric parenteral fluid sheet should be kept at the bedside of infants and small children to record the observed flow rate, the amount of fluid absorbed each hour, the amount of fluid left in the bottle, and the appearance of the infusion site. Such frequent observations and notations greatly reduce the risks of excessive fluid administration and undetected infiltration.[34] Obviously, fluid monitoring is a major aspect of pediatric nursing.

APPROACHES FOR ORAL FLUID REPLACEMENT

When infants and children are able to take fluids by mouth and retain them, fluid replacement by the oral route is preferred over the parenteral route. Parenterally administered fluids pass directly into the circulation, whereas fluids taken into the GI tract are absorbed slowly. Thus, there is less risk of fluid overload with oral fluid replacement. Also, the child's freedom of movement is not impaired with oral replacement as it is with parenteral replacement.

Oral electrolyte solutions that are available as commercial products are listed in Table 24-1. These solutions are indicated for children who have mild or moderate fluid and electrolyte imbalances and for children who are recovering from acute imbalances that have been treated by parenteral therapy.

Infants and children who are able to take and retain oral fluids may not be willing to do so. Illness often makes them irritable and anorexic, and they cannot understand why they are sick, why their distress cannot be alleviated promptly, and why they need to drink. Children who have gastroenteritis and those who have acute respiratory infections are usually restricted to clear liquids. They may react with frustration when an oral electrolyte solution is offered because they expect and want milk. The phrase "force fluids" is often used in hospital settings, but fluids should *never* be forced on a child. Attempts to force a child to drink will only increase the child's distress and decrease the likelihood that the child will take and retain the fluid.

Efforts to encourage infants and children to take oral fluids should be gentle and persistent; the process requires patience, perseverance, and creativity. Some recommended approaches for meeting the oral fluid needs of infants and young children are listed below.

- Talk with the child's parents and learn about the child's usual experience in taking fluids at home. What type of fluids does the child usually drink? What amount? What temperature? How often? What method (bottle, cup, or special glass)? What are favorite fluids?
- Plan with the parents to meet the child's fluid needs and involve them in encouraging fluids, measuring amounts, and recording the intake accurately.
- Offer small amounts of fluids in small containers at frequent intervals (at least every hour).
- Use measured containers for precise determination of intake and record the intake accurately.
- Promote the child's comfort before offering fluids. Make certain the child is clean and dry and the upper airway is clear of mucus. (A rubber syringe can be used to remove mucus from the nares.)
- Continue to offer fluids on a regular schedule even though the infant or child may refuse to drink.
- Hold infants before and after offering fluids. Toddlers and preschool children may prefer to sit on the nurse's lap and hold the cup or glass.
- Toddlers may respond positively to a routine, such as offering a drink to a stuffed animal before offering the child a drink. Toddlers might also respond to the opportunity to feed themselves bite-sized pieces of frozen Popsicle or fruit juice.
- Young children like stories and may respond to the power of suggestion in stories about thirsty boys or girls who are looking for a drink.
- Some young children will drink if they have some solid food to hold or mouth, such as a saltine cracker or a vanilla wafer.
- Infants and children who are required to fast before surgery or diagnostic tests should have extra fluids just before the period of fasting to

prevent dehydration. A pacifier helps relieve the distress that infants experience while oral feedings are withheld.

Nurses who are patient, perseverant, and creative will be successful in meeting the oral fluid needs of infants and children who are able to take and retain oral fluids.

CASE STUDY

24-1. Ms. H. brought her 10-month-old son to the emergency department of a children's hospital. She stated that she was worried about her baby, Casey, because he looked so sick and had diarrhea that was getting worse. In response to the nurse's questions, Ms. H. explained that Casey had not been "acting right" for nearly a week. He had been cranky and then began vomiting after his feedings. His irritability increased and it was difficult to soothe him. When his diarrhea started 3 days ago, he acted as if he had "stomach cramps." Ms. H. stopped giving Casey milk and, for the past 12 hrs, had been offering him sugar water in a bottle. His vomiting stopped, but his diarrhea "got worse." In the initial assessment, the nurse noted the following: Casey's color was pale, his anterior fontanelle was slightly sunken, his skin felt very dry and tented when pinched, his mucous membranes were pale and dry, and his extremities felt cool. His apical heart rate was 170 beats/min, his peripheral pulses were weak, and his blood pressure was normal. He became irritable when his blood pressure was measured and made efforts to resist the nurse. Ms. H. stated that she thought Casey was urinating normally because his soiled diapers were "so watery." Casey's weight in the emergency department was 9 kg.

COMMENTARY: This baby's deficit is in the high range of moderate dehydration. He requires immediate fluid replacement to prevent the development of shock. This estimate is based on the assessment findings of dry skin and mucous membranes, poor skin turgor, pallor, a sunken fontanelle, tachycardia, and weak peripheral pulses. The assessment findings indicate that Casey has a fluid volume deficit of at least 8%.

After an intravenous line was established, Casey received a bolus infusion of 180 mL of Ringer's lactate solution. A urine collection bag was placed, and a blood sample was sent to the laboratory for serum electrolytes. A second infusion of 180 mL of Ringer's lactate solution was administered over the next 30 min. Casey's vital signs, appearance, and behavior were monitored closely. After the second infusion, Casey voided, his heart rate was 160 beats/min, and his peripheral pulses were strong. He became more active and wanted his mother to hold him. He passed a large amount of liquid, watery stool. In addition to fluid replacement requirements in the first 8 hrs of treatment, maintenance requirements needed to be met.

Recall the general formula for calculating daily fluid maintenance requirements: 100 mL/kg/24 hrs for the first 10 kg. Casey's maintenance requirement is 300 mL in the first 8 hrs (900 mL/24 hrs).

After Casey's status improved, an oral electrolyte solution was offered to him in a bottle. The amount that he takes and retains needs to be deducted from the IV fluid maintenance total. Accuracy in calculating, monitoring, and documenting parenteral and oral fluids is a major responsibility in pediatric nursing practice.

Because oral liquids that are high in sugar content and low in sodium exert an osmotic pull in the intestine that increases fluid volume loss through diarrhea this baby's condition worsened when given sugar water. Nurses who care for children have many opportunities to talk with parents about the prevention of diarrhea and the prevention of dehydration when diarrhea does occur. The early administration of an oral electrolyte solution can prevent the potentially devastating consequences of fluid volume deficit.

REFERENCES

1. Robson A: Pathophysiology of body fluids. In: Behrman R (ed): Nelson Textbook of Pediatrics, 14th ed, p 176. Philadelphia, WB Saunders, 1992

2. Yared A, Foose J, Ichikawa I: Disorders of Osmoregulation. In: Ichikawa I (ed): Pediatric Textbook of Fluids and Electrolytes, p 185. Baltimore, Williams & Wilkins, 1990
3. Ichikawa I, Narins RG, Harris HW Jr: Regulation of acid–base homeostasis. In: Ichikawa I (ed): Pediatric Textbook of Fluids and Electrolytes, p 84. Baltimore, Williams & Wilkins, 1990
4. Robson A: Tetany. In: Behrman R (ed): Nelson Textbook of Pediatrics, 14th ed, p 212. Philadelphia, WB Saunders, 1992
5. Ibid
6. Wong DL: Whaley & Wong's Nursing Care of Infants and Children, 5th ed, p 1218. St. Louis, Mosby-Year Book, 1995
7. Pestana C: Fluids and Electrolytes in the Surgical Patient, 4th ed, p 47. Baltimore, Williams & Wilkins, 1989
8. Ibid
9. Avner ED, et al: Fluid and electrolyte abnormalities in the stressed neonate. In: Ichikawa I (ed): Pediatric Textbook of Fluids and Electrolytes, p 403. Baltimore, Williams & Wilkins, 1990
10. Guy J, Haley R, Zuspan S: Use of intraosseous infusion in the pediatric trauma patient. J Pediatr Surg 28:158,1993
11. Manley L, Haley R, Dick M: Intraosseous infusion: rapid vascular access for critically ill or injured infants and children. J Emerg Nurs 14:63,1988
12. Robson A: Parenteral fluid therapy. In: Behrman R (ed): Nelson Textbook of Pediatrics, 14th ed, p 206. Philadelphia, WB Saunders, 1992
13. Cusson, RM: Rice-based oral rehydration fluid in the treatment of infant diarrhea. J Pediatr Nurs 7:414,1992
14. Robson, p 204
15. Ibid
16. Ibid
17. Ibid, p 205
18. Rice KH: Oral rehydration therapy: A simple, effective solution. J Pediatr Nurs 9:349,1994
19. Myers A: Fluid and electrolyte therapy for children. Curr Opin Pediatr 6:303,1994
20. Fayad IM, Hashem M, Duggan C, Refat M, Bakir M, Fontaine O, Santosham M: Comparative efficacy of rice-based and glucose-based oral rehydration salts plus early reintroduction of food. Lancet 342(8874):772,1993
21. Cusson, p 415
22. Rice, p 354
23. Kokko J, Tannen R: Fluids and Electrolytes, 2nd ed, p 166. Philadelphia, WB Saunders, 1990
24. Keating JP, Schears GJ, Dodge PR: Oral water intoxication in infants. Am J Dis Child 145:985,1991
25. Bennett J, Wagner T, Fields A: Acute hyponatremia and seizures in an infant after a swimming lesson. Pediatrics 73:125,1983
26. Kokko, Tannen, p 166
27. Robson, p 209
28. Ibid
29. Medani C: Seizures and hypothermia due to dietary water intoxication in infants. South Med J 80:421,1987
30. Feld L, Kaskel F, Schoeneman M: The approach to fluid and electrolyte therapy in pediatrics. In: Barness et al (eds): Advances in Pediatrics, vol 35, p 508. Chicago, Year Book Medical Publishers, 1988
31. Robson, p 203
32. Miccolo MA: Intraosseous infusion. Crit Care Nurs 10(10):35,1990
33. Rosovsky M, Fitzpatrick M, Goldfarb C, Finestone H: Bilateral osteomyelitis due to intraosseous infusion: case report and review of the English-language literature. Pediatr Radiol 24:72,1994
34. Handler EG: Superficial compartment syndrome of the foot after infiltration of intravenous fluid. Arch Physical Med Rehab 71:58,1990

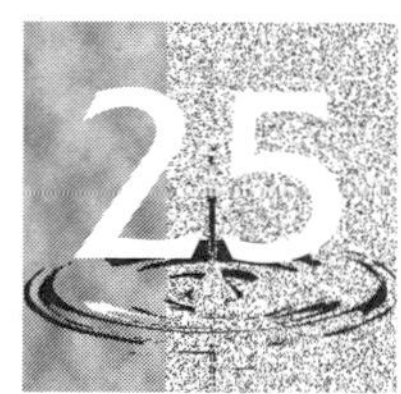

Fluid Balance in the Elderly Patient

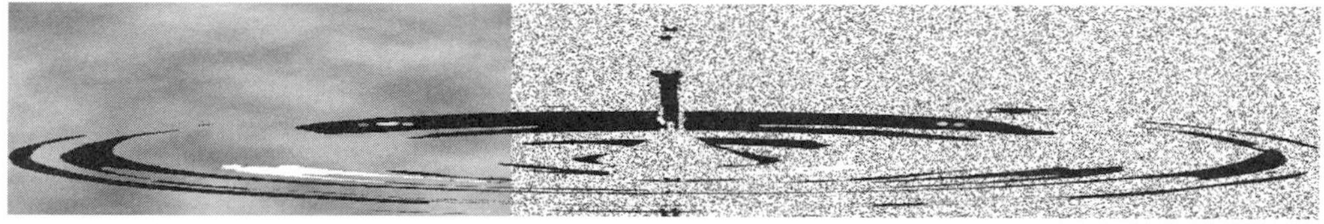

CHANGES IN WATER AND ELECTROLYTE HOMEOSTASIS ASSOCIATED WITH AGING

Because the percentage of elderly in the population is increasing, nurses in all settings must be aware of the risk of fluid and electrolyte imbalances in the elderly. Fluid balance in the elderly is marginal at best because of physiological changes associated with aging. Under normal conditions, elderly people can usually maintain homeostasis; however, they may require more time to return to normal when deficits or excesses are imposed by disease or environmental stress.[1] Elderly people do not possess the fluid reserves or ability to adapt readily to rapid changes. Alterations in fluid and electrolyte balance frequently accompany acute illness, particularly in aged persons. These alterations may delay recovery, prolong hospitalization, and result in loss of independence.[2,3]

Normal aging changes that affect fluid and electrolyte balance are summarized in Table 25-1. Included also are nursing implications related to these changes.

Renal structural changes associated with aging result in a decreased glomerular filtration rate (GFR) and a decrease in the older person's ability to concentrate urine when fluid intake is restricted. The nurse must remain alert to this when aged patients are subjected to fluid restriction for any reason. It is also an important consideration when patients are disoriented and unaware of fluid needs, or are unable to provide for their own fluid needs.

Aged kidneys have a slower response to sodium and potassium imbalances. For example, half-time for reduction in urinary sodium after salt restriction is 17 hr in young people but increases to 31 hr in elderly people. Hyponatremia may occur in an older patient who is placed on a strict sodium-restricted diet. Hyperkalemia has been shown to develop quickly in the aged when intravenous (IV) potassium is administered.[4]

Cardiovascular and respiratory changes combine to contribute to a slower response to stress in the aged. As a result, the aged person cannot respond as quickly to blood loss, fluid depletion, shock, and acid–base imbalances.

Current research indicates that thirst sensation diminishes with aging.[5,6] In a comparison of 24-hr water deprivation in two age groups, the elderly group reported a lack of thirst sensation after the 24-hr period.[7] In another study comparing thirst sensation in normotensive young adults with that in healthy older adults, the older group failed to develop thirst after the administration of a hypertonic saline solution.[8] Decreased thirst has been demonstrated in elderly subjects with normal mental status, ability to communicate needs, and ability to physically obtain water. Ratings of thirst did not change despite laboratory changes indicating dehydration.[9–11] Thus, the studies indicate that reduced sensitivity of the thirst mechanism to osmotic stimuli may be a problem in elderly persons. The elderly patient, therefore, may fail to drink sufficient amounts, even when fluids are readily available. It is important for the nurse to assess the adequacy of fluid intake in all elderly patients, but especially in those with an altered mental status because this may significantly interfere with the ability to recognize thirst.[12] Adding to the problem of decreased thirst is the conscious restriction of fluid by urinary-incontinent elderly patients in an effort to limit involuntary urination.

Elderly patients experience a decreased acuity for the taste of salt; thus, they may salt food heavily in an attempt to satisfy this taste sensation. For all of the above reasons, the aged are at risk for dehydration (hypernatremia) and hyperosmolarity.[13]

In summary, one should be aware that the elderly are often slow in adapting to change and may lack the physiological reserves to respond adequately to stress.

ASSESSMENT OF THE ELDERLY PATIENT

Fluid imbalances, particularly dehydration (hypernatremia), are seen quite frequently in aged clients in all settings. To make accurate nursing diagnoses, a thorough physical and functional assessment must be done.

CORRELATION OF PHYSICAL FINDINGS WITH LABORATORY DATA

There is a sparse amount of research that correlates laboratory values indicative of dehydration with physical signs. One study correlated laboratory values

TABLE 25–1

Normal Aging Changes Affecting Fluid Balance: Related Nursing Implications

PHYSIOLOGICAL COMPONENT	NORMAL AGING CHANGES	NURSING IMPLICATIONS
Total body water	Approximately 6% reduction in total body water Decrease in ratio of intracellular fluid	Increased risk for fluid volume deficit
Renal function	Reduction in weight by 50 g between ages 40 and 80 Loss of 30% to 50% of glomeruli by age 70 Thickening of glomerular and tubular basement membranes 46% decrease in glomerular filtration rate from age 20 to 90 Decrease in ability to concentrate urine (maximum ability to concentrate urine is 1.022–1.026)	Greater difficulty in eliminating heavy solute loads (drugs, glucose, protein, electrolytes) Slower conservation of fluids in response to fluid restriction
Regulatory functions	Decrease in secretion of aldosterone from adrenal cortex Decreased response of zona glomerulosa Decreased response of distal tubule to vasopressin Decreased ability to form and excrete ammonia Decreased glucose tolerance Decreased sensation of thirst	Diminished ability to conserve sodium and excrete potassium Reduced ability to correct an acid–base imbalance Increased risk for hyperglycemia and osmotic diuresis Decreased ability to recognize a fluid deficit
Skin changes	Decreased skin elasticity Atrophy of sweat glands Diminished capillary bed	Skin turgor is a poor indicator of state of hydration Skin is less effective in cooling body temperature
Cardiovascular function	Decreased baroreceptor sensitivity Decreased cardiac output (1% per year from age 20–80) Decreased stroke volume (0.7% per year from age 20–80) Decrease in renal plasma flow from 600 mL/min in 2nd decade to 300 mL/min by 8th decade Decreased elasticity of arteries Increased vascular rigidity causing increased peripheral resistance	Diminished ability to manage hypotension associated with shock Increased frequency of peripheral edema Increased risk for orthostatic hypotension, dizziness, falls
Respiratory function	Decreased compliance of chest wall Decreased elasticity of lung tissue Decreased number of alveoli Decreased strength of expiratory muscles Decreased normal partial pressure of oxygen	Increased difficulty in regulation of pH if experiencing major illness, surgery, burns, or trauma
Gastrointestinal function	Decreased volume of saliva Decreased volume of gastric juice Decreased calcium absorption	Mouth may be dryer Increased risk for hyponatremia and hypokalemia during vomiting and gastric suction Increased need for dietary calcium and vitamin D

Adapted from Burnside I: Nursing and the Aged, pp 83–94. New York, McGraw-Hill, 1988; Kenney R: Physiology of Aging, pp 13–121. Chicago, Year Book Medical Publishers, 1989.

Garner B: Guide to changing lab values in elders. Geriatr Nurs: 10: 144, 1989.

with tongue dryness, longitudinal tongue furrows, dryness of mucus membranes of the mouth, upper body weakness, confusion, speech difficulty, and sunken eyes.[14] If using these measures, one must be aware of the older adult's usual upper body strength, mental status, and speech patterns and check for any medications that may be contributing to the oral dryness.

SKIN TURGOR

Usual measures for assessing fluid balance may need to be altered for the elderly; for example, testing skin turgor on the forearm is not a valid measure for the elderly as skin loses elasticity with age. Skin turgor can best be observed in the older patient by tenting the tissue on the forehead or over the sternum because alterations in skin elasticity are less marked in these areas.

RATE OF VEIN FILLING

Rate and degree of filling of small veins in the foot has been used to assess hydration status. A dorsal foot vein can be occluded by finger pressure at a distal point and emptied of its blood by stroking proximally with another finger. In a well-hydrated patient, the vein will fill instantly when the pressure is released. In a volume-depleted patient, the vein will fill slowly, over a period longer than 3 s. Researchers using this measure found that changes in the rapidity and degree of foot vein filling provided the best means for evaluating changes in hydration of elderly subjects.[15]

INTAKE AND OUTPUT

Although intake and output (I&O) records are often crucial in managing patients with fluid imbalances, research has indicated that frequent inaccuracies make these records less than reliable. According to Pflaum,[16] daily weights may be a more accurate measure of a patient's fluid status. However, one must be aware that inaccuracies also occur in measuring body weights. Therefore, *both* I&O and weight records should be maintained to monitor fluid status. In general, a gain or loss of 1 kg body weight in a short period is equivalent to a gain or loss of 1 L of fluid.

BLOOD PRESSURE

Monitoring for positional changes in blood pressure is another measure that is helpful in assessing hydration. Research has indicated that a drop of at least 15 mmHg in the systolic pressure and 10 mmHg in the diastolic pressure occurs when volume-depleted patients are quickly shifted from a lying to a standing position.[17]

BODY TEMPERATURE

In younger individuals, a temperature elevation above normal (37 °C [98.6 °F]) may be an indicator of dehydration (hypernatremia). However, when assessing aged patients, it is important to remember that their normal body temperature is often lower than 37 °C (98.6 °F), possibly closer to 36.1 °C (97 °F). Thus, a temperature of 37 °C (98.6 °F) may represent a significant elevation in an aged patient.

ABILITY TO OBTAIN FLUIDS

Functional assessment of an aged client's ability to obtain fluids is essential before determining nursing diagnoses and appropriate interventions. For example, one should assess the patient's ability to ambulate and use the arms and hands to obtain fluids. Also, is the patient able to swallow? Is he or she mentally clear? Is he or she able to participate independently in interventions to meet goals set up in the nursing care plan? Also, what are his or her fluid preferences?[18]

DELIRIUM

Development of delirium is a common complication of hospitalization of the elderly. A study was recently conducted to develop and validate a predictive model that would identify on admission those elders at risk for development of delirium.[19] Of 107 elderly medical patients 70 years or older, 27 (25%) developed delirium during their hospital stay. A predictive model was developed and validated. Results identified four independent baseline risk factors for delirium:

1. Vision impairment
2. Severe illness

3. Cognitive impairment
4. Dehydration (blood urea nitrogen [BUN]/creatinine >18:1)

SPECIAL PROBLEMS IN THE ELDERLY PATIENT

Elderly patients with specific problems can be identified as having a potential for fluid imbalances. The care plans for these patients should include a nursing diagnosis reflecting this potential. Interventions should be used to monitor for these imbalances and prevent them from occurring when possible.

HYPERNATREMIA RELATED TO POOR INTAKE OR INCREASED WATER LOSS

Hypernatremia associated with a decreased extracellular fluid (ECF) volume is a common problem in the elderly. It may be induced by free-water losses from diuresis, diarrhea, vomiting, and hyperglycemia. Usually it will not occur unless oral intake is restricted.[20,21]

Synder et al.[22] found a 1.1% prevalence of serious hypernatremia (42% mortality rate) in elderly hospitalized patients. The causes were primarily treatment related.

According to Campbell,[23] the prevalence of dehydration may be as high as 25% in long-term care residents. O'Neill et al.[24] found that hyperosmolality was a marker for increased mortality in long-term care. Residents are often unable to ambulate, pour their own fluids, or express feelings of thirst. A study comparing fluid intake practices of institutionalized and noninstitutionalized elderly found that the average daily intake for institutionalized persons was 1507 mL, as compared with 2115 mL for those not confined to institutions.[25] In addition, those not confined to institutions tended to consume water in greater amounts than the institutionalized subjects. Another interesting finding was that subjects outside institutions had greater access to very cold and very hot liquids; the extent to which this influenced fluid intake is not known.

A study by Himmelstein et al.[26] examined the frequency of hypernatremia in patients admitted from long-term care. When reviewing circumstances under which hypernatremia developed, no evidence of vomiting, diarrhea, or refusal of fluids was found. The researchers concluded that with adequate observation and provision of fluids, this condition could have been prevented.

A number of research studies have attempted to identify risk factors for dehydration in elders in long-term care. Result of these studies indicate that those elderly at risk for dehydration are over 80 years old, women, and suffer from multiple chronic diseases. The role of mental status and functional status as predictors of dehydration in long-term care remains inconclusive.[27–32]

The role of the caregiver in preventing hypernatremia by early recognition of inadequate fluid intake and provision of needed fluids cannot be overemphasized.[33] Functional elders can be made aware of their fluid needs and can actively participate in attaining those goals. Hoffman[34] suggests that prescriptions be given to these elders to consume a certain number of glasses of fluid. The elderly resident simply marks on the glass the level of the fluid consumed (see Fig. 25-1).

Maintaining fluid intake is sometimes an enormous challenge for the nurse providing care to a frail elder or an elderly person suffering from dementia. As dementia progresses, muscle rigidity increases and positioning becomes difficult. Although 2000 mL is the recommended intake goal, a more reasonable, attainable goal of 1500 mL may be set for these persons.[35] Medicine cups and adaptive devices such as spouted cups may be helpful.

For those residents whose muscle rigidty prevents the normal tilting of the head with drinking, a semi-circle can be cut from the rim of a paper cup. This allows space for the nose as the cup is tipped. Offering fluids with a syringe should be considered a last resort. The ability to eat and drink may be the only remaining functional ability. Replacing this with syringe feeding may destroy the last element of dignity. Before being syringe-fed, the elder should be examined by a speech pathologist to determine that there is an intact pharyngeal stage. The elder should be seated at a 90-degree position with the chin tipped downward. The caregiver must get the elder's attention, tell him or her what liquid is being offered, and deposit 5 mL of fluid on the side of the tongue in the front one-third of the mouth.[36,37]

The older adult suffering from Alzheimer's dis-

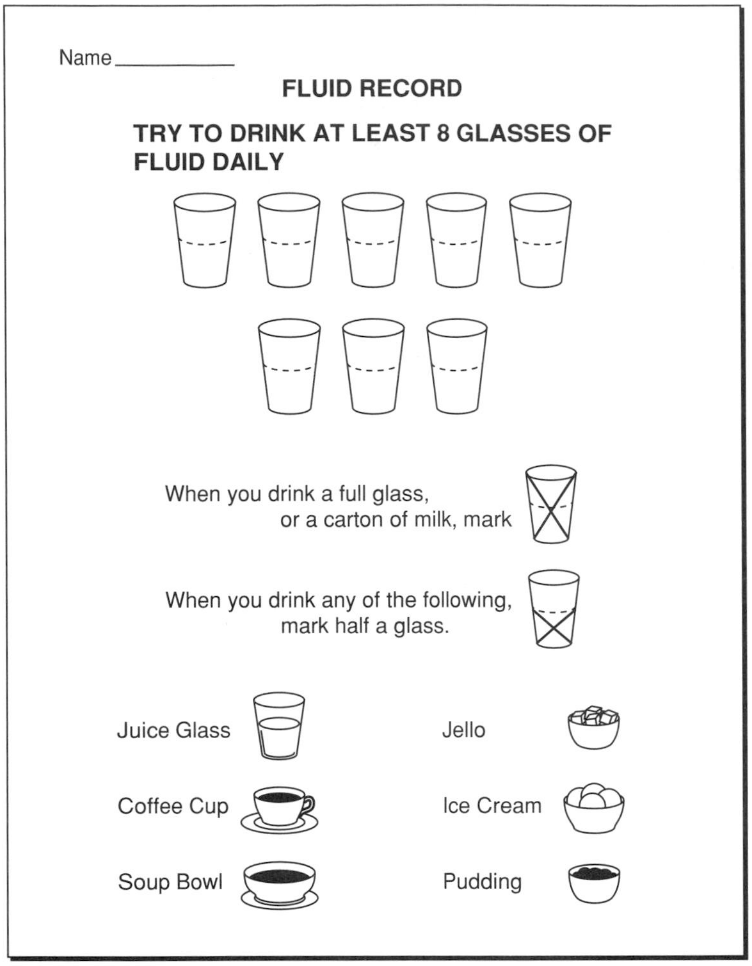

Name__________

FLUID RECORD

TRY TO DRINK AT LEAST 8 GLASSES OF FLUID DAILY

When you drink a full glass, or a carton of milk, mark

When you drink any of the following, mark half a glass.

Juice Glass

Coffee Cup

Soup Bowl

Jello

Ice Cream

Pudding

Figure 25–1. Decatur Memorial Hospital Patient Fluid Record. Developed by Sherry Robinson, RNCS, MSN(R), 1994.

ease presents a special challenge. This elder may fail even to recognize a glass of water and frequently will not remember how to get the glass of water from the table to the mouth. To get the resident to drink, the nurse may have to prompt each step. For example,"Put your hand around this cup. Lift the cup to your mouth. Tip the cup so that you can get a drink." In addition, elders who have Alzheimer's disease frequently wander around the facility much of the day. Nurses must be alert that this older adult is losing additional fluids through increased metabolism and insensible loss.

As evidenced by the above, fluid intake is a special concern in the long-term care setting. Hydration programs using a multidisciplinary approach must be instituted. Nurses should encourage elders to consume a full glass of water with medications. The diet should insure that residents are receiving foods with high fluid content. Fluids should be incorporated into daily activities. A fluid cart, stocked with a variety of fluids, should make regular and frequent rounds.

Development of hypernatremia as a result of high-protein (hypertonic) tube feedings is not as common today because of the widespread use of isotonic tube feedings. However, fluid balance of tube-fed aged patients should be closely monitored as extra fluid may be needed even when isotonic feedings are used. Recall that elderly individuals are not as able to concentrate urine as their younger counterparts because of changes in renal structure. (See Chapter 12 for further discussion of this topic.)

Hypernatremia, superimposed on volume depletion, is one of the more common etiological factors related to the acute confusional states that are common in the aged. When an elderly client in any setting experiences a change in mental status, the nurse should immediately assess fluid status. The frequency of this problem is supported by research. When fluid is limited for any reason, there is an increase in serum sodium concentration and mental functioning can be impaired. Using the case study method, Jana and Jana[38] studied four confused elderly dehydrated (hypernatremic) patients. With restoration of fluid volume, all subjects became oriented and cooperative. Seymour et al.[39] examined 71 patients older than age 70 admitted to a hospital in acute confusional states. Assessment of mental status and fluid status was done on admission and 1 week later after measures to restore hydration. Results indicated a significant relationship between mental scores on admission and degree of dehydration. Because of the large number of subjects, the study provides strong evidence for the relationship between confusion and dehydration (hypernatremia). Another study found a significant change in mental status in elderly patients depleted of fluids in preparation for diagnostic procedures.[40] Clinical Tip: Mini-Mental State Examination (MMSE) is an example of a mental status questionnaire.

In a study of 71 hospitalized elderly medical patients, it was found that one-third of them developed confusion.[41] The researchers found that hypernatremia, as well as hypokalemia, hypotension, elevated creatinine, and elevated BUN, were among the 10 factors significantly associated with confusion. Another study of 90 confused hospitalized patients found fluid and electrolyte imbalances to be confirmed, probable, or possible causes of confusional states in 20 patients.

A care plan for an elderly client with a nursing diagnosis of altered mental status related to inadequate fluid intake is shown in Clinical Tip: Nursing Care Plan for an 80-Year-Old Woman With a Nursing Diagnosis of Alteration in Thought Process Related to Inadequate Fluid Intake.

Older adults should be cautioned not to use sodium bicarbonate antacids. These are readily absorbed and can result in hypernatremia.[43]

IMBALANCES ASSOCIATED WITH USE OF DIURETICS

Diuretics are the most frequently prescribed drugs for treatment of hypertension and congestive heart failure in the elderly. Both thiazides and furosemide (Lasix) are potassium-losing diuretics, and they have a greater tendency to induce hypokalemia in the aged than in the younger adult. Remember that hypokalemia potentiates the action of digitalis and can precipitate toxic symptoms. Use of a potassium-sparing diuretic, such as spironolactone (Aldactone) or triamterene (Dyrenium), has been shown to produce a higher incidence of hyperkalemia in the aged.[44]

Hyponatremia has also been attributed to thiazide diuretic use. Persons of small body mass, low fluid intake, or excessive intake of low-sodium nutritional supplements are at greater risk for effects of fluid and electrolyte imbalance caused by diuretics.[45]

Because of the orthostatic hypotension associated with diuretic-induced *fluid volume deficit* (FVD), an older patient may become dizzy on position change and experience a fall. Indeed, use of diuretics has been identified as a characteristic of patients at risk for falls.[46]

Patients on diuretic therapy should be weighed daily. Serum electrolyte levels should be determined at regular intervals. In addition, older patients should be monitored closely for signs of weakness, lethargy, and postural hypotension. One should also monitor for confusion, thirst, and muscle cramps.[47]

IMBALANCES RELATED TO CONSTIPATION AND LAXATIVE ABUSE

Reduced motility of the intestinal tract and a lessened sense of the need to eliminate can lead to chronic constipation with laxative and enema dependency. Prolonged use of strong laxatives predisposes to hypokalemia and FVD. Metabolism of drugs by the aged person is generally slower than in a younger person. Abnormal prolongation of the effect of some "over-the-counter" laxatives containing phenolphthalein has been seen. There is an increase in the half-life of the drug and therefore, diarrhea may result as the drug's action continues.

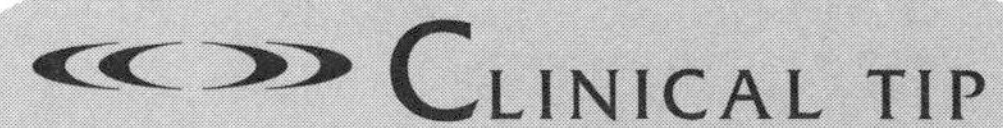

Mini-Mental State Examination (MMSE)

QUESTIONS	POINTS
1. What is the: Year? Season? Date? Day? Month?	5
2. Where are we: State? County? Town or City? Hospital? Floor?	5
3. Name three objects (Apple, Penny, Table), taking one second to say each. Then, ask the patient to tell you the three objects. Repeat the answers until the patient learns all three.	3
4. Serial 7s. Subtract 7 from 100. Then, subtract 7 from that number, etc. Stop after five answers.	5
5. Ask for the names of the three objects learned in #3.	3
6. Point to a pencil and a watch. Have the patient name them as you point.	2
7. Have the patient repeat "No ifs, ands, or buts."	1
8. Have the patient follow a three-stage command: "Take the paper in your right hand. Fold the paper in half. Put the paper on the floor."	3
9. Have the patient read and obey the following: "CLOSE YOUR EYES." (Write in large letters.)	1
10. Have the patient write a sentence of his or her own choice.	1
11. Have the patient copy the following design (overlapping pentagons).	1

Total points = 30

Scoring
24–30 = No cognitive impairment
18–23 = Mild cognitive impairment
0–17 = Severe cognitive impairment

Folstein M, Folstein S, McHugh P: MiniMental Mental State. A practical method for grading the cognitive state of patients for the clinician. Psychiat 12:189–198, 1975. With permission.

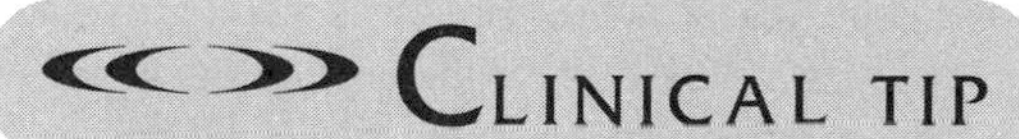

Nursing Care Plan for an 80-Year-Old Woman With a Nursing Diagnosis of Alteration in Thought Process Related to Inadequate Fluid Intake

ASSESSMENT	GOAL	INTERVENTIONS	EVALUATION CRITERIA
Disoriented Score on MMSE is 18 (normal is 24) Behavior changes Skin turgor poor on forehead Tongue dry and furry No pool of saliva under tongue BP 160/80 (supine), 128/62 (standing) Foot vein fills in 6 seconds Oral intake 900 mL/day Able to swallow Unable to pour fluids due to arthritis in hands Favorite fluids • Water • Lemonade • Orange juice	Restore normal mental status	Increase oral intake to 2000 mL/day **Follow this schedule:** 8:00 breakfast 300 mL 9:00 water 120 mL 10:00 lemonade 120 mL 11:00 water 120 mL 12:00 lunch 300 ml 1:00 water 120 mL 2:00 water 120 mL 3:00 orange juice 120 mL 4:00 water 120 mL 5:00 water 120 mL 6:00 supper 300 mL 7:00 water 120 mL 8:00 water 120 mL Continue assessment of fluid and mental status every shift	Score on Mental Status Questionnaire will improve Behavior will improve Oral intake will reach 2000 mL in 24 hours Physical assessment will reveal improved skin turgor, pool of saliva under tongue, normal vein filling, and absence of marked postural hypotension on position change

MMSE, Mini-Mental State Examination.

It has been reported that persons over 70 years take laxatives twice as often as those in the 40- to 50-year-old age group. In addition to decreased gastrointestinal (GI) motility with aging, certain drugs, such as anticholinergics and antacids containing calcium carbonate or aluminum hydroxide, predispose to constipation. Unfortunately, use of laxatives in the aged often becomes habit-forming, requiring larger and more frequent doses to achieve results.[48]

Increased fluid and bulk intake, in addition to regular exercise, should be encouraged to correct constipation. Stool softeners are useful physiological tools, and a glass of warm water or hot coffee first thing in the morning can stimulate the evacuation reflex. Natural laxative mixtures composed of raisins, currants, prunes, figs, and dates have also proven to be effective.[49] These nursing interventions are preferable to drugs in reducing the constipation problem and thereby preventing fluid and electrolyte problems associated with laxatives and enemas.

IMBALANCES ASSOCIATED WITH PREPARATION FOR DIAGNOSTIC TESTS

Standard colon-cleansing techniques for diagnostic studies usually include dietary restrictions (liquid diet several days before, NPO after midnight the day before the test), purgatives (such as castor oil, magnesium citrate, Dulcolax), and numerous cleansing enemas. These techniques constitute a threat to elderly persons who are only marginally hydrated. Studies have indicated that the rigorous catharsis associated with this kind of preparation leads to significant shifts of fluid among body compartments. If the shifts occur rapidly in an elderly person with cardiovascular disease, the results can be dangerous. Computed tomography had been recommended rather than a barium enema for the initial investigation of the large bowel in frail elderly.[50]

In a study of elderly persons undergoing preparation for a barium enema, a significant number of indicators of fluid volume depletion were detected on nursing assessment.[51] In addition, there was a slowed response to restore fluid balance.

Elderly persons undergoing rigorous bowel preparation should be observed closely for adverse reactions. On the basis of current research, it is most appropriate to include a nursing diagnosis in the care plan that reflects the potential for fluid volume depletion related to bowel preparation. The need for close observation is reflected in the care plan in Clinical Tip: Nursing Care Plan for an 84-Year-Old Man With a Nursing Diagnosis of at Risk for Hypernatremia With Fluid Volume Depletion Related to X-Ray Preparation. Care should be taken to perform the procedure correctly the first time to avoid the need for repeated radiographs, requiring more cathartics, more enemas, and more fluid restrictions. The elderly can ill afford to undergo one test after another without a "rest period";

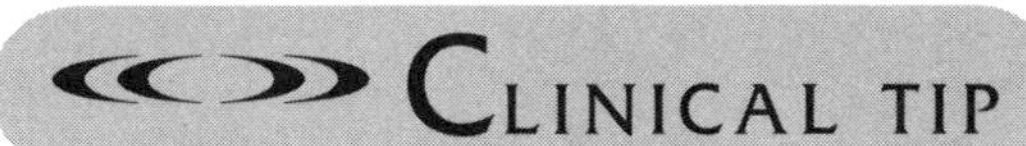

Nursing Care Plan for an 84-Year-Old Man With a Nursing Diagnosis of at Risk for Hypernatremia With Fluid Volume Depletion Related to X-Ray Preparation

ASSESSMENT	GOAL	INTERVENTIONS	EVALUATION CRITERIA
To receive rigorous colon preparation on Tuesday Fluid restriction (NPO) after midnight Tuesday Decreased renal function, related to advanced age Alert and functionally able to obtain own fluids Baseline physical assessment of fluid balance within normal limits	To prevent hypernatremia with fluid volume depletion	Physical assessment of fluid balance every shift 2000 to 3000 mL of fluid orally the day before X ray; give 150 mL/hr from 8:00 a.m. to 10:00 pm. Obtain order for IV fluids if unable to drink above amount Force fluids (150 mL/hr) after X ray until HS Explain need for fluids to patient; give schedule to him; assist as needed	Intake exceeds 2000 mL/day on day before X ray Intake exceeds 2000 mL/ day after X ray No change in baseline physical assessment parameters

HS, hour of sleep (bedtime).

it is frequently up to the nurse to intervene in this area on the patient's behalf.

It should be noted that the radiocontrast agents used in diagnostic radiology (such as intravenous [IV] pyelography) are sodium-rich. Because of the already reduced GFR, the older patient has difficulty excreting the increased solute load. This may cause osmotic diuresis and thus, increased fluid loss.[52] The aged patient undergoing GI radiographs should probably receive IV fluids during the preparation period of reduced oral intake and increased fluid loss by catharsis and enemas.

OSTEOPOROSIS

Calcium deficiency has been associated with osteoporosis development in the elderly. Hip fracture associated with falls is the leading cause of accidental death among elderly women. Annually, 1.5 million fractures (mainly of the spine, wrist, and hip) are attributed to osteoporosis. The risk of developing osteoporosis increases with age. Postmenopausal osteoporosis is most common in small-framed white women older than 50 years. Obesity appears to offer some protection against osteoporosis. Stress on the skeleton due to added weight and the increased serum estrogen concentrations in fat tissue may increase skeletal mass.[53] Back pain is the most frequent symptom, and spinal deformity is the most common sign. "Dowager's hump" (a hunchback posture due to severe loss of anterior vertebral height) is a common finding. The patient's height may be 1 to 6 inches shorter than the arm span if multiple wedge-compression fractures have occurred. Loss of 2 inches in height has been found to be an accurate screening mechanism to detect osteoporosis. Involutional bone alterations may reduce cortical bone mass of the femurs by a factor of 30% to 50%.[54]

It should be noted that serum concentrations of calcium, phosphate, and alkaline phosphatase are normal, although deficits of total body calcium, phosphate, and nitrogen exist.

Reduced calcium intake seems to play a role in the development of postmenopausal osteoporosis. Also implicated are diminished physical activity, impaired intestinal calcium absorption, increased renal calcium loss, increased parathyroid hormone (PTH) effect, and reduced secretion of estrogen. Increased PTH secretion in postmenopausal osteoporosis may be related to a slightly decreased ionized calcium level owing to a number of hepatic, renal, and intestinal changes that accompany aging.[55]

Research has indicated that no single treatment is effective in preventing osteoporosis. Calcium supplements alone, even in amounts of 2000 mg/day, were not effective in protecting against accelerated trabecular bone loss of the spine and wrist. However, calcium in combination with estrogen or exercise did result in decreased bone loss.[56]

It seems that oral calcium, vitamin D, and estrogen can reverse negative calcium balance related to menopause and probably delay or prevent the onset of clinical osteoporosis. Women should consume at least 1500 mg/day of elemental calcium and 400 IU of vitamin D to increase calcium absorption and bone formation. If the elderly person is housebound, vitamin D may be increased to 800 IU.[57] An ongoing longitudinal study has identified that vitamin D malnutrition is prevalent among patients admitted to long-term care facilities. The researchers hypothesize that vitamin D supplements may reduce the incidence of osteoporotic fractures in nursing home residents.[58]

There are now numerous studies that have drawn similar conclusions: estrogen intervention reduces the rate of loss of skeletal tissue by reducing bone remodeling. All routes of administration (oral, transdermal, or subcutaneous) are equally effective. To protect the endometrium, women who have not had a hysterectomy are given progestin. It should be remembered, however, that large daily doses of estrogen have been shown to be associated with sodium retention, hypertension, myocardial infarction, and increased risk of endometrial carcinoma. Many physicians believe that the anticatabolic effect of estrogen, which reduces bone resorption, outweighs the risk of these untoward effects.[59] Recent investigations are focusing on the role of vitamin K and bone health.[60]

Because of the lack of longitudinal studies, the exact relationship of exercise and the skeleton remain incompletely defined. There are numerous benefits, including increased strength, coordination, and flexibility that may in themselves prevent falls and the resultant fractures.[61] Education in the areas of nutrition, proper exercise, and safety must be included in the care plans of patients with osteoporosis.

Nutrition

1. Encourage the intake of adequate calcium in the diet. One quart of skim milk daily is recommended; whole milk or cheese products may be used if the patient's physical condition allows. (Some sources recommend 1000–1500 mg of calcium for postmenopausal women and elderly men.)
2. Encourage adequate protein intake. For the older adult, the recommendation is 1 g of protein per kilogram of body weight.
3. Encourage intake of sufficient calories to maintain normal body weight.
4. For those unable to consume adequate calcium in the diet, consider use of calcium supplements. Caution elderly patients to take calcium 1 hr before or 2 hr after meals to ensure absorption.

Exercise

After assessing for abilities and disabilities, consider the following interventions:

1. Encourage patients who swim, golf, or bicycle to continue to do so. Jogging should be avoided because of the possibility of joint damage.
2. Teach individuals who have been habitually sedentary to avoid strenuous exercise. (Research indicates that simple exercises will help decrease bone mass loss.) The heart rate should not increase more than 60 beats/min over baseline.
3. Suggest the following exercises for sedentary individuals:
   A. Arm circles
      I. Sit erect, arms extended
         ii. Form circles by moving arms backward and then forward
   B. Angle stretch
      I. Lie on bed (not floor), legs straight, feet together, and arms at side
         ii. Slide arms and legs to a spread-eagle position and return
   C. Stationary rocking
      I. Sit erect on chair, feet flat on floor, arms at side
         ii. Lean forward and press floor with toes
         iii. Lean back to upright position and press floor with heels
4. Recommend extension and isometric abdominal exercises for those diagnosed with spinal osteoporosis. Teach them to avoid any flexion exercises of the spine as this action may cause compression/fractures.[62]

Safety

1. Teach the patient to avoid sudden bending, twisting, lifting, or carrying of heavy objects.
2. Teach the patient to use assistive devices, such as canes or walkers, if needed, to prevent falls.
3. Teach the patient to wear well-fitted, low-heeled shoes (athletic shoes should be suggested).
4. Teach the patient to use long-handled utensils and cleaning tools if needed.
5. Assess the patient's environment. Make sure the home is well lighted and has non-skid rugs. Look for objects that might cause falls.

HYPERTHERMIA

The greatest number of cases of heatstroke occur in the elderly. Sweating, the major mechanism for heat dissipation, is altered in the aged. Not only is the number of operative sweat glands decreased in aged persons, it takes longer for them to begin sweating, and they produce less sweat than in their younger years. Loss of subcutaneous adipose tissue reduces the effectiveness of the skin as an insulator and enhances water loss from the deeper tissues.

Elderly persons seem to have an impaired sense of warmth perception. Also, the elderly exhibit little change in cardiac output in response to heat stress. The circulatory system cannot dissipate efficiently the heat through peripheral vasodilatation and evaporation of perspiration.[63] In addition, a number of medications frequently prescribed for aged patients can interfere in some way with thermoregulation (eg, diuretics, antiparkinsonian drugs, propranolol, antihistamines, phenothiazines, tricyclic antidepressants). Other risk factors for hyperthermia in the elderly include recent diarrheal or febrile illness, obesity, sleep deprivation, and dehydration.[64]

Mortality related to heat stress increases progressively in those older than 70 years. Because of their greater susceptibility to heat stress, it is important to teach these individuals to take the following precautions during a heat wave:

- Avoid excessive physical activity.
- Wear light-colored cotton fabrics to facilitate sweating.
- Increase dietary consumption of carbohydrates and fluids.
- Use air conditioners or fans when available.
- Contact health provider if cessation of sweating occurs.[65]

The nurse must be cautious when assessing the older person for heat stress. Normal body temperature decreases with age; as such, the older adult may be experiencing heat stress with a temperature of 37.2 °C (99 °F).

SPECIAL CONSIDERATIONS RELATED TO PERIOPERATIVE PERIOD

Elderly persons tolerate major surgery and its complications less well than younger adults; therefore, preoperatively, every effort should be made to treat conditions likely to cause postoperative problems. Cardiac complications are a common cause of postoperative mortality; pneumonia and atelectasis also occur frequently.[66] Conscientious preoperative preparation often means the difference between success or failure of surgery in the aged as the decreased body homeostatic adaptability of these patients predisposes to difficulty when they are exposed to stress.

The following facts apply to the aged surgical patient:

- Moderate FVD and decreased circulating blood volume are not uncommon in the elderly *before* surgery. The patient probably has been NPO since midnight, may be on diuretic therapy, or may have had a preoperative problem with nausea and vomiting. Fluid volume deficit predisposes to renal insufficiency, particularly in elderly individuals. Administration of adequate IV fluids before surgery improves renal blood flow and renal function; in contrast, administration of the same fluids after induction of anesthesia will have only minimal effect in increasing renal blood flow. It is important that parenteral fluids be started before surgery and an adequate urine volume established before induction of anesthesia. Urine flow should be at least 50 mL/hr (preferably 75–100 mL/hr).[67]
- In the operating room, the older patient is at risk for hypothermia. In addition to the cool environment, the patient is rapidly infused with cool IV fluids and possibly blood. Rinsing the skin with cool solutions also increases the risk of hypothermia. Use of a cap, warm gown, stockinette on unaffected limbs, and warmed flannelette blankets are recommended.[68–70]
- Because diminished respiratory function interferes with carbon dioxide elimination, many aged patients are in a state of impending respiratory acidosis. Because of this decline in pulmonary function, the nurse must help the aged patient achieve maximal ventilation. This can be accomplished by keeping the respiratory tract free of excessive secretions, providing maximal allowed activity, turning the bed-fast patient from side to side at regular intervals, and avoiding restrictive clothing and chest restraints.
- Because renal response to pH disturbances is not as efficient in the aged, imbalances occur faster. There is a tendency toward metabolic acidosis as a result of decreased renal function. It behooves the health care team to detect imbalances early and to intervene early.
- Changes in pH are less well tolerated in the aged. In addition to decreased renal and pulmonary reserves, presence of anemia, with its decreased hemoglobin, depletes one of the major buffer systems. Blood should be administered as needed to correct anemia, preferably several days before the operation. Emphysema is not uncommon in the aged and also disrupts pH control. Measures to improve pulmonary function should also be used preoperatively.
- Hypotension is poorly tolerated by the aged and, unless corrected quickly, is frequently complicated by renal damage, stroke, or myocardial infarct. Shock becomes irreversible earlier than in young patients.
- The aged patient will develop sodium deficit faster than younger adults; thus, the nurse should be particularly alert for this imbalance when the patient is losing body fluids containing sodium. Hyponatremia is particularly apt to occur when there is a free intake of water

orally or when excessive volumes of 5% dextrose in water are administered IV.

- Hyponatremia may also result from excessive water retention associated with the stress of hospitalization and anticipation of surgery. Stress mediates the release of antidiuretic hormone (ADH). Research has shown that relocation and separation from loved ones, as occur with hospitalization, cause greater stress in the aged. This stress has been shown to contribute to the development of water intoxication (dilutional hyponatremia).[71]
- Malnutrition is more common in aged than in younger adults and contributes to the increased incidence of postoperative complications. Preoperative dietary management is particularly important. Optimal nutrition helps the aged patient withstand the electrolyte deficits and pH changes occurring with surgery. If the patient is unable to eat, tube feedings or parenteral nutrients are indicated to meet nutritional needs and build up operative reserves. (Tube feedings are discussed in Chapter 12 and parenteral nutrition is discussed in Chapter 11.)
- Ambulation and activity improve appetite and sleep and prevent the complications of bedrest. Bedrest in the preoperative period can be damaging to the aged patient because it predisposes to negative nitrogen balance, osteoporosis, muscle weakness, pneumonia, phlebitis, pressure ulcers, bladder and bowel dysfunction, decrease in myocardial reserve, and diminished pulmonary ventilation and tidal volume.

Intravenous therapy for treatment of fluid imbalances is on the rise in both long-term care and the community setting.[72] Coulter[73] recommends the use of a small 22- to 24-gauge catheter and a rehydration rate of 80 to 100 mL/hr. In maintaining patency of the IV site in a restless elderly person, restraints should be avoided. Use of restraints creates anxiety and agitation, as well as respiratory and cardiovascular problems. IV tubing can be hidden under long sleeve shirts or covered with flexible elastic netting. Turtle neck shirts can be used to protect central lines from manipulation by confused elders. Because of the older person's increased skin fragility, a skin protectant should be applied before tape application, excessive tape should be avoided in securing the IV site, and extreme care should be taken when removing the tape to prevent skin tears.[74]

HYPEROSMOLAR HYPERGLYCEMIC NONKETOTIC SYNDROME

Most patients who develop hyperosmolar hyperglycemic nonketotic syndrome (HHNS) are elderly with relatively mild (perhaps not-yet-detected) diabetes mellitus. Unconscious patients may present in the emergency room with a history of days or weeks of polyuria and increased thirst. Precipitating factors in the diabetic elderly may include medications such as osmotic diuretics, phenytoin sodium (Dilantin), steroids, immunosuppressive agents, infections such as pneumonia, hyperosmolar tube feedings, and high carbohydrate infusion loads (as in total parenteral nutrition).[75] Normal aging changes affecting kidney function create a greater potential for fluid imbalance in the older diabetic. Monitoring fluid intake adequacy in the elderly diabetic is an important nursing assessment that can lead to earlier detection of HHNS. A thorough discussion of HHNS is presented in Chapter 18.

CASE STUDY

25-1. Mr. D. is an 89-year-old gentleman who has been admitted to the hospital with a diagnosis of hypernatremic dehydration (sodium, 150 mEq/L; BUN, 54 mg/dL; creatinine, 1.5 mg/dL; BUN/creatinine ratio, 36:1). Mr. D. also has Alzheimer's disease and has been residing in a long-term care facility for approximately 1 year. Mr. D. is disoriented and does not recognize his wife who accompanies him to your unit. He is restless, combative, and very anxious. The emergency room personnel inserted an IV into his right arm and secured Mr. D's hands with wrist restraints.

COMMENTARY: There are several alternatives to wrist restraints that could be used to maintain IV fluids. Due to Mr. D's usual state of dementia, the restraints will only make nursing management more difficult. Ask his wife to stay with him if possible. Ask her to hold his left hand, gently stroke his arm and reminisce with him about their earlier life together (He may have retained some long-term memory and thinking about something familiar is usually comforting and quieting.) If she cannot stay, there are still some other alternatives. Disguise the IV by running the IV tubing along his arm and by placing a long sleeve shirt on him. If this option is not effective, Posey mitts or Nerf balls placed in each hand and secured with burn net may be beneficial. By using these options, his arms can remain free and he will probably be less restless.

The patient's mental status should improve, although he will always have some cognitive deficits. In this situation, we have dementia (a chronic confusional state) compounded by delirium (acute confusional state). The dehydration, the elevated sodium, the elevated BUN, the restraints, and relocation to a strange environment are all contributing to the acute confusional state aggravating the chronic confusional state.

Because of his age, the IV fluids should not be infused too rapidly (no more than 120 mL/hr). During any calm periods, approach Mr. D. gently, place a glass of water in his hand and gently help him to raise it to his lips. Remember that a person with Alzheimer's disease may no longer be able to recognize a glass of water and may have forgotten how to bring the glass to his lips and drink it. Also, provide him with fresh fruit slices like oranges to improve hydration. When Mr. D. is rehydrated, approach the doctor about discontinuing the IV fluids and returning him to long-term care. It is very important to return the patient with Alzheimer's disease to his normal routine and environment as soon as possible. The staff in the long-term care facility must be extremely attentive to his fluid needs. As most people with Alzheimer's will wander within the facility, the long-term care nurse must recognized the increased fluid needs required by the increased metabolism and constant movement of the wanderer. Every staff member should be alerted to offer him frequent drinks and finger foods high in fluids.

REFERENCES

1. Hoffman A: Dehydration in the elderly: Insidious and manageable. Geriatrics 46(6):35,1991
2. Kositzke J: A question of balance: Dehydration in the elderly. J Gerontol Nurs 16(5):4,1990
3. Miller M: Fluid and electrolyte balance in the elderly. Geriatrics 42(11):65,1987
4. Cape R, Coe R, Rossman I: Fundamentals of Geriatric Medicine, p 71–74. New York, Raven Press, 1983
5. Porth C, Erickson M: Physiology of thirst and drinking: Implications for nursing practice. Heart Lung 21(3):273,1992
6. Rolls B, Phillip P: Aging and disturbances in thirst and fluid balance. Nutrition Rev 48(3):137,1990.
7. Phillips et al: Reduced thirst after water deprivation in elderly healthy men. N Engl J Med 311:753,1984
8. Menully G: Thirst threshold changes pose dehydration risk. Geriatrics 40(12):91,1985
9. Miller et al: Hypodipsia in geriatric patients. Am J Med 72:354,1982
10. Forsling M, Rolls B, Phillips P, Ledingham J, Smith R: Altered water excretion in healthy elderly. Age Aging 16:285,1987
11. Silver A, Morley J: Role of the opioid system on hypodipsia of aging. Clin Res 37:90a,1989
12. Michaelsson E: Assessment of thirst among severely demented patients in the terminal phase of life: Exploratory interviews with ward sisters and enrolled nurses. Int J Nurs Stud 24(2):87,1987
13. Matteson M, McConnel E: Gerontological Nursing: Concepts and Practice, p 323. Philadelphia, WB Saunders, 1988
14. Gross C, Lindquist R, Wooley A, Granieri R, Allard K, Webster B: Clinical indicators of dehydration severity in elderly patients. J Emerg Med 10:267,1992
15. Robinson S, Demuth P: Diagnostic studies for the aged: What are the dangers? J Gerontol Nurs 11(6):6,1985
16. Pflaum S: Investigation of intake-output as a means of assessing body fluid balance. Heart Lung 8:495,1979
17. Wolanin M, Phillips L, Confusion: Prevention and Care, p 117. St. Louis, CV Mosby, 1981.
18. Adams F: How much do elders drink? Geriatr Nurs 9(4):218,1988
19. Inouye S, Viscoli C, Horwitz R, Hurst L, Tinetti M: A predictive model for delirium in hospitalized elderly medical patients based on admission characteristics. Ann Intern Med 119:474,1993
20. Beck L, Lavizzo-Maurey R: Geriatric hypernatremia. Ann Intern Med 107:768,1987
21. Sadat A, Paulman P, Mathews M: Hypernatremia in the elderly. Fam Pract 40:125,1989
22. Snyder N, Feigal D, Arieff A: Hypernatremia in elderly patients: A heterogenous, morbid, and iatrogenic entity. Ann Intern Med 107:309,1987

23. Campbell S: Maintaining hydration status in elderly persons: Problems and solutions. Support Line 24(3):7,1992
24. O'Neill P, Faragher E, Davies I, Wears R, McLean K, Fairweather D: Reduced survival with increasing plasma osmolality in elderly continuing care patients. Age Ageing 14:68,1990
25. Adams, p 218
26. Himmelstein D, Jones A, Wollhander S: Hypernatremic dehydration in nursing home patients: An indicator of neglect. J Am Geriatr Soc 31(8):466,1983
27. Adams, p 218
28. Dontas A, Paraskaki I, Petrikkos G, Giamarellou H: Diuresis bacteriuria in physically dependent elderly women. Age Ageing 16: 215,1987
29. Gaspar P: What determine how much patients drink? Geriatr Nurs 9(4):221,1988
30. Lavizzo-Maurey R, Johnson J, Stotley P: Risk factors for dehydration among elderly nursing home residents. J Am Geriatr Soc 36(3):213,1988
31. Long C, Martin P, Bayer A, Shetty H, Pathy M: J Postgrad Med 25:118,1991
32. Snyder, p 309
33. Aaronson L, Seaman L: Managing hypernatremia in fluid deficient elderly. J Gerontol Nurs 15(7):29,1989
34. Hoffman A: Dehydration in the elderly: Insidious and manageable. Geriatrics 46(6):35,1991
35. Alford D: Tips on promoting food and fluid intake in the elderly. J Gerontol Nurs 17(7):44,1991
36. Soriano R: Syringe feeding: Current clinical practice and recommendations. Geriatric Nurs 15(2):85,1994
37. Yen P: When swallowing is a problem. Geriatric Nurs 12:313,1991
38. Jana D, Jana L: Hypernatremic psychoses in the elderly: Case reports. J Am Geriatr Soc 31(10):473,1983
39. Seymour et al: Acute confusional states and dementia in the elderly: The role of dehydration/volume depletion, physical illness, and age. Age Ageing 9:137,1980
40. Robinson, DeMuth, p 6–9
41. Foreman M: Confusion in the hospitalized elderly: Incidence, onset, and associated factors. Res Nurs Health 12(2):21,1989
42. Francis J, Martin D, Kapoor W: A prospective study of delirium in hospitalized elderly. JAMA 263: 1097,1990
43. Todd B: Antacid alert. Geriatr Nurs 10(6):278,1989
44. Todd B: Diuretics' danger. Geriatr Nurs 10(4):212, 1989
45. Sonnenblick J, Friedlander Y, Rosin A: Diuretic-induced severe hyponatremia. Chest 103(2):601,1993
46. Watson M, Mayhew P: Identifying fall risk factors in preparation for reducing the use of restraints. Medsurg Nurs 3(1):25,1994
47. Todd B: p 212
48. Yakaborwich M: Prescribe with care: the role of laxatives in the treatment of constipation. J Gerontol Nurs 16(7):7,1990
49. Beverly L, Travis I: Constipation: Proposed natural laxative mixtures. J Gerontol Nurs 18(10):5,1992
50. Day J, Freeman A, Coni N, Dixon A: Barium enema or computed tomography for the frail elderly patient? Clin Radiol 48(1):48,1993
51. Robinson, DeMuth, p 8–9
52. Cape et al, p 74
53. Levin R: Osteoporosis: Prevention is key to management. Geriatrics 48(suppl 1):18,1993
54. Reed A, Burge S: Screening for osteoporosis. J Gerontol Nurs 14(7):18,1988
55. Holm K, Walker J: Osteoporosis: Treatment and prevention update. Geriatr Nurs 11(3):140,1990
56. Heaney R: Bone mass, nutrition, and other lifestyle factors. Am J Med 95(suppl 5a):29s,1993
57. Heaney, p 29s
58. Komar L, Nieves J, Cosman F, Rubin A, Shen V, Lindsay R: Calcium homeostasis of an elderly population upon admission to a nursing home. J Am Geriatr Soc 42(10):1057,1993
59. Lindsay R: Hormone replacement therapy for prevention and treatment osteoporosis. Am J Med 95(suppl 5a):5a–375,1993
60. Heaney, p 30s
61. Chesnut C: Bone mass and exercise. Am J Med 95(suppl 5a):34s,1993
62. Aisenbrey J: Exercise in the prevention and management of osteoporosis. Phys Ther 67:1100,1987
63. Robbins A: Hypothermia and heat stroke: Protecting the elderly. Geriatrics 44(1):73,1989
64. Delaney K: Heatstroke: Underlying processes and lifesaving management. Postgrad Med 91(4):379,1992
65. Robbins, p 73
66. Latz P, Wyble R: Elderly patients perioperative nursing implications. AORN J 46(2):238,1987
67. Saleh K: The elderly patient in the post-anesthesia care unit. Nurs Clin North Am 28(3):507–517,1993
68. Jackson M: High risk surgical patient. J Gerontol Nurs 14(1):8,1988
69. White H, Thurston N, Blackmore K, Green S, Hannah K: Body temperature in elderly surgical patient. Res Nurs Health 10:317,1987
70. Moddeman G: The elderly surgical patient-a high risk for hypothermia. AORN 53(5):1270,1991
71. Booker J: Severe symptomatic hyponatremia in elderly outpatients. J Am Geriatr Soc 33(2):108,1985
72. Baldwin D: Provision of intravenous therapy in a skilled nursing facility. J Intravenous Nurs 14(6):366, 1991
73. Coulter K: Intravenous therapy for the elder patient: Implications for the intravenous nurse. J Intravenous Nurs 15(suppl 2):s18,1992
74. Mellema S, Ponialawski B: Geriatric I.V. therapy. J Intravenous Ther 11(1):56,1988
75. Butts D: Fluid and electrolyte disorders associated with diabetic ketoacidosis and hyperglycemic hyperosmolar nonketotic coma. Nurs Clin North Am 22(4):827,1987

Index

Index